PHEROMONES

NORTH-HOLLAND RESEARCH MONOGRAPHS

FRONTIERS OF BIOLOGY

VOLUME 32

Under the General Editorship of

A. NEUBERGER

London

and

E. L. TATUM

New York

NORTH-HOLLAND PUBLISHING COMPANY
AMSTERDAM · LONDON

PHEROMONES

Edited by

Martin C. BIRCH

Department of Entomology and Nematology,
University of California at Davis,
Davis, California, U.S.A.

1974

NORTH-HOLLAND PUBLISHING COMPANY - AMSTERDAM • LONDON
AMERICAN ELSEVIER PUBLISHING COMPANY, INC. – NEW YORK

Library of Congress Catalog Card Number: 73-88157

North-Holland ISBN: 0 7204 7133 8
American Elsevier ISBN: 0 444 10604 9

PUBLISHERS:

NORTH-HOLLAND PUBLISHING COMPANY – AMSTERDAM
NORTH-HOLLAND PUBLISHING COMPANY, LTD. – LONDON

SOLE DISTRIBUTORS FOR THE U.S.A. AND CANADA:

AMERICAN ELSEVIER PUBLISHING COMPANY, INC.
52 VANDERBILT AVENUE, NEW YORK, N.Y. 10017

PRINTED IN THE NETHERLANDS

General preface

The aim of the publication of this series of monographs, known under the collective title of '*Frontiers of Biology*', is to present coherent and up-to-date views of the fundamental concepts which dominate modern biology.

Biology in its widest sense has made very great advances during the past decade, and the rate of progress has been steadily accelerating. Undoubtedly important factors in this acceleration have been the effective use by biologists of new techniques, including electron microscopy, isotopic labels, and a great variety of physical and chemical techniques, especially those with varying degrees of automation. In addition, scientists with partly physical or chemical backgrounds have become interested in the great variety of problems presented by living organisms. Most significant, however, increasing interest in and understanding of the biology of the cell, especially in regard to the molecular events involved in genetic phenomena and in metabolism and its control, have led to the recognition of patterns common to all forms of life from the bacteria to man. These factors and unifying concepts have led to a situation in which the sharp boundaries between the various classical biological disciplines are rapidly disappearing.

Thus, while scientists are becoming increasingly specialized in their techniques, to an increasing extent they need an intellectual and conceptual approach on a wide and non-specialized basis. It is with these considerations and needs in mind that this series of monographs, '*Frontiers of Biology*' has been conceived.

The advances in various areas of biology, including microbiology, biochemistry, genetics, cytology, and cell structure and function in general will be presented by authors who have themselves contributed significantly to these developments. They will have, in this series, the opportunity of bringing together, from diverse sources, theories and experimental data, and of integrating these into a more general conceptual framework. It is unavoidable, and probably even desirable, that the special bias of the individual authors will become evident in their contributions. Scope will also be given for presentation of new and challenging ideas and hypotheses for which complete evidence is at present lacking. However, the main emphasis will be on fairly complete and objective presentation of the more important and more rapidly advancing aspects of biology. The level will be advanced, directed primarily to the needs of the graduate student and research worker.

Most monographs in this series will be in the range of 200–300 pages, but on occasion a collective work of major importance may be included somewhat exceeding this figure. The intent of the publishers is to bring out these books promptly and in fairly quick succession.

It is on the basis of all these various considerations that we welcome the opportunity of supporting the publication of the series '*Frontiers of Biology*' by North-Holland Publishing Company.

E. L. TATUM

A. NEUBERGER, *Editors*

Preface

Previous books on pheromones have either emphasized the chemistry of pheromones, practical utilization of chemical determinants of behavior, or a variety of topics in the area of chemoreception. None has primarily emphasized the biology of pheromones throughout the animal kingdom or attempted to cover animal pheromones as a single topic. The study of pheromones demands an involvement with the behavior of animals, but that involvement has usually been kept to a minimum. There has been a strong tendency with the insect work to concentrate on chemical isolation, identification and synthesis, and the technology of field deployment – the behavior of compounds rather than the behavior of insects. Mammalian pheromone research has had a somewhat different approach. Partly due to the greater complexities of the secretions involved, chemistry has lagged behind here: behavior has had more emphasis, although, as with the insect work, it has for the most part been restricted to laboratory animals in situations that cannot easily be translated to natural populations.

The current situation merely reveals how little we know about the way pheromones actually influence the behavior and population dynamics of animals. The biological basis for pheromone research needs a much greater input, especially since pheromones are currently being heralded as one of the most promising new tools for management of pest populations. They are clearly going to be used with, or without, a sound knowledge of the underlying biology.

Hence, this book is concerned with the biology of pheromones, avoiding techniques, chemistry and cataloguing of identifications, all of which are indispensable but have tended to crowd out the biology. The book concentrates on the two main groups studied to date – the insects and the mammals (plus fish). Where chemistry and technology intrude, the paucity of the behavioral research is merely emphasized. This book will have served its purpose if it can indicate where research on pheromone mediated behavior is weak and can indicate and stimulate research into new or weak areas.

The editor is very grateful to Barbara Barr, Linda Birch, Stanley Caveney, Charles David, Lewis Edson, Dorothy van Emden, Doug Light, Henry Moeck, David

Moscioni, Curtis Pantle and Susie Wong for their help in various ways with editing many of the chapters, to H. A. Bern, H. van Emden and J. C. Young for valuable help with the introduction, and to R. van den Bosch and J. Diekman for reading the introductory section to Ch. 22. The book could never have been put together without Professor David Wood's support during the time I was with his research group at the University of California, Berkeley; I am very grateful to him. Marian Merrill provided excellent administrative help throughout the organization and editing. The editor is particularly indebted to Barbara Zelwer for typing the entire final draft and to Linda Birch for the arduous task of compiling the index.

C. J. Sanders – Canadian Forestry Service, Great Lakes Forest Research Centre, P. O. Box 490, Sault Ste. Marie, Ontario P6A 5M7, Canada *(ch. 22)*

H. H. Shorey – Division of Toxicology anf Physiology, Department of Entomology, University of California, Riverside, California 92502, U.S.A. *(chs. 4, 5, 22)*

D. Michael Stoddart – Department of Zoology, University of London, King's College, The Strand, London WC2R 2LS, England *(ch. 15)*

James P. Tette – Pheromone Field Research and Development, Zoëcon Corporation, Palo Alto, California 94304, U.S.A. (present address: Pheromone Systems, Box 260 D, R.D. 1, Stanley, New York 14561, U.S.A. *(ch. 21)*

Kenneth Trammel – New York State Agricultural Experiment Station, Cornell University, Geneva, New York 14456, U.S.A. *(ch. 22)*

J. Weatherston – Canadian Forestry Service, Insect Pathology Research Institute, P. O. Box 490, Sault Ste.Marie, Ontario P6A 5M7, Canada *(ch. 2)*

David L. Wood – Department of Entomological Sciences, University of California, Berkeley, California 94720, U.S.A. *(ch. 22)*

Contents

Section III. Pheromones in manipulation of populations

CHAPTER 1

Introduction

Martin BIRCH

Pheromones are one channel of biological communication. However, the concept of communication in animals has consistently resisted definition. Burghardt (1970a) defines it as 'the phenomenon of one organism producing a signal that, when responded to by another organism, confers some advantage or probability of advantage to the signaller or his group'. When 'group' is equated with species this definition adequately covers pheromones, for they are restricted to chemical signals within a species, but other chemical interactions – such as those between predator and prey or competing species – are often more difficult to characterize. Law and Regnier (1971) incorporate all chemicals acting as messages between organisms as semiochemicals. Those chemical interactions which affect the growth, health, behavior or population biology of individuals ~~of other~~ species have been termed allelochemical interactions (Whittaker and Feeny 1971). Under this umbrella term: allomones are allelochemicals which confer adaptive advantage to the producing organism (sender), such as repellent secretions or venoms; kairomones give the adaptive advantage to the receiving organism and include food attraction stimuli or secretions from a prey species that attract predators; depressants may inhibit the receiver without any apparent advantages to the releaser. Within species the chemical interactions are either autotoxins, auto-inhibitors or pheromones.

The term pheromone was first proposed and defined by Karlson and Lüscher (1959) to refer to a group of biologically active substances resembling hormones in some respects, yet which could not be included among them as they evidently did not come from endocrine glands. Karlson and Lüscher's definition is still appropriate: 'pheromones are substances which are secreted to the outside by an individual and received by a second individual of the same species in which they release a specific reaction, for example, a definite behavior or developmental process'. The derivation of the word from the Greek *pherein* (to transfer) and *hormon* (to excite) was initially criticized etymologically, but the term has become so universally adopted as to be firmly established.

Characteristics of pheromones: Pheromones are generally active in minute quantities. They may evoke a behavioral response with a single compound or a mixture. In either case, the complex of compounds or the single compound is by definition a pheromone if it stimulates a behavioral reaction in the receiving organism(s). Individual components of a mixture which are inactive by themselves are not pheromones per se, but may synergize with other singly inactive or active compounds to evoke the response. If the behavioral response is rigorously applied as a definition, such terms as pheromone-bouquet, pheromone-medley or pheromone complex are redundant to describe a pheromone comprised of several component chemicals.

The information carried by chemical means may not be as restricted as is usually supposed. Wilson's (1968, 1970) lucid conceptual analysis of the chemical channel indicates that the quantity and rate of information transfer by this means can be very great. Some of the ways in which information is maximized are through use of multiple gland sources, complex chemicals or mixtures of chemicals, changes in concentration evoking different responses, response patterns changing rapidly and precisely with diel or annual periodicity, use of natural currents (wind or water) and differences in fade-out time achieved by manipulating volatility, reactivity or stability of the pheromone. Certainly in many insect species this mode of communication is more widely used than either vision or sound.

Karlson (1960) originally separated olfactory and gustatory pheromones. Wilson (1963) more usefully distinguished primer and releaser effects. Releaser pheromones appear to act directly on the central nervous system to evoke an immediate and reversible change in behavior; for example, female sex pheromones attracting males in insects; alarm substance in fish. Primer pheromones, on the other hand, trigger permanent physiological changes in the receiver. There may be no immediate change in behavior, but the organism develops new response potentials which can be evoked by new stimuli. Examples are pheromones stimulating sexual maturation in insects and mammals or controlling caste differentiation in insects.

More recently pheromones, at least those of insects, have been classified on the basis of their biological function (Butler 1967, 1970) or the kind of behavior they evoke (Shorey 1973). Although the two classifications are commonly confused, they are not necessarily convergent (Kennedy 1972). Classified on the basis of behavior in the receiving animal, insect pheromones release aggregation, trail-following, dispersion, sexual behavior, oviposition, alarm and specialized behavior in the regulation of social insect colonies (Blum 1969; Jacobson 1972; Wilson 1972; Shorey 1973, inter alia and chs. 2–13). In mammals, pheromones are involved in, for example, social hierarchies, territorial behavior, individual imprinting and primer reproductive effects (e.g, Gleason and Reynierse 1969; Cowley and Wise 1970; Whitten and Bronson 1970; Ralls 1971; inter alia, and chs. 15–20). Such classifications of behavior appear to be straightforward, but some pheromones have different functions in different contexts. Thus, aggregation and release of sexual behavior may be triggered by the same pheromone in bark beetles, or the pheromone of one insect may be used as a kairomone by its predator (Borden ch. 8)*. Such pheromone parsimony (multiplicity of effects) is nowhere better seen than with the pheromones of the honey bee (Gary ch. 11) and is common in social insects generally (Blum ch. 10).

The above terminology is also strained when applied to pheromone-mediated behavior in mammals, where interactions are clearly on a more individual basis. Recognition of an individual's pheromone pattern is the rule rather than the exception in dominance interactions, leadership, territorial behavior and parent-offspring relationships. The contrast between the stereotyped responses of insects and those of mammals, which are flexible and vary in the light of experience, reflects the general differences in their behavior and nervous systems. In addition, although research on mammalian pheromones is in its infancy, chemical studies so far have clearly shown that we are dealing with far greater complexities of active secretion than the few precise components which evoke the full response repertoire of the insect. These characteristics create problems in analyzing pheromone-mediated behavior in mammals. A specific behavior pattern may be evoked by a combination of inputs from the visual, auditory, tactile and olfactory senses; any one of which can possibly be blocked without noticeably affecting the behavior, since this relies more heavily on the remaining senses. Thus, the concept of a definite pheromone is difficult to apply experimentally, i.e. quantitative and qualitative pheromone characteristics change so readily that isolation of the active components may be impossible. Bronson (1971) suggests that the term pheromone be restricted to those situations where there is a good chance of isolating and chemically identifying specific compounds (see also Bronson ch. 18).

In contrasting the insect and mammalian systems it is very easy to lose sight of some considerable similarities. Thus, the same general dichotomy of primer and releaser effects can usefully be applied to both groups. Both may be utilizing pheromones in similar functional strategies, for example, to ensure mutual sexual receptivity or to modify reproductive physiology. Although mammalian pheromones possess more individuality, even in the insects certain *types* of individual (e.g. queens) can be pheromonally recognized. In their social units, where individual colony odors are behaviorally distinguished, insect pheromones approach the complexity and uniqueness of their mammalian counterparts.

It is now clear that pheromone-mediated behavior is ubiquitous throughout the animal kingdom (and also in fungi and algae), with the possible striking exception of the birds. The vast majority of research effort has involved the insects and more recently the mammals, as is strongly reflected in the two major sections of this book. Fish and amphibia are the exceptions which broaden the treatment to that of

* Such chemical interactions may be between very diverse groups. A fascinating example of a kairomone is a pheromone-like factor from newborn baby rabbits, which boosts impregnation, sperm transfer and maturation in rabbit fleas. The active airborne stimulus may be a cortisol metabolite in the urine of 1–8-day old rabbits (Rothschild and Ford 1970; Rothschild 1971).

vertebrates in general. Chemical perception by reptiles has only recently become experimental (see Burghardt 1970b, for background).

Research on pheromones of non-insectan invertebrates and all aquatic (including marine) organisms represents a relatively unexplored field. Even the non-insectan terrestrial arthropods have been neglected*. Wilson's (1970) review gives a valuable summary of pheromone-mediated behavior in the principal invertebrate phyla, fungi and algae, and is referred to as an excellent background to the subject. Pheromone research has recently begun to diversify rapidly into this area, at such a rate that any attempt to treat pheromones of other invertebrates would be premature and of little value by the time of publication. However, one new area where exciting progress is being made is with pheromones of marine organisms. For example, a pheromone has now been chemically identified that attracts male gametes of a brown alga, *Ectocarpus* sp., to the female (Muller et al. 1971). Pheromones have also been described from the marine Hydrozoa (Miller 1972), Mollusca (Dinter and Manos 1972) and Amphipoda (Dahl et al. 1970), and recently crustecdysone, the crustacean molting hormone, has been shown to have sex pheromone activity for several species of crabs (Decapoda) (Kittredge et al. 1971), although it has not been proven to be the pheromone.

In the scheme proposed by Kittredge and Takahashi (1972), the development of pheromonal capabilities (release and reception) in a molting hormone may have been the origin of pheromone communication in the Arthropoda. Haldane (1955) had earlier argued another scheme, that chemical contact was probably the first form of communication between living things and further that chemical communication between acellular organisms would have been a necessary pre-requisite to the development of metazoan animals. Wilson (1970) extended this to argue that hormones and pheromones are 'linearly' related; i.e. hormones appeared after pheromones as the intercellular equivalent of pheromones which had mediated behavior in the single-celled organisms. Although these two schemes take opposite positions, they are clearly not mutually exclusive since the position of the first Metazoa and Arthropoda in evolution are so different and chemicals may have changed their function more than once. Whatever their precise evolutionary route, it is clear that pheromones have become a fundamental biological means of communication.

Treatment in this volume: It is impossible to cover all the important aspects of pheromone knowledge in one volume while still including enough recent discoveries and interpretations to be of any value to researchers in the field. The major restriction placed on the subject matter in this book has been to limit it to the biology of pheromones. Biological and chemical methods in insect pheromone research have developed their own technology, which often threatens to dominate study of the behavior and functioning of the organisms these methods have been developed to investigate. There are several quite adequate reviews of the methods of biological,

* Only recently has the first tick pheromone been identified (Berger 1972).

chemical and physical analysis of pheromone systems. An excellent introduction to both biological and chemical technology in the study of chemical communication systems is given by Young and Silverstein (1974). Both biological and chemical methods for insects are also extensively treated in Wood et al. (1970), Beroza (1970) and Jacobson (1972). Physical constraints on the system are well discussed by Wilson (1968, 1970), who analyzes the information capacity of the chemical channel. Treatment of the various theories of odor are excluded for reasons of space and unity of subject matter. Biosynthesis of pheromones is an unexplored field and only for that reason is omitted.

The book is divided into three sections. The first and second of these deal with insect pheromone systems (chs. 2–13) and vertebrate pheromone systems (chs. 14–20). Differences mentioned earlier make it more convenient that they receive separate treatment. In the insect system, production, release and reception of pheromones, interpretation of the message and the environmental and physiological factors influencing pheromone behavior are discussed first (chs. 2–4). This leads into an analysis of the mechanisms by which insects orient to and arrive at a distant odor source (ch. 5). Sex pheromones of Lepidoptera and Coleoptera are extensively treated (chs. 6 and 9), since they are now being shown to be intimately involved in the processes of speciation and evolution of these two groups. Two more specialized types of pheromone behavior are also discussed: courtship pheromones (ch. 7) and the aggregation pheromones of bark beetles (ch. 8). Communication in the social insects involves additional concepts since in many species the entire social order and cohesion appears chemically controlled (ch. 10). The honey bee (ch. 11) and other social Hymenoptera (ch. 12) are extensively treated here; their sociality and economic importance has made them favorite experimental insects, though worldwide it is apparent that termite societies may be found to rely even more completely on this form of social regulation (ch. 13).

Among non-mammalian vertebrates, fright and alarm pheromones have been found to be widespread in the fish and amphibia (ch. 14). Within the mammals, pheromone communication has probably been investigated more thoroughly in the rodents than in any other single group (chs. 15 and 18). Throughout the mammals olfaction has been found to be important in the recognition of species, groups and individuals (ch. 16). Primer effects have also been discovered in which pheromones have long-term effects on the reproductive processes (ch. 18) and affect the population dynamics of the animals (ch. 17). Although the primates are not macrosmatic (well-developed sense of smell) like most mammals, pheromones have been found to be prevalent in sexual processes here too (ch. 19), and the occurrence of pheromones in man has become more than a possibility (ch. 20).

The practical uses of pheromones and their success is examined in the third section (chs. 21 and 22). Those infected by the optimism, which accompanied the development of 'routine' chemical identification and synthesis of pheromones, claimed that pheromones would be the panacea for many of the ills incurred by the effects of intensive agricultural practices on pest problems. Few spectacular successes have yet been established, but the applied use of pheromones is still a rapidly expanding field. It is time to take stock and analyze what has actually been accomplished in this area.

References

Berger, R. S. (1972) 2,6-dichlorophenol, sex pheromone of the lone star tick. Science 177, 704–705.

Beroza, M., ed. (1970) Chemicals Controlling Insect Behavior (Academic Press, New York) 170 pp.

Blum, M. S. (1969) Alarm pheromones. Ann. Rev. Entomol. 14, 57–80.

Bronson, F. H. (1971) Rodent pheromones. Biol. Reprod. 4, 344–357.

Burghardt, G. M. (1970a) Defining 'communication'. *In*: Advances in Chemoreception, I; eds.: J. W. Johnston Jr., D. G. Moulton and A. Turk (Appleton-Century-Crofts, New York) pp. 5–18.

Burghardt, G. M. (1970b) Chemical perception in reptiles. *In*: Advances in Chemoreception, I; eds.: J. W. Johnston Jr., D. G. Moulton and A. Turk (Appleton-Century-Crofts, New York) pp. 241–308.

Butler, C. G. (1967) Insect pheromones. Biol. Rev. Cambridge Phil. Soc. 42, 42–87.

Butler, C. G. (1970) Chemical communication in insects: behavioral and ecologic aspects. *In*: Advances in Chemoreception, I; eds.: J. W. Johnston Jr., D. G. Moulton and A. Turk (Appleton-Century-Crofts, New York) pp. 35–78.

Cowley, J. J. and D. R. Wise (1970) Pheromones, growth and behavior. *In*: Chemical Influences on Behavior; eds. R. Porter and J. Birch. CIBA Fdn. Study Gp. No. 35 (Churchill, London) pp. 144–170.

Dahl, E., H. Emanuelsson and C. von Mechlenburg (1970) Pheromone transport and reception in an amphipod. Science 170, 739–740.

Dinter, J. and P. J. Manos (1972) Evidence for a pheromone in the marine periwinkle, *Littorina littorea* Linnaeus. Veliger 15, 45–47.

Gleason, K. K. and J. H. Reynierse (1969) The behavioral significance of pheromones in vertebrates. Psychol. Bull. 71, 58–73.

Haldane, J. B. S. (1955) Animal communication and the origin of human language. Sci. Progr. (London) 43 (171), 385–401.

Jacobson, M. (1972) Insect Sex Pheromones (Academic Press, New York) 382 pp.

Karlson, P. (1960) Pheromones. Ergebn. Biol. 22, 212–225.

Karlson, P. and M. Lüscher (1959) Pheromones: a new term for a class of biologically active substances. Nature (London) 183, 55–56.

Kennedy, J. S. (1972) The emergence of behaviour. J. Australian Entomol. Soc. ll, 168–176.

Kittredge, J. S. and F. T. Takahashi (1972) The evolution of sex pheromone communication in the Arthropoda. J. Theor. Biol. 35, 467–471.

Kittredge, J. S., T. Michelle and F. T. Takahashi (1971) Sex pheromone activity of the molting hormone, crustecdysone, on male crabs (*Pachygrapsus crassipes, Cancer antennarius* and *C. anthonyi*) Fishery Bull. 69, 337–343.

Law, J. H. and F. E. Regnier (1971) Pheromones. Ann. Rev. Biochem. 40, 533–548.

Miller, R. L. (1972) Gel filtration of the sperm attractants of some marine hydrozoa. J. Exptl. Zool. 182, 281–297.

Muller, D. G., L. Jaenicke, M. Donike and T. Akintobi (1971) Sex attractant in a brown alga: chemical structure. Science 171, 815–817.

Ralls, K. (1971) Mammalian scent marking. Science 171, 443–449.

Rothschild, M. (1971) Coating the antennae of the rabbit flea: its effect on maturation and impregnation. Proc. Roy. Entomol. Soc. London Ser. C 36, 19, 25–26.

Rothschild, M. and B. Ford (1970) (exhibit) Proc. Roy. Entomol. Soc. London Ser. C. 35, 11.

Shorey, H. H. (1973) Behavioral responses to insect pheromones. Ann. Rev. Entomol. 18, 349–380.

Whittaker, R. H. and P. P. Feeny (1971) Allelochemics: chemical interactions between species. Science 171, 757–770.

Whitten, W. K. and F. H. Bronson (1970) The role of pheromones in mammalian reproduction. *In*: Advances in Chemoreception, I, eds.: J. W. Johnston Jr., D. G. Moulton and A. Turk (Appleton-Century-Crofts, New York) pp. 309–325.

Wilson, E. O. (1963) Pheromones. Sci. Amer. 208, 100–114.

Wilson, E. O., (1968) Chemical systems. *In*: Animal Communication: Techniques of Study and Results of Research; ed.: T. A. Sebeok (Univ. of Indiana Press) pp. 75–102.

Wilson, E. O. (1970) Chemical communication within animal species. *In*: Chemical Ecology; eds.: E. Sondheimer and J. B. Simeone (Academic Press, New York) pp. 133–155.

Wilson, E. O. (1972) The Insect Societies (Harvard Univ. Press, Cambridge) 548 pp.

Wood, D. L., R. M. Silverstein and M. Nakajima, eds. (1970) Control of Insects by Natural Products (Academic Press, New York) 345 pp.

Young, J. C. and R. M. Silverstein (1974) Biological and chemical methodology in the study of animal communication systems. *In*: Methods in Olfactory Research; eds.: D. G. Moulton, J. W. Johnston Jr. and A. Turk (Academic Press, London) (in press).

Section I

Insect pheromone systems

CHAPTER 2

Gland structure and pheromone production in insects*

J. E. PERCY and J. WEATHERSTON

2.1. *Introduction*

The types and locations of the exocrine glands which produce insect pheromones are as varied as the many functions attributed to the pheromones. Although much interdisciplinary research has been directed towards a better understanding of pheromonal systems there is a paucity of knowledge of the relationships between gland structure and pheromone production in insects.

Pheromones are usually produced by glandular modifications of the epidermal cells of the integument, which may be situated in almost any area of the insect. In this chapter discussion of the glands will be with respect to the particular modifications involved. Admittedly this concept does not encompass individual variations. However, most pheromone producing glands can be discussed under the following headings.

2.2. *Individual secretory cells irregularly dispersed throughout the epidermis*

Mature male *Schistocerca gregaria* Forskäl possess individual secretory cells interpersed among the unspecialized epidermal cells of the head, thorax, legs, and the second to seventh abdominal sternites and tergites. The cells are particularly evident in males which have been crowded but a few have been observed in mature crowded females (Thomas 1970). The function of these cells is suggested to be the production of a maturation pheromone by mature crowded males which hastens the maturation of both males and females (Thomas 1970 and references therein). It has been further suggested that a similar system may be involved in the production of the sex pheromone in females of those species of cockroaches where the location of the pheromone production site is unknown (Barth 1968).

* Contribution No. 251. Insect Pathology Research Institute, Canadian Forestry Service, P.O. Box 490, Sault Ste. Marie, Ontario, Canada.

The secretory cells are found between and beneath the epidermal cells. A small apical vacuole is present in cells of immature males. The vacuole increases in size with ageing: in mature yellow males the enlargement is so great that it is difficult to discern the nucleus of the cell (Thomas 1970). A ductule arises in the vicinity of the vacuole, meanders through the epidermal cells and opens on the surface of the cuticle (Strong 1971).

2.3. *Modified intersegmental membranes*

These glands are usually confined to the production of sex attractants primarily in females of the order Lepidoptera. They have also been noted in species representative of the orders Mecoptera and Coleoptera, where they produce sex attractants and assembling scents respectively. Longitudinal folds increase the surface area of the modified intersegmental membrane over that of undifferentiated membranes (Roelofs and Feng 1968; Weatherston and Percy 1970). In addition the glands are sometimes deeply invaginated dorsally, ventrally or laterally within the body cavity; these modifications having been used by Urbahn (1913) and later workers to systematize female lepidopterous scent glands (Götz 1951; Jefferson et al. 1968; Percy and Weatherston 1971; Thibout 1972).

Eversion of the glands is assumed to be due to changes in haemolymph pressure. Retraction is brought about by muscular action which may also be a factor in gland eversion. The muscles involved in the case of the moths either insert or originate on or near the posterior and/or anterior apophyses (Jefferson et al. 1966, 1968; Percy, unpublished). In a few cases it has also been reported that the muscles insert directly on the cuticle of the gland (Steinbrecht 1964a; Jefferson et al. 1968; Crossley and Waterhouse 1969).

Innervation of the glands does not seem to have been well studied although in *Harpobittacus australis* (Klug) axons invested with many laminae, and neurosecretory-type axons were seen in thin sections of the glandular cells (Crossley and Waterhouse 1969).

2.3.1. *Ductless cells*

This sub-group is restricted to glands which produce sex pheromones in female Lepidoptera and the assembling scent in female *Trogoderma granarium* Everts. The secretory cells are hypertrophied epidermal cells which may be squamous, cuboidal, columnar or goblet shaped. Histological studies have revealed that the cells contain a large nucleus, many vacuoles and, some studies mention an 'apical zone' or brush border. The cuticle overlying the cells consists of a thick laminar endocuticle and a thin epicuticle, which may contain epicuticular projections or spikes. For more detailed information with respect to particular species the reader is referred to the following papers: Dickens 1936; Götz 1951; Steinbrecht 1964a; George 1965; Barnes et al. 1966; Jefferson et al. 1966; 1968, 1971; El Sawaf et al. 1968; Roelofs and Feng 1968; Weatherston and Percy 1968; Jefferson and Rubin 1970; Stanic et al. 1970; Percy and Weatherston 1971; Percy et al. 1971; Thibout 1972.

The presence of vacuoles appears to be a characteristic feature of these secretory cells. In *Choristoneura fumiferana* (Clem.) the vacuoles are of two types. Near the base of the cell there are one or two large vacuoles which on the basis of histochemical tests contain glycogen. Most of the other vacuoles are smaller and randomly distributed throughout the cell. These vacuoles absorb oil red O in water soluble wax sections indicating that they contain lipids. The number and presence of these small vacuoles cannot be correlated with the diurnal cycle of attractiveness in virgin female *C. fumiferana* (Weatherston and Percy, unpublished). Steinbrecht (1964a) carried out detailed histochemical tests on the vacuoles in *Bombyx mori* L., and determined that, although they contained unsaturated, neutral lipids (which would not exclude the sex attractant bombykol) it was unlikely that the lipids represent the final secretion. This hypothesis is based on three observations. First, the total volume of lipid droplets per cell is estimated to be 10 μg while the total amount of bombykol per insect is 0.8–2.5 μg. Second, there is no decrease in the number of lipid droplets with age – as in *Trichoplusia ni* (Hübner) (Jefferson et al. 1966) – or following insemination even though bombykol production declines in both cases. Finally, it is concluded from physiological tests (Steinbrecht 1964b) that in attractive insects most of the pheromone has been transported to an area where it can easily evaporate.

There have been very few ultrastructural studies of gland cells (*Bombyx mori* – Steinbrecht 1964a; Waku and Sumimoto 1969; *Plodia interpunctella* (Hübner) – Smithwick 1970; *Choristoneura fumiferana* – Percy, unpublished). In all three species, smooth tubular endoplasmic reticulum predominates in the adult from the time of emergence, whereas before eclosion rough endoplasmic reticulum is typical. Agranular endoplasmic reticulum is indicative of lipid synthesizing cells. Occasionally vesicles with electron dense contents are seen near the apex of the cell in *Bombyx mori* and *Plodia interpunctella.* Mitochrondria are numerous, as are lipid droplets. The apical zone (brush border) consists of many microvilli in *Trichoplusia ni* (Miller et al. 1967), *Plodia interpunctella* and *Choristoneura fumiferana.* In the latter two, the microvilli contain a central canal which in *C. fumiferana* appears continuous with the smooth endoplasmic reticulum. In *Bombyx mori* the apical membrane appears microvillate, but closer inspection reveals that it is folded to produce a tightly packed lamellar border.

The cuticle overlying the gland, following the terminology of Filshie (1970) consists, in *B. mori* and *Choristoneura fumiferana*, of lamellate endocuticle, protein epicuticle, a thin electron dense cuticulin layer, and outer epicuticle (figs. 2.1a and b). Running through the endocuticle lamellae are epicuticular filaments which in *C. fumiferana* originate at or near the tips of the microvilli. In both species these filaments form large masses beneath the protein epicuticle and some penetrate this layer and the cuticulin. The cuticle of an undifferentiated intersegmental membrane is similar, except that there are fewer epicuticular filaments. Absence of pore canals or similar structures in the cuticle led Steinbrecht (1964a) to propose that a diffusion process took place whereby a gradient across the cuticle is maintained by evaporation of the pheromone from the gland surface. It is further postulated that the epicuticular filaments play a role in the passage of secretion, but is it not possible at this point to elaborate on the exact mechanism.

The filaments do not appear to be composed entirely of pheromone, pheromone precursors, or lipids; this conclusion may be deduced from a comparison with

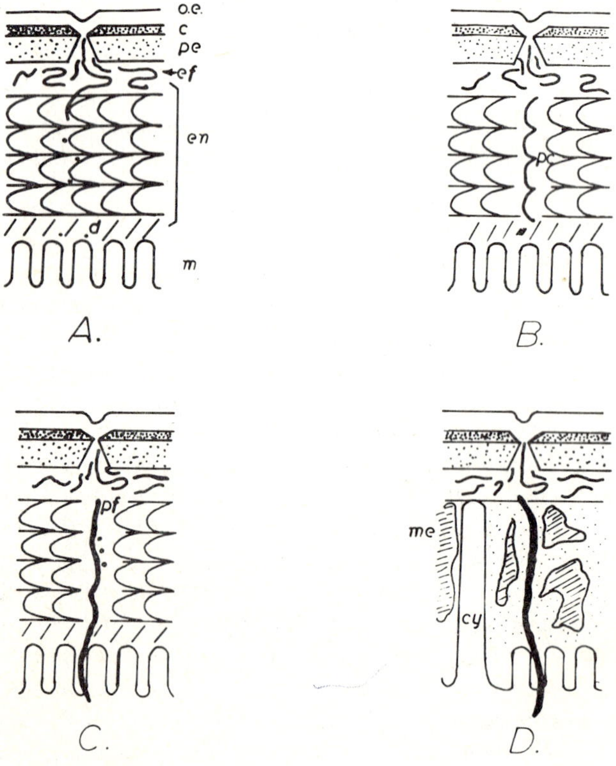

Fig. 2.1. Diagrammatic representation of structures observed in the cuticle overlying pheromone glands in which the cells are ductless (for explanation see text). a) *Bombyx mori* (after Steinbrecht 1964a); b) *Choristoneura fumiferana*; c) *Kalotermes flavicollis* (after Quennedey 1971b); d) *Trinervitermes germinatus* (after Quennedey 1972). *c* – cuticulin; *cy* – cytoplasmic projection (only observed in the Termitidae); *d* – dense granule; *ef* – epicuticular filament; *en* – lamellate endocuticle; *m* – microvilli; *me* – mesocuticle; *oe* – outer epicuticle; *pc* – pore canal; *pf* – pore canal filament (= axial filament); *pe* – protein epicuticle.

filaments in specialized and unspecialized regions of the cuticle in larvae of *Calpodes ethlius* (Stahl) (Locke 1961, 1964, 1966, 1969; Filshie 1970). Locke's earlier studies suggested that the filaments represent lipid/water liquid crystals, possibly continuous with outer epicuticle. It appears unlikely that the filaments are solely lipid, at least in the cuticle of the wax secreting gland of *C. ethlius* and certain termites (sect. 2.4.1), because of the inability of lipid solvents to extract them from the cuticle (Filshie 1970). Possibly part of the filament is proteinaceous, i.e. the structures originated as protein/lipid liquid crystals and later became stabilized to form channels for the transport of lipid-soluble materials (Locke and Krishnan 1971). This protein may consist in part of enzymes; several reports have indicated the presence of esterases and phenoloxidases in cuticle (Locke 1960; Quennedey and Noirot 1968; Locke and Krishnan 1971).

In other words the filaments may represent channels for the transport and possible modification of pheromone substances passing through the cuticle. These ideas will remain conjectural until it can be shown that enzymes associated with the elaboration of a pheromone of known chemical structure are localized in the cuticle.

2.3.2. Cells associated with ducts

In the only representative of this type, *Harpobittacus australis*, modifications of secretory cells are very similar to those described for some defensive mechanism glands (Eisner et al. 1964; Happ et al. 1966; Filshie and Waterhouse 1968; Schnepf et al. 1969). Immediately beneath the cuticle is a layer of cuticle-secreting squamous epithelial cells. Beneath this layer are the two cells which comprise the secretory 'organule': the secretory duct cell and the secretory cell (Crossley and Waterhouse 1969). The secretory duct opening to the exterior is formed by a tubular invagination of cuticle secreted by the enveloping secretory duct cell (fig. 2.2), which is itself completely surrounded by the upper half of the larger secretory cell. On leaving the base of the duct cell the cuticular duct enlarges slightly so that it resembles a funnel. The secretory cell, whose invaginated portion encompasses the duct cell, is also enlarged in this area and its surface is microvillate. Lying within the duct opening, and originating at or near the tips of the microvilli, are numerous filaments remarkably similar in size and structure to the epicuticular filaments described above. Modification of the surface of secretory cells, its association with filaments, and the presence of a cuticular duct, were first described ultrastructurally by Mercer and Brunet (1959) in their studies of the left colleterial gland of a cockroach. For the specialized structural modifications they coined the term 'end apparatus'. It should be noted, as described for spermathecal gland cells (Gupta and Smith 1969), that the duct is not intracellular, there being no permanent gap in the plasma membrane of the secretory cell. The secretory cells rest on a basement membrane above which the basal plasma membrane of the cell is deeply

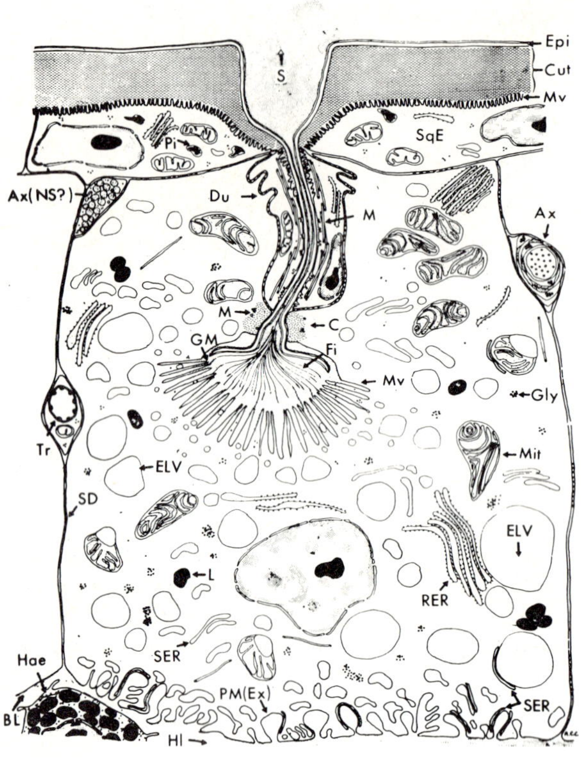

Fig. 2.2. Diagram of secretory epithelium illustrating glandular cells of type 3.2. *AX(NS?)* – neurosecretory axon (?); *BL* – basement membrane; *Cut* – endocuticle; *C* – fibrous collar; *Du* – secretory duct cell; *Epi* – epicuticle; *ELV* – electron lucid vacuole; *Fi* – filaments of end apparatus; GM – granular mass of end apparatus; *Gly* – glycogen; *Hae* – haemocyte; *Hl* – haemolymph; *L* – lysosome; *M* – microtubules; *Mit* – mitochondrion; *Mv* – microvilli; *Pi* – pigment granule; *PM(Ex)* – infolds of basal plasma membrane; *RER* – rough surfaced endoplasmic reticulum; *SER* – smooth surfaced endoplasmic reticulum; *SD* – septate desmosome; *S* secretion; *Sq.E* – squamous epidermal cell; *Tr* – trachea. (Permission to reproduce this diagram from Crossley and Waterhouse 1969 was obtained from the Editor of Tissue and Cell.)

convoluted. The cytoplasm contains moderately well developed granular and agranular endoplasmic reticulum, together with granules which are probably glycogen. The mitochondria are massive with whorled cristae. Numerous electron lucid, membrane bound vacuoles are seen; they vary in number and size but those near the end apparatus are generally smaller. These may represent a precursor of the pheromone. Although in electron micrographs secretion is visualized within the duct, no similar material is seen within the filaments, microvilli or cellular cytoplasm. From such observations it is concluded that the secretion is converted to pheromone in the end apparatus. The filaments may function in the final stages of the synthesis by supplying enzymes and/or mixing the components of the secretion.

2.4. *Modified abdominal sternites*

These are integumentary glands represented by modifications of one or more sternites and occur in at least two orders, the Isoptera and Coleoptera. The glands of the termites are structurally the most complex of the pheromone secreting glands. They are represented by an unpaired medial thickening of the epidermis and are not eversible. In all species they produce trail pheromones, the chemical structures of which are largely unknown. In a few species there are indications that these glands are involved in sex pheromone production (Stuart 1969; Quennedey 1971a; Pasteels 1972). In the lower termites of the families Kalotermitidae, Hodotermitidae and Rhinotermitidae the sternal glands are situated, in the genera so far studied, on either sternite four or five. In the higher termites (Termitidae) the gland is always located on the fifth sternite. These glands are present in all castes but slight modifications with polymorphism have been observed in some species (Noirot 1969). A peculiarity of the termite sternal gland is the presence of campaniform sensilla.

Within the Coleoptera the sternal glands producing sex pheromones have been described for six species of dermestid beetles of the genus *Trogoderma* (Hammack et al. 1973).

2.4.1. *Sternal glands with ductless cells*

In representatives of the Kalotermitidae, Termitidae and Hodotermitidae the glands are similar in that more than one type of modified epidermal cell is involved in secretion production. In the former two families there are two types of cells and these have been designated a) intercalary cells and b) gland cells (Noirot 1969; Quennedey 1971a, b, 1972). *Intercalary cells* extend from the basement membrane to the cuticle and they are structurally very similar to the cells in sect. 2.3.1 which possess microvilli. The cells of the Termitidae have large finger-like cytoplasmic protrusions of the apical membrane which partially penetrate the cuticle (fig. 2.1d). *Gland cells* are located in the intercellular spaces between adjacent intercalary cells. Large numbers of lipid droplets associated with the mitochondria (Kalotermitidae) and enlarged modified mitochondria (Termitidae) make the ultrastructure distinct from that of the intercalary cells. There are unique modifications of the basal plasma membrane of the gland cells.

Within the Kalotermitidae differences in size and cytoplasmic contents are seen between the cells of the anterior and posterior regions of the gland, and in addition nervous efferent fibers are observed between the cells of the anterior region (Quennedey 1969). In both regions pore canals, pore canal filaments and epicuticular filaments are present. The only structures that extend through the cuticulin are epicuticular filaments in the anterior region (fig. 2.1c) and pore canals containing the epicuticular filaments in the posterior region (Quennedey 1971b). A positive test for esterase was obtained only in the anterior region of the gland (Quennedey and Noirot 1968). In the Termitidae the cuticle overlying the gland is similar to that described for the posterior region of the Kalotermitidae.

In the Hodotermitidae there are three types of cells and these have been designated columnar, glandular and basal cells (Satir and Stuart 1965; Stuart and Satir 1968). *Columnar cells* are similar in position and function to the intercalary cells, but unlike them do not reach the basement membrane. Their basal plasma membranes possess long extensions which interdigitate among the underlying glandular cells. *Glandular cells* contain peculiar intracellular membrane bound channels lined with microvilli. These channels appear to be derived from vacuoles lying near the Golgi complex and at times they contain a secretory product. *Basal cells* are undifferentiated and are situated between the glandular cells and the basement membrane.

The cuticle overlying the sternal gland of this type is similar to that described in sect. 2.3.1. The function and inter-relationships of the intercalary (columnar) and glandular cells in the sternal glands of the three termite families under discussion, is thought to be that the secretion is synthesized in the glandular cells and transported to the intercalary or columnar cells where it may be modified or a lipoidal component added. The epicuticular filaments are again involved, in some yet undescribed manner, in the transport of the secretion to the outside.

2.4.2. Sternal glands in which the cells are associated with ducts

Within the Rhinotermitidae the sternal gland is even more complex. Superficially, the gland has anterior and posterior regions separated by a constricted middle region. There are six cell types in the epidermis, four of which appear to be secretory. Of the four, two possess secretory ductules (Quennedey 1971a). a) *Glandular cells of the anterior region* reach the cuticle and possess apical microvilli. b) *Intercalary cells of the anterior region* are elongate and although they surround the glandular cells they also reach the cuticle. Extensive apical microvilli are observed but they are of uneven length thus forming a reservoir-like space beneath the cuticle of the middle region. The space contains a secretion. c) *Glandular cells immediately anterior and posterior to the constriction* contain extensive agranular endoplasmic reticulum. A well developed 'end apparatus' leads to the cuticle-lined ductule which passes through the space of the intercalary cell and penetrates the cuticle in the middle region. d) *Glandular cells of the posterior region* contain granular endoplasmic reticulum and well-developed Golgi complexes. Again, a well-developed 'end apparatus' leads to a cuticle-lined ductule, which penetrates the cuticle in the same manner as described for the glandular cells (c). A layer of squamous epithelial cells lies between the glandular cells and the cuticle of the posterior region. Apart from a thickening in the middle region around the opening of the ductules, the structure of the cuticle is similar to that of the Termitidae.

The chemical structures of the pheromones secreted by the Rhinotermitidae are not known. It is likely, however, that variable secretory activity of the glandular cell types is reflected in the variations of development observed within the castes (Quennedey 1971a).

In the dermestid beetles, the cells of the sternal glands are columnar or goblet shaped and each possesses a secretory ductule. Cells are separated from the overlying cuticle by a layer of squamous epithelial cells. Vacuoles, whose numbers increase with age, are present in the cytoplasm. Generally the secretory cells are not present in males (Hammack et al. 1973).

2.5. *Modification of abdominal tergites*

There are three representatives of tergal glands: the glands producing the sex pheromone in some Isoptera, the cast differentiation pheromone of the queen honey bee, and the Nassanoff secretion of worker bees. The functions of these non-eversible glands differ in each case and for this reason they are considered separately.

In the Isoptera the number of modified tergites varies within families. Where they are present the glands are possessed by either the female alone or by both sexes. The glands possess two cell types, intercalary cells and secretory cells (Noirot 1969). The intercalary cells are similar to those of the sternal glands. The secretory cells lie between the intercalary cells and each has a secretory ductule. A scanning electron microscope study of the surface of the cuticle overlying the gland in *Kalotermes flavicollis* Fabr. has revealed several modifications including the presence of numerous pores. It has been suggested that these pores represent the openings of the secretory ducts (Lebrun 1971).

The function of the Nassanoff gland and the nature of its secretion have been well studied in workers of the honey bee. The pheromone may attract foragers over a distance or may serve as a short range orientation factor for confused bees. The pheromones are neither race nor colony specific (Renner 1960; Butler 1967; Wells and Wenner 1971).

The eversible gland is located in the anterior part of the seventh abdominal tergite which in the resting insect lies beneath the posterior sixth tergite. The gland is arc-shaped with a concave anterior face. When not exposed it forms a slight plateau above the integument. Posteriorly a transverse chitinous rod forms the wall of the plateau; anteriorly the wall is steeper and at its base is located the apodeme of the seventh segment. Adjacent and anterior to the apodeme the intersegmental membrane forms a groove which follows the contours of the concave face of the gland and is therefore nearly a closed space.

The glandular cells are separated from the overlying cuticle by a layer of squamous epithelial cells. Each glandular cell possesses a secretory ductule which terminates at a large vacuole near the nucleus (this presumably represents a type of 'end apparatus'). The ducts, which are sometimes quite long, all penetrate the cuticle in the anterior wall. In this way the groove formed by the intersegmental membrane becomes a reservoir for the secretion (Renner 1960).

The honey bee queen secretes a pheromone from the mandibular glands which enables her to inhibit ovarian development in the workers and maintain her dominating position in the hive. A queen deprived of mandibular glands is still capable of exerting this influence. It has been suggested that glands located in the second, third and fourth abdominal tergites are responsible for the secretion involved (Velthuis 1970). The groups of glandular cells implicated in this ability are medially located in the space between the posterior part of the tergite and the anterior extending part of the intersegmental membrane. Each cell possesses a long secretory ductule which opens through either the tergite or the intersegmental membrane (Renner and Baumann 1964).

2.6. Localized integumentary modifications with disseminating mechanisms

This type of gland includes the tergal glands found in many species of male cockroaches and the scent apparatus of male Lepidoptera. The secretions function as sex pheromones. In both cases, the glands possess scent scales or hairs; however, the glandular cells of the cockroaches have ducts whereas those of the male Lepidoptera are hypertrophied trichogen cells at the base of the scales.

2.6.1. Secretory cells associated with ducts

The location of these tergal glands in male cockroaches and the evolutionary significance of positional variation has recently been extensively reviewed (Barth 1968; Roth 1969, 1971). The number of tergal glands found within a species can range from one to five and the glands vary in complexity even within the same insect when the species has more than one gland. The glandular modifications are located medially on the tergite, the secretory portion forming a depression. In some species this depression is slight while in others it is completely inverted within the segment, essentially forming an internal sac-like reservoir which is not eversible. The disseminating mechanism consists of setae which differ in number, form and distribution between species but are always in the vicinity of the secretory portion.

The secretory cell possesses a secretory apparatus and ductules. The ductules open either on the tergal cuticle or into the cuticle-lined sac. Between the secretory cells and the cuticle is a layer of squamous epithelial cells (Roth 1952; Stay 1957).

2.6.2. Secretory units are hypertrophied trichogen cells

In contrast to the sex pheromone producing glands of female Lepidoptera, the glandular apparatus of the males is exceedingly more complex. Arbitrary division by location is difficult because in several cases the glandular portion may be located in one body region while the disseminating apparatus is located in another. In most cases the active secretions are thought to be aphrodisiacs (see Birch, ch. 7). Within the butterflies, demonstration of function is easier than in the moths where there is the lack of overt behavioral response in the female. In the Pyralidae, two examples are known where the male-produced pheromone functions as a sex attractant. It is also known, at least in some species, that the male is capable of perceiving his own secretion (Schneider and Seibt 1969; Grant 1970). This ability may stimulate the male, in some manner, during courtship (Grant 1970).

·The scent scales are often distinguished from clothing scales by their extreme length. They vary considerably in shape: in many insects they closely resemble and are thus called 'hairs'. (For the purpose of this discussion the disseminating structure will be called a scale when it is flattened in cross-section, otherwise it will be referred to as a hair.)

A considerable proportion of the earlier reports concerning pheromone apparatus, mainly in tropical Lepidoptera, results from the work of Barth during the years 1937 to 1961. Recently an exhaustive survey of these studies and other relevant literature was reported (McColl 1969). Resulting from this survey, a system of classification for the types of male pheromone glands was derived. This classification scheme is designed to indicate the increasing complexity of the glands. Although not indicating an evolutionary tendency with respect to systematics, the scheme, according to McColl, emphasizes the development of the glands in a manner which reduces unnecessary evaporation of the secretion. The large number of species in which the males have a scent apparatus necessitates restricting the detailed discussion to representatives of those groups in which the pheromones have been isolated and characterized.

As the scent apparatus becomes more complex so does the method of its eversion. Retractor muscles at the base of the scent scales or pencils have been reported for many species (Dickens 1936; Barth 1955, 1957; Brower et al. 1965; Weatherston and Percy 1969; Birch 1970; Pliske and Salpeter 1971; inter alia). For some species possessing tubular shaped glands it has been suggested that they are everted by the entrance of air into a complex tracheal system at their bases (Barth 1956). One of the most complicated methods of eversion occurs in those species of noctuids which have an anterior 'brush organ'. This organ, in part, consists of a cuticular fold stretching posteriorly from ventral abdominal segment four. The posterior portion of the fold, in the resting insect, forms a pocket for the distributing brush (pencil). The scent hairs comprising the brush originate in the anteriorly projecting portion of the 'lever', the sclerotized arm of the posterior portion of the second sternite. The triangular base of the 'lever' is attached to the main sternite by a less sclerotized area, thus forming a 'hinge'. Eversion of the brush is brought about by a contraction of several muscles attached to the 'lever', the 'hinge', and the anterior apodeme of the third segment (Birch 1970).

The development of the scent scales or hairs is similar to that of clothing scales (Dixey 1931; Overton 1966; Pliske and Salpeter 1971). Briefly, each scale arises as an outgrowth of a trichogen cell in the early pupa; shortly thereafter cuticle secretion begins. When the scale reaches adult size sculpting of the cuticle takes place. In the late pupae the cellular cytoplasm retracts from the scale and inverts to form a vesicle which is continuous with the lumen of the scale. Trichogen cells which produce clothing scales atrophy shortly after emergence of the adult, while those which produce the scent scales usually remain large and seem active. In the latter cells the vesicles become long and distended and occupy a considerable volume of the cells. The vesicles are bordered by microvillate projections from the cytoplasm (Barth 1938; Brower et al. 1965; Birch 1970; Grant 1970, 1971; Pliske and Salpeter 1971; Grant and Eaton 1973).

In the noctuid *Trichoplusia ni*, the scent apparatus arises from the eighth abdominal sternite. Although the trichogen cells of the scent hairs atrophy within two days of emergence, cells of small fanshaped scales lining the pocket do not atrophy (Grant 1970, 1971) (fig. 2.3). These structural relationships are also observed in the sphingid *Manduca sexta* (L.) (Grant and Eaton 1973). It is not known whether the cells of the pocket scales alone produce the pheromone (Grant 1970). Perhaps some explanation can be derived from the results of studies on other noctuids. Similarly in these species, trichogen cells of small flattened scales lining the pocket (see below) do not atrophy. However, these cells by themselves do not produce the odor which characterizes the pheromone. It has been suggested that they produce a substance, possibly an enzyme, which converts, within the pocket, an inactive precursor to the active form. The inactive precursor in these moths is secreted by Stobbe's glands (fig. 2.4). These paired glands are formed by invaginated tubes between the 'hinge' and the unmodified second sternite (see above). Each gland consists of a cluster of extremely large secretory trichogen cells, each of which possesses a very fine apical hair similar to a scent hair except there are no pores. The hairs extend the length of the invaginated tubes and terminate near the bases of the scent brushes. Upon emergence of the adult insect the cells are very distended, the vesicle occupying almost the entire volume of the cell. The large basal nucleus is consequently flattened and branched. Later the size of the central cavity decreases, presumably indicating the discharge of the secretion. After a few days the entire gland has collapsed, atrophies and is no longer functional. The secretion travels the lumina of the fine hairs, penetrates the cuticle in an undescribed manner, and is converted to the active secretion in the pocket (Birch 1970; Clearwater and Sarafis, 1973).

It is possible that the secretory cells of the scent hairs in *T. ni* function similarly

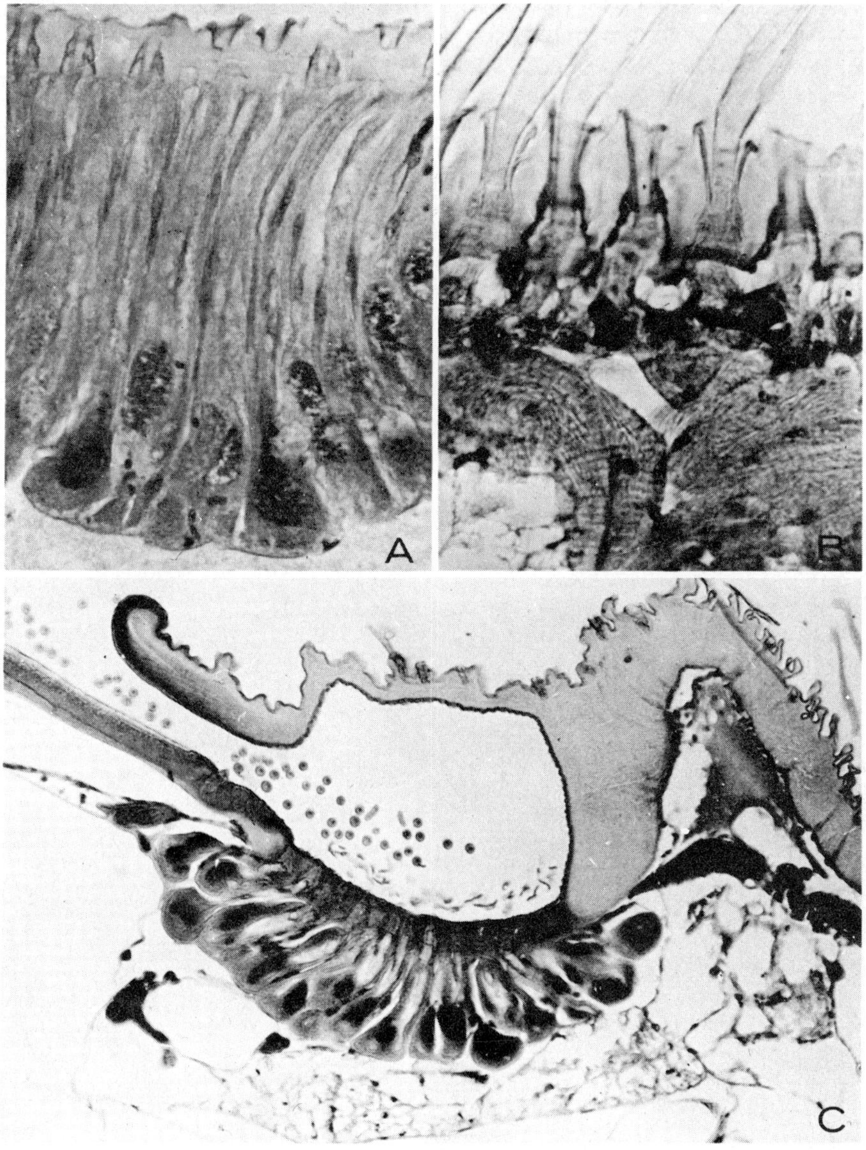

Fig. 2.3. Illustrations indicative of cell type 6.2. a) longitudinal section through glandular epithelium of the large scent brush of a newly emerged male cabbage looper (Grant 1971); b) the same gland from a two-day old male (Grant 1971); c) glandular cell at base of pocket scale of a male tobacco hornworm (Grant and Eaton 1973). (Acknowledgement for permission to reproduce these photographs is made to the Entomological Society of America.)

to those of Stobbe's gland, i.e. the trichogen cells of the scent hairs produce the precursor. On the other hand, in noctuids with anterior brush organs, atrophied trichogen cells at the base of the scent hairs do not produce the precursor. This has been shown by mixing these scent hairs with Stobbe's glands: the resulting mixture does not produce the odor of the pheromone. This is in contrast to the result obtained when the pocket scales are mixed with Stobbe's gland (Birch 1970).

The pheromone producing glands have also been well studied in the family Nymphalidae, particularly the Danainae. In most species the scent apparatus consists primarily of a pair of scent pencils formed by lateral invaginations of the intersegmental membrane between the eighth and ninth abdominal segments. The

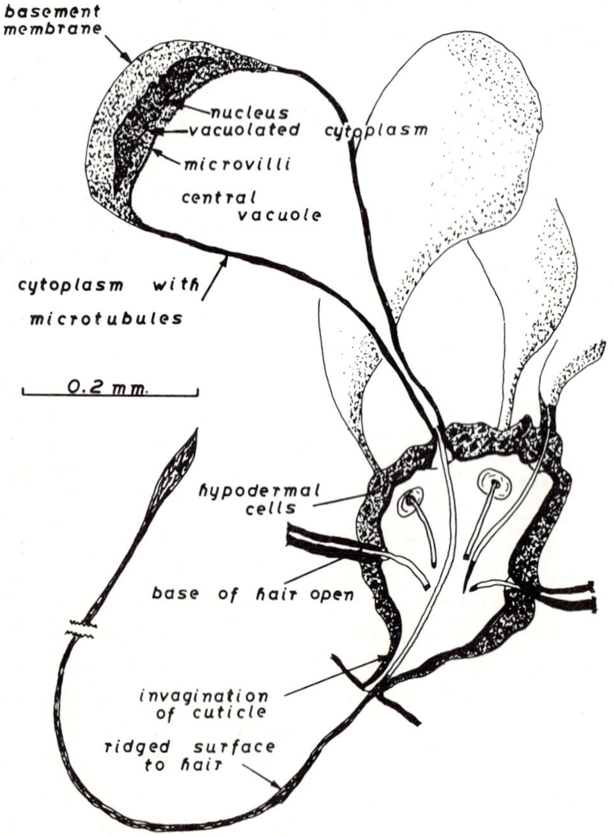

Fig. 2.4. Diagrammatic representation illustrating cells of type 6.2. Section through part of Stobbe's gland from a late pupa of a male *Phlogophora meticulosa* (L) (Birch 1970). (Reproduced by permission of the Royal Entomological Society of London.)

structure and function of the scent apparatus and its secretion have been most completely studied in *Danaus gilippus berenice* (Cramer), the Queen butterfly. Males identify females by sight, and during flight as a female is overtaken by a male the scent pencils are everted whereupon they disseminate particles of 'dust'. In some species the 'dust' particles are absent, but when present they coat the antennae and body of the female, and this is a prerequisite for mating (Brower et al. 1965; Pliske and Eisner 1969; see Birch ch. 7). The bulk of a 'dust' particle, in the case of the Queen butterfly, consists of an inner core of protein – the carrier; an alkaloidal ketone – the active compound; and a diol – the adhesive substance (Meinwald et al. 1969; Pliske and Eisner 1969).

The development of a scent hair resembles that of a clothing scale except during the early stages of cuticle deposition following the formation of the cuticulin. Masses of amorphous material occur between the plasma membrane and the overlying cuticulin. After a gradual protrusion from the surface of the hair, the masses, with the cuticulin surrounding them, separate from the surface. These immature 'dust' particles do not possess aphrodisiac properties (Pliske and Eisner 1969; Schneider and Seibt 1969). They remain in the intersegmental pocket adjacent to the scent hairs. The trichogen cell at the base does not atrophy in the adult. A few days after adult emergence the large nucleus becomes branched, the vesicle becomes elongate and twisted. At this stage the cells are presumed to synthesize and release the ketone and the diol (Pliske and Salpeter 1971).

Glandular complexes are also located on the hind wings and in these insects are a distinctive sexual characteristic. Observations on the behavior of several species indicate that the male occasionally everts the hairpencils and bends the abdomen so that the pencils are inserted into these wing pockets. The function of the wing pockets in the communication system is not fully understood, although several hypotheses have been proposed (Brower and Jones 1965; Pliske and Eisner 1969; Myers 1972).

In the pyralid moths *Galleria mellonella* L. and *Achroia grisella* Fab. it has been shown that the pheromone is actually an attractant. The behavior of the females upon receiving the stimulus is similar to that normally observed in other moths during bioassay for female-produced sex attractants (Röller et al. 1968; Dahm et al. 1971). In both species the gland is located on the underside and near the base of the forewing. It appears as a swelling which is actually an invaginated pocket whose duct opens away from the base of the wing. The pocket is lined with hairs originating from enlarged trichogen cells located on the dorsal and lateral sides of the pocket (Barth 1938).

2.7. *Internally located glands with cuticular lined reservoirs*

Within this category are several glands of the Hymenoptera and one from the Isoptera. Compounds originating in the glands are intricately involved in the behavior of the complex inter-relationships of the social insects. The chemicals can function as alarm, trail, sex or caste-regulating pheromones.

Each gland possesses an internal reservoir for storage and a reservoir duct which transfers the secretion to the site of dispersion. The glands may be divided into two groups with respect to the location of the secretory cells.

2.7.1. *Gland cells form part of the reservoir wall*

Dufour's gland in the formicine ants produces alarm pheromones, while in those myrmicine ants, where the function is known, it produces trail pheromones.

In the formicines, where the sting apparatus has all but disappeared, the reservoir duct forms part of the poison funnel. The reservoir is a bilobed sac of variable size. In the myrmicines the sting apparatus is present though it may be modified and, at its base, the duct from the single lobed reservoir enters the sting bulb. Muscles associated with the poison gland close the duct from Dufour's gland so that its secretion can be ejected separately. No such mechanism has been described for the formicines (Wheeler 1913; Whelden 1957, 1960; Callahan et al. 1959; Hermann and Blum 1967; Bergström and Löfqvist 1972).

The reservoirs are cuticle-lined, this lining thickening in the duct. External to the cuticle of the reservoir is a single layer of cuboidal to columnar epithelial cells. Two layers of cells were observed in *Solenopsis saevissima* (Fr. Smith). No further modifications of the cells have been described; an external layer of striated muscle may be present (Wheeler 1913; Callahan et al. 1959; Hermann and Blum 1967).

Pavan's gland is found in several species of dolichoderine ants where it is the site of production of the trail pheromone. The unpaired gland is located immediately beneath the central portion of the fourth sternite of the gaster. Its duct lies in a longitudinal ridge at the posterior edge and opens at the anterior edge of the fifth sternite. The structure of the single lobed reservoir is similar to that described for Dufour's gland with the addition of peculiar internal hexagonal projections of the cuticle (Pavan and Ronchetti 1955; Gabba 1967).

Tibial glands on the posterior legs of *Crematogaster* workers produce trail pheromones. The gland is a modified tendon, its enlarged groove forming a reservoir which opens via a pore located in the articulating membrane between the last tarsomere and tarsus. The epithelial cells of the tendon are cuboidal as compared to the squamous epithelial cells of smaller unmodified tendons of other legs. The release of the pheromone is probably controlled by the action of the associated muscle (Pasteels et al. 1970).

A frontal gland found in the termites produces alarm pheromones in soldiers of the family Termitidae (Moore 1969). The gland structure has been best studied in the Nasutiterminae, where it consists of a large pear-shaped reservoir with an extremely long duct opening at the extremity of the rostrum. The cuticle-lined reservoir is enclosed by a single layer of cells comprised of two types, columnar and glandular. The columnar cells have an obvious apical brush border whereas the glandular cells possess a secretory ductule. Glandular cells are especially abundant in the duct and anterior portion of the reservoir. The function of each cell type is unknown. Muscles are associated with the anterior part of the reservoir (Noirot 1969).

2.7.2. *Glands in which the cells form a secretory aggregate distinct from but connected to the reservoir*

The mandibular glands as a source of pheromones have been well studied. In the ants the secretion is often a mixture and usually functions as an alarm pheromone (Blum 1969, 1970; Wilson 1971; Wilson and Regnier 1971). Various functions have been ascribed to the mandibular gland secretions of bees including use as aerial trail pheromones in male bumble bees and solitary bees; alarm pheromones, when emitted in high concentrations by *Apis* species; sex pheromones; also inhibitors of queen rearing and ovarian development in queen honey bees (Butler 1967; Blum 1969; Wilson 1971).

The paired glands are located in the head capsule at the base of the mandibles. Each gland consists of an aggregate of secretory cells and a reservoir with its associated efferent duct. Each of the secretory cells possesses a ductule which opens into the apical portion of the reservoir either singly or through a cribellum. The efferent duct terminates in a slit-like pore mesally located at the base of the mandible. The opening and closing of the duct is accomplished by chitinous plates which are in turn controlled by apodemes (Wheeler 1913; Whelden 1957, 1960; Butler and Simpson 1958; Nedel 1960).

Unmodified squamous epithelial cells are the only type observed beneath the cuticle of the reservoir. It is therefore probable that the only secretory cells are those of the aggregate. Brief discussions of the histology and an ultrastructural study of the secretory cells indicate that they resemble those described in sect. 2.3.2. During the ultrastructural description of the bumble bee mandibular gland an attempt was made to determine the relationship of cytoplasmic structures in the secretory cells to the final product. A developmental sequence from secretory granules to 'vakuolenähnliche Bildungen' was proposed by Stein (1962). Unfortunately these 'vakuolenähnliche Bildungen' bear a remarkable resemblance to the schizonts of protozoan parasites of the order Microsporida. These parasites often occur in insect cells and since Stein's report their ultrastructure has frequently been described (Youssef and Hammond 1971 and references therein; Percy 1973).

The anal gland is present only in dolichoderine ants where it produces alarm pheromones. Situated dorsally in the gaster it consists of paired aggregates of secretory cells and paired reservoirs. The secretory cells possess ductules and probably resemble those of the mandibular glands. It has been reported that the secretory ductules join to form a single duct before entering each reservoir. The efferent ducts from the reservoirs join to form a common duct which opens between the fourth and fifth tergites. The reservoir walls have an external layer of muscles (Wheeler 1913; Pavan and Ronchetti 1955).

The poison gland in the formicine ants also produces an alarm pheromone; in the myrmicine ants this gland elaborates the trail pheromones, sometimes as trace constituents in a mixture of protein and amino acids.

The scelerotized portions of the sting apparatus are present in the non-stinging myrmicines, but are modified to function in trail laying. The poison gland consists of aggregates of secretory cells and a reservoir which narrows to form an efferent duct. This duct in the myrmicines enters the sting bulb adjacent to the duct from Dufour's gland, whereas in the formicine ants it is joined by the duct from Dufour's gland – the common duct forming the poison funnel.

The secretory portion of the gland is formed by paired free filaments and a convoluted gland. The free filaments may be very long and ramify throughout the gaster. They terminate near the reservoir where they join and become continuous with the gland which lies on the surface of the reservoir but invaginated within it. The entire reservoir is surrounded by a sheath of striated muscle.

A free filament is composed of a central cuticle-lined duct ensheathed by a single layer of cuboidal to low columnar cells. The filament ducts join to form convoluted gland ducts where the filaments become continuous with the convoluted gland. Each of the cells of the convoluted gland contains a secretory ductule opening into the larger ducts which eventually penetrate the cuticle lining the reservoir. Unmodified squamous epithelial cells form a single layer beneath the cuticle. Only the cells of the free filaments and convoluted gland are thought to participate in elaboration of secretion. Since the convoluted gland is invaginated within the reservoir the secretory cells are limited by cuticle on both sides. This could be of vital importance in those cases where the final secretion is extremely toxic (Wheeler 1913; Blum and Ross 1965; Hermann and Blum 1966, 1967; Hermann et al. 1970).

2.8. *Glandular source associated with internal organs whose prime function is not pheromone production*

The scarcity of data relating to the location and structure of these glands precludes any generalized statements. Pheromones from such structures occur in the Orthoptera, Isoptera, Hymenoptera, Coleoptera and Diptera. Areas of the hindgut have been implicated in the production of aggregating, caste differentiation and trail pheromones in some species of Orthoptera, Isoptera and Hymenoptera respectively (Ishii and Kuwahara 1967; Wilson 1971). Considerable effort has been devoted to the isolation and characterization of the aggregating pheromones of the boll weevil and various bark beetles. Again the hindgut has been implicated as the site of elaboration but no conclusive evidence has as yet been reported (Pitman et al. 1965; Schneider and Rudinsky 1969; Hardee 1970; Rudinsky 1970). The colleterial glands of *Costelytra zealandica* (White) contain symbiotic bacteria which are apparently capable of producing a sex attractant of this beetle (Hoyt et al. 1971).

In *Dacus tryoni* (Frogg.) (Diptera) the sex pheromone is produced by the male in a secretory sac which arises ventrally to the point where the anal tube leaves the rectum. The secretion is stored in a reservoir which lies ventrally to the secretory sac. In newly emerged males both the walls of the secretory sac and those of the reservoir contain enlarged, irregularly shaped cells covered by thin cuticle. As the fly matures the secretion accumulates in the secretory sac and the reservoir; eventually the reservoir becomes distended with secretion. At this stage the reservoir walls contain squamous epithelial cells. Both the secretory sac and the reservoir are surrounded by a longitudinal and a circular muscle layer which enables the reservoir, in particular, to expel the pheromone to the anus where it is discharged with the feces (Fletcher 1969).

2.9. Conclusion

Within recent years large numbers of pheromones have been isolated, chemically identified and their functions established. The morphology and histology of various glands is also well documented. Careful choice of a gland could now provide insight into the synthesis and release of pheromones, accomplished by a thorough investigation of the ultrastructure as related to the biochemistry of the cell and cuticle. Such a study may be especially revealing in those insects where one gland produces a variety of compounds e.g. the mandibular glands. It is quite likely that some secretions consist of a mixture of precursors and product, both of which are biologically active. However, the possibility exists that, within an individual gland, the cells, although histologically similar, differ from each other either by the compounds secreted or by the time during which a particular component is synthesized.

These are only a few of the unsolved problems concerning gland structure and pheromone production. Solutions to such problems will undoubtedly provide us with a better insight into the many interesting aspects of chemical communication.

References

Barnes, M. M., D. M. Peterson and J. J. O'Connor (1966) Sex pheromone gland in the female codling moth, *Carpocapsa pomonella* (Lepidoptera: Olethreutidae). Ann. Entomol. Soc. Am. 59, 732–734.

Barth, R. (1938) Bau und Funktion der Flügeldrüsen einiger Mikrolepidopteren. Untersuchungen an den Pyraliden: *Aphomia gularis, Galleria mellonella, Plodia interpunctella, Ephestia elutella* und *E. kuhniella*. Z. Wiss. Zool. 150, 1–37.

Barth, R. (1955) Maennliche Duftorgane Brasilianischer Lepidopteren. 10. Mitteilung *Hemiceras prosimata* Dogm. (Notodontidae). An. Acad. Brasil. Cienc. 27, 539–545.

Barth, R. (1956) Os sukos abdominais des machos de algunas Arctiidae e Ctenuchidae do Brasil. Mem. Inst. Oswaldo Crus 54, 499–515.

Barth, R. (1957) O órgão odórifero masculino de una espécie de gènere *Episimus* (Lepidoptera: Olethreutidae). Mem. Inst. Oswaldo Crus 55, 113–126.

Barth, R. H. Jr. (1968) The comparative physiology of reproductive processes in cockroaches. Part 1. Mating behaviour and its endocrine control. *In*: Advances in Reproductive Physiology, Vol. 3; ed.: A. McLaren (Academic Press, New York) pp. 167–207.

Bergström, G. and J. Löfqvist (1972) Similarities between the Dufour gland secretions of the ants *Camponotus ligniperda* (Latr.) and *Camponotus herculeanus* (L.) (Hym.). Entomol. Scand. 3, 225–238.

Birch, M. C. (1970) Structure and function of the pheromone-producing brush-organs in males of *Phlogophora meticulosa* (L.) (Lepidoptera; Noctuidae). Trans. Roy. Entomol. Soc. London 122, 277–292.

Blum, M. S. (1969) Alarm pheromones. Ann. Rev. Entomol. 14, 57–80.

Blum, M. S. (1970) The chemical basis of insect sociality. *In*: Chemicals Controlling Insect Behavior; ed.: M. Beroza (Academic Press; New York and London) pp. 61–94.

Blum, M. S. and G. N. Ross (1965) Chemical releasers of social behaviour, V. Source, specificity, and properties of the odour trail pheromone of *Tetramorium guineense* (F.) (Formicidae: Myrmicinae) J. Insect Physiol. 11, 857–868.

Brower, L. P., J. v. Z. Brower and F. P. Cranston (1965) Courtship behavior of the Queen butterfly, *Danaus gilippus berenice* (Cramer). Zoologica (New York) 50, 1–39.

Brower, L. P. and M. A. Jones (1965) Precourtship interaction of wing and abdominal sex glands in male *Danaus* butterflies. Proc. Roy. Entomol. Soc. London 40, 147–151.

Butler, C. G. (1967) Insect pheromones. Biol. Rev. Cambridge Phil. Soc. 42, 42–87.

Butler, C. G. and J. Simpson (1958) The source of the queen substance of the honey bee (*Apis mellifera* L.). Proc. Roy. Entomol. Soc. London 33, 120–122.

Callahan, P. S., M. S. Blum and J. R. Wallace (1959) Morphology and histology of the poison glands and sting of the imported fire ant (*Solenopsis saevissima V. richteri* Forel). Ann. Entomol. Soc. Am. 52, 573–590.

Clearwater, J. R. and V. Sarafis (1973) The secretory cycle of a gland involved in pheromone production in the noctuid moth, *Pseudaletia separata*. J. Insect Physiol. 19, 19–28.

Crossley, A. D. and D. F. Waterhouse (1969) The ultrastructure of a pheromone-secreting gland in the male scorpion-fly *Harpobittacus australis* (Bittacidae: Mecoptera). Tissue and Cell 1, 273–294.

Dahm, K. H., D. Meyer, W. E. Finn, V. Reinhold and H. Röller (1971) The olfactory and auditory mediated sex attraction in *Achroia grisella* (Fabr.). Naturwissenschaften 58, 265–266.

Dickens, G. R. (1936) The scent glands of certain Phycitidae (Lepidoptera). Trans Roy. Entomol. Soc. London 85, 331–362.

Dixey, F. A. (1931) Development of wings in Lepidoptera. Trans. Roy. Entomol. Soc. London 79, 365–393.

Eisner, T., F. McHenry and M. M. Salpeter (1964) Defense mechanisms of arthropods. XV. Morphology of the quinone-producing glands of a tenebrionid beetle (*Eleodes longicollis* LeC.) J. Morphol. 115, 355–399.

El-Sawaf, B. M., A. H. Kaschef and A. A. Soliman (1968) Development and histology of the scent gland in the cotton leafworm, *Prodenia litura* F. and the pink bollworm, *Pectinophora gossypiella* S. (Lepidoptera). Z. Angew. Entomol. 61, 229–239.

Filshie, B. K. (1970) The resistance of epicuticular components of an insect to extraction with lipid solvents. Tissue and Cell 2, 181–190.

Filshie, B. K. and D. F. Waterhouse (1968) The fine structure of the lateral scent glands of the green vegetable bug, *Nezara viridula* (Hemiptera, Pentatomidae). J. Microscop. 7, 231–244.

Fletcher, B. S. (1969) The structure and function of the sex pheromone glands of the male Queensland fruit fly. J. Insect Physiol. 15, 1309–1322.

Gabba, A. (1967) Aspetti dell'organizzazione negli insetti sociali 2. La sostanza della traccia nei Formicidae. Natura (Milano) 58, 150–172.

George, J. A. (1965) Sex pheromone of the oriental fruit moth *Grapholitha molesta* (Busch) (Lepidoptera: Tortricidae). Can. Entomol. 97, 1002–1007.

Götz, B. (1951) Die Sexualduftstoffe an Lepidopteren. Experientia 7, 406–418.

Grant, G. G. (1970) Evidence for a male sex pheromone in the noctuid, *Trichoplusia ni.* Nature (London) 227, 1345–1346.

Grant, G. G. (1971) Scent apparatus of the male cabbage looper, *Trichoplusia ni.* Ann. Entomol. Soc. Am. 64, 347–352.

Grant, G. G. and J. L. Eaton (1973) Scent brushes of the male tobacco hornworm, *Manduca sexta* (Lepidoptera, Sphingidae). Ann. Entomol. Soc. Am. (in press).

Gupta, B. L. and D. S. Smith (1969) Fine structural organization of the spermatheca in the cockroach, *Periplaneta americana.* Tissue and Cell 1, 295–324.

Hammack, L., W. E. Burkholder and M. Ma (1973) Sex pheromone localization in females of six *Trogoderma* species. Ann. Entomol. Soc. Am. 66, 545–550.

Happ, G. M., J. D. Strandberg and C. M. Happ (1966) The terpene-producing glands of a phasmid insect. Cell morphology and histochemistry. J. Morphol. 119, 143–160.

Hardee, D. D. (1970) Pheromone production by male boll weevils as affected by food and host factors. Contrib. Boyce Thompson Inst. 24, 315–321.

Hermann, H. R. Jr. and M. S. Blum (1966) The morphology and histology of the hymenopterous poison apparatus. I. *Paraponera clavata* (Formicidae). Ann. Entomol. Soc. Am. 59, 397–409.

Hermann, H. R. and M. S. Blum (1967) The morphology and histology of the hymenopterous poison apparatus. II. *Pogonomyrmex badius* (Formicidae). Ann. Entomol. Soc. Am. 60, 661–668.

Hermann, H. R., J. C. Moser and A. N. Hunt (1970) The hymenopterous poison apparatus. X Morphological and behavioral changes in *Atta texana.* Ann. Entomol. Soc. Am. 63, 1552–1558.

Hoyt, C. P., G. O. Osborne and A. P. Mulcock (1971) Production of an insect sex attractant by symbiotic bacteria. Nature (London) 230, 472.

Ishii, S. and Y. Kuwahara (1967) An aggregation pheromone of the German cockroach *Blatella germanica* L. (Orthoptera: Blatellidae). 1. Site of the pheromone production. Appl. Entomol. Zool. 2, 203–217.

Jefferson, R. N. and R. E. Rubin (1970) Sex pheromones of noctuid moths. XVII. A clarification of the description of the female sex pheromone gland of *Prodenia litura.* Ann. Entomol. Soc. Am. 63, 431–433.

Jefferson, R. N., H. H. Shorey and L. K. Gaston (1966) Sex pheromones of noctuid moths. X. The morphology and histology of the female sex pheromone gland of *Trichoplusia ni* (Lepidoptera: Noctuidae). Ann. Entomol. Soc. Am. 59, 1166–1169.

Jefferson, R. N., H. H. Shorey and R. E. Rubin (1968) Sex pheromones of noctuid moths. XVI. The morphology of the female sex pheromone glands of eight species. Ann. Entomol. Soc. Am. 61, 861–865.

Jefferson, R. N., L. L. Sower and R. E. Rubin (1971) The female sex pheromone gland of the pink bollworm, *Pectinophora gossypiella* (Lepidoptera: Gelechiidae). Ann. Entomol. Soc. Am. 64, 311–312.

Lebrun, D. (1971) Glandes tergales et surfaces cuticulaires correspondantes chez le termite, *Calotermes flavicollis* Fabr. C. R. Acad. Sci. (Paris) 272, 3162–3164.

Locke, M. (1960) The cuticle and wax secretion in *Calpodes ethlius* (Lepidoptera, Hesperiidae). Quart. J. Microscop. Sci. 101, 333–338.

Locke, M. (1961) Pore canals and related structures in insect cuticle. J. Biophys. Biochem. Cytol. 10, 589–618.

Locke, M. (1964) The structure and formation of the integument in insects. *In*: Physiology of Insecta, Vol. 3; ed.: M. Rockstein (Academic Press, New York) pp. 379–470.

Locke, M. (1966) The structure and formation of the cuticulin layer in the epicuticle of an insect, *Calpodes ethlius* (Lepidoptera, Hesperiidae). J. Morphol. 118, 461–494.

Locke, M. (1969) Structure of an epidermal cell during the development of the protein epicuticle and the uptake of moulting fluid in an insect. J. Morphol. 127, 7–40.

Locke, M. and H. Krishnan (1971) The distribution of phenoloxidases and polyphenols during cuticle formation. Tissue and Cell 3, 103–126.

McColl, H. P. (1969) The sexual scent organs of male Lepidoptera, M. Sc. thesis (Univ. Coll. Swansea, Wales) pp. 1–214.

Meinwald, J., Y. C. Meinwald and P. H. Mazzocchi (1969) Sex pheromone of the Queen butterfly: Chemistry. Science 164, 1174–1175.

Mercer, E. H. and P. C. J. Brunet (1959) The electron microscopy of the left colleterial gland of the cockroach. J. Biophys. Biochem. Cytol. 5, 257–262.

Miller, T., R. N. Jefferson and W. W. Thompson (1967) Sex pheromones of noctuid moths. XI. The ultra-structure of the apical region of cells of the female sex pheromone gland of *Trichoplusia ni*. Ann. Entomol. Soc. Am. 60, 707–708.

Moore, B. P. (1969) Biochemical studies in termites. *In*: Biology of Termites, Vol. 1; eds.: K. Krishna and F. M. Weisner (Academic Press, New York) pp. 407–432.

Myers, J. (1972) Pheromones and courtship behavior in butterflies. Am. Zool. 12, 545–551.

Nedel, J. C. (1960) Morphologie und Physiologie der Mandibeldrüse einiger Bienen-Arten (Apidae). Z. Morphol. Oekol. Tiere 49, 139–183.

Noirot, Ch. (1969) Glands and secretions. *In*: Biology of Termites, Vol. 1: eds.: K. Krishna and F. M. Weisner (Academic Press, New York), pp. 89–123.

Overton, J. (1966) Microtubules and microfibrils in morphogenesis of the scale cells of *Ephestia kühniella*. J. Cell Biol. 29, 293–305.

Pasteels, J. M. (1972) Sex-specific pheromones in a termite. Experientia 28, 105–106.

Pasteels, M., R. M. Crewe and M. S. Blum (1970) Etude histologique et examen aux microscope électronique à balayage de la glande sécrétant la phéromone de piste chez deux *Crematogaster* Nord-americains (Formicidae, Myrmicinae). C. R. Acad. Sci. (Paris) 271, 835–838.

Pavan, M. and G. Ronchetti (1955) Studi sulla morfologia esterna e anatomia interna dell'operaia di *Iridomyrmex humilis* Mayr e ricerche chimiche e biologiche sulla iridomirmecina. Atti Soc. Ital. Sci. Nat. 94, 379–477.

Percy, J. (1973) The intranuclear occurrence and fine structural details of schizonts of *Perezia fumiferanae* (Microsporida: Nosematidae) in cells of *Choristoneura fumiferana* (Clem.) (Lepidoptera: Tortricidae). Can. J. Zool. 51, 553–554.

Percy, J. and J. Weatherston (1971) Studies of physiologically active arthropod secretions. IX. Morphology and histology of pheromone producing glands of some female Lepidoptera. Can. Entomol. 103, 1733–1739.

Percy, J., E. J. Gardiner and J. Weatherston (1971) Studies of physiologically active arthropod secretions. VI. Evidence for a sex pheromone in female *Orgyia leucostigma* (Lepidoptera: Lymantridae). Can. Entomol. 103, 706–712.

Pitman, G. B., R. A. Klieforth and J. P. Vité (1965) Studies on the pheromone of *Ips confusus* (LeConte) II. Further observations on the site of production. Contrib. Boyce Thompson Inst. 23, 13–17.

Pliske, T. E. and T. Eisner (1969) Sex pheromone of the Queen butterfly; Biology. Science 164, 1170–1172.

Pliske, T. E. and M. M. Salpeter (1971) The structure and development of the hairpencil glands in males of the Queen butterfly, *Danaus gilippus berenice*. J. Morphol. 134, 215–242.

Quennedey, A. (1969) Innervation de type neurosécréteur dans la glande sternale de *Kalotermes flavicollis* (Isoptera). Etude ultrastructurale. J. Insect Physiol. 15, 1807–1814.

Quennedey, A. (1971a) Les glandes exocrines des Termites. II. Organisation de la glande sternale des Rhinotermitidae. Etude ultrastructurale préliminaire. C. R. Acad. Sci. (Paris) 273, 376–379.

Quennedey, A. (1971b) Les glandes exocrines des termites. I. Etude histochimique et ultrastructurale de la glande sternale de *Kalotermes flavicollis* Fab. (Isoptera, Kalotermitidae). Z. Zellforsch. Mikroskop. Anat. 121, 27–47.

Quennedey, A. (1972) Les glandes exocrines des termites. III. Structure fini de la glande sternale de *Trinervitermes germinatus* Wasman (Termitidae, Nasutitermitinae). Z. Zellforsch. Mikroskop. Anat. 130, 205–218.

Quennedey, A. and C. Noirot (1968) Esterase cuticulaire dans la glande sternale de *Calotermes flavicollis* F. (Isoptera, Termitidae). Etude histochémique. C. R. Acad. Sci. (Paris) 266, 2456–2458.

Renner, M. (1960) Das Duftorgan der Honigbiene und die Physiologische Bedeutung ihres Lockstoffes. Z. Vergl. Physiol. 43, 411–468.

Renner, M. and M. Baumann (1964) Über Komplexe von subepidermalen Drüsenzellen (Duftdrüsen?) der Bienenkönigin. Naturwissenschaften 3, 68–69.

Roelofs, W. L. and K. C. Feng (1968) Sex pheromone specificity tests in the Tortricidae – an introductory report. Ann. Entomol. Soc. Am. 61, 312–316.

Röller, H., K. Biemann, J. S. Bjerke, D. W. Norgard and W. H. McShan (1968) Sex pheromones of pyralid moths. 1. Isolation and identification of the sex attractant of *Galleria mellonella* L. (greater waxmoth). Acta Entomol. Bohemslov. 65, 208–211.

Roth, L. M. (1952) The tergal gland of the male cockroach, *Supella supellictilium*. J. Morphol. 91, 469–477.

Roth, L. M. (1969) The evolution of male tergal glands in the Blattaria. Ann. Entomol. Soc. Am. 62, 176–208.

Roth, L. M. (1971) Additions to the oothecae, uricose glands, ovarioles and tergal glands of Blattaria. Ann. Entomol. Soc. Am. 74, 127–141.

Rudinsky, J. A. (1970) Sequence of Douglas fir beetle attraction and its ecological significance. Contrib. Boyce Thompson Inst. 24, 311–314.

Satir, P. and A. M. Stuart (1965) A new apical micro-tubule-associated organelle in the sternal glands of *Zootermopsis nevadensis* (Hagen) Isoptera. J. Cell Biol. 24, 277–283.

Schneider, D. and M. Seibt (1969) Sex pheromone of the Queen butterfly: Electroantennogram response. Science 164, 1173–1174.

Schneider, I. and J. A. Rudinsky (1969) The site of pheromone production in *Trypodendron lineatum* (Coleoptera: Scolytidae): Bioassay and histological studies of the hindgut. Can. Entomol. 101, 1181–1186.

Schnepf, E., W. Wenneis and H. Schildknecht (1969) Über Arthropoden Abwehrstoffe XLI. Zur Explosionschemie der Bombadierkäfer (Coleoptera, Carabidae). Z. Zellforsch. Microskop. Anat. 96, 582–599.

Smithwick, E. E. B. (1970) Development of the sex pheromone gland and of the production of the sex pheromone in the Indian meal moth. Ph. D. thesis (Univ. Georgia, Athens, Ga.) pp. 1–185.

Stanic, V., E. Zlotkin and A. Shulov (1970) Localization of pheromone excretion in females of *Trogoderma granarium* (Dermestidae). Entomol. Exptl. Appl. 13, 342–351.

Stay, B. (1957) The sternal scent gland of *Eurycotis floridana*. Ann. Entomol. Soc. Am. 50, 514–519.

Stein, G. (1962) Uber den Feinbau der Mandibeldrüse von Hummelmännchen. Z. Zellforsch. Mikroskop. Anat. 57, 719–736.

Steinbrecht, R.A. (1964a) Feinstruktur und Histochemie der Sexualduftdrüse des Seidenspinners *Bombyx mori* L. Z. Zellforsch. Mikroskop Anat. 64, 227–261.

Steinbrecht, R. A. (1964b) Die Abhängigkeit der Lochwirkung des Sexualduftorgans weiblicher Seidenspinner von Alter und Kopulation. Z. Vergl. Physiol. 48, 341–356.

Strong, L. (1971) Intracellular ducts in the epidermis of the male desert locust. J. Insect Physiol. 17, 1823–1831.

Stuart, A. M. (1969) Social behavior and communication. *In*: Biology of Termites, Vol. 1; eds.: K. Krishna and F. M. Weisner (Academic Press, New York) pp. 193–232.

Stuart, A. M. and P. Satir (1968) Morphological and functional aspects of an insect epidermal gland. J. Cell Biol. 36, 527–549.

Thibout, E. (1972) Glandes exocrines males et femelles intervenant dans le comportement de pariade d'*Acrolepia assectella* (Lepidoptère: Plutellidae). Ann. Soc. Entomol. Fr. (N.S.) 8, 475–480.

Thomas, J. G. (1970) Probable pheromone-secreting cells in the epidermis of mature males of *Schistocerca gregaria* Forskäl (Orthoptera: Acrididae). Proc. Roy. Entomol. Soc. London Ser. A. 45, 125–135.

Urbahn, E. (1913) Abdominale Duftorgane bei weiblichen Schmetterlingen. Jena. Z. Naturwiss. 59, 277–355.

Velthuis, H. H. W. (1970) Queen substances from the abdomen of the honey bee queen. Z. Vergl. Physiol. 70, 210–222.

Waku, Y. and K. Sumimoto (1969) Ultrastructure and secretory mechanism of the alluring gland cell in the silkworm, *Bombyx mori* L. (Lepidoptera: Bombycidae). Appl. Entomol. Zool. 4. 135–146.

Weatherston, J. and J. E. Percy (1968) Studies of physiologically active arthropod secretions. I. Evidence for a sex pheromone in *Vitula edmandsae* (Lepidoptera: Phycitidae). Can. Entomol. 100, 1065–1070.

Weatherston, J. and J. E. Percy (1969) Studies of physiologically active arthropod secretions. II. Some observations on the scent pencils of male *Vitula edmandsae* (Lepidoptera: Phycitidae). Can. Entomol. 101, 280–285.

Weatherston, J. and J. E. Percy (1970) Studies of physiologically active arthropod secretions. IV. Topography of the sex pheromone producing gland of the eastern spruce budworm, *Choristoneura fumiferana* (Clem.) (Lepidoptera: Tortricidae). Can. J. Zool. 48, 569–571.

Wells, P. H. and A. M. Wenner (1971) The influence of food scent of foraging honey bees. Physiol. Zool. 44, 191–209.

Wheeler, W. M. (1913) Ants, Their Structure, Development and Behavior. Columbia Univ. Biol. Series IX (Columbia Univ. Press.) 663 pp.

Whelden, R. M. (1957) Notes on the anatomy of *Rhytidoponera convexa* ('Violacea' Forel) (Hymenoptera: Formicidae). Ann. Entomol. Soc. Am. 50, 271–282.

Whelden, R. M. (1960) The anatomy of *Rhytidoponera metallica* F. Smith (Hymenoptera: Formicidae). Ann. Entomol. Soc. Am. 53, 793–808.

Wilson, E. O. (1971) The Insect Societies (Belknap Press, Harvard Univ. Press, Cambridge, Mass.) 548 pp.

Wilson E. O. and F. E. Regnier (1971) The evolution of the alarm-defense system in the formicine ants. Amer. Nat. 105, 279–289.

Youssef, N. N. and D. M. Hammond (1971) The fine structure of the developmental stages of the microsporidian *Nosema apis* Zander. Tissue and Cell 3, 283–294.

CHAPTER 3

Pheromone perception

Thomas L. PAYNE

3.1. *Introduction*

Olfaction in insects has received considerable attention in recent years due, in part, to the increased interest in the role of insect (pheromones) and host-produced odors in insect behavior. Recently there has been an excellent review of insect olfaction in general (Kaissling 1971). This chapter is not intended as a general review. It will deal only with pheromones, from the physiological response of the receptors to the whole organism behavioral response.

The olfactory perception of insects is highly sensitive, especially to important stimuli in the insect's environment such as food source, habitat and mate. Certainly pheromones are some of the most important olfactory cues in the insect's environment and insects have evolved a highly developed olfactory sense for them. The role pheromones play in host selection and in communication leading to species propagation is absolutely essential to the existence of many, if not all, insects. Pheromones may be ubiquitous throughout the class Insecta, and probably the entire animal kingdom (see ch. 1).

The importance of pheromones to insect life, coupled with the fact that they are released in such minute amounts, necessitates that insects be equipped with an exceptionally efficient mechanism to collect air-borne pheromone molecules and to subsequently decipher the molecule-bound information. The mechanism must also have a high degree of selectivity for a narrow range of compounds because of the complexity of odors in the environment, and must be able to handle the perception of a single pheromone in some species, mixtures of pheromones in others, or mixtures of pheromones and host odors in still others.

3.2. *Methods of investigation*

Investigations of pheromone perception in insects have been carried out at both the behavioral (whole organism) and physiological levels.

Most behavioral investigations involve activity or attraction bioassays. These bioassays provide important insights into the role of various biological factors in pheromone perception, such as; pheromone molecular structure; specificity as to species, sex, age, virginity and developmental stage; location of the organ(s) of pheromone perception and others. In addition the bioassays provide insights on the effects of various environmental influences on perception, such as time of day, light intensity and so on.

The use of behavioral bioassays alone to study pheromone perception cannot lead to the fullest understanding. In some cases, the absence of a behavioral response to stimulation by a pheromone does not necessarily mean the insect does not perceive the pheromone. In addition, the intricacies of pheromone receptors require more detailed investigation than is possible through behavioral study alone. It is essential therefore, that additional methods be employed to investigate pheromone perception.

Antennal excision experiments and electrophysiological investigations of antennal olfactory responsiveness show that, for the most part, the olfactory sense in insects is a function of the antennae in general and specifically of certain antennal sensilla.

Neurologically the olfactory receptors of insects are primary neurons (sense cells) consisting of dendrites, cell bodies and axons. Once the receptor site (thought to be on the membrane of the dendrite of a receptor: Schneider 1970; Steinbrecht and Kasang 1972), is stimulated by pheromone, a series of electrophysiological events result (Wolbarsht 1963). First, a receptor potential (slow, graded potential, which may be intra- or extracellular) occurs at the receptor site of the stimulus. Second, a generator potential (also a slow, graded potential) results in the dendritic process. If the generator potential is of sufficient intensity to overcome the threshold of the cell body, fast rising, short duration impulses (action potentials or spikes) are generated from the proximal region of the cell body. The intensity or height of the receptor potential is directly dependent upon the strength of the olfactory stimulus (Boeckh et al. 1965; Stürckow 1965; Payne et al. 1970; Payne 1971). In turn, the intensity of the receptor potential determines the frequency of the subsequent spikes (Priesner, unpublished in Boeckh et al. 1965).

Modern electrophysiological and histological techniques have been employed to investigate pheromone perception at the antennal receptor level. Measurements of antennal olfactory responsiveness are possible through use of the 'electroantennogram (EAG)' technique (Schneider 1955, 1957a, b; Schneider and Hecker 1956), which consists of a measurement of the summated receptor potentials of several olfactory receptors responding simultaneously to a stimulus (Boeckh et al. 1965). In general, EAGs can be recorded by placing a recording electrode over or in the distal end of the antenna and an indifferent electrode in the proximal end (fig. 3.1) (for details see Schneider 1957a, Stürckow 1965; Payne et al. 1970). There are, however, limitations and difficulties in the use of the EAG and care must be taken to ensure that proper controls are carried out (Schneider 1957a,b; Stürckow 1970; Adler 1971; Birch 1971).

A more intricate technique involves the measurement of olfactory perception in a single receptor sensillum. In this technique the recording electrode is placed at the base of an olfactory sensillum and the indifferent electrode is situated in the haemolymph space of the antenna (fig. 3.1) (for details see Boeckh 1962; Lacher 1964; Schneider et al. 1964; Kafka 1970). In this way it is possible to measure the spikes generated by an individual receptor.

Information on pheromone perception obtained through the use of electrophysiological techniques enhances the knowledge gained from behavioral studies. For example, studies of antennal olfactory responsiveness can provide information on whether various biological and environmental factors affect pheromone perception at the peripheral receptor level, or possibly work through some central integration process. Single cell investigations of olfactory receptors provide information on receptor specificity and the effects of inhibitors and synergists on perception. In conjunction with histological studies of olfactory sensilla, electrophysiological in-

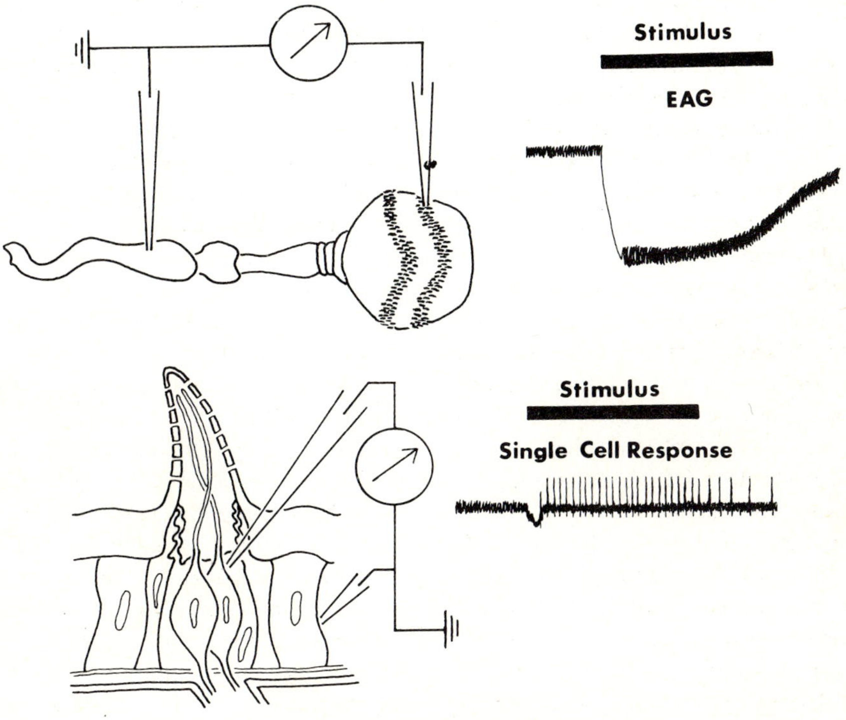

Fig. 3.1. Schematic diagram of the electroantennogram (EAG) and single cell recording techniques.

vestigations have been essential in providing insights on how pheromone molecules reach the insect's nervous system and on the thresholds of electrophysiological and behavioral response to pheromone.

Electrophysiological recordings are also possible from the olfactory center located in the deutocerebrum of the insect brain. The recording electrode is implanted in various areas of the deutocerebrum while the indifferent electrode is situated in the haemolymph of the head capsule (for details see Yamada et al. 1970; Yamada 1971). To date, knowledge of the neurological activity of the olfactory center is limited. However, the potential exists through this technique for obtaining information on how incoming signals from peripheral olfactory receptors are integrated and, possibly, relayed to effector organs.

3.3. *Structures used for pheromone perception*

3.3.1. *The antennae*

Insect antennae possess several characteristics critical to pheromone perception and to insect behavior in general, such as antennal shape and size relative to their function and the general behavior of the insect, and the type, abundance and location of the sensilla on the antennae. In a recent review on insect olfaction Kaissling (1971) provides considerable detail on the morphology of insect antennae with respect to their efficiency as 'odor filters'. In summary, he explains that the efficiency of the antenna as an odor filter is defined by several factors, most of which are dependent upon the external geometry of the antenna. Certain saturniid moths have large, multi-branched antennae, endowed with numerous sensilla that have considerable overlapping 'diffusion spaces'. Mathematical calculations for some of these antennae indicate that they 'sieve' almost all odor molecules from the air stream. Antennae with a less diffuse form are likely to be less efficient as odor filters.

The antennal form and arrangement of sensilla appear to be well adapted to the open or confined habitat of a particular species in nature and the importance of pheromone perception to that species. For example, the cabbage looper moth (*Trichoplusia ni* (Hübner)) commonly occurs in open habitats, on the surfaces of leaves, or hovering over host plants. Its antennae are setiform with a large number of flagellar segments (Jefferson et al. 1970). All but a few basal segments are heavily endowed with sensilla, including those sensilla believed to be important in pheromone perception (Payne et al. 1970). Most of the sensilla are situated on the ventral surface of the antenna. When the antennae are moved forwards from the resting position along the wings, the ventral surfaces face forwards and the sensilla are maximally exposed to sample odor-carrying air.

In the cabbage looper moth, and many other lepidopterous species, the female-produced sex pheromone evokes a behavioral response only from males of the species and electrophysiological investigations show the antennae of the female to be void of the pheromone receptors (Schneider and Hecker 1956; Schneider 1957a, b; Schneider et al. 1964; Payne et al. 1970). However, male and female cabbage looper moths appear to have morphologically identical sensilla in relatively the same numbers. Other insect species show sexual dimorphism in the presence or absence of pheromone receptor sensilla as well as in overall antennal form and size. For example, females of the saturniid moth (*Antheraea pernyi* Guérin-Méneville) not only lack the ability to perceive their pheromone, but their antennae lack the sensilla identified as pheromone receptors on the male (Schneider et al. 1964). In addition, the antennae of the male are about five times larger in outline area than those of the female (Kaissling 1971). Olfactory sensilla make up the majority of the sensilla on the antennae of the male and 60 to 70 percent are specialized receptors for the female sex pheromone (Schneider et al. 1964).

The leaf-cutting ant (*Atta texana* Buckley) operates in at least two distinct habitats. It can be found in the open following pheromone trails and also inhabits an underground nest and fungus garden. The antennae of the insect enable the ant to maneuver within the confines of its subterranean habitat and still be poised to perceive important olfactory cues. Above ground, the elbowed antennae and location of pheromone receptor sensilla on the distally expanded flagella enable the insect to scan closely over the surface in following its trail pheromone. Antennal excision and electrophysiological investigations show that alarm and trail pheromone receptors occur primarily on the distal two antennal segments (Payne and Moser 1972, unpublished).

The bark beetle spends only a small part of its life cycle in the open; most of the time it is found tunneling in the confines of its host tree. The beetle is equipped with short seven- to nine-segmented, club-shaped antennae within all sensilla, except a few mechanoreceptors being located on the enlarged terminal segment – the club (Payne et al. 1973). The antennal form and localization of the sensilla on the club provide the beetle with a concentrated mass of pheromone receptors for perception of aggregation pheromones during the aggregation phase of its behavior (see ch. 8). In addition, the antennal form enables the beetle to hold the antennae close to the head capsule and prevent physical damage to sensilla through abrasions or resin coating as the insect tunnels in the host tree.

3.3.2 The sensilla

Based on electrophysiological evidence Schneider and Steinbrecht (1968) considered four types of sensilla to be olfactory. They are: (1) sensilla trichodea (Lepidoptera): (2) sensilla basiconica (Lepidoptera, Diptera, Coleoptera, Hymenoptera); (3) sensilla placodea (Hymenoptera); and (4) sensilla coeloconica (Orthoptera, Hymenoptera) (fig. 3.2). These sensilla vary in size. For example, the hair-like sensilla trichodea and basiconica vary in length from 45 to 370 microns and 8 to

40 microns respectively. In addition, varying numbers of sense cells are found associated with one type of sensillum for a given insect species (see table 1 in Schneider and Steinbrecht 1968). In the silk moth (*Bombyx mori* L.) for example, there are one to two sense cells per sensillum trichodium and one to three per sensillum basiconicum. In contrast, the migratory locust (*Locusta migratoria* R. and F.) has 25 to 45 sense cells per sensillum basiconicum.

Investigations of the reaction spectra of the various sense cells associated with the olfactory sensilla led to the terms 'odor generalists' and 'odor specialists' (Boeckh et al. 1965). Odor generalists are cells, each of which has a unique odor spectrum, but the spectra of different cells overlap to a great degree. Sense cells of

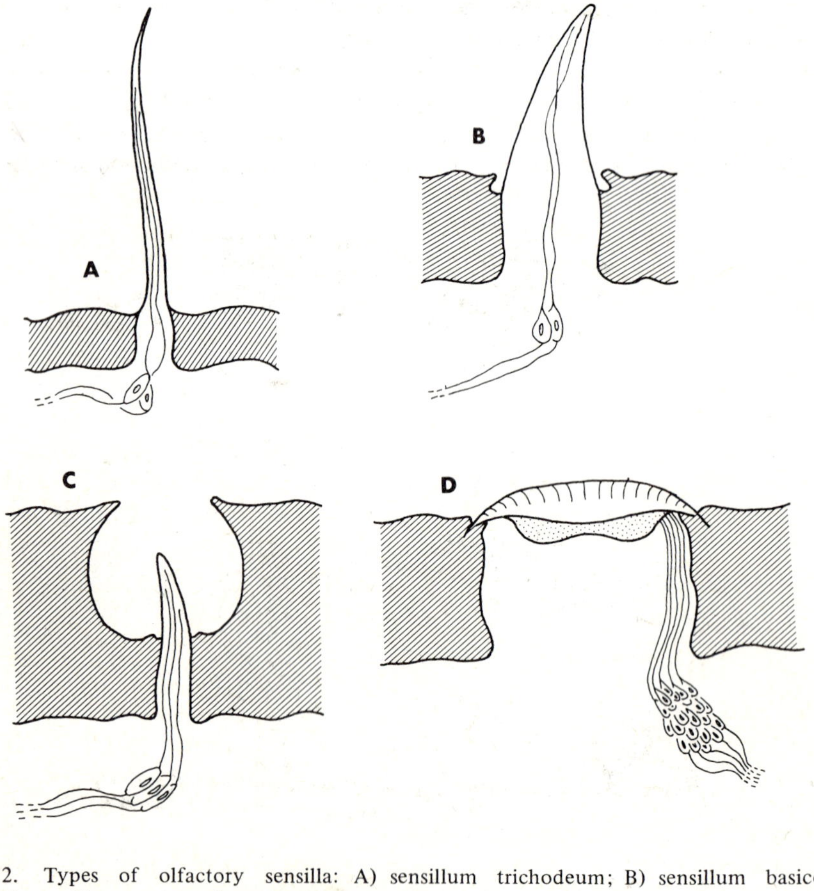

Fig. 3.2. Types of olfactory sensilla: A) sensillum trichodeum; B) sensillum basiconicum; C) sensillum coeloconicum; and D) sensillum placodeum (after Schneider and Steinbrecht 1968). Sensillum hairs and cells are not drawn to scale.

For example, the southern pine beetle (*Dendroctonus frontalis* Zimmerman), a scolytid, is preyed upon by a checkered clerid beetle (*Thanasimus dubius* F.). Field investigations (Vité and Williamson 1970) have shown that the clerid beetle is attracted to a southern pine beetle aggregation pheromone, frontalin (Kinzer et al. 1969), a compound unlikely to be produced by the clerid beetle. It is apparent that both the southern pine beetle and its predator have receptors for the aggregation pheronome, the information transferred and the resulting behaviors being the same. The absence of species specificity in pheromone perception for some lepidopterous species has been found to accompany the production of a common pheromone by these species and to result in the same whole organism behavioral response by these species (Brady et al. 1971; Kuwahara et al. 1971). In this case, it appears that perception of the same pheromone results in identical information transfer for each species. In general, however, the occurrence or possible occurrence, of a common pheromone and the resulting identical behavioral responses have been restricted to closely related species (Brady et al. 1971; Kuwahara et al. 1971; Shorey et al. 1965).

Varying degrees of specificity in pheromone perception also exist within any species. In many species sex is often a factor determining the capability for perception. As mentioned earlier, in many moths only the males are capable of perceiving the female-released sex pheromone (Schneider 1957a, b; Payne et al. 1970). In some cases the incapacity is because of a lack of specific olfactory sensilla (Schneider et al. 1964); in other cases it results from a lack of pheromone receptors, even though both males and females have the same sensilla (Boeckh et al. 1965; Payne et al. 1970).

The ability of a given sex to perceive a pheromone does not necessarily mean it will display a stereotyped behavioral response or respond at all. For example, in the American cockroach only the adult male was found to respond behaviorally to the female sex pheromone extract (Yamada et al. 1968). However, investigation of antennal olfactory responsiveness showed that adult females as well as adult males could perceive the extract. The information derived from the pheromone molecules might not be interpreted in the same way by each sex and/or may come from different receptors, thus accounting for the presence or absence of behavioral response. Differences may also occur between the sexes in the neural integrative and/or motor pathways responsive to pheromone-related inputs.

The age and development stage of an insect are also important in its capability to perceive pheromone (see also ch. 4). The adult male cabbage looper does not respond maximally on a behavioral level to the female sex pheromone (Berger 1966) until it is about 2.5 days post eclosion (Shorey and Gaston 1964). Few individuals respond at less than one day post eclosion, although their pheromone receptors are functional much earlier. EAGs recorded from male pupae showed significant response to pheromone as early as 6–12 hr before adult emergence (Payne et al. 1970). In comparison, southern pine beetles are not responsive to pheromone at the behavioral level until they are essentially through the callow adult stage, about three days after the pupal stage. EAG investigations did not show antennal olfactory responsiveness to occur significantly earlier (Payne 1972, unpublished).

Specificity associated with pheromone perception also occurs in social insects. Here reference is made to a caste specific pheromone. Hölldobler and Maschwitz (1965) reported the presence of a male-produced pheromone in the carpenter ant (*Camponotus herculeanus* L.), which stimulated young females into flight. The pheromone had a slight excitatory effect on the workers and males did not react. A compound with similar effects has been isolated and identified from *C. pennsylvanicus* DeG.) (Brand et al. 1973). EAGs were recorded from males, females and workers to the pheromone (Payne and Blum 1972, unpublished). EAGs and behavioral responses in the laboratory to the pheromone were large in the females and workers, but comparatively low, although present, in the males. It is apparent that the three castes have receptors for the pheromone although the effects of the pheromone on their behavior are different. Specificity in response to the pheromone is absent at the receptor level between the castes on a response–no response basis. However, there is specificity at the behavioral level in the type or degree of response elicited from a given case.

Investigations of the effects of pheromone molecular structure on activity have provided insights into specificity at the receptor level. Schneider et al. (1967) found that, for the silk moth, the geometrical isomers of bombykol were required in 100-fold greater amounts than bombykol in order to elicit comparable responses at both the peripheral receptor and behavioral levels. Similarly, structural modifications of the cabbage looper pheromone resulted in varying degrees of reduced behavioral response depending upon the extent of the modification (Berger and Canerday 1968; Jacobson et al. 1968; Toba et al. 1970; Gaston et al. 1972).

Electrophysiological (EAG) and behavioral investigations of the response of the male cabbage looper to compounds (parapheromones) systematically modified in structure from that of the pheromone show the importance of carbon chain length and site of unsaturation to the activity of the pheromone and show their importance in the specificity of the pheromone receptor (Payne 1969; Gaston et al. 1972). The more a parapheromone differs in structure from the natural pheromone, either in carbon chain length or site of unsaturation, the greater is the concentration required to elicit responses comparable to those elicited by the pheromone (figs. 3.4 and 3.5). Similar evidence of pheromone receptor specificity for molecular shape has been found through electrophysiological (EAG and single cell) and behavioral investigations of the silk moth (Priesner 1969; Kasang and Kaissling 1972) and other lepidopterous species (Roelofs and Comeau 1971a; Roelofs et al. 1971; Payne et al. 1973).

Perception of a pheromone and parapheromones may take place through the same or different receptor sites on the dendrites of the receptors. It may be that the pheromone-specific receptor site can accommodate different structures. A high concentration of parapheromone is necessary in order that sufficient molecules are present for a few to be in the correct configuration, alignment, etc. to stimulate the receptor site. Parapheromones may stimulate different receptor sites than does the pheromone. The receptor sites may occur in small numbers thus requiring a high concentration of parapheromone to insure stimulation. However, the fact that parapheromones elicit the same behavioral response as pheromone, although at higher concentrations, is evidence that they probably stimulate the same receptor. In fact, for the silk moth, Priesner (1969) found that all compounds (other pheromones, parapheromones, nonpheromones all in higher concentrations) which stimulated the bombykol receptor elicited the sexual behavior response. No compound could be found to elicit that behavior without having stimulated the pheromone receptor. These findings indicate that for straight-chain pheromones the receptors can be

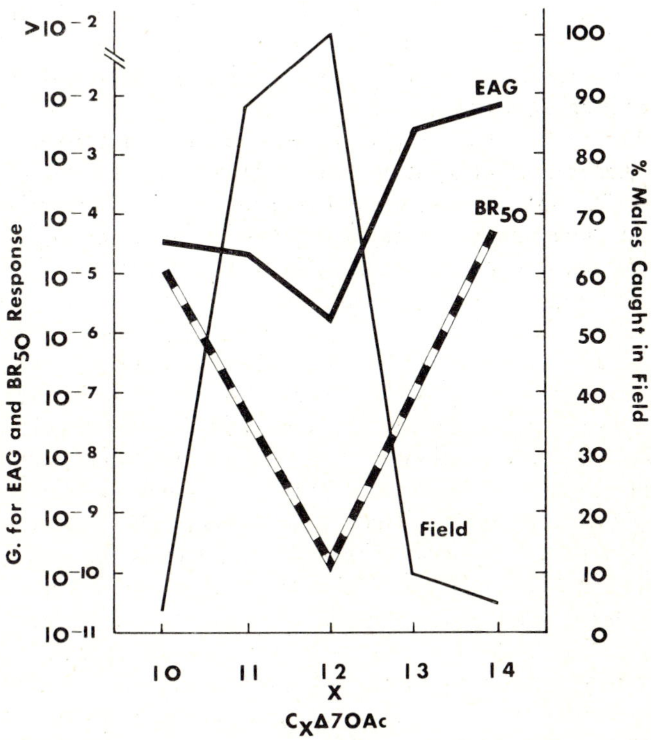

Fig. 3.4. The response of male cabbage looper moths to the female sex pheromone, *cis*-7-dodecenyl acetate ($C_{12}\Delta 7OAc$) and parapheromones. Amount of material on filter paper necessary for a significant EAG (▬); amount of material on filter paper necessary for a 50% behavioral response (▬); % of males caught in field relative to $C_{12}\Delta 7OAc$ (———). C_X = carbon chain length. (Gaston et al. 1972).

quite specific in the range of molecular structures to which they will respond. It can be said that the pheromone receptor functions as a molecular filter for molecules important in the life of the insect.

The effects of pheromone structure on perception is not limited to the straight-chain compounds found in Lepidoptera. The effects on perception of pheromone structural modifications have been investigated in insects which produce pheromones with cyclic structures and which are therefore chemically more complex than lepidopterous pheromones. Nevertheless, parapheromones of cyclic pheromones were generally much less effective in eliciting pheromone-associated, stereotyped behavioral responses than were the pheromones. For example, out of over 30 compounds modified from the trail pheromone (methyl 4-methyl pyrrole-2-carboxylate, Tumlinson et al. 1971) of the leaf-cutting ant, only 11 were found to

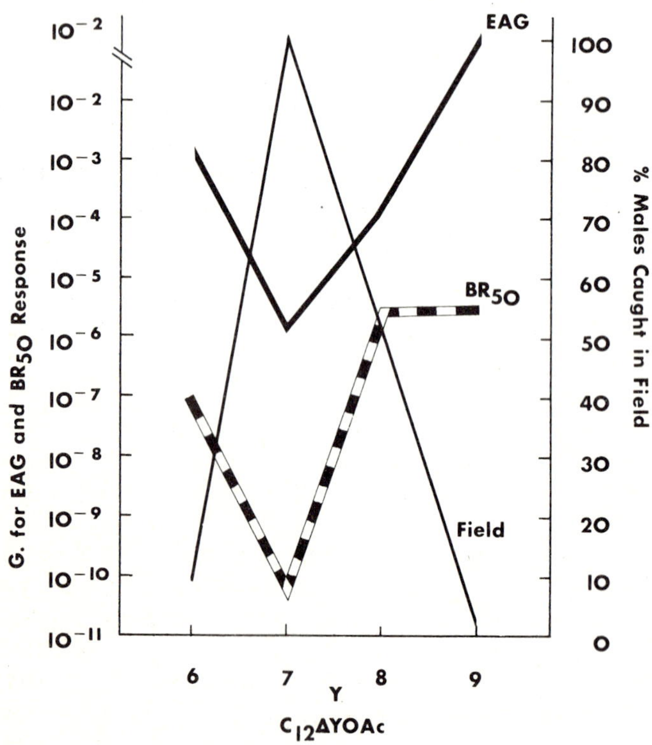

Fig. 3.5. The response of male cabbage looper moths to the female sex pheromone, *cis*-7-dodecenyl acetate ($C_{12}\Delta 7OAc$) and parapheromones. Amount of material on filter paper necessary for a significant EAG (▬▬); amount of material on filter paper necessary for a 50% behavioral response (▬▭▬); % of males caught in the field relative to $C_{12}\Delta 7OAc$ (———). ΔY = site of unsaturation. (Gaston et al. 1972).

elicit a positive response (Sonnet and Moser 1972). All but one of the 11 compounds were required in amounts 10^2 to 10^4 times greater than the pheromone to elicit a response. Information is not, however, available on the effects of the parapheromones at the antennal receptor level.

For the southern pine beetle, all but one of 10 parapheromones of frontalin (1,5-dimethyl-6, 8-dioxabicyclo [3.2.1.] octane) were completely inactive in field tests (Renwick 1970). The parapheromone 5,7-dimethyl-6, 8-dioxabicyclo [3.2.1.] octane had a slight additive effect on the field response of female southern pine beetles to frontalin and the host tree terpene α-pinene. Eight of the parapheromones were investigated for their effects at the receptor level (Payne 1970, unpublished). All of the compounds were active in undiluted form (table 3.1). However, serial dilutions were not tested, so thresholds of response relative to frontalin are unavailable.

In comparison with lepidopterous species, a decrease or absence of behavioral response by the bark beetle is not necessarily correlated with the degree of difference in structure between the parapheromone and the pheromone or electrophysiological response from the antenna. It is possible that different receptors are involved in the perception of the pheromone and the various parapheromones, thus accounting for the absence of behavioral response and the presence of receptor response. However, there is strong evidence that only one receptor is involved. EAGs from the southern pine beetle are nearly identical to frontalin and *exo*-brevicomin (*exo*-7-ethyl-5-methyl-6, 8-dioxabicyclo [3.2.1.] octane: Silverstein et al. 1968), an aggregation pheromone of the western pine beetle, *Dendroctonus brevicomis* LeConte, and essentially a parapheromone of frontalin. The response to frontalin can be completely eliminated by saturation of the receptors with a previous exposure to *exo*-brevicomin (Payne 1971, unpublished). The effect is reversible and prior exposure to frontalin will prevent response to *exo*-brevicomin. In addition, while antennal receptors for these compounds are adapted, response can still be elicited from exposure to unrelated compounds such as host tree terpenes, thus indicating that all receptors on the antenna are not blocked by saturation with one compound (table 3.2).

It is apparent that the correlation of pheromone structure to behavioral response is more difficult in bark beetles than other insects because in these beetles a mixture of compounds (pheromone(s) and host odors) is necessary to elicit behavioral responses. A beetle produced compound alone can be essentially inactive, but become active in the presence of host tree terpene (Kinzer et al. 1969). However, at the antennal level both the pheromone and host tree terpene can be independently effective (Payne 1970). In comparison to some lepidopterous species it appears that stimulation of a given receptor in bark beetles does not mean that a given behavioral response will result. Apparently initiation of a behavioral response requires the integration of information from different receptors.

Table 3.1

EAG activity of frontalin and parapheromones on the southern pine beetle*

Compound	Activity
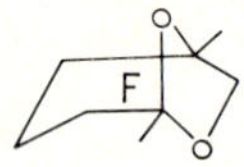 (Frontalin) 1,5-dimethyl-6,8-dioxabicyclo [3.2.1] octane	+
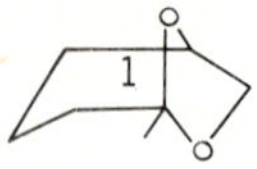 5-methyl-6,8-dioxabicyclo [3.2.1] octane	+
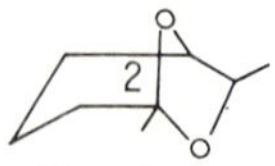 5,7-dimethyl-6,8-dioxabicyclo [3.2.1] octane	+
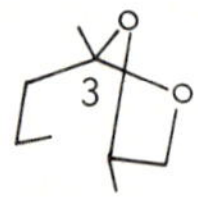 2-propyl-2,5-dimethyl-1,3-dioxalane	+
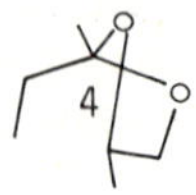 2-ethyl-2,5-dimethyl-1,3-dioxalane	+
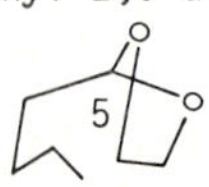 2-butyl-1,3-dioxalane	+
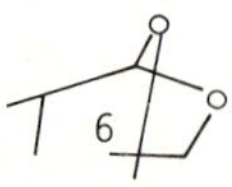 2-isopropyl-5,5-dimethyl-1,3-dioxalane	+
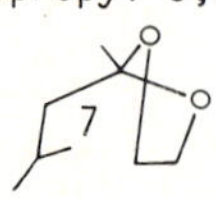 2-isobutyl-2-methyl-1,3-dioxalane	+
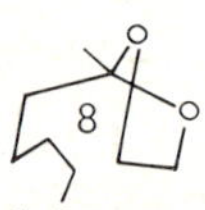 2-amyl-2-methyl-1,3-dioxalane	+

* Compounds provided through the courtesy of Dr. J. P. Vité, Boyce Thompson Institute. >95% purity by GLC.

TABLE 3.2

EAG activity of compounds on the southern pine beetle during period of adaptation to previous compounds.

Stimulus compound	Adapted compound	Activity
frontalin	frontalin	0
exo-brevicomin	*exo*-brevicomin	0
α-pinene	α-pinene	0
3-carene	3-carene	0
frontalin	*exo*-brevicomin	0
exo-brevicomin	frontalin	0
α-pinene	frontalin	+
frontalin	α-pinene	+
3-carene	frontalin	+
frontalin	3-carene	+
α-pinene	*exo*-brevicomin	+
exo-brevicomin	α-pinene	+
3-carene	*exo*-brevicomin	+
exo-brevicomin	3-carene	+
3-carene	α-pinene	+
α-pinene	3-carene	+

Stimulus compound delivered $<$10 msec after adaptation to previous compound.

3.4.4. Attractant mixtures

The perception of a single pheromone, or stimulation of a specific receptor which results in a stereotyped behavior pattern, may appear rather straight forward. When mixtures of compounds are necessary to elicit the behavioral response, the events which might take place can be more complicated.

In a number of different species, mostly Coleoptera, pheromone-associated behavior is only released in response to a mixture of naturally occurring compounds. The aggregation pheromone of the boll weevil for example, consists of four compounds (Tumlinson et al. 1969) and the aggregation behavior of various bark beetle species is mostly elicited by mixtures of pheromones and host tree terpenes (Bedard et al. 1969; Kinzer et al. 1969). In all of these cases anything less than the complete mixture results in substantial reduction or total elimination of the behavioral response.

Perception of attractant mixtures may result through stimulation of a common receptor. If this is the case it is unlikely that the receptor relays the same information to the central nervous system for each compound of the mixture. However, if that were so, it would be logical to expect that any one compound which stimulated the receptor would elicit the given behavior, as mentioned earlier for the silk moth (Priesner 1969). Where attractant mixtures occur, stimulation of a common receptor is likely to result in different information relayed for each compound.

There is evidence that a pheromone receptor can be stimulated by individual compounds, or mixtures of compounds of different structure, and relay different information. O'Connell (1972) found that the two pheromone receptors of the sensilla trichodea on the red-banded leaf roller (*Argyrotaenia velutinana* Walker) not only responded to the sex pheromone, *cis*-11-tetradecenyl acetate (Roelofs and Arn 1968), but also to an inhibitor – *trans*-11-tetradecenyl acetate, a synergist – dodecenyl acetate (Roelofs and Comeau 1971b) and their mixtures. Each compound, alone and in mixtures, elicited a different response from the receptors.

It is also possible that perception of attractant mixtures results from stimulation of different receptors. Evidence for this was found in the southern pine beetle, as mentioned earlier, in which adaptation of antennal receptors indicates that aggregation pheromones and host tree terpenes stimulate separate receptors (Payne 1971, unpublished).

In general it appears that both common and independent receptors can function in the perception of attractant mixtures. For a given species, compounds with closely related structures (e.g. the pheromone(s) alone) may stimulate a common receptor, either alone or in mixture, but elicit the transfer of different information. Compounds of dissimilar structure (e.g. pheromones and terpenes) may stimulate independent receptors. Behavioral response may result from a single line of information generated by a mixture of compounds at one receptor or by the integration of different lines of information in the CNS.

3.4.5. Inhibitors and synergists

Pheromone perception in some species has been found to be influenced by inhibitors and synergists. The chemical structure of these compounds is closely related in some cases to a given pheromone (Roelofs and Comeau 1971b; Vité and Renwick 1971) and not so closely related in others (Bedard et al. 1969, 1970; Kinzer et al. 1969; Pitman 1969; Renwick and Vité 1969). The effects of these compounds may take place at the peripheral receptor level or through integration in the CNS.

Peripherally, inhibitors might block the pheromone receptor sites. It is also possible that an inhibitor could stimulate different receptors from those for a pheromone. In that way information from the pheromone and the inhibitor would be transferred independently to the CNS. The inhibitory effect would originate at the level of the brain. However, recent information from behavioral and electrophysiological investigations indicates that inhibition of response to pheromone in some insects results through active interaction of the inhibitor with the pheromone receptor. O'Connell (1972) found that an inhibitor of the red-banded leaf roller sex pheromone (see sect. 3.4.4) stimulates the receptors for the sex pheromone. When presented with the sex pheromone, the inhibitor significantly reduced the electrical output of the cells. These findings correlate well with the effect the inhibitor has in reducing the attractiveness of the pheromone in behavioral tests (Roelofs and Comeau 1968, 1971b). In the southern pine beetle *endo* and *exo*-brevicomin have been reported to reduce the attractiveness of frontalin and α-pinene to the beetles (Vité and Renwick 1971). The fact that *exo*-brevicomin and frontalin are believed to stimulate the same receptors (see sect. 3.4.3) suggests that an active type of inhibition also occurs in the southern pine beetle.

There is evidence to suggest that synergists can affect perception by stimulating a common receptor with the pheromone or by stimulating different receptors. O'Connell (1972) found that the synergistic effect of dodecenyl acetate on the sex pheromone of the red-banded leaf roller occurs through a common receptor. The synergist alone had little effect on the output of the cell, but when presented with the sex pheromone, it significantly increased the output over response to the sex pheromone alone.

Host tree terpenes are known to have a synergistic effect on bark beetle aggregation pheromones (Bedard et al. 1969, 1970; Pitman 1969; Renwick and Vité 1969). There is evidence to suggest that the terpenes stimulate different receptors from those stimulated by pheromone (Payne 1971, unpublished – see discussion sect. 3.4.3); it is therefore likely that the terpenes exert their synergistic effects via integration in the CNS and not through modification of the pheromone-derived information at the receptor level.

It is not clear whether or not an inhibitor or synergist which affects the same receptor as a pheromone also reacts with the same receptor site. The mechanism whereby the compounds affect perception of the pheromone is also not understood. The compounds might possibly have their effects through facilitation of hyper- or de-polarization along the receptor membrane. It does appear that where separate receptors are involved, the inhibitor or synergist affects perception through neural integrations is the CNS. However, information on any such integrations is lacking.

3.4.6. Environmental influences

Variables within the insect's environment such as light, time of day and previous exposure to pheromone have been found to have effects on pheromone perception at the whole organism level, but not at the peripheral receptor level.

Shorey and Gaston (1964) found that male cabbage looper moths were most sensitive to pheromone at a light intensity near moon light (ca. 0.3 lumens/M^2). In light of greater intensity significant responses could only be elicited with greater amounts of pheromone. In a 12 : 12 hr light–dark photoperiod the moths were most responsive to pheromone during the 6–12 hr period after beginning of the dark phase. Responses at any other time required greater concentrations of pheromone. Moths previously exposed to pheromone were found to be insensitive (habituated) to the pheromone for several min or even hr (Shorey and Gaston 1965).

By comparison, Payne et al. (1970) found that antennal olfactory responsiveness of male moths to pheromone remained essentially constant to the above mentioned variables (figs. 3.6 and 3.7). Adaptation of antennal receptors lasted only seconds and could not account for the longer times of habituation.

While environmental factors obviously affect pheromone perception at the behavioral level, it is apparent that the effects are mediated via neural integration beyond the peripheral receptors. Other environmental factors such as season of the year (Silverstein et al. 1968) and temperature (Vité et al. 1964) may affect pheromone perception at the behavioral level, but they have not been investigated at the peripheral receptor level.

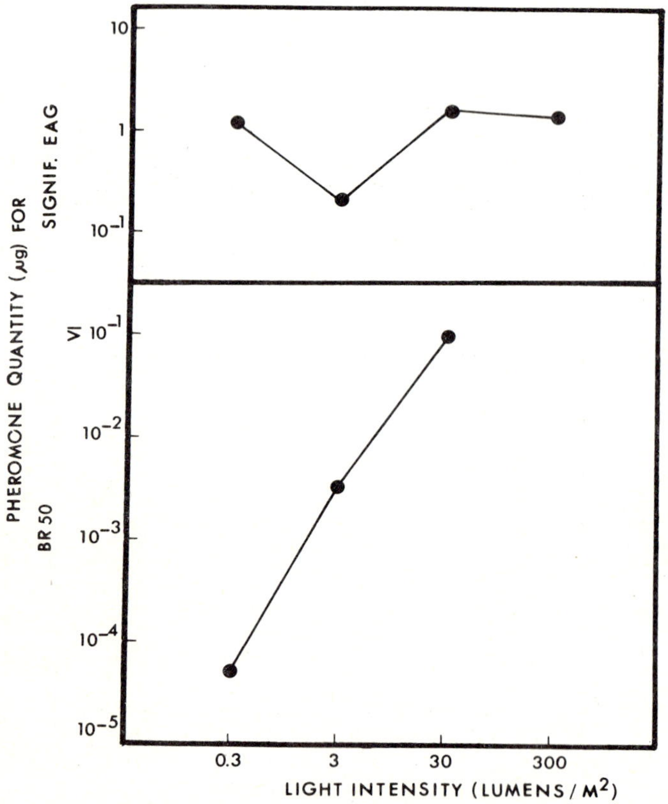

Fig. 3.6. Effect of light intensity on the quantity of female pheromone on filter paper necessary for a significant EAG vs. a 50% behavioral response (Shorey and Gaston 1964) in male cabbage looper moths (Payne et al. 1970).

3.4.7. *Odor discrimination and information coding*

Pheromone odor specialists enable the insect (at least in some Lepidoptera: Boeckh et al. 1965) to discriminate pheromone molecules from other odor molecules in its environment. Molecule-bound information is decoded through the pheromone receptor sites and transferred to the cell body of the neuron as the intensity of the generator potential. The cell body transforms the information into a frequency of action potentials which is relayed via the axon to the deutocerebrum of the insect's brain. Pheromone quality is discriminated through the specificity of the receptor sites and the frequency of action potentials (see sect. 3.4.4). However, pheromonal quantity is coded in the intensity of the generator potentials and the frequency of action potentials. For example, increases in pheromone concentration elicit generator potentials of increased intensity and action potentials of increased frequency (Priesner, unpublished, in Boeckh et al. 1965). However, O'Connell (1972) has

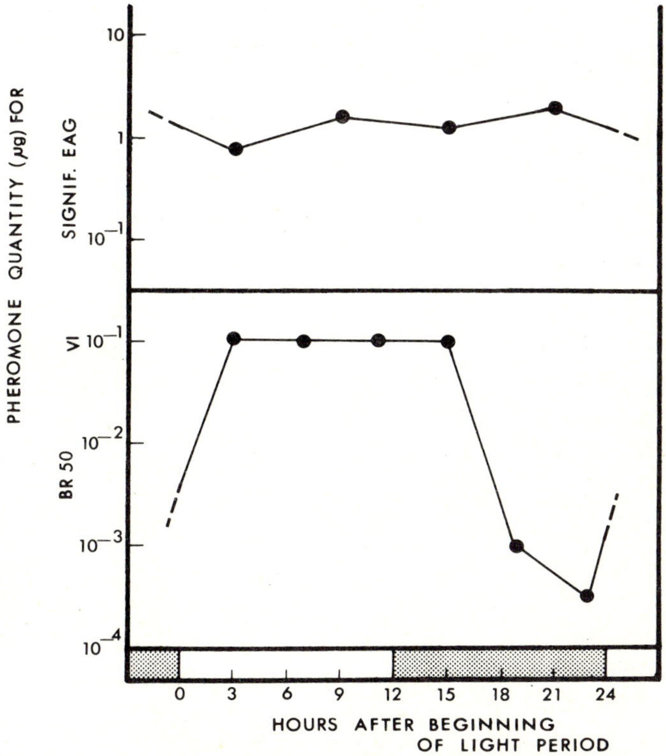

Fig. 3.7. Effect of time of day on the quantity of female sex pheromone on filter paper necessary for a significant EAG vs a 50% behavioral response (Shorey and Gaston 1964) in male cabbage looper moths (Payne et al. 1970).

shown that at high concentration sex pheromone can reduce the frequency of action potentials. This might account for the fact that at high concentration, pheromone becomes less attractive for some insect species (Sonnet and Moser 1972; Kaae et al. 1973).

The events that take place in the deutocerebrum and between the receptors and the deutocerebrum are not at all understood. Yamada et al. (1968, 1970) and Yamada (1971), have reported the presence of neurons in the deutocerebrum of the American cockroach specific for 'prepurified sex attractant'. Such specific neurons may be where the first stages of central integration of incoming peripheral information occur.

Discrimination of all compounds important in pheromone perception may not take place through odor specialists. Some compounds may stimulate odor generalists. In such cases, information is no longer coded through receptors sending the same information. Information coding may result from the responses of several receptors in the form of various combinations of excitatory, inhibitory or no response (Boeckh 1969). Information from the various receptors would be integrated in the CNS and would eventually end in a given behavioral response.

3.5. Concluding remarks

The pheromone perceiving insect is indeed equipped with a morphologically and physiologically efficient mechanism for collecting molecule-bound information and transforming it into important behavioral responses. Integrative circuits appear to be present which enable important environmental factors to modify pheromone perception at the behavioral level.

Although the knowledge of pheromone perception is somewhat detailed it is far from complete. All but a few investigations have dealt with perception at the peripheral and behavioral levels. The vast middle ground of events which take place in second order and third order neural transmissions is virtually unexplored. This unknown must be explored before there can be an understanding of pheromone perception at all levels.

Acknowledgments

Original research supported by McIntire-Stennis Project 1525. Texas Agricultural Experiment Station Paper No. 10354. The author thanks Dr. E. R. Hart, Department of Entomology, Texas A & M University, for assistance in preparation of the figures; Dr. C. R. Pantle, Division of Entomology and Parasitology, University of California, Berkeley, and Mr. W. E. Finn, Department of Biology, Texas A & M University, for review of the manuscript.

Priesner, E. (1969) A new approach to insect pheromone specificity. *In*: Proceedings of the Third International Symposium on Olfaction and Taste, New York 1968; ed.: C. Pfaffmann (Rockefeller University Press, New York) pp. 235–240.

Renwick, J. A. A. (1970) Chemical aspects of bark beetle aggregation. (Symposium on population attractants) Contrib. Boyce Thompson Inst. 24, 337–341.

Renwick, J. A. A. and J. P. Vité (1969) Bark beetle attractants; mechanism of colonization by *Dendroctonus frontalis*. Nature (London) 224, 1222–1223.

Renwick, J. A. A. and J. P. Vité (1970) Systems of chemical communication in *Dendroctonus*. Symposium on population attractants. Contrib. Boyce Thompson Inst. 24, 283–292.

Riddiford, L. M. (1970) Antennal proteins of saturniid moths – their possible role in olfaction. J. Insect Physiol. 16, 653–660.

Roelofs, W. L. and H. Arn (1968) Sex attractant of the red-banded leaf roller. Nature (London) 219, 513.

Roelofs, W. L. and A. Comeau (1968) Sex pheromone perception. Nature (London) 220, 600–601.

Roelofs, W. L. and A. Comeau (1971a) Sex attractants in Lepidoptera. Proceedings of the Second International Congress of Pesticide Chemistry, Tel Aviv, Israel pp. 91–112.

Roelofs, W. L. and A. Comeau (1971b) Sex pheromone perception: Synergists and inhibitors for the red-banded leaf roller attractant. J. Insect Physiol. 17, 435–448.

Roelofs, W. L., A. Comeau, A. Hill and G. Milecevic (1971) Sex attractants of the codling moth: characterization with electroantennogram technique. Science 174, 297–299.

Schneider, D. (1955) Mikro-Elektroden registrieren die elektrischen Impulse einzelner Sinnesnervenzellen der Schmetterlingsantenne. Industrie-Elektronik (Hamburg) 5, 3–7.

Schneider, D. (1957a) Elektrophysiologische Untersuchungen von Chemo- und Mechanorezeptoren der Antenne des Seidenspinners *Bombyx mori* L. Z. Vergl. Physiol. 40, 8–41.

Schneider, D. (1957b) Electrophysiological investigation on the antennal receptors of the silk moth during chemical and mechanical stimulation. Experientia 31, 89–91.

Schneider, D. (1962) Electrophysiological investigation on the olfactory specificity of sexual attracting substances in different species of moths. J. Insect Physiol. 8, 15–30.

Schneider, D. (1970) Olfactory receptors for the sexual attractant (Bombykol) of the silk moth. *In*: The Neurosciences: Second Study Program: ed.: F. Schmith (Rockefeller University Press, New York) pp. 511–518.

Schneider, D. and E. Hecker (1956) Zur Elektrophysiologie der Antenne des Seidenspinners *Bombyx mori* bei Reizung mit angereicherten Extrakten des Sexuallockstoffes. Z. Naturforsch. 11b, 121–124.

Schneider, D. and R. A. Steinbrecht (1968) Checklist of insect olfactory sensilla. Symp. Zool. Soc. London. 23, 279–297.

Schneider, D., V. Lacher and K. E. Kaissling (1964) Die Reactionsweise und das Reaktionsspektrum von Riechzellen bei *Antheraea pernyi* (Lepidoptera: Saturniidae). Z. Vergl. Physiol. 48, 632–662.

Schneider, D., B. C. Block, J. Boeckh and E. Priesner (1967) Die Reaktion der Männlichen Seidenspinner auf Bombykol und seine Isomeren: Elektroantennogram und Verhalten. Z. Vergl. Physiol. 54, 192–209.

Shorey, H. H. and L. K. Gaston (1964) Sex pheromones of noctuid moths. III. Inhibition of male responses to the sex pheromone in *Trichoplusia ni* (Lepidoptera: Noctuidae). Ann. Entomol. Soc. Am. 57, 775–779.

Shorey, H. H. and L. K. Gaston (1965) Sex pheromones of noctuid moths. V. Circadian rhythm of pheromone responsiveness in males of *Autographa californica*, *Heliothis virescens*, *Spodoptera exigua*, and *Trichoplusia ni* (Lepidoptera: Noctuidae). Ann. Entomol. Soc. Am. 58, 597–600.

Shorey, H. H., L. K. Gaston and J. S. Roberts (1965) Sex pheromones of noctuid moths. VI. Absence of behavioral specificity for the female sex pheromones of *Trichoplusia ni* versus *Autographa californica*, and *Heliothis zea* versus *H. virescens* (Lepidoptera: Noctuidae). Ann. Entomol. Soc. Am. 58, 600–603.

Shorey, H. H., L. K. Gaston and R. N. Jefferson (1968) Insect sex pheromones. *In*: Advances in Pest Control Research; ed.: R. Metcalf (Interscience, New York) pp. 57–126.

Silverstein, R. M., R. G. Brownlee, T. E. Bellas, D. L. Wood and L. E. Browne (1968) Brevicomin: principal sex attractant in the frass of the female western pine beetle. Science 159, 889–891.

Slifer, E. H. (1967) Thin-walled olfactory sense organs on insect antennae. *In*: Insects and Physiology; eds.: J. Beament and J. Treherne (Oliver and Boyd, Edinburgh – London) pp. 232–245.

Slifer, E. H. and S. S. Sekhon (1964) Fine structure of the sense organs on the antennal flagellum of a flesh fly, *Sarcophaga argyrostoma* R-D. (Diptera: Sarcophagidae). J. Morphol. 114, 185–208.

Slifer, E. H., J. J. Prestage and H. W. Beams (1959) The chemoreceptors and other sense organs on the antennal flagellum of the grasshopper (Orthoptera: Acrididae). J. Morphol. 195, 145–191.

Sonnet, P. E. and J. C. Moser (1972) Synthetic analogs of the trail pheromone of the leafcutting ant, *Atta texana* (Buckley). J. Agr. Food Chem. 20, 1191–1194.

Steinbrecht, R. A. (1969a) Comparative morphology of olfactory receptors. *In*: Proceedings of the Third International Symposium on Olfaction and Taste, New York 1968; ed.: C. Pfaffmann (Rockefeller University Press, New York) pp. 3–21.

Steinbrecht, R. A. (1969b) On the question of nervous syncytia: lack of axon fusion in two insect sensory nerves. J. Cell Sci. 4, 39–53.

Steinbrecht, R. A., (1970) Zur Morphometrie der Antenne des Seidenspinners, *Bombyx mori* L.: Zahl und Verteilung der Riechsensillen (Insecta, Lepidoptera). Z. Morphol. Tiere. 68, 93–126.

Steinbrecht, R. A. and B. Müller (1971) On the stimulus conducting structures in insect olfactory receptors. Z. Zellforsch. 117, 570–575.

Steinbrecht, R. A. and G. Kasang (1972) Capture and conveyance of odour molecules in an insect olfactory receptor. *In*: Proceedings of the Fourth International Symposium on Olfaction and Taste. Seewiesen, Germany 1971; ed.: D. Schneider (Wissenschaftliche Verlagsgesellschaft MBH Stuttgart) pp. 193–199.

Stürckow, B. (1965) The electroantennogram (EAG) as an assay for the reception of odours by the gypsy moth. J. Insect Physiol. 11, 1573–1584.

Stürckow, B. (1970) Responses of olfactory and gustatory receptor cells in insects. *In*: Advances in Chemoreception, vol. I Communication by Chemical Signals; eds.: J. Johnston, D. Moulton and A. Turk (Appleton-Century-Crofts, New York) pp. 107–158.

Toba, H. H., N. Green, A. N. Kishaba, M. Jacobson and J. W. DeBolt (1970) Responses of the male cabbage looper to 15 isomers and cogeners of the looper pheromone. J. Econ. Entomol. 63, 1048–1051.

Tumlinson, J. H., D. D. Hardee, R. C. Gueldner, A. C. Thompson, P. A. Hedin and J. P. Minyard (1969) Sex pheromone produced by male boll weevil. Science 166, 1010–1012.

Tumlinson, J. H., J. C. Moser, R. M. Silverstein, R. G. Brownlee and J. M. Ruth (1971) Identification of the trail pheromone of a leafcutting ant, *Atta texana*. Nature (London) 234, 348–349.

Vité, J. P. and J. A. A. Renwick (1971) Inhibition of *Dendroctonus frontalis* response to frontalin by isomers of brevicomin. Naturwissenschaften 8, 418.

Vité, J. P. and D. L. Williamson (1970) *Thanasimus dubius*: Prey perception. J. Insect Physiol. 16, 233–239.

Vité, J. P., R. I. Gara and H. D. von Scheller (1964) Field observations on the response to attractants of bark beetles infesting southern pines. Contrib. Boyce Thompson Inst. 22, 261–270.

Wolbarsht, M. L. (1963) Electrical signs of chemoreception. *In*: Proceedings of the Sixteenth International Congress of Zoology (Washington) 3, 107–110.

Wright, R. H. (1964) Odor and molecular vibration: The far infra-red spectra of some perfume chemicals. Acad. Sci. Ann. N. Y. 116, 552.

Wright, R. H. (1969) Olfactory specificity. *In*: Proceedings of the Ninth International Congress of Oto-Rhino-Laryngology. Mexico, D. F. pp. 3–11.

Yamada, M. (1971) A search for odour encoding in the olfactory lobe. J. Physiol. 214, 127–143.

Yamada, M., S. Ishii and Y. Kuwahara (1968) Preliminary report on olfactory neurons specific to the sex pheromone of the American cockroach. Botyu-Kagaku 33, 37–39.

Yamada, M., S. Ishii and Y. Kuwahara (1970) Odour discrimination: 'Sex pheromone specialists' in the olfactory lobe of the cockroach. Nature (London) 227, 855.

CHAPTER 4

Environmental and physiological control of insect sex pheromone behavior

H. H. SHOREY

4.1. Introduction

Sex pheromones are produced by specialized glands in insects of one sex and elicit a behavioral response in the opposite sex. In most cases, the producing sex does not release the pheromone continuously throughout its adult life. Nor does the responding sex typically display a constant degree of responsiveness to the pheromone. Instead, certain physiological factors within the insects themselves and certain properties of the environment in which the insects live control the occurrence and the timing of pheromone communication.

The manner in which sex pheromones are used in the premating communication between a male and female may vary considerably from one species to the next. Males of many species, perceiving the sex pheromone released from conspecific females, exhibit a sequence of behavioral steps, in a hierarchical manner. For instance, the female sex pheromone of many species of Lepidoptera and Coleoptera may cause: 1) activation of a resting male; 2) his oriented approach toward the pheromone source; and 3) various short-range behavioral reactions, often termed 'courtship', that serve to stimulate the female to mate (Shorey 1973). Most investigators of the influence of environmental and physiological variables on pheromone behavior have not examined the effect of these factors on each step in the behavioral hierarchy. Rather, most experiments designed to evaluate pheromone responsiveness as influenced by these variables have been conducted using laboratory bioassays, which mainly measure the activation reaction, or pheromone-baited traps, which measure the oriented approach reaction. Experiments evaluating the influence of the variables on the pheromone-producing sex are also often conducted under conditions far removed from the natural situation. Despite the necessary artificiality of most experiments, the accumulating published data are starting to show how adaptive – how appropriate to the conditions existing in and around them – is the sex pheromone communication system of insects.

Three aspects of pheromone communication have been investigated with regard to the controlling influence of environmental and physiological variables: 1) production; and 2) release of pheromone by the sex which initiates the communication sequence; and 3) response to the pheromone by a member of the opposite sex. Unfortunately, investigators have often failed to differentiate the first two aspects, and experiments demonstrating the amount or timing of release of pheromone are often erroneously claimed to give the amount or timing of pheromone produced. Where possible, quantitative changes in levels of these three aspects, as influenced by changes in the controlling variables, will be considered in this chapter.

The relative level of responsiveness by the sex receiving the pheromone can be determined for many species by laboratory bioassay techniques. The relative level of pheromone production can also be determined quantitatively by extracting the pheromone glands or even the entire bodies of the producing insects in an appropriate solvent, followed by bioassay or gas chromatographic analyses. The level of pheromone release, however, is often not determined. Rather, the extrusion of a pheromone gland or the attraction of members of the opposite sex to the releasing individual are commonly used as all-or-none indications of the occurrence of releasing behavior.

4.2. *Environmental variables*

Certain environmental factors control sex pheromone communication of insects in two different ways (Bartell and Shorey 1969). Firstly, each factor may operate directly, influencing the intensity at which the pheromone activity will be expressed. Examples of these direct effects are given in the following four sections. Secondly, the daily fluctuations of certain environmental factors, particularly light intensity, may control the timing of pheromone activity by phase-setting of circadian rhythms. This cyclic recurrence of pheromone behavior will be discussed later (sect. 4.3.1).

4.2.1. Light intensity

Light intensity, varying between > 100,000 lux at midday and < 0.01 lux on a moon-less night, is one of the most pronounced and most predictable of the environmental factors that fluctuate on a daily basis. It is little wonder, then, that light intensity is a major factor controlling whether insect sex pheromone activity will occur and, sometimes, the intensity at which it will occur. Thus, females of the Queensland fruit fly, *Dacus tryoni* (Froggatt), which normally approach males and mate at dusk, were maximally responsive to the male-produced sex pheromone when held in a 'dim' light intensity of 8 lux (Fletcher and Giannakakis 1973). Female responsiveness decreased at both higher and lower light intensities. In another insect that typically mates at dusk, the light-brown apple moth, *Epiphyas postvittana* (Walker), light intensities greater than 3.5 lux suppressed the responsiveness of males exposed to the female sex pheromone (Bartell and Shorey 1969). On the other hand, the cabbage looper moth, *Trichoplusia ni* (Hübner), typically communicates and mates during the hours of darkness; light intensities greater than that equivalent to full moonlight (0.3 lux) inhibited male responses to female sex pheromone (Shorey and Gaston 1964). A 10,000-fold increase in pheromone concentration was required at a light intensity of 30 lux to cause males to exhibit the same level of responsiveness seen at 0.3 lux. The relative pheromone responsiveness of cabbage looper males has not been evaluated at intensities lower than 0.3 lux. However, Saario et al. (1970) found that the males were attracted to pheromone-emitting traps in the field as readily on nights having a full moon as they were on nights having no moonlight (< 0.01 lux).

No studies could be found indicating whether the *production* of sex pheromone is influenced by the prevailing light intensity. Also, little research has been conducted on the control of sex pheromone *release* by light intensity. Probably pheromone release will be found to be as strongly controlled by this environmental factor as is pheromone responsiveness. For instance, Sower et al. (1970) observed that cabbage looper females everted their glands and released pheromone more readily with increasing darkness. Release behavior became maximal at the same 0.3-lux intensity found most suitable for male responsiveness.

Batiste (1970) and Batiste et al. (1973) studied the attraction of male codling moths, *Carpocapsa pomonella* (L.), to female-baited traps in the field. Captures of males in the traps provided evidence that light intensity did not inhibit either male responsiveness nor female pheromone release. Mating activity in this species typically begins well before sunset. Correspondingly, males approached the traps when the light intensity was as high as 50,000 lux, as long as the other controlling factors such as temperature and time-of-day were not limiting.

4.2.2. Temperature

Insects have narrow bands of temperature for optimal growth and reproduction. Likewise, the temperatures at which certain species of insects respond to sex pheromone emitted from a potential mating partner have been found to fall in narrow bands (introduced pine sawfly, *Diprion similis* (Hartig), (Casida et al. 1963); codling moth (Batiste 1970; Batiste et al. 1973); gypsy moth, *Porthetria dispar* (L.), (Collins and Potts 1932); European corn borer moth, *Ostrinia nubilalis* (Hübner), (Klun 1968); cabbage looper moth (Shorey 1966)). The temperature ranges allowing optimal pheromone responsiveness would be expected to be appropriate to the way-of-life of the particular species. Thus males of the gypsy moth, which mate in the daytime, never responded to female sex pheromone sources in the field at temperatures below 21 °C; they approached the sources in increasing numbers as temperatures rose to 32 °C (Collins and Potts 1932). On the other hand, males of the night-active European corn borer moth gave greater responses to female sex pheromone extracts when the laboratory temperature was maintained at 20–23 °C than when it was maintained at 27 °C (Klun 1968). These pheromone studies with the European corn borer support the observations of Sparks (1963) that cool temperatures typical of night are more conducive to mating than warmer temperatures.

Although little research has been conducted on the control of pheromone release by temperature, it appears likely that for any given species, optimal release would occur in the same range of temperature that is conducive to pheromone responsiveness by the opposite sex. Thus, the minimum temperature for pheromone release by females of the cabbage looper moth (Sower et al. 1971) and for pheromone responsiveness by males of this species (Shorey 1966) is near 12 °C.

4.2.3. Air velocity

Air velocity is an important controlling factor for those insect species using sex pheromones for communication over distances greater than a few cm. Velocities lower than some minimum value may prevent the responding sex from approaching the pheromone source because: 1) the pheromone may not be carried far from its source; and/or 2) the resulting, slowly formed, aerial trail may be so disrupted or otherwise improperly constructed that the responding insects cannot orient along it to the source. High air velocities may inhibit successful response because: 1) the wind speed may exceed the flight speed of the responding insects; and/or 2) the aerial trail may be improperly constructed for normal orientation behavior.

Examples of air velocities that do or do not allow approaches by the responding sex are discussed in ch. 5. Unfortunately, few experiments have been conducted to determine whether high air velocities prevent approach responses because of physical impediments as outlined above, or whether in some cases the responding insect is inhibited from even initiating an orientation reaction when it senses the improper velocity. A behavioral effect of air velocity on the responding sex has been documented in two cases: 1) honey bee drones, *Apis mellifera* L., mate with queens while in flight. The altitude at which drones tend to fly in response to visual lures releasing pheromone decreases as air velocity increases from 15 m at a velocity of 1.4 m/sec down to 8 m at 7.3 m/sec (Butler and Fairey 1964). 2) Kaae and Shorey (1973) placed traps releasing pink bollworm, *Pectinophora gossypiella* (Saunders), female sex pheromone at various elevations above the ground in cotton fields. Most males approached traps located near foliage tops on relatively calm nights (air velocity 0–3 m/sec) and near foliage bottoms on windy nights (8–12 m/sec). Females of this species must be affected by wind velocity in a similar manner, because most mating pairs were found high on cotton plants on calm nights and at lower levels on windy nights. Presumably females settled in these locations before releasing pheromone.

Sower et al (1972) found that sex pheromone evaporated more rapidly from articificially extruded pheromone glands of female cabbage loopers held in an air stream moving 100 cm/sec than in one moving 10 cm/sec. Enhancement of evaporation rate with increasing air velocities may be one of the factors that has led to the behavior, seen in many lepidopterous species, of a female vibrating her wings while extruding the sex pheromone gland.

Virgin cabbage looper females spent more time per night releasing pheromone when exposed to air velocities in the range 0.3 to 1.0 m/sec than in higher or lower velocities (Kaae and Shorey 1972). Apparently, females have evolved a behavioral reaction causing them to minimize the release of pheromone when wind conditions for pheromone dispersal or for male response flights are not favorable.

4.2.4. Host substrate

The immature forms of some insect species are restricted to feeding on only one or a few host plant species. For certain of these monophagous or oligophagous insect species, mechanisms have evolved which cause males and females to aggregate at the larval feeding sites prior to mating. A number of investigators have found that traps baited with females of a given insect species attract and capture large numbers of males only when located on or near the larval host plants (Holbrook et al. 1960; Riddiford 1967; Riddiford and Williams 1967a,b; Sharma et al 1971; Aliniazee and Stafford 1972). However, most of these studies do not distinguish whether: 1) males and females aggregated at the larval host *before* pheromone communication occurred; 2) females were able to emit pheromone only after they had been stimulated by the larval host; or 3) males were only able to respond to pheromone when simultaneously stimulated by the larval host. Riddiford (1967) and Riddiford and Williams (1967a,b) examined the host specificity of pheromone communication by the polyphemus moth, *Antheraea polyphemus* (Cramer), the larvae of which feed only on oak leaves. The chemical *trans*-2-hexenal, which is released from oak leaves, must be perceived by the female moth before she will release her pheromone. Although leaves of many plant species contain *trans*-2-hexenal also, species other than oak release 'masking' odors which prevent the female moth from performing her pheromone releasing behavior.

Some insect species are more general in their feeding habits. Cabbage looper larvae are fairly polyphagous and traps baited with virgin female moths of this species captured large numbers of males irrespective of the presence or absence of larval hosts in the vicinity (Saario et al. 1970).

4.3. Physiological variables

A number of physiological factors may operate simultaneously in insects to control the occurrence and the intensity of expression of pheromone production, pheromone release and pheromone responsiveness.

4.3.1. Time of day and circadian rhythms

Animals are seldom active at all times of day. Instead, their behavioral activities are often partitioned into characteristic time-periods of the 24-hr cycle. Thus, most insect species can be characterized as mating during night, day, or crepuscular periods. One factor that influences time of mating activity is light intensity, discussed earlier in sect. 4.2.1. However, it would seem efficient for a system to have evolved that causes the *tendency* to communicate for mating to be higher at an appropriate time of day. This indeed seems to be the case in a number of insect species which have been examined, with either release of sex pheromone, or responsiveness to pheromone, or both being highest at a characteristic time of the day or night (Rau and Rau 1929; Kettlewell 1942, 1946; Götz 1951; Casida et al. 1963; Gentry et al. 1964; Perez and Long 1964; Shorey and Gaston 1964, 1965a; George 1965; Solomon and Morris 1966; Wellso 1966; Jacklin et al. 1967; Bartell and Shorey 1969; Fletcher 1969; Jacklin and Yonce 1969; Sanders, 1969; Batiste 1970; Saario et al. 1970; Sower et al. 1970, 1971; Traynier 1970b; Lange et al. 1971; Sharma et al. 1971; Wong et al. 1971a, b; Batiste et al. 1973; Burkholder et al. 1973). In each species for which pheromone release and pheromone responsiveness have been examined separately, these two phenomena correspond closely in timing. For species that use sex pheromones to communicate over long distances, it would seem reasonable to assume the exact time of mating would be determined by the releasing sex. The process of pheromone release presumably initiates the premating communication sequence. Thus, when female cabbage loopers maintained on one time-of-day schedule were paired with males entrained to a light : dark periodicity four hr out of phase, the mating time approximated that expected by the female cycle (Shorey 1966).

The mechanism controlling the time of occurrence of sex pheromone communication has been examined in several species of Lepidoptera (Mediterranean flour moth, *Anagasta kühniella* (Zeller) (Traynier 1970b), oriental fruit moth, *Grapholitha molesta* (Busck) (George 1965), cabbage looper moth (Shorey and Gaston 1965a; Sower et al. 1970, 1971)). A circadian rhythm of pheromone-behavior has been found in each of these species. The phase of the rhythm is reset each day, occurring at some specific time with relation to the light : dark periodicity. In the absence of the normal entraining light : dark cues, the rhythm re-occurs at an approximately 24-hr periodicity. Furthermore, in studies of the time of pheromone release by females of the Mediterranean flour moth, or the time of pheromone responsiveness by males of the cabbage looper moth or the Mediterranean flour moth, when the timing of the light : dark cycle was abruptly shifted by 12 hr, the timing of the behavioral rhythm became re-entrained to its 'normal' phase with relation to the new cycle within 48 hr.

A seasonal shift in the characteristic time of night at which males become responsive to pheromone has been observed in two lepidopteran species, the cabbage looper (Saario et al. 1970) and the pink bollworm (Sharma et al. 1971). In both species, the time when most males approached pheromone-baited traps in the field advanced as the season progressed, from after midnight in midsummer to early evening by October. Sower et al. (1971) examined the interaction of temperature and light : dark periodicity on the time of pheromone release by cabbage looper females in the laboratory. When females were conditioned in cool temperatures. the mean time of sex pheromone release occurred earlier in the dark period than when they were conditioned in warmer temperatures. Perhaps this phenomenon will be found to be very common, with the re-occurrence of pheromone behavior at a 24-hr periodicity being controlled by the light : dark periodicity, but with the exact phase of expression of the behavior relative to dawn or dusk being controlled by the temperature. Presumably, the forward phase shifts in timing of pheromone communication behavior correlated with reduced conditioning temperatures have adaptive significance. As the season progresses from summer to fall and the nights become cooler, those insects that complete their premating communication before the temperature falls too low for normal activity would have a selective advantage.

Some insects do not seem to have their pheromone release or response behavior partitioned into a particular time of day (Götz 1951; Steinbrecht 1964b; Brady and Smithwick 1968). For instance, females of the silkworm moth, *Bombyx mori* (L.), expose their sex pheromone glands shortly after emergence from the pupal case and keep them in that state until they copulate or deposit unfertilized eggs (Steinbrecht 1964b).

Few studies have been conducted to determine whether pheromone production, as indicated by the content of pheromone in the glands, is correlated with time of day. Of three species of Lepidoptera that have been examined, two (the cabbage looper (Shorey and Gaston 1965b; Sower et al. 1972) and the Mediterranean flour moth (Traynier 1970b)) showed no tendency toward higher glandular content at certain times of day. In the third species, the smaller tea tortrix, *Adoxophyes fasciata* Walsingham (Nagata et al. 1972), two maxima in glandular content were found during each 24-hr period. One maximum corresponded to the time of mating, near dawn, and the other occurred eight hr later. Also, females of the dermestid beetle *Trogoderma glabrum* (Herbst), exhibited a daily rhythm of pheromone synthesis, the extractable quantity being highest at that time of day when pheromone release and mating occurred (Burkholder et al. 1973).

4.3.2. Age

For each insect species studied, the systems for pheromone responsiveness, pheromone production, and pheromone release mature and become operative at characteristic ages. Presumably, the timing of maturation of each of these essential components of the total pheromone communication system is closely correlated with the maturation of the other physiological processes of the insect associated with mating. Thus, silkworm moth females, which are reproductively mature and capable of laying viable eggs shortly after emergence from the pupa, contained a maximum quantity of sex pheromone at emergence. Pheromone release, mating, and oviposition occurred within a few hours following emergence (Steinbrecht 1964a, b). However, females of certain noctuid moth species neither matured their eggs nor contained detectable sex pheromone in their glands until some time following emergence (Shorey et al. 1968a).

Because maturation of the system for pheromone responsiveness implies mating readiness, this system would be expected to become operative after the other physiological systems necessary for mating. Males of most of the eight noctuid moth species studied by Shorey et al. (1968b) were not reproductively mature at emergence. Movement of sperm bundles from the testes into the ductus ejaculatorius duplex, from which position they can be transferred into the female during mating, occurred an average of 1.3 days before maturation of the behavioral system for pheromone responsiveness. A similar situation was observed in the Queensland fruit fly; only females containing some mature eggs in the ovarian follicles responded to sex pheromone released by males (Fletcher and Giannakakis 1973).

4.3.3. Mating history

Males of most insect species can mate with many females during their adult lives. If the males respond to female-produced pheromones as part of a premating communication sequence, then they must maintain (or regain) their pheromone responsiveness in order to mate again.

In many species, females also mate more than once. In a number of such species studied in which the female is the pheromone producer, no pronounced decrease in pheromone content in the gland occurred following mating (Shorey and Gaston 1965b; Brady and Smithwick 1968; Shorey et al. 1968a). Also, after a characteristic refractory period, the female must release pheromone again, since it is this release which leads to further mating behavior.

In other species, the female seldom, if ever, mates twice. Of course, these females do not tend to release pheromone again (Perez and Long 1964; Wellso 1966). Also, females of these species may exhibit a rapid reduction in pheromone content in the glands following mating (Collins and Potts 1932; Steinbrecht 1964b).

An intermediate situation has been observed in a number of species, with pheromone production, pheromone release, or pheromone responsiveness being reduced for long or short periods of time following mating (Brady and Smithwick 1968; Adeesan et al. 1969; Hardee et al. 1969; Minks and Noordink 1971; Nagata et al. 1972; Burkholder et al. 1973; Fletcher and Giannakakis 1973). In most of these cases, it is not yet clear how the reduced level of pheromone behavior correlates with the subsequent sexual behavior of the particular species.

Certain insects such as cockroaches exhibit repetitive cycles of mating and maturation of eggs. Pheromone behavior is also cyclic in these species, as discussed below in sect. 4.3.8.

4.3.4. *Previous exposure to pheromone*

When animals are exposed to constant or repetitive stimulation of their olfactory, visual, or auditory sensory systems, their responsiveness to the stimulus characteristically decreases. This lowered responsiveness, which is usually seen following pheromone stimulation, may be due to an interaction of two nervous system phenomena. One of these is sensory adaptation; a sensory neuron exposed to a constant level of stimulation increases its response threshold. It then ceases or decreases the transmission of action potentials that indicate the presence of pheromone to the central nervous system. Olfactory sensory adaptation is a transitory event. Quantitative investigations of silkworm (Boeckh et al. 1965; Schneider 1969) and cabbage looper (Payne et al. 1970) male moths indicate that olfactory sensory neurons on the male's antennae recover from sensory adaptation, caused by exposure to the female sex pheromone, within 60 sec following removal of the pheromone stimulus.

The second cause of a decrease in responsiveness following sensory stimulation is habituation. Olfactory habituation appears to involve an inhibition occurring at one or more sites in the central nervous system. In general, habituation is probably a valuable reaction of animals, since it decreases their tendency to respond to a stimulus that is repeatedly or continuously presented, when the response does not lead to some appropriate 'reward' such as mating or feeding. In contrast to sensory adaptation, the time required for complete recovery from habituation may be many minutes or hours. Elevated thresholds for male response to female sex pheromones following previous pheromone stimulation and apparently caused by habituation have been recorded for a number of insect species (Wharton et al. 1954a, b; Ignoffo et al. 1963; Shorey and Gaston 1964; Kliewer et al. 1966; Bartell and Shorey 1969; Traynier 1970a; Bartell and Lawrence 1973; Bartell and Roelofs 1973).

Based on research with the Mediterranean flour moth and the cabbage looper moth, Traynier (1970a) proposed that male habituation to the female sex pheromone is an all-or-none phenomenon, with its intensity not being correlated to the initially perceived pheromone concentration providing the concentration caused a behavioral response. However, Bartell and Lawrence (1973) later experimented with individually caged males of the light-brown apple moth and could not confirm Traynier's hypothesis. More research is necessary to aid our understanding of the physiological basis of pheromone habituation. This research area is of considerable current interest because of possible applications in the control of insect pests by interfering with their ability to perceive pheromones.

4.3.5. *Population density*

Population density may have a profound effect on insect behavior. This factor probably should be considered in interpreting the results of many field and laboratory studies in which pheromone production, release, or responsiveness are determined. For instance, male boll weevils, *Anthonomus grandis* (Boheman), released more pheromone, as indicated by an increased attractancy to other boll weevils, when isolated individually than when confined together in groups (Hardee et al. 1969). On the other hand, female yellow mealworm beetles, *Tenebrio molitor* (L.), released more sex pheromone in the presence of other females than when isolated individually (Happ and Wheeler 1969).

Populations of the Virginia-pine sawfly, *Neodiprion pratti* (Dyar), typically have outbreaks lasting two to three years, followed by a rapid decline in population size. Bobb (1964, 1972) found that sawfly females released relatively high levels of sex pheromone during outbreak years and little pheromone during low population years. He proposed that the lack of female attractancy was the factor leading to a lack of mating and, therefore, to the population decline. Although no evidence is available, perhaps the crowding during the outbreak years operated as the control factor, resulting in female offspring that had a reduced tendency to produce or release sex pheromone.

4.3.6. *Nutrition*

The influence of diet on subsequent sex pheromone behavior has received little attention. In the few species studied, prior exposure to a sub-optimal food source has led to a decrease in sex pheromone release (California red scale females *Aonidiella aurantii* (Maskell) (Rice and Moreno 1969), boll weevil males (Hardee et al 1970), Australian sheep blowfly females *Lucilia cuprina* (Wied.) (Bartell et al. 1969)). The influence of nutrition on pheromone responsiveness has been investigated only in the Australian sheep blowfly. Males provided a protein food were more responsive when exposed to female sex pheromone than were non protein-fed males (Bartell et al. 1969). None of the above experiments have evaluated whether the appropriate food had a selective controlling action on pheromone behavior, or whether the observed effects occurred in conjunction with many other behavioral and physiological effects as a result of an increased vigor due to the proper nutrition.

4.3.7. *Laboratory strains*

Different habitats or laboratory rearing conditions may place different selection pressures on insects of any one species, in some cases leading to changes in behavioral traits. For instance, rearing of adult moths in small cages might select against females that release relatively large amounts of pheromone and males that are stimulated to fly vigorously when they perceive the pheromone. The confined conditions might confer a reproductive advantage on those individuals whose premating behavior is more adapted to the small available space. Females of the summer fruit tortrix moth, *Adoxophyes orana* (F. von R.), from a laboratory strain that had been inbred for four to five years exhibited a lower level of pheromone production than females from a strain that had been inoculated yearly with insects taken from the field (Minks 1971). Also, screw-worm fly females, *Cochliomyia hominivorax* (Coquerel), of a 'Florida' strain were responsive to sex pheromone released from male flies, whereas females of a 'Mexican' strain were not. This difference in responsiveness was attributed to possible differences in the selection pressures of mass rearing placed on the two colonies. The Mexican strain was apparently held at higher densities, making distance communication stimulated by the sex pheromone a disadvantageous trait (Fletcher et al. 1968).

Despite the above indications of strain differences, a number of studies have shown pheromone release rate to be as high among insects that had been raised for a number of generations in the laboratory as it was among feral populations of the same species (lesser peach tree borer moth *Synanthedon pictipes* (G. and R.) (Wong et al. 1969), boll weevil (Hardee et al. 1969), and the almond moth, *Cadra cautella* (Walker), (Sower et al. 1973)). Likewise, for both the peach tree borer moth (Wong et al. 1969) and the almond moth (Sower et al. 1973), males of laboratory strains were as responsive to sex pheromone as males of wild strains.

Considerable heterogeneity in pheromone-behavior has been observed in a few species, giving a possible basis for the rapid selection of different strains. Female codling moths used individually as bait in traps exhibited a large variability in attractancy to males, presumably indicating a corresponding variability in pheromone release rate (Butt and Hathaway 1966). Also female cabbage looper moths had a large variability in individual pheromone release rates, from less than one to more than 21 ng/minute; the content of pheromone in individual cabbage looper female glands also varied, from less than 0.2 to 2.8 μg (Sower et al. 1972).

Investigators should use caution in expressing research results that seem to indicate a difference in the level of pheromone-behavior between two different strains. Sower et al. (1972) found that unexplained population variation over several weeks and months caused large changes in the content of pheromone in glands and the release rate of pheromone from glands of female cabbage loopers. Probably colonies of many insect species exhibit considerable daily, monthly, or seasonal variations in levels of pheromone content, release rate, or responsiveness. The determination of these pheromone-behavior levels during the 'highpoint' of one colony but the 'lowpoint' of another could give rise to faulty conclusions concerning strain differences.

4.3.8. Hormones

Females of certain insect species are long-lived in the adult stage and have repeated reproductive cycles. Mating occurs only during some defined portion of each cycle. Barth (1965) proposed that for such insects one might reasonably expect to find the timing of pheromone production to be under hormonal control. This is known to be the case in the cockroaches *Byrsotria fumigata* (Guerin) and *Pycnoscelus surinamensis* (L.) (Barth 1961, 1962; Bell and Barth 1970) and in the yellow mealworm beetle (Menon 1970). For each of these species, the corpora allata are necessary for the maintenance of high pheromone levels. In *Byrsotria fumigata*, corpora allata hormone selectively controls pheromone production and/or release, and does not control other aspects of female sexual behavior; allatectomized females artificially coated with pheromone accepted the males attracted to them and mated normally (Barth 1962, 1963; Roth and Barth 1964).

.Barth (1965) also proposed that insects that are short-lived as adults – that mate, lay their eggs, and die within a few days – might not require hormonal control of pheromone-behavior; the communication system for mating might advantageously be built into the adult development process such that it appears automatically when the adult stage is reached. Short-lived, non-feeding adults of the silkworm moth (Steinbrecht 1964a, b), the greater wax moth, *Galleria mellonella* (L.) (Röller et al. 1963), and the Chinese silkmoth, *Antheraea pernyi* (Guerin) (Barth 1965) do not have their pheromone production and/or release systems under control of the corpora allata hormone. In proposing his hypothesis regarding the probable presence vs absence of hormonal control in long-lived (with cyclic reproductive periods) vs short-lived insects, respectively, Barth (1965) recognized that only the extreme cases of life style have been examined. Data are needed concerning insects, such as many Lepidoptera, that feed as adults and do not exhibit pheromone behavior or mate until several days following emergence from the pupa.

Recently, White et al. (1972) maintained isolated sex pheromone glands of sugarcane borer female moths *Diatraea saccharalis* (F.), in organ culture for over two months. Adults of this species are fairly short-lived and, in the laboratory, normally mate, lay their eggs, and die within one week following emergence. Juvenile hormone was needed for the successful maintenance of the isolated gland tissue. However, the possible role of the hormone in pheromone production by the gland was not determined, and these results neither support nor refute Barth's (1965) hypothesis.

Barth's hypothesis may be limited to a consideration of the role of the corpora allata hormone only, in the production or release of sex pheromone. Recently, Riddiford and Williams (1971) studied the effect of a hormone from the corpora cardiaca on the release of sex pheromone from females of two short-lived lepidopterous species, the polyphemus moth and the cecropia moth, *Hyalophora cecropia* (L.). Environmental signals determine the timing of release of pheromone in each of these species. In the polyphemus moth, release only occurs when the female senses the chemical message emanating from the appropriate host plant (sect. 4.2.4). In the cecropia moth, release only occurs at a specific time of day, governed by the environmental light : dark periodicity (sect. 4.3.1). For each species, the brain presumably responds to the appropriate environmental signals by stimulating release of the hormone from the corpora cardiaca. The hormone then acts directly on the abdominal nervous system to cause eversion of the sex pheromone gland.

4.3.9. Sterilization

A number of entomological laboratories are exploring the potentials for release of sterile insects of certain pest species into the environment. Copulation of wild, potentially fertile insects with sterile mates would result, at the minimum, in wastage of gametes. In the case of female insects that are restricted to only a single mating during their life, union with a sterile partner has obvious adverse consequences.

The released, sterile insects should be competitive with wild insects in communicating for potential mates. Therefore, investigations have been conducted to determine whether pheromone production, release, or responsiveness were affected by the sterilizing treatment. Few data are available on sex pheromone production; however, production by female beetles of the yellow meal worm was not affected by a sterilizing dose of gamma irradiation (Menon and Nair 1972).

In a variety of studies of sex pheromone release, insects sterilized by gamma irradiation appeared competitive with non-sterilized individuals in their attraction of the opposite sex (boll weevil (Bartlett et al. 1968; Hardee et al 1969), gypsy moth (Statler 1970), cabbage looper moth (Stimmann et al. 1972), American cockroach *Periplaneta americana* (L.), (Wharton and Wharton 1957)). In fact, sterilized American cockroach females released more pheromone than normal females. Chemical sterilization with apholate also did not cause a reduction in release of sex pheromone by boll weevil males (Hardee et al. 1969).

Pheromone responsiveness of those insects that have been assayed following gamma-irradiation appears to be unimpaired (female boll weevils (Bartlett et al. 1968), male yellow meal worm beetles (Menon and Nair 1972), male cabbage looper moths (Stimmann et al. 1972)). Cabbage looper males sprayed with the chemical sterilant tepa were fully responsive to the female sex pheromone; however, males fed with tepa exhibited a reduced level of pheromone responsiveness (Henneberry et al. 1966).

4.3.10. Insecticides

Brady and Finley (1969) found that males of the Indian-meal moth *Plodia inter-*

punctella (Hübner), that survived an LD_{50} dose of the insecticide Bidrin® were as responsive to the female sex pheromone as were non-treated males. More studies of this type are needed to determine how pheromones can be used in conjunction with other agents of insect control in pest management programs.

4.3.11. *Anesthetization*

Many investigators routinely anesthetize insects at one time or another during their adult life to facilitate differentiation of sexes, for transfer to fresh containers, or for various surgical operations. The possible effect of such anesthetization on pheromone behavior is rarely questioned. However, Brady and Smithwick (1968) found that treatment of female Indian meal moths with nitrogen, carbon dioxide, or ether vapors suppressed sex pheromone release for up to nine hours. Holding the females at a cold temperature of 8 °C, which resulted in a high degree of immobilization, had no effect on subsequent pheromone releasing behavior.

4.4. *Interrelation of variables*

The control of sex pheromone-behavior obviously is not simple. Pheromone-behavior, like most other insect behavior, is probably precoded in a manner somewhat analogous to a computer program within a pheromone-behavior 'center' located in the central nervous system. Most of the time the behavior is not expressed because inhibitory messages arrive at the center over nervous system channels from some of the other, competing nervous system centers (such as the 'feeding behavior center' or 'escape behavior center'). Also, most of the time inhibitory messages will arrive over some of the sensory channels that communicate the state of the outside environment and of the internal physiology of the insect. The details of the degree of control of pheromone-behavior exerted by each of the environmental and physiological variables discussed in this chapter vary from one species to the next. Some species exhibit pheromone-behavior under a wide range of variables and others may be restricted to a narrow range. The simultaneous action of the variables can be appreciated by a summary of some of the information presented in this chapter concerning male pheromone responsiveness in one species, the cabbage looper moth. Males respond optimally to female sex pheromone: 1) during a few specific hours of the night; 2) at a light intensity equivalent to moonlight or darker; 3) at a temperature above 12 °C; 4) when the wind velocity is below male flight speed (about 3 m/sec); 5) when the male has reached the physiological age (about 2 days after emergence) so that sperm is available for mating; 6) when he has not mated already during that same dark period; and 7) when he has not been recently exposed to a high level of the pheromone. Any one of these restrictive conditions alone can entirely prevent his response to pheromone during some potential reproductive periods, as when the temperature does not exceed 12 °C at the appropriate time of night. The female's behavior of releasing pheromone is presumably controlled by similar levels of the same variables. Thus, both sexes will automatically be synchronized in the expression of their pheromone communication behavior.

References

Adeesan, C., G. W. Rahalkar and A. J. Tamhankar (1969) Effect of age and previous mating on the response of Khapra beetle males to female sex pheromone. Entomol. Exptl. Appl. 12, 229–234.

Aliniazee, M. T. and E. M. Stafford (1972) Sex pheromone studies with the omnivorous leafroller *Platynota stultana* (Lepidoptera: Tortricidae): Effect of various environmental factors on attraction of males to the traps baited with virgin females. Ann. Entomol. Soc. Am. 65, 958–961.

Bartell, R. J. and L. A. Lawrence (1973) Reduction in responsiveness of males of *Epiphyas postvittana* (Lepidoptera) to sex pheromone following previous brief pheromonal exposure. J. Insect Physiol. (in press).

Bartell, R. J. and W. L. Roelofs (1973) Inhibition of sexual response in males of the moth *Argyrotaenia velutinana* by brief exposures to synthetic pheromone or its geometrical isomer. J. Insect Physiol. 19, 655–661.

Bartell, R. J. and H. H. Shorey (1969) A quantitative bioassay for the sex pheromone of *Epiphyas postvittana* (Lepidoptera) and factors limiting male responsiveness. J. Insect Physiol. 15, 33–40.

Bartell, R. J., H. H. Shorey and L. Barton Browne (1969) Pheromonal stimulation of the sexual activity of males of the sheep blowfly *Lucilia cuprina* (Calliphoridae) by the female. Anim. Behav. 17, 576–585.

Barth, R. H., Jr. (1961) Hormonal control of sex attractant production in the Cuban cockroach. Science 133, 1598–1599.

Barth, R. H., Jr. (1962) The endocrine control of mating behavior in the cockroach *Byrsotria fumigata* (Guérin). Gen. Comp. Endocrinol. 2, 53–69.

Barth, R. H., Jr. (1963) Endocrine-exocrine mediated behavior in insects. Proc. 16th Int. Congr. Zool. 3, 3–5.

Barth, R. H., Jr. (1965) Insect mating behavior: Endocrine control of a chemical communication system. Science 149, 882–883.

Bartlett, A. C., P. A. Hooker and D. D. Hardee (1968) Behavior of irradiated boll weevils. I. Feeding, attraction, mating and mortality. J. Econ. Entomol. 61, 1677–1680.

Batiste, W. C. (1970) A timing sex-pheromone trap with special reference to codling moth collections. J. Econ. Entomol. 63, 915–918.

Batiste, W. C., W. H. Olson and A. Berlowitz (1973) Codling moth: The influence of temperature and daylight intensity on the periodicity of daily flight in the field. J. Econ. Entomol. (submitted for publication).

Bell, W. J. and R. H. Barth, Jr. (1970) Quantitative effects of juvenile hormone on reproduction in the cockroach *Byrsotria fumigata*. J. Insect Physiol. 16, 2303–2313.

Bobb, M. L. (1964) Apparent loss of sex attractiveness by the female of the Virginia-pine sawfly, *Neodiprion pratti pratti*. J. Econ. Entomol. 57, 829–830.

Bobb, M. L. (1972) Influence of sex pheromones on mating behavior and populations of Virginia-pine sawfly. Environmental Entomol. 1, 78–80.

Boeckh, J., K.-E. Kaissling and D. Schneider (1965) Insect olfactory receptors. Cold Spr. Harbor Symp. Quant. Biol. 30, 263–280.

Brady, U. E. and L. H. Finley (1969) Behavioral response of Bidrin®-treated male Indian meal moths to the female sex pheromone. J. Econ. Entomol. 62, 1117–1118.

Brady, U. E. and E. B. Smithwick (1968) Production and release of sex attractant by the female Indian-meal moth, *Plodia interpunctella*. Ann. Entomol. Soc. Am. 61, 1260–1265.

Burkholder, W. E., L. Hammack, J. E. Gorman and M. Ma (1973) Calling behavior of Dermestidae and its relation to pheromone production. J. Econ. Entomol. (submitted for publication).

Butler, C. G. and E. M. Fairey (1964) Pheromones of the honey bee: Biological studies of the mandibular gland secretion of the queen. J. Apic. Res. 3, 65–76.

Butt, B. A. and D. O. Hathaway (1966) Female sex pheromone as attractant for male codling moths. J. Econ. Entomol. 59, 476–477.

Casida, J. E., H. C. Coppel and T. Watanabe (1963) Purification and potency of the sex attractant from the introduced pine sawfly, *Diprion similis*. J. Econ. Entomol. 56, 18–24.

Collins, C. W. and S. F. Potts (1932) Attractants for the flying gypsy moths as an aid in locating new infestations. U. S. Dept. Agric. Tech. Bull. 336, 1–43.

Fletcher, B. S. (1969) The structure and function of the sex pheromone glands of the male Queensland fruit fly, *Dacus tryoni*. J. Insect Physiol. 15, 1309–1322.

Fletcher, B. S. and A. Giannakakis (1973) Factors limiting the response of females of the Queensland fruit fly *Dacus tryoni* to the sex pheromone of the male. J. Insect Physiol. (submitted for publication).

Fletcher, L. W., H. V. Claborn, J. P. Turner and E. Lopez (1968) Difference in response of two strains of screw-worm flies to the male pheromone. J. Econ. Entomol. 61, 1386–1388.

Gentry, C. R., F. R. Lawson and J. D. Hoffman (1964) A sex attractant in the tobacco budworm. J. Econ. Entomol. 57, 819–821.

George, J. A. (1965) Sex pheromone of the oriental fruit moth *Grapholitha molesta*-Busck (Lepidoptera, Tortricidae). Can. Entomol. 97, 1002–1007.

Götz, B. (1951) Die Sexualduftstoffe an Lepidopteren. Experientia 7, 406–418.

Happ, G. M. and J. Wheeler (1969) Bioassay, preliminary purification, and effect of age, crowding, and mating on the release of sex pheromone by female *Tenebrio molitor*. Ann. Entomol. Soc. Am. 62, 846–851.

Hardee, D. D., W. H. Cross, E. B. Mitchell, P. M. Huddleston, H. C. Mitchell, M. E. Merkl and T. B. Davich (1969) Biological factors influencing responses of the female boll weevil to the male sex pheromone in field and large-cage tests. J. Econ. Entomol. 62, 161–166.

Hardee, D. D., T. C. Cleveland, J. W. Davis and W. H. Cross (1970) Attraction of boll weevils to cotton plants and to males fed on three diets. J. Econ. Entomol. 63, 990–991.

Henneberry, T. J., H. H. Shorey and A. H. Kishaba (1966) Mating frequency and copulatory aberrations, response to female sex pheromone, and longevity of male cabbage loopers treated with TEPA. J. Econ. Entomol. 59, 573–576.

Holbrook, R. F., M. Beroza and E. D. Burgess (1960) Gypsy moth (*Porthetria dispar*) detection with the natural female sex lure. J. Econ. Entomol. 53, 751–756.

Ignoffo, C. M., R. S. Berger, H. M. Graham and D. F. Martin (1963) Sex attractant of cabbage looper, *Trichoplusia ni* (Hübner). Science 141, 902–903.

Jacklin, S. W. and C. E. Yonce (1969) Induced shift of the diurnal emergence and calling of the peach tree borer. J. Econ. Entomol. 62, 21–22.

Jacklin, S. W., C. E. Yonce and J. P. Hollon (1967) The attractiveness of female to male peach tree borers. J. Econ. Entomol. 60, 1291–1293.

Kaae, R. S. and H. H. Shorey (1972) Sex pheromones of noctuid moths. XXVII. Influence of wind velocity on sex pheromone releasing behavior of *Trichoplusia ni* females. Ann. Entomol. Soc. Am. 65, 436–440.

Kaae, R. S. and H. H. Shorey (1973) Sex pheromones of Lepidoptera. XLIV. Influence of environmental conditions on the location of pheromone communication and mating in *Pectinophora gossypiella*. Ann. Entomol. Soc. Am. (submitted for publication).

Kettlewell, H. B. D. (1942) The assembling scent of *Arctia villica* and *Parasemia plantaginis*. Entomol. Record 54, 62–63.

Kettlewell, H. B. D. (1946) Female assembling scents with reference to an important paper on the subject. Entomologist 79, 8–14.

Kliewer, J. W., T. Miura, R. C. Husbands and C. H. Hurst (1966) Sex pheromones and mating behavior of *Culiseta inornata* (Diptera: Culicidae). Ann. Entomol. Soc. Am. 59, 530–533.

Klun, J. A. (1968) Isolation of a sex pheromone of the European corn borer. J. Econ. Entomol. 61, 484–487.

Lange, R., D. Hoffmann and M. Weissinger (1971) Untersuchungen über das Flugverhalten männlicher Falter von *Rhyacionia buoliana* (Lep., Tortricidae). Oecologia 6, 156–163.

Menon, M. (1970) Hormone-pheromone relationships in the beetle, *Tenebrio molitor*. J. Insect Physiol. 16, 1123–1139.

Menon, M. and K. K. Nair (1972) Sex pheromone production and reproductive behaviour in gamma-irradiated *Tenebrio molitor*. J. Insect Physiol. 18, 1323–1331.

Minks, A. K. (1971) Decreased sex pheromone production in an in-bred stock of the summerfruit tortrix moth, *Adoxophyes orana*. Entomol. Exptl. Appl. 14, 361–364.

Minks, A. K. and J. Ph. W. Noordink (1971) Sex attraction of the summerfruit tortrix moth, *Adoxophyes orana*: evaluation in the field. Entomol. Exptl. Appl. 14, 57–72.

Nagata, K., Y. Tamaki, H. Noguchi and T. Yushima (1972) Changes in sex pheromone activity in adult females of the smaller tea tortrix moth *Adoxophyes fasciata*. J. Insect Physiol. 18, 339–346.

Payne, T. L., H. H. Shorey and L. K. Gaston (1970) Sex pheromones of noctuid moths: factors influencing antennal responsiveness in males of *Trichoplusia ni*. J. Insect Physiol. 16, 1043–1055.

Perez, R. and W. H. Long (1964) Sex attractant and mating behavior in the sugarcane borer. J. Econ. Entomol. 57, 688–690.

Rau, P. and N. Rau (1929) The sex attraction and rhythmic periodicity in giant saturniid moths. Trans. Acad. Sci., St. Louis 26, 83–221.

Rice, R. E. and D. S. Moreno (1969) Comparative production of pheromone by the California red scale reared on lemons and potatoes. J. Econ. Entomol. 62, 958–959.

Riddiford, L. M. (1967) Trans-2-hexenal: mating stimulant for polyphemus moths. Science 158, 139–141.

Riddiford, L. M. and C. M. Williams (1967a) Volatile principle from oak leaves: role in sex life of the polyphemus moth. Science 155, 589–590.

Riddiford, L. M. and C. M. Williams (1967b) Chemical signaling between polyphemus moths and between moths and host plant. Science 156, 541.

Riddiford, L. M. and C. M. Williams (1971) Role of the corpora cardiaca in the behavior of saturniid moths. I. Release of sex pheromone. Biol. Bull. 140, 1–7.

Röller, H., H. Piepho and I. Holz (1963) Zum Problem der Hormonabhängigkeit des Paarungsverhaltens bei Insekten. Untersuchungen an *Galleria mellonella* (L.). J. Insect Physiol. 9, 187–194.

Roth, L. M. and R. H. Barth, Jr. (1964) The control of sexual receptivity in female cockroaches. J. Insect Physiol. 10, 965–975.

Saario, C. A., H. H. Shorey and L. K. Gaston (1970) Sex pheromones of noctuid moths. XIX. Effect of environmental and seasonal factors on captures of males of *Trichoplusia ni* in pheromone-baited traps. Ann. Entomol. Soc. Am. 63, 667–672.

Sanders, C. J. (1969) Extrusion of the female sex pheromone gland in the eastern spruce budworm, *Choristoneura fumiferana* (Lepidoptera: Tortricidae). Can. Entomol. 101, 760–762.

Schneider, D. (1969) Insect olfaction: Deciphering system for chemical messages. Science 163, 1031–1037.

Sharma, R. K., R. E. Rice, H. T. Reynolds and H. H. Shorey (1971) Seasonal influence and effect of trap location on catches of pink bollworm males in sticky traps baited with hexalure. Ann. Entomol. Soc. Am. 64, 102–105.

Shorey, H. H. (1966) The biology of *Trichoplusia ni* (Lepidoptera: Noctuidae). IV. Environmental control of mating. Ann. Entomol. Soc. Am. 59, 502–506.

Shorey, H. H. (1973) Behavioral responses to insect pheromones. Ann. Rev. Entomol. 18, 349–380.

Shorey, H. H. and L. K. Gaston (1964) Sex pheromones of noctuid moths. III. Inhibition of male responses to the sex pheromone in *Trichoplusia ni* (Lepidoptera: Noctuidae). Ann. Entomol. Soc. Am. 57, 775–779.

Shorey, H. H. and L. K. Gaston (1965a) Sex pheromones of noctuid moths. V. Circadian rhythm of pheromone-responsiveness in males of *Autographa californica*, *Heliothis virescens*, *Spodoptera exigua*, and *Trichoplusia ni* (Lepidoptera: Noctuidae). Ann. Entomol. Soc. Am. 58, 597–600.

Shorey, H. H. and L. K. Gaston (1965b) Sex pheromones of noctuid moths. VII. Quantitative aspects of the production and release of pheromone by females of *Trichoplusia ni* (Lepidoptera: Noctuidae). Ann. Entomol. Soc. Am. 58, 604–608.

Shorey, H. H., S. U. McFarland and L. K. Gaston (1968a) Sex pheromones of noctuid moths. XIII. Changes in pheromone quantity, as related to reproductive age and mating history, in females of seven species of Noctuidae (Lepidoptera). Ann. Entomol. Soc. Am. 61, 372–376.

Shorey, H. H., K. L. Morin and L. K. Gaston (1968b) Sex pheromones of noctuid moths. XV. Timing of development of pheromone-responsiveness and other indicators of reproductive age in males of eight species. Ann. Entomol. Soc. Am. 61, 857–861.

Solomon, J. D. and R. C. Morris (1966) Sex attraction of the carpenter-worm moth. J. Econ. Entomol. 59, 1534–1535.

Sower, L. L., H. H. Shorey and L. K. Gaston (1970) Sex pheromones of noctuid moths. XXI. Light : dark cycle regulation and light inhibition of sex pheromone release by females of *Trichoplusia ni*. Ann. Entomol. Soc. Am. 63, 1090–1092.

Sower, L. L., H. H. Shorey and L. K. Gaston (1971) Sex pheromones of noctuid moths. XXV. Effects of temperature and photoperiod on circadian rhythms of sex pheromone release by females of *Trichoplusia ni*. Ann. Entomol. Soc. Am. 64, 488–492.

Sower, L. L., H. H. Shorey and L. K. Gaston (1972) Sex pheromones of Lepidoptera. XXVIII. Factors modifying the release rate and extractable quantity of pheromone from females of *Trichoplusia ni* (Noctuidae). Ann. Entomol. Soc. Am. 65, 954–957.

Sower, L. L., D. W. Hagstrum and J. S. Long (1973) Comparison of the female pheromones of a wild and a laboratory strain of *Cadra cautella*, and male responsiveness to the pheromone extracts. Ann. Entomol. Soc. Am. 66, 484–485.

Sparks, A. (1963) Preliminary studies of factors influencing mating of the European corn borer. Proc. N. Centr. Br. Entomol. Soc. Am. 18, 96.

Statler, M. W. (1970) Effects of gamma radiation on the ability of the adult female gypsy moth to attract males. J. Econ. Entomol. 63, 163–164.

Steinbrecht, R. A. (1964a) Feinstruktur und Histochemie der Sexualduftdrüse des Seidenspinners *Bombyx mori* L. Z. Zeitforschung 64, 227–261.

Steinbrecht, R. A. (1964b) Die Abhängigkeit der Lockwirkung des Sexualduftorgans weiblicher Seidenspinner (*Bombyx mori*) von Alter und Kopulation. Z. Vergleich. Physiol. 48, 341–356.

Stimmann, M. W., W. W. Wolf and H. H. Toba (1972) Pheromone response of γ-irradiated cabbage loopers in the field. J. Econ. Entomol. 65, 1496–1498.

Traynier, R. M. M. (1970a) Habituation of the response to sex pheromone in two species of Lepidoptera, with reference to a method of control. Entomol. Exptl. Appl. 13, 179–187.

Traynier, R. M. M. (1970b) Sexual behaviour of the Mediterranean flour moth, *Anagasta kühniella*: some influences of age, photo-period, and light intensity. Can. Entomol. 102, 534–540.

Wellso, S. G. (1966) Sexual attraction and biology of *Xenorhipis brendeli* (Coleoptera: Buprestidae). J. Kans. Entomol. Soc. 39, 242–245.

Wharton, D. R. A., G. L. Miller and M. L. Wharton (1954a) The odorous attractant of the American cockroach, *Periplaneta americana* (L.). J. Gen. Physiol. 37, 461–469.

Wharton, D. R. A., G. L. Miller and M. L. Wharton (1954b) The odorous attractant of the American cockroach, *Periplaneta americana* (L.) II. A bioassay method for the attractant. J. Gen. Physiol. 37, 471–481.

Wharton, M. L. and D. R. A. Wharton (1957) The production of sex attractant substance and of oothecae by the normal and irradiated American cockroach, *Periplaneta americana* L. J. Insect Physiol. 1, 229–239.

White, M. R., R. L. Amborski, A. M. Hammond, Jr. and G. F. Amborski (1972) Organ culture of the terminal abdominal segment of an adult female lepidopteran. In Vitro 8, 30–36.

Wong, T. T. Y., M. L. Cleveland and D. G. Davis (1969) Sex attraction and mating of lesser peach tree borer moths. J. Econ. Entomol. 62, 789–792.

Wong, T. T. Y., M. L. Cleveland, D. F. Ralston and D. G. Davis (1971a) Virgin female traps to determine activity and population of red-banded leaf roller. J. Econ. Entomol. 64, 132–134.

Wong, T. T. Y., M. L. Cleveland, D. F. Ralston and D. G. Davis (1971b) Time of sexual activity of codling moths in the field. J. Econ. Entomol. 64, 553–554.

CHAPTER 5

Mechanisms of orientation to a distant pheromone source

S. R. FARKAS and H. H. SHOREY

5.1. Introduction

Insects of many species utilize sex pheromones for recruiting mates. The pheromone is emitted by one sex, the sender, and transported through the air to a prospective mate, the receiver. If the receiver perceives an above threshold concentration of the pheromone, it initiates a series of responses which eventually bring it to the vicinity of the source of the chemical. The mechanisms by which an insect finds the source of a chemical located many meters away appear to be very different from those used for locating the source of a visual or mechanical stimulus. If the organism is suitably equipped, visual and mechanical stimuli yield information about the direction of the source (Fraenkel and Gunn 1961; Erulkar 1972); the individual orients its body in line with the stimulus and moves toward the source. On the other hand, except within a few cm of the source (Wright 1958; Shorey and Gaston 1967), chemical cues are non-directional and do not relay information about the exact location of the stimulus. An insect must therefore utilize other sensory cues, in addition to the chemical stimulus, to determine the direction of a chemical source located many cm or m away.

This chapter will be devoted mainly to a discussion of probable mechanisms used by flying insects in orienting to a distant pheromone source. Since much work has been done on insect attraction to hosts and food through olfactory cues, information will be freely drawn from these non-pheromone related studies.

5.2. Physical nature of chemical trails

Pheromones may be emitted directly into the air, forming aerial trails, or deposited on the ground, creating terrestrial trails (Butler 1970). Aerial trails are characteristically used by flying insects when orienting toward odor sources; terrestrial trails are used by ants and termites in their ground-based chemical communication systems. The similarities and differences of these two types of trails are worth noting, for the mechanisms used by insects in following either one may be analogous.

5.2.1. Aerial trails

The transmission of a chemical signal in air is dependent upon the rate of diffusion of the chemical and the directional flow of the medium. Dispersal of a chemical by diffusion alone occurs very slowly with time; in a static environment the molecules become distributed in a concentration gradient radiating out from the source. With the introduction of air movement, any existing concentration gradient is disrupted and the relative importance of diffusion in the dispersal of molecules is minimal. The chemical is carried downwind forming an elongate aerial trail, and the distance over which the signal is transmitted is greatly increased (Bossert and Wilson 1963). Bossert and Wilson (1963) designated the active space as that zone around or downwind from the odor that contains a density of molecules at or above the behavioral threshold concentration.

The behavior of aerial chemical trails has been studied using visible smoke and mathematical models (Wright 1958; Kellogg et al. 1962; Bossert and Wilson 1963; Wilson and Bossert 1963; Fuchs 1964; Traynier 1968; Farkas and Shorey 1972). These studies indicate that the aerial trails are not a uniform mass of molecules, but are filamentous in structure (fig. 5.1). The filaments readily change shape, break up, and radiate out from the longitudinal axis of the trail while they are being carried

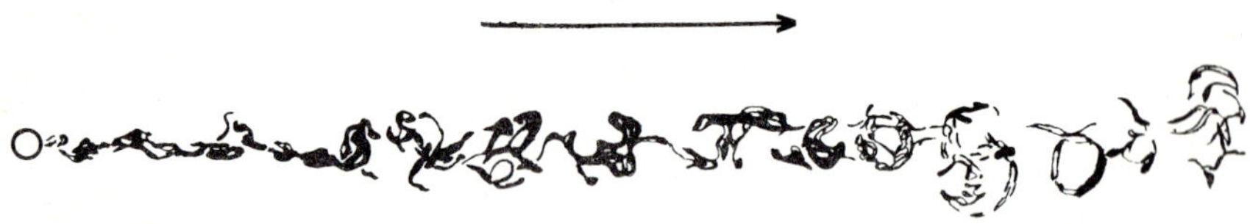

Fig. 5.1. Artist's representation of an aerial chemical trail based on an actual photograph of a trail of visible smoke. Circle indicates source of smoke. Arrow indicates direction of wind.

downwind. The amount of disruption of the trail is dependent upon the degree of atmospheric turbulence. The diameter of the trail therefore increases as the distance from the source increases and the molecular density is, on the average, greater near the longitudinal axis of the trail than near the periphery. Speculatively (for no factual evidence is at hand), the insect detects a series of separate pulses of pheromone as it flies through a chemical trail; the highest density of pulses and the highest molecular concentration per pulse being located near the longitudinal axis of the trail and near the source (Wright 1958).

5.2.2. Terrestrial trails

Workers of many species of ants and termites deposit chemical trails on the ground. In several species of ants, these trails are deposited in discontinuous streaks or spots (Carthy 1951; Wilson 1962, 1971; Hangartner 1969). Wilson (1971) indicates that the trail which is actually followed is not the streak deposited on the substrate, but rather is a 'vapor tunnel' produced by evaporation of the molecules into the air. Analysis of trails of the imported fire ant, *Solenopsis saevissima* (Fr. Smith), demonstrates that this vapor tunnel of pheromone has an effective active space radius of about one cm (Wilson 1963; Wilson and Bossert 1963). A concentration gradient is also present through the cross section of the vapor tunnel (Hangartner 1967; Wilson 1971). Thus, in the case of terrestrial trails, diffusion becomes the mode of transporting molecules from the source (the trail) to the olfactory receptors. This is in contrast to directional air movement, which is the main transporting means for aerial trails.

An ant following a terrestrial trail is subjected to an elongate active space similar to that present in aerial trails; however, a main difference is that the width of a terrestrial trail is narrower relative to the size of the insect.

5.3. Mechanisms

The approach of a flying insect to a chemical source involves a complex sequence of behavioral events, including: initiation of flight, directed movement along or through the chemical trail, arrestment of locomotion and landing. These events may involve various types of kinesis and taxis mechanisms and are probably regulated by the perceived concentration of the pheromone and by visual stimuli.

5.3.1. Initiation of flight

When a receptive insect at rest perceives a concentration of pheromone above the threshold level, it may be stimulated to initiate the flight response that will eventually bring it to the vicinity of the source of the chemical. Sower et al. (1971), working with males of the cabbage looper moth, *Trichoplusia ni* (Hübner), showed that the threshold concentration of pheromone for eliciting behavioral activation (wing vibration) or flight is in the order of 10 mols/mm^3. The behavioral threshold concentration for the activation of the silkworm moth, *Bombyx mori* (L.), is likewise approximately 10 mols/mm^3 (Kaissling and Priesner 1970). Sensory adaptation must also be considered, since the threshold concentration required for activation may be raised when prior exposure to the chemical has occurred (Shorey and Gaston 1964; Boeckh et al. 1965; Shorey et al. 1967; Bartell and Lawrence 1973).

Behavioral activation or initiation of flight may be rapid following perception of the pheromone molecules. In *B. mori*, males repond by vibrating their wings within two seconds of exposure to sex pheromone (Kaissling and Priesner 1970). Take-off response for *Ips paraconfusus* Lanier (=*confusus* LeConte) bark beetles likewise appears rapid when they are exposed to the species aggregation pheromone (Gara 1963). Ambient temperature may have a marked effect on the response time for initiation of flight. In some insect species, a warm-up period is necessary in preparation for flight when the ambient temperature and thus body temperature are low; muscular activity, in part via wing vibration, serves to raise the body temperature to an optimum temperature for flight activity (Heath and Adams 1967; Adams 1969).

5.3.2. Locomotion toward the source

Within a few cm of the odor source, where a relatively steep concentration gradient might persist, an insect may use chemoklinotaxis or chemotropotaxis in determining the direction of the origin of the chemical. In employing chemoklinotaxis, the insect swings its antennae from side to side and makes successive comparisons of the chemical concentration on each side of its body (Shorey 1973). In using chemotropotaxis, the individual simultaneously compares the chemical concentration on each side of its body with its two antennae (Shorey 1973). In either tactic reaction the insect turns toward the side of highest stimulation (if the chemical is an attractant) and, in this way, becomes oriented toward the stimulus source. Tactic reactions only imply steering per se and a chemo-orthokinetic reaction – speed of locomotion dependent on chemical concentration (Fraenkel and Gunn 1961) – maintains forward progress toward the source (Janders 1963).

At our present level of knowledge it appears that two different components of orientation may function simultaneously to enable the insect to approach a distant odor source. The first component allows the insect to determine which direction to follow along the trail so as to arrive at, as opposed to move away from, the odor source. The second component is superimposed on the first and enables the insect to make lateral correcting movements so as to remain near the central longitudinal axis of the trail.

Several mechanisms have been proposed by which an insect can determine the first component – the actual direction of an odor source. These include: 1) anemotaxis; 2) use of an elongate gradient of odor filaments; and 3) use of an elongate gradient of molecular density. To what extent these mechanisms are actually used is a matter of conjecture. Therefore, the discussion that follows is largely hypothetical.

An anemotactic response occurs when the insect orients its body axis parallel with the direction of movement of an air current (Fraenkel and Gunn 1961). If the insect were in physical contact with the substratum, the direction of an air current could, in principle, be determined by the direction of deflection of mechanoreceptors on the body (Weis-Fogh 1948, 1949; Camhi 1969a, b, 1970). However, flying insects cannot rely entirely upon mechanoreception in obtaining this directional information. The following example will illustrate this point. Suppose that a weightless, blind insect is free-floating in a current of air. When the insect is not flying, both the direction in which it is carried and its velocity are equal to the direction and velocity of the air current. Its mechanoreceptors can only detect that it is motionless with respect to the air mass within which it is carried. Now, if the insect begins to fly, its mechanoreceptors may sense movement, but the sensation of direction is relative to the current rather than to the substratum over which it is passing. Therefore, contact with the substratum or other fixed objects in the environment must be maintained in order to sense the true direction of a flowing medium. Kennedy (1939) reported that the yellow-fever mosquito, *Aedes aegypti* (L.), uses visual contact with the substratum to maintain an upwind flight direction and he hypothesized that the steering mechanism involved both the speed and the direction at which objects passed below the eye. The apparent direction and velocity of these images are dependent upon the air velocity, the flight speed of the insect, and the angle at which the insect is flying with respect to the wind. Upwind flight must produce a lower apparent velocity of images passing beneath the eyes than downwind flight, and the apparent direction of the substrate objects must be from fore to aft, parallel to the body axis. Crosswind flight causes a sideslippage of the insect's body with relation to the substrate that results in substrate objects moving at an apparent oblique angle to the eye. Upon sensing this sideslippage information, the individual is supposed to make compensatory turning responses in order to maintain upwind flight. The ability of an insect to detect sideslippage when it flies at an angle to the wind then becomes a determining factor in utilizing anemotaxis. Later studies on *A. aegypti* and on the vinegar fly, *Drosophila melanogaster* (Meigen), have further demonstrated the need for visual contact with the substratum in maintaining an anemotactic orientation (Kellogg et al. 1962; Wright 1962, 1964).

The effect of air velocity on anemotaxis has been examined in several species of insects. Field observations often indicate that the number of individuals arriving at a pheromone source decreases as the wind velocity decreases below some threshold value. In the scarabaeid beetle, *Rhopaea magnicornis* (Blackburn), males exposed to sex pheromone flew at random when winds of less than 135 cm/sec were present, but with an increase in wind velocity to 225 cm/sec, males were observed flying toward the source (Soo Hoo and Roberts 1965). Butler and Fairey (1964) noted that when drones of the honey bee, *Apis mellifera* L., hovered around a queen or a synthetic pheromone source suspended in air, they dispersed when the wind velocity became low or lacking. Drones re-appeared when the air velocity increased to above 50 cm/sec. In the introduced pine sawfly, *Diprion similis* (Hartig), large numbers of males were observed flying to a female sex pheromone source when wind velocities were above 90 cm/sec; fewer males approached the source at velocities less than this value (Casida et al. 1963). The decreased number of individuals reaching the pheromone source when air velocities were low might be attributed to the insects' inability to detect sideslippage visually, since lower wind velocities result in less relative sideslippage when the insects' flight speed remains constant.

The hypothetical anemotactic orientation sequence is as follows. The anemotactic response is initiated when the insect perceives an above threshold concentration of molecules. The insect continues to fly upwind as long as it remains within the active space of the aerial trail. When the insect moves out of the active space, upwind flight ceases and crosswind or downwind flights are made until the chemical trail is regained (Kellogg et al. 1962; Wright 1964; Traynier 1968).

Insects of many species make prominent crosswind casts while flying along a chemical trail. This results in a zigzag flight pattern (Dethier 1947; Steiner 1953; Danzer 1956; Kellogg et al. 1962; Rudinsky and Daterman 1964; Traynier 1968; Cole 1970; Farkas and Shorey 1972), the probable function of which will be discussed below. For some species, the zigzag flight pattern may be eliminated when the chemical aerial trail is artificially disrupted and the insect is exposed to an air flow carrying a near uniform cross-sectional distribution of molecules (Kellogg et al. 1962; Wright 1964; Traynier 1968; Dahm et al. 1971). In such cases, the pheromone-stimulated insect may fly upwind in a fairly direct manner, presumably by means of anemotaxis.

Recently, Farkas and Shorey (1972) have demonstrated that males of the pink bollworm moth, *Pectinophora gossypiella* (Saunders), utilize a mechanism other than anemotaxis in steering to a sex pheromone source. Interference with possible visual cues from the substratum failed to inhibit individuals from flying to the pheromone source. Likewise, when a chemical aerial trail was presented to the moths in a flight tunnel and the air movement then eliminated, the insects were able to fly along the motionless trail to the vicinity of the source. Thus, mechanisms other than anemotaxis must be considered that can be used by the insect to determine the direction of the source.

Wright (1958) proposed a mechanism by which a flying insect could steer toward a distant chemical source without the use of anemotaxis. His hypothesis is based upon observations of the physical nature of a chemical trail. Wright noted that the spaces between the odorous filaments of the trail are positively correlated with the distances from both the odor source and the longitudinal axis of the odor plume. He proposed that an insect downwind from the source perceives a series of discontinuous chemical signals in the form of pulses as it flies through a sequence of filaments. When the insect is headed in the direction of the source, it senses a decrease in the time between pulses and is inhibited from turning. If the insect is headed away from the source, or if the insect approaches the outer boundary of the trail (thus sensing an increase in the time between pulses), it is stimulated to initiate a zigzag flight pattern until it once again senses a decrease in the time between pulses and is thus flying toward the odor source. Wright then tested his hypothesis on *Drosophila melanogaster* and found that this species did not fit his model but apparently utilized anemotaxis as its steering mechanism (Wright 1964).

A similar mechanism for detecting the direction of an odor source may be based on utilization of an elongate concentration gradient. Bossert and Wilson (1963) state that at the downwind limit of its theoretical communication distance (1820 m) a male gypsy moth, *Porthetria dispar* (L.), could not conceivably detect a behaviorally significant difference in odor concentration by flying one meter either upwind or downwind. At that distance, the average concentration difference in one meter would be only 0.013%. However, if conditions are examined closer to the source, an insect may be able to detect a difference in concentration over *time*.

Fig. 5.2 illustrates the theoretical concentration gradient of pheromone emitted by a female cabbage looper moth, *Trichoplusia ni*, in a wind velocity of 25 cm/sec. Flight by the male toward the source from six m downwind would result in an increase in concentration of approximately 41% over a one-m distance. A 25% decrease in concentration would occur during a one-m flight away from the source. Thus, a mechanism allowing detection of the elongate, average concentration gradient over time could work within a few meters of the source to indicate the direction toward the source. Flight toward the source would result in a detectable average increase in concentration over some period of time: the insect would, perhaps, not then be stimulated to change course. Flight away from the source would result in a detectable decrease in concentration; perhaps the insect would then be stimulated to turn and fly in the opposite direction. Thus, the elongate gradient would provide the polarization of the trail, informing the insect as to which direction to fly along it in order to reach the source. Similar mechanisms for orientation toward a chemical source have been proposed by Macnab and Koshland (1972) for the bacterium, *Salmonella typhimurium*, and by Wensler (1972) for

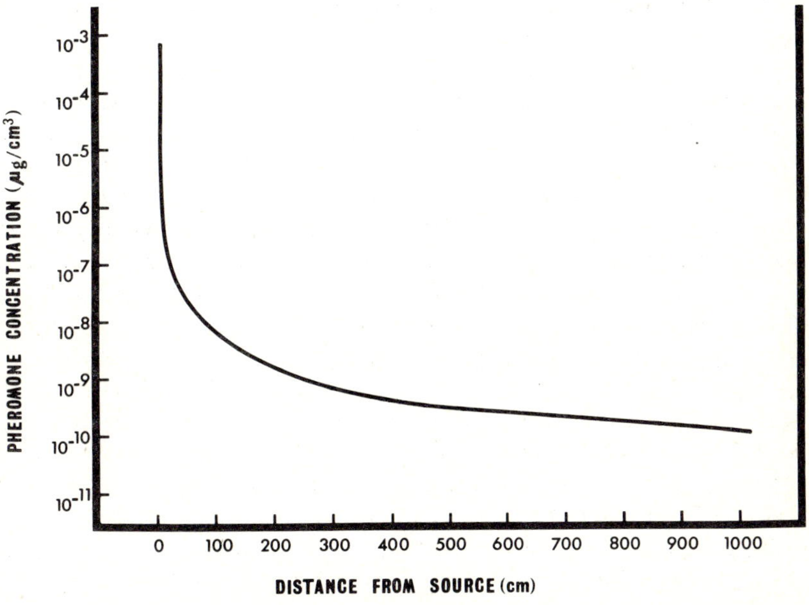

Fig. 5.2. Average concentration, measured at the central axis of the odor trail, at various distances from a female *Trichoplusia ni* releasing pheromone in a wind velocity of 25 cm/sec. Calculations based on Sower et al. (1971).

Aedes aegypti. They indicate that such a time-dependent mechanism must involve a memory system; i.e. the organism must remember what concentration of chemical it was previously exposed to in order to initiate the appropriate response when it detects a higher or lower concentration.

The second proposed component of orientation behavior, that which enables the insect to remain within the aerial trail, involves the correction of lateral deviation from the central axis of the trail. Farkas and Shorey (1972) reported that males of *Pectinophora gossypiella*, as well as males or females of many other insect species, exhibit a lateral zigzag flight pattern in approaching a sex pheromone source. Visual and photographic analysis of the flight tracks of males of *P. gossypiella* indicated that the lateral amplitude of the zigzag approximates the lateral dimension of the trail. Analysis of the nature of the stimuli that are responsible for turns made during this zigzag flight behavior has been attempted only superficially. Such analysis may be of utmost importance in further understanding the mechanism by which lateral corrections are made. Working with *Aedes aegypti*, Daykin et al. (1965) found that the tendency to execute a turn was greater when the mosquitoes left the active space than when they entered it. Using photographic techniques, Kellogg et al. (1962) found that a similar turning response for *Drosophila melanogaster* occurred 0.1–0.2 sec after losing the odor. Perttunen et al. (1968) also found a greater tendency to turn when individuals of the scolytid beetle *Blastophagus piniperda* L. walked from an area containing an odorous attractant to an area without the chemical. Farkas et al. (1974) found that male moths of *Pectinophora gossypiella* executed their turns at slightly sharper angles as they encountered higher concentrations of female sex pheromone. Correlating the typical zigzag flight pattern with the physical nature of the chemical trail, Farkas and Shorey (1972) speculated that these turns are probably initiated near the boundaries of the active space by either a drop in molecular concentration or a decreased frequency at which odor filaments are perceived. In this way the insect is able to reorient continually toward the longitudinal axis of the trail. The direction in which the insect turns near the boundaries of the active space may possibly be regulated by: 1) detection of the direction of visual sideslippage during its anemotactic response (Kennedy 1939); 2) chemotaxis mechanisms (Martin 1965); 3) a pre-programmed zigzag flight pattern in which right and left turns are alternately executed; 4) detection of an elongate concentration gradient of odor molecules or filaments (Wright 1958); or 5) a combination of these four.

Certain aspects of the behavior displayed by an insect in flying toward a chemical source along an aerial trail appear similar to those exhibited by insects that follow chemical terrestrial trails. Many species of ants characteristically follow a terrestrial trail in a zigzag pattern (Carthy 1951; Wilson 1962; Wilson and Bossert 1963; Hangartner 1967). Hangartner (1967) presents strong evidence that the zigzag turning exhibited by workers of *Lasius fuliginosus* Latr. in following terrestrial pheromone trails is the result of the ant using chemotropotaxis. As the ant moves along the trail and senses a lower concentration from the right than from the left antenna, it responds by turning to the left, and vice versa. Thus, orientation along the longitudinal axis of the trail is maintained. This occasional loss of contact from the trail by each antenna may be of additional value in preventing prolonged sensory adaptation (Wilson and Bossert 1963). Although the ant is thus considered able to determine the position of the longitudinal axis of the trail, there is no evidence for the existence of polarity and the actual direction in which the trail was deposited cannot be determined via olfactory cues (Carthy 1951; Dethier 1957; Wilson 1962; Wilson and Bossert 1963).

Recently, an ability to follow a terrestrial chemical trail has been demonstrated in a moth which normally flies toward a sex pheromone source by following an aerial trail (Shorey and Farkas 1973). Wingless males of the moth *Trichoplusia ni* were observed to follow a trail of pheromone drawn on a horizontal substrate. Although terrestrial trail following by this species may be an artifact of the laboratory, the fact that it does occur lends further support to the hypothesis that both terrestrial and aerial chemical trail following may be regulated by similar mechanisms.

5.3.3. Arrestment of locomotion

Arrestment of locomotion for a flying insect involves both a reduction in flight speed and an initiation of landing. These two responses are not independent of each other and both appear to be regulated by a number of stimuli, including chemical concentration and visual cues.

A chemo-orthokinesis reaction often seems to operate near the pheromone source, causing a reduction in flight speed as the pheromone concentration increases (Casida et al. 1963; Traynier 1968). When exposed to a high concentration of pheromone, many members of the family Scolytidae (Vité and Pitman 1967; Borden and Bennett 1969; Bennett and Borden 1971) and the scarabaeid beetle, *Geotrupes stercorarius* De G. (Steiner 1953) respond by reducing their flight speed and terminating flight. Also, when exposed to a high concentration of female sex pheromone, male moths of *Pectinophora gossypiella* reduce their flight speed and land on objects within the active space (Farkas et al. 1974). Similarly, males of the ichneumonid wasp, *Apanteles medicaginis* Muesebeck, appear to be stimulated to alight when they perceive a high pheromone concentration, and landing normally occurs 10 cm downwind from a single hidden female (Cole 1970). Osborne and Hoyt (1970) observed that males of the scarabaeid beetle, *Costelytra zealandica* (White), land 30 to 60 cm downwind of a source releasing a high concentration of female sex pheromone, but they alight on the source when it releases a lower concentration of pheromone.

Male insects, stimulated by female sex pheromone, are often seen to utilize visual cues from the female in orienting their landing or hovering response. Shorey and Gaston (1970) demonstrated that male moths of *Trichoplusia ni* visually orient and hover adjacent to a model of a female, even when the model is located two cm to one side of a pheromone source. When a female moth of *Porthetria dispar*, that is not emitting pheromone, is placed 15 cm upwind from a hidden sex pheromone source, males are unable to locate her, even though they may overshoot the source and pass but a few cm from her (Doane 1968). A similar female located 15 cm downwind from the source is readily located by the males and landing and attempted copulation occur.

5.4. *Effective distances for chemical communication*

The maximum distance over which a 'receiver' insect can orient to pheromone emitted by a 'sender' insect depends upon many factors including: 1) pheromone emission rate of the sender; 2) behavioral threshold for response to the pheromone by the receiver; 3) wind velocity; 4) length of time the sender releases pheromone; 5) flight speed of the receiver. The first three factors establish the foundation for estimating the theoretical maximum distance of pheromonal chemical communication (Bossert and Wilson 1963; Wilson and Bossert 1963). Less obvious are the factors of length of time the pheromone is released and flight speed of the receiver (Sower et al 1973). The latter variables will not affect the theoretical maximum communication distance if the sender emits pheromone for an indefinitely long, continuous period and the wind velocity is ideal for upwind flight by the receiver. Such ideal conditions probably often occur for some species. However, female moths of *Trichoplusia ni* release pheromone for an average period of only 20 min at any one time (Sower et al. 1971), the length of this release period decreasing even further with increased wind velocity (Kaae and Shorey 1972). The maximum distance for communication, then, is limited by the ability of the receiver to reach the chemical source before pheromone emission ceases.

Using data on pheromone release rates, male response thresholds and formulae concerning the dispersion of odor molecules in moving air, Sower et al. (1971) calculated that with a wind velocity of 50 cm/sec the mean maximum communication distance for *T. ni* is 20 m. However, due to the high individual variability of both female release rates and male threshold concentrations, a range of distances from one to approximately 100 m appears realistic.

Males have been reported in the literature to fly exceptionally long distances (0.8 to 4.5 km) to reach a pheromone source (Rau and Rau 1929; Collins and Potts 1932; Holbrook et al. 1960; Teale 1961). Determinations of these long distances were based on captures of marked male moths released at various distances from female-baited traps. Because of possible upwind movement by the males prior to encountering an above threshold concentration of pheromone, these determinations should not be used as a basis for estimating the absolute maximum distance of communication; such estimates may be greatly exaggerated and unreliable (Collins and Potts 1932; Dethier 1957; Shorey and Gaston 1967; Shorey et al. 1968; Shorey 1970; Sower et al. 1971).

5.5. *An integrated system*

The above information can be integrated to establish a proposed system for the behavior of a hypothetical flying insect in response to a pheromone (fig. 5.3). When the insect perceives an above threshold concentration of pheromone it may either be resting on a substrate or flying. If the individual is stationary, it is stimulated to initiate flight. Once airborne, the insect steers its body upwind (if anemotaxis is used) and flies in the general direction of the source. If the insect is many meters downwind and the active space is several meters wide and contains a low concentration of molecules, the insect steers more or less in a straight line, turning only when it is in the vicinity of the boundaries of the active space. As the insect flies nearer to the source, the concentration increases and the active space becomes narrower. The angle at which each turn is executed is decreased and a zigzag flight pattern results. The turning response, which results in the zigzag pattern, is possibly accomplished in the following manner. As the insect flies across the chemical trail, toward the boundary of the active space, it perceives a decrease in either the chemical concentration or number of filaments; it is then stimulated to turn back toward the center of the trail. The direction in which it turns may be regulated by: 1) chemotactic mechanisms; 2) an anemotactic response; 3) detection of a concentration gradient of odor molecules or odor-filament pulses over time; 4) a preprogrammed turning response in which right turns are alternated with left turns; or 5) a combination of these factors. As the insect progresses along the length of the trail there

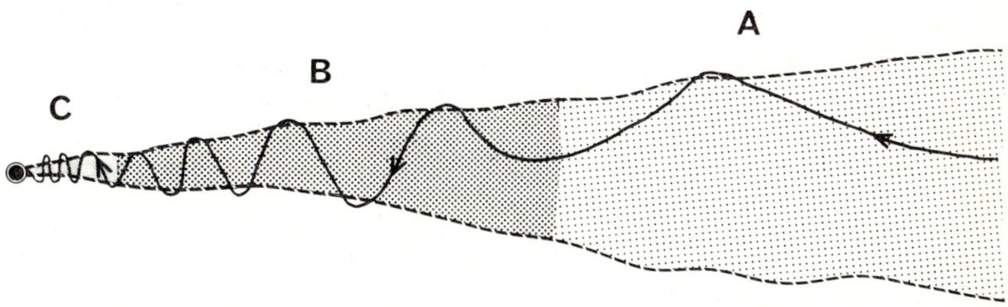

Fig. 5.3. Proposed flight path of a hypothetical insect flying in a schematic representation of an aerial trail of pheromone. A) area of low concentration and extremely wide active space relative to size of insect: anemotaxis or possibly other mechanisms involved for determining polarity of trail; relatively straight flight path; high flight speed. B) area of medium concentration and narrow active space relative to size of insect: anemotaxis, following of elongate gradient, or other mechanisms involved for determining polarity of trail; determination of lateral boundaries of trail by zigzag flight pattern; decrease in flight speed. C) area of high pheromone concentration and extremely narrow active space relative to size of insect: activation of visual orientation; arrestment of flight and landing.

is a decrease in 1) its flight speed; 2) the angle of each turn; and 3) the lateral amplitude of the zigzag pattern. When the insect perceives a high concentration of odor (occurring in the vicinity of the emitting insect) it is stimulated to arrest its forward progress and either alight or visually search for the emitting insect or for another appropriate object.

This hypothetical integrated system is based on bits and pieces of information gathered from observations of many different species of insects. It is not our intent to infer that only one mechanism is used by a species under all conditions. Even though it has been demonstrated that a particular species can orient along an odor trail without using anemotaxis, it would be a fallacy to assert that that species does not use anemotaxis under certain environmental conditions. On the contrary, many insects may have a wide potential repertoire of orientation mechanisms. The mechanisms (singly or in combination) are likely to have evolved in a way that allows them to be varied according to the sensory input arising from the many different internal and external stimuli perceived.

Knowledge of how insects use olfactory orientation mechanisms is still rudimentary. Still other mechanisms have, undoubtedly, yet to be uncovered. The way in which the mechanisms integrate into the complex scheme of orientation for any one species is strictly hypothetical at this time. Many more questions need to be answered before we can accumulate enough information to understand just one integrated system for guidance of an insect to its pheromone-releasing mate.

References

Adams, P. A. (1969) How moths keep warm. Discovery 4, 83–88.

Bartell, R. J. and L. A. Lawrence (1973) Reduction in responsiveness of males of *Epiphyas postvittana* (Lepidoptera) to sex pheromone following previous brief pheromonal exposure. J. Insect Physiol. 19, 845–855.

Bennett, R. B. and J. H. Borden (1971) Flight arrestment of tethered *Dendroctonus pseudotsugae* and *Trypodendron lineatum* (Coleoptera: Scolytidae) in response to olfactory stimuli. Ann. Entomol. Soc. Am. 64, 1273–1286.

Boeckh, J., K.-E. Kaissling and D. Schneider (1965) Insect olfactory receptors. Cold Spring Harbor Symp. Quant. Biol. 30, 263–280.

Borden, J. H. and R. B. Bennett (1969) A continuously recording flight mill for investigating the effect of volatile substances on the flight of tethered insects. J. Econ. Entomol. 62, 782–785.

Bossert, W. H. and E. O. Wilson (1963) The analysis of olfactory communication among animals. J. Theoret. Biol. 5, 443–469.

Butler, C. G. (1970) Chemical communication in insects: behavioral and ecological aspects. *In*: Advances in Chemoreception, vol. I: Communication by Chemical Signals; eds.: J. Johnston, Jr., D. G. Moulton and A. Turk (Appleton-Century-Crofts, New York) pp. 35–78.

Butler, C. G. and E. M. Fairey (1964) Pheromones of the honey bee: biological studies of the mandibular gland secretion of the queen. J. Apicult. Res. 3, 65–76.

Camhi, J. M. (1969a) Locust wind receptors. I. Transduced mechanics and sensory response. J. Exptl. Biol. 50, 335–348.

Camhi, J. M. (1969b) Locust wind receptors. II. Interneurons in the cervical connective. J. Exptl. Biol. 50, 349–362.

Camhi, J. M. (1970) Yaw-correcting postural changes in locusts. J. Exptl. Biol. 52, 519–531.

Carthy, J. D. (1951) The orientation of two allied species of British ants. II. Odour trail laying and following in *Acanthomyops* (*Lasius*) *fuliginosus*. Behaviour 3, 304–318.

Casida, J. E., H. C. Coppel and T. W. Watanabe (1963) Purification and potency of the sex attractant from the introduced pine sawfly, *Diprion similis*. J. Econ. Entomol. 56, 18–24.

Cole, L. R. (1970) Observations on the finding of mates by male *Phaeogenes invisor* and *Apanteles medicaginis* (Hymenoptera: Ichneumonoidae). Anim. Behav. 18, 184–189.

Collins, C. W. and S. F. Potts (1932) Attractants for the flying gypsy moth as an aid in locating new infestations. U. S. Dept. Agric. Tech. Bull. 336, 1–43.

Dahm, K. H., I. Richter, D. Meyer and H. Röller (1971) The sex attractant of the Indian-meal moth *Plodia interpunctella* (Hübner). Life Sci. Part II, 10, 531–539.

Danzer, A. (1956) Die Duftorientierung von *Geotrupes silvaticus* im Natürlichen Biotop. Z. Vergl. Physiol. 39, 76–83.

Daykin, P. N., F. E. Kellogg and R. Wright (1965) Host-finding and repulsion of *Aedes aegypti* Can. Entomol. 97, 239–263.

Dethier, V. G. (1947) The role of the antennae in the orientation of carrion beetles to odors. J. New York Entomol. Soc. 55, 285–293.

Dethier, V. G. (1957) Chemoreception and the behavior of insects, *In*: Survey of Biological Literature; ed.: B. Glass (Academic Press, Inc., New York) pp. 149–183.

Doane, C. C. (1968) Aspects of mating behavior of the gypsy moth. Ann. Entomol. Soc. Am. 61, 768–773.

Erulkar, S. D. (1972) Comparative aspects of spatial localization of sound. Physiol. Rev. 52, 237–360.

Farkas, S. R. and H. H. Shorey (1972) Chemical trail-following by flying insects: a mechanism for orientation to a distant odor source. Science 178, 67–68.

Farkas, S. R., H. H. Shorey and L. K. Gaston (1974) Sex pheromones of Lepidoptera. XLV. Influence of pheromone concentration, and visual cues on aerial odor trail following by males of *Pectinophora gossypiella*. Ann. Entomol. Soc. Am. (submitted for publication).

Fraenkel, G. S. and D. L. Gunn (1961) The Orientation of Animals. (Dover Publications, Inc., New York, N. Y.) 376 pp.

Fuchs, N. A. (1964) The Mechanics of Aerosols. (The Macmillan Company, New York, N. Y.) 408 pp.

Gara, R. I. (1963) Studies on the flight behavior of *Ips confusus* (LeC.) (Coleoptera: Scolytidae) in response to attractive material. Contrib. Boyce Thompson Inst. 22, 51–66.

Hangartner, W. (1967) Spezifität und Inaktivierung des Spurpheromons von *Lasius fuliginosus* Latr. und Orientierung der Arbeiterinnen im Duftfeld. Z. Vergl. Physiol. 57, 103–136.

Hangartner, W. (1969) Trail laying in the subterranean ant, *Acanthomyops interfectus*. J. Insect Physiol. 15, 1–4.

Heath, J. E. and P. A. Adams (1967) Regulation of heat production by large moths. J. Exptl. Biol. 47, 21–33.

Holbrook, R., M. Beroza and E. Burgess (1960) Gypsy moth (*Porthetria dispar*) detection with the natural female sex lure. J. Econ. Entomol. 53, 751–756.

Janders, R. (1963) Insect orientation. Ann. Rev. Entomol. 8, 95–114.

Kaae, R. S. and H. H. Shorey (1972) Sex pheromones of noctuid moths. XXVII. Influence of wind velocity on sex pheromone releasing behavior of *Trichoplusia ni* females. Ann. Entomol. Soc. Am. 65, 436–440.

Kaissling, K.-E. and E. Priesner (1970) The olfactory threshold of the silk moth. Naturwissenschaften 57, 23–28.

Kellogg, F. E., D. E. Frizel and R. H. Wright (1962) The olfactory guidance of flying insects. IV. *Drosophila*. Can. Entomol. 94, 884–888.

Kennedy, J. S. (1939) The visual responses of flying mosquitoes. Proc. Zool. Soc. London, Ser. A 109, 221–242.

Macnab, R. M. and D. E. Koshland, Jr. (1972) The gradient-sensing mechanism in bacterial chemotaxis. Proc. Natl. Acad. Sci. 69, 2509–2512.

Martin, H. (1965) Osmotropotaxis in the honey bee. Nature (London) 208, 59–63.

Osborne, G. O. and C. P. Hoyt (1970) Phenolic resins as chemical attractants for males of the grass grub beetle, *Costelytra zealandica* (Coleoptera: Scarabaeidae). Ann. Entomol. Soc. Am. 63, 1145–1147.

Perttunen, V., E. Kangas and H. Oksanen (1968) The mechanism by which *Blastophagus piniperda* L. (Col., Scolytidae) reacts to the odour of an attractant fraction isolated from pine phloem. Ann. Entomol. Fenn. 34, 205–222.

Rau, P. and N. Rau (1929) The sex attraction and rhythmic periodicity in giant saturniid moths. Trans. Acad. Sci. St. Louis 26, 83–221.

Rudinsky, J. A. and G. E. Daterman (1964) Field studies on flight patterns and olfactory responses of ambrosia beetles in Douglas-fir forests of western Oregon. Can. Entomol. 96, 1339–1352.

Shorey, H. H. (1970) Sex pheromones of Lepidoptera, *In*: Control of Insect Behavior by Natural Products; eds.: D. L. Wood, R. M. Silverstein and M. Nakajima (Academic Press, New York, N. Y.) pp. 244–284.

Shorey, H. H. (1973) Behavioral responses to insect pheromones, Ann. Rev. Entomol. 18, 349–380.

Shorey, H. H. and S. R. Farkas (1973) Terrestrial odor-trail following by pheromone-stimulated male moths. Ann. Entomol. Soc. Amer. (in press).

Shorey, H. H. and L. K. Gaston (1964) Sex pheromones of noctuid moths. III. Inhibition of male responses to the sex pheromone in *Trichoplusia ni* (Lepidoptera: Noctuidae). Ann. Entomol. Soc. Am. 57, 775–779.

Shorey, H. H. and L. K. Gaston (1967) Pheromones. *In*: Pest Control; eds.: W. W. Kilgore and R. L. Doutt (Academic Press, New York) pp. 241–265.

Shorey, H. H. and L. K. Gaston (1970) Sex pheromones of noctuid moths. XX. Short-range visual orientation by pheromone-stimulated males of *Trichoplusia ni*. Ann. Entomol. Soc. Am. 63, 829–832.

Shorey, H. H., L. K. Gaston and R. N. Jefferson (1968) Insect sex pheromones. *In*: Advances in Pest Control Research, Vol. 8; ed.: R. L. Metcalf (Interscience, New York) pp. 57–126.

Shorey, H. H., L. K. Gaston and C. A. Saario (1967) Sex pheromones of noctuid moths. XIV. Feasibility of behavioral control by disrupting pheromone communication in cabbage loopers. J. Econ. Entomol. 60, 1541–1545.

Soo Hoo, C. F. and R. J. Roberts (1965) Sex attraction in *Rhopaea* (Coleoptera: Scarabaeidae). Nature (London) 205, 724–725.

Sower, L. L., L. K. Gaston and H. H. Shorey (1971) Sex pheromones of noctuid moths. XXVI. Female release rate, male response threshold, and communication distance for *Trichoplusia ni*. Ann. Entomol. Soc. Am. 64, 1448–1456.

Sower, L. L., R. S. Kaae and H. H. Shorey (1973) Sex pheromones of Lepidoptera. XLI. Factors limiting potential distance of sex pheromone communication in *Trichoplusia ni*. Ann. Entomol. Soc. Am. 66, 1121–1122.

Steiner, G. (1953) Zür Duftorientierung fliegender Insekten. Naturwissenschaften 40, 514–515.

Teale, E. W. (1961) The Insect World of J. Henri Fabre. (Dodd, Mead and Co., New York) 333 pp.

Traynier, R. M. M. (1968) Sex attraction in the Mediterranean flour moth, *Anagasta kühniella*: location of the female by the male. Can. Entomol. 100, 5–10.

Vité, J. P. and G. B. Pitman (1967) Concepts in research on bark beetle attraction and manipulation. Proc. XIV Intern. Union Forest Res. Organ. Section 24, pp. 683–701.

Weis-Fogh, T. (1948) An aerodynamic sense organ in locusts. Int. Cong. Entomol. 8, 584–588.

Weis-Fogh, T. (1949) An aerodynamic sense organ stimulating and regulating flight in locusts. Nature (London) 164, 873–874.

Wensler, R. (1972) The effect of odors on the behavior of adult *Aedes aegypti* and some factors limiting responsiveness. Can. J. Zool. 50, 415–420.

Wilson, E. O. (1962) Chemical communication among workers of the fire ant *Solenopsis saevissima* (Fr. Smith), 1. The organization of massforaging. Anim. Behav. 10, 134–147.

Wilson, E. O. (1963) The social biology of ants. Ann. Rev. Entomol. 8, 345–368.

Wilson, E. O. (1971) The Insect Societies. (The Belknap Press of Harvard University Press, Cambridge, Mass.) 548 pp.

Wilson, E. O. and W. H. Bossert (1963) Chemical communication among animals. *In*: Recent Progress in Hormone Research, vol. XIX. Proceedings of the 1962 Laurentian Hormone Conference; ed.: G. Pincus (Academic Press, New York) pp. 673–716.

Wright, R. H. (1958) The olfaction guidance of flying insects. Can. Entomol. 90, 81–89.

Wright, R. H. (1962) The attraction and repulsion of mosquitoes. World Rev. Pest Control 1, 2–12.

Wright, R. H. (1964) The Science of Smell. (George Allen and Unwin Ltd., London) 164 pp.

CHAPTER 6

Sex pheromones in the reproductive isolation of lepidopterous species

Wendell L. ROELOFS and Ring T. CARDÉ

6.1. Introduction

Throughout millions of metamorphoses, evolutionary processes in the Lepidoptera have resulted in many differences in morphology, biology and behavior; not the least subtle of these changes being in the chemical communication systems developed by the various species. Most moth species utilize chemical emanations as a primary stimulus in their specialized mating behavior and the evidence is increasing that in many instances these specialized olfactory cues can also serve as important behavioral barriers to interspecific matings. Although premating mechanisms that operate at close range, such as visual and tactile stimuli, and recognition and stimulatory pheromones (for example, those from abdominal hair pencils), could help effect reproductive isolation, the main premating mechanisms appear to involve circadian and seasonal cycles, habitat preference, geographical distribution and the pheromonal systems. Unique pheromonal systems would be of increased importance in those sympatric species for which the other isolating mechanisms are not very effective.

Situations for which some type of ecobiotic isolation is required are particularly evident in the lepidopterous family Tortricidae. The phylogenetic relationships evident in the Tortricidae have been discussed quite thoroughly by Powell (1964) and there is also an excellent account of the bionomics of apple-feeding tortricids (Chapman 1973). It is thought that the two major subfamilies, Olethreutinae and Tortricinae, evolved from a single olethreutoid stock, which deposited eggs singly, was a wood borer and had a well-defined annual life cycle. The Tortricinae represent an early divergence from this stock and became external feeders. Some tortricines later developed the habit of depositing eggs in overlapping groups or masses, a habit which resulted in different dispersal activities of the newly hatched larvae and a widening of host plant range for species in the subfamily Tortricinae. The olethreutines did not evolve along a single line and so some continue to be borers, utilizing the stems, seeds and fruits of their hosts, whereas others are external feeders or semi-internal feeders. The olethreutines do continue the ancestral habit of laying their eggs singly, and have not developed the wide host range found among the Tortricinae.

Throughout the evolutionary processes described above, reproductive separation of the various populations was effected by many factors, but we presently find many tortricid species with broadly overlapping mating cycles co-occurring in nature (Roelofs and Feng 1968; Comeau and Roelofs 1973). Chemical specificity in stimulating premating behavior could, therefore, be particularly important for reducing cross-attractancy. Investigations to date have revealed interesting pheromone structural relationships between and within the two tortricid subfamilies (table 6.1). The accumulated evidence shows that compounds attractive to olethreutine species are usually unsaturated 12-carbon chain acetates, aldehydes or alcohols, whereas attractants for tortricine species are generally found to be 14-carbon chain compounds with unsaturation in the 11-position. Exceptions to this trend are found, however, with *Argyrotaenia quadrifasciana* (Fernald) (Tortricinae), which is attracted to *cis*-10-dodecenyl acetate, and with the *Zeiraphera diniana* (Guenée) (Olethreutinae) attractant, *trans*-11-tetradecenyl acetate.

6.2. *Reproductive isolation with one compound systems*

It is obvious that many species could achieve reproductive isolation because they employ different pheromone compounds. In the Tortricidae (table 6.1), structural variation, as known to date, is obtained by changing the functional moiety (acetate, alcohol or aldehyde), the double-bond position (7 to 11), configuration (*cis* or *trans*), or number (one or two sites of unsaturation), or carbon-chain length (12 or 14 carbons). Most of the known lepidopterous attractants in other families are similar compounds (Roelofs and Comeau 1971b), with the exception of: 1) a hydrocarbon, 2-methylheptadecane, in some tiger moth species (Roelofs and Cardé 1971); 2) an epoxy-hydrocarbon, *cis*-7,8-epoxy-2-methyloctadecane for the gypsy moth, *Porthetria dispar* (L.) (Bierl et al. 1970); and 3) a branched ester, *cis*-dec-5-en-1-yl 3-methylbutanoate for the pine emperor moth, *Nudaurelia cytherea* (F.) (Henderson and Warren 1972). Although recent data suggest that many species actually use a main attractant and small percentages of secondary components in their natural pheromonal system, consideration of just the main attractant indicates an important role for pheromones in the reproductive isolation of some species. This was first reported (Roelofs and Comeau 1969) for two morphologically similar gelechiid species, *Bryotropha similis* (Stainton) and *B.* sp. They exhibit identical four-dot wing patterns, but the former species appears grayish and the latter more yellowish. They co-occur in nature and have broadly overlapping diel mating cycles, but each is attracted to a different geometrical isomer of *cis*- and *trans*-9-tetradecenyl acetates. A mixture of the two isomers attracts males of neither species, suggesting that females of one species would actually inhibit attraction of males of the other species, thus effecting complete reproductive isolation.

Another case was found for two sympatric New York populations of the noctuid *Amathes c-nigrum* (L.). The populations were previously considered conspecific, but they possess subtle differences in size, coloration, and morphology. The larger species, however, is attracted to *cis*-7-tetradecenyl acetate and the smaller species to the geometrical isomer, *trans*-7-tetradecenyl acetate, allowing the co-occurring populations to be reproductively isolated in nature (Roelofs and Comeau 1970).

In the Tortricidae, two closely-related apple-feeding Olethreutinae species, *Grapholitha prunivora* (Walsh) and *G. packardi* Zeller, with essentially the same life cycle would not be cross-attracted because the former is lured to *cis*-8-dodecenyl acetate and the latter to *trans*-8-dodecenyl acetate. In the genus *Choristoneura*, a complex of closely-related species in North America (Freeman 1967) has been the subject of an interesting sex pheromone specificity study (Sanders 1971a, 1971b). Reclassification of the species *C. fumiferana* (Clemens) (Freeman 1953, 1967) re-

TABLE 6.1

Sex attractants in the Tortricidae.

Olethreutinae species	Attractants (ratio of components) (references)
Epinotia zandana (Kearfott)	c7–12:Ac (1,2)
Epinotia atistriga Clarke	c7–12:Ac (1,2)
Cryptophlebia leucotreta (Meyrick)	t7–12:Ac (3,4)
Aphania infida (Heinrich)	c8–12:Ac (1,2)
Epiblema desertana (Zeller)	c8–12:Ac (1,2)
Grapholitha funebrana (Treitschke)	c8–12:Ac (2,5)
Grapholitha molesta	c8–12:Ac (6) + 12:OH(1:4) (7)
Grapholitha prunivora	c8–12:Ac (2,6)
Laspeyresia sp.	c8–12:Ac (1,2)
Pseudexentera maracana (Kearfott)	c8–12:Ac (1,2)
Epiblema scudderiana (Clemens)	c8–12:OH (1,2)
Ecdytolopha insiticiana (Zeller)	t8–12:Ac (1,2)
Grapholitha packardi	t8–12:Ac (2,6)
Hedia chionosema (Zeller)	t8–12:Ac + t8–12:OH (2:1) (1,2)
Laspeyresia pomonella (L.)	t8, t10–12:OH (8)
Thiodia sp.	t8, t10–12:OH (2,23)
Episimus argutanus (Clemens)	c9–12:Ac (1,2)
Paralobesia viteana	c9–12:Ac (9)
Dichrorampha sp.	t9–12:Ac or t9–12:OH (1,2)
Thiodia alterana Heinrich	t10–12:Ac (2,23)
Zeiraphera diniana	t11–14:Ac (10)

Table 6.1 (continued)

Tortricinae species	
Argyrotaenia quadrifasciana	*c*10–12:Ac (2,21)
Choristoneura rosaceana	*c*11–14:Ac (11)
Argyrotaenia velutinana	*c*11–14:Ac (12) + 12:Ac (2:3) (13)
Adoxophyes orana	*c*9–14:Ac + *c*11–14:Ac (9:1) (14)
Adoxophyes fasciata (Walsingham)	*c*9–14:Ac + *c*11–14:Ac (4:1) (15)
Clepsis spectrana	*c*9–14:Ac + *c*11–14:Ac (1:3) (16)
Clepsis melaleucana	*c*11–14:Ac + *c*11–14:OH (1:1) (1,2)
Archips rosanus (L.)	*c*11–14:Ac + *c*11–14:OH (2:3) (17)
Choristoneura fractivittana	*c*11–14:OH (1,2)
Sparganothis niveana groteana (Fernald)	*c*11–14:OH (1,2)
Choristoneura viridis	*t*11–14:Ac (18)
Cnephasia sp.	*t*11–14:Ac (2,19)
Platynota stultana (Walsingham)	*t*11–14:Ac (4,20)
Sparganothis sulfureana (Clemens)	*t*11–14:Ac (1,2)
Sparganothis albicaudana (Busck)	*t*11–14:Ac (1,2)
Platynota idaeusalis	*t*11–14:OH + *t*11–14:Ac (1:1) (1,21)
Choristoneura fumiferana	*t*11–14:Ald (22)
Choristoneura biennis	*t*11–14:Ald (18)
Choristoneura occidentalis	*t*11–14:Ald (22)

(1) Roelofs and Comeau 1971b
(2) Found by field screening studies
(3) Read et al. 1968
(4) Field attractancy not reported
(5) Granges and Baggiolini 1971
(6) Roelofs et al. 1969
(7) Synergist found by field studies, Roelofs et al. 1973
(8) Roelofs et al. 1971b
(9) Roelofs et al. 1971c
(10) Roelofs et al. 1971a
(11) Roelofs and Tette 1970
(12) Roelofs and Arn 1968
(13) Synergist found by field studies, Roelofs and Comeau 1968
(14) Tamaki et al. 1971b; Meijer et al. 1972
(15) Tamaki et al. 1971a
(16) Minks et al. 1973
(17) Roelofs and Madsen, unpublished
(18) Sanders et al. 1973
(19) Klun and Robinson 1972
(20) Hill, Cardé and Roelofs, unpublished
(21) Comeau 1971
(22) Weatherston et al. 1971
(23) This paper. We thank Drs. R. Hodges, D. Davis (U.S.N.M., Washington) and J. Franclemont (Cornell) for the identifications.

sulted in four new species in the west and two species, *C. fumiferana*, eastern spruce budworm, and *C. pinus* Freeman, jack-pine budworm, in the east. The last two species are sympatric for part of their ranges (Freeman 1953; Stehr 1967). They will hybridize when confined in cages and produce fertile offspring. In the field the potential for hybridization is reduced by ecological and temporal isolation, but even when these barriers are ineffective, no hybrid matings occur (Smith 1954). Differences in the mating periodicity are not sufficient to prevent the possibility of hybridization, but there is evidence that the two species use different sex pheromone systems. The attractant for *C. fumiferana* was identified as *cis*-11-tetradecenal (Weatherston et al. 1971) and preliminary information indicates that the main attractant for *C. pinus* is not an aldehyde, but rather an acetate. Additionally, attractancy of the females is species-specific in the field and crude female extracts are species-specific in laboratory bioassays. Two of the western species, *C. biennis* Freeman and *C. occidentalis* Freeman, use the same aldehyde attractants as the eastern species, *C. fumiferana*, but hybridization is apparently reduced by ecological and temporal isolation. The other western species, *C. orea* Freeman, and *C. viridis* Freeman, appear to utilize the same or similar acetate chemical as the eastern species, *C. pinus*, although *C. viridis* is attracted to *trans*-11-tetradecenyl acetate alone, while *C. pinus* is not (Sanders et al. 1973).

6.2.1. Release rates

Although the use of different main attractants is the most obvious method of achieving reproductive isolation, many species apparently employ the same attractant system. In these cases rate of pheromone release from the female may be a species-specific cue. Particular pheromone concentrations may be required to elicit male attraction, close-range searching behavior and copulatory attempts. Hierarchies of behavioral responses (antennal movement, wing fluttering, anemotaxis, etc.) in which each successive step necessitates a specific concentration have been demonstrated in laboratory assays with several Lepidoptera (Schwinck 1955; Traynier 1968; Bartell and Shorey 1969). In the Tortricidae attraction response to synthetic pheromone often requires a specific release rate. The larch bud moth, *Zeiraphera diniana* was found to be attracted to very low concentrations of *trans*-11-tetradecenyl acetate (10^{-3} to 10^{-6} mg per lure as compared to 10 mg per lure for redbanded leafroller attractancy); high release rates were completely unattractive (Roelofs et al. 1971a). In a similar case, the grape berry moth, *Paralobesia viteana* (Clemens) was best lured to 10^{-1} to 10^{-2} mg of attractant per dispenser while 1 and 10^{-3} mg treatments were largely ineffective (Roelofs et al. 1974).

In Iowa, Klun and Robinson (1972) have reported another apparent example of male discrimination among various release rates. *Cis*-11-tetradecenyl acetate was found to be most attractive to males of the obliquebanded leafroller, *Choristoneura rosaceana* (Harris), at high release rates, such as 10^{-1} mg per lure, whereas the pyralid European corn borer, *Ostrinia nubilalis* (Hübner), was most attracted to dispensers containing about 10^{-3} mg of this chemical and not attracted at all to the high release rates, such as one mg.

Kaae et al. (1973a) demonstrated the importance of pheromone concentration on a reproductive isolating mechanism between two closely allied noctuids, *Trichoplusia ni* (Hübner) (the cabbage looper) and *Autographa californica* (Speyer) (the alfalfa looper), both of which overlap widely in geographical distributions, seasonal cycles and diel mating rhythms. These species apparently use the same male attractant, *cis*-7-dodecenyl acetate (*c*7-12 : Ac). This chemical was identified as a sex pheromone for *Trichoplusia ni* (Berger 1966) and based on gas chromatography, bioassays and electroantennogram responses, *Autographa californica* also appears to employ the same pheromone (Kaae et al. 1973a). Observations in a heterogeneous population of both species showed that *Trichoplusia ni* males tended to be attracted to release rates of *c*7-12 : Ac that were 10 to 100 times greater than the most attractive release rates for *Autographa californica* (see fig. 6.1). These high release rates were essentially unattractive to *A. californica* males. Such findings indicate that one important isolating mechanism is differing rates of pheromone release from the female. Field trapping tests utilizing virgin females support this hypothesis: *Trichoplusia ni* females attract only conspecific males, whereas *Autographa californica* females lure males of both species, but are less attractive to *Trichoplusia ni* males than are conspecific females. Presumably the *Autographa californica* females would not release sufficient *c*7-12 : Ac to elicit copulatory attempts from *Trichoplusia ni* males. Although the discriminatory powers of the males to detect different release rates can play a role in the isolation of species, it is possible that other differences exist in their use of pheromones to help reduce fruitless long-

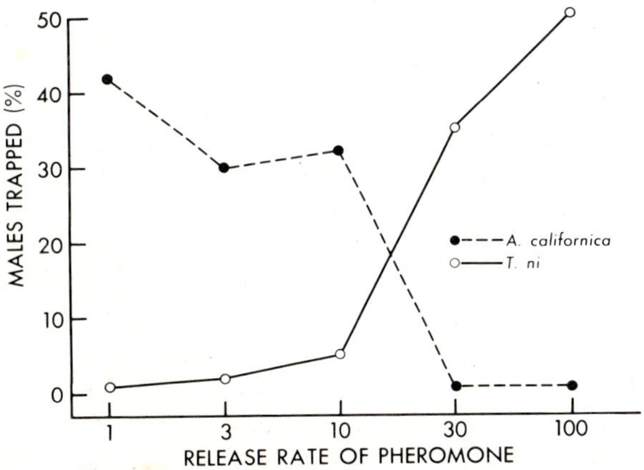

Fig. 6.1. Male catches of two noctuid species with various relative release rates of *c*7-12 : Ac (Kaae et al. 1973a) (Copyright 1973; American Association for the Advancement of Science).

distance orientation behavior by males. It would be inefficient for males responding to low release rates to orient to fast pheromone-releasing females of another species, only to reach a critical concentration, which elicits searching behavior for a phantom female.

6.2.2. *Circadian rhythms*

Differing circadian mating rhythms can also be important for the partitioning of fully sympatric Lepidoptera that use the same chemical communication system. In most Lepidoptera, the female secretes pheromone (calls) and is receptive to mating only during a relatively brief period during the day or night. As might be expected, the periodicity of male response is roughly coincident with the rhythm of female attractiveness. Long before the first sex attractant structure was elucidated, the potential importance of mating periodicity as a reproductive isolating mechanism was recognized. In a now classic series of experiments with saturniids, Rau and Rau (1929) demonstrated that silkworm moths could possess vastly different mating rhythms: for example, *Callosamia promethea* (Drury), was noted to attract and mate from 3 p.m. to 7 p.m. compared to 9 p.m. to 5 a.m. for *Samia cynthia* (Drury).

Indeed it now appears that such variation in mating periodicity isolates certain sympatric saturniids. *C. promethea, C. angulifera* (Walker) and *C. securifera* (Maassen) are all sympatric in South Carolina, where recent studies by Dominick and Edwards (Ferguson 1971–2) have shown that *C. securifera* commenced calling about 10 a.m. while males ceased flying between 3 and 4 p.m. At about this time, females of the second diurnal species, *C. promethea*, initiated calling and male response, which continued until sunset. Finally, *C. angulifera* has an entirely nocturnal cycle, reported to occur between dusk and midnight (Collins and Weast 1961; Ferguson 1971–2). At least two of the species, *C. promethea* and *angulifera*, are known to cross-attract (Collins and Weast 1961).

Exclusive mating cycles also appear to function in maintaining separation of two closely related lymantriids, the gypsy moth (*Porthetria dispar*) and the nun moth (*Lymantria monacha* (L.)), both of which co-occur widely from Europe to Japan. The gypsy moth sex attractant pheromone is *cis*-7,8-epoxy-2-methyloctadecane (Bierl et al. 1970) and the nun moth has recently been shown to be lured to this chemical (Schönherr 1972). In Europe the nun moth's mating periodicity occurs from about 6 p.m. until 1 a.m. (Ambros 1940), while the gypsy moth's cycle is apparently diurnal (Jacentovský 1932, 1934). The gypsy moth was introduced into North America in New England in 1868 or 1869 and various investigations there on its mating periodicity showed this interval to be 9 a.m. to 3 or 4 p.m. in 1896 (Forbush and Fernald), 9 a.m. to 6 p.m. in 1932 (Collins and Potts) and 9 a.m. to 8 p.m. in 1974 (Cardé et al.). Thus, in North America the gypsy moth appears to have evolved a lengthened mating periodicity in response to lessened communication interference in the absence of the nun moth.

Although the evolution of distinct mating rhythms among closely-related species suggests that these differences constitute important isolating mechanisms, such variations may be only of minor importance. Smith (1954) thought that differences in mating periodicity were a primary barrier to natural hybridization of sympatric populations of the tortricid budworms *Choristoneura fumiferana* and *pinus*, but it is now known that these species are isolated by different chemical communication systems (Sanders 1971b). In the same way, disparate diel mating periodicity seems to isolate certain sibling species of the arctiid *Holomelina aurantiaca* (Hübner) complex. All species in this group investigated to date produce 2-methylheptadecane and attraction to this pheromone has been demonstrated for five species: *H. aurantiaca, H. immaculata* (Reakirt), *H. rubicundaria* (Hübner), *H. lamae* (Freeman) and an undescribed species (Roelofs and Cardé 1971). In Nova Scotia *H. aurantiaca* and *H. lamae* fly within sight of each other in distinct but contiguous habitats (Ferguson 1953) and exclusive female calling periodicity suggests that mechanism would effectively partition these species. Females of *H. lamae* call at midday, whereas females of *H. aurantiaca* call in the early evening. In the field *H. lamae* males are attracted to 2-methylheptadecane at midday, but *H. aurantiaca* males exhibit a rather indiscriminate response as they are lured to the synthetic from 10 a.m. until 10 p.m. Apparently isolation must be achieved through additional chemical specificity. Males of *H. aurantiaca* are attracted to 2-methylheptadecane at a variety of release rates (10 to 10^{-3} mg per lure), but *H. lamae* males are usually lured only to within a meter or so of the pheromone source, indicating that a secondary component is needed for complete attraction.

This rather unspecific diel response of *H. aurantiaca* males further suggests that mating periodicity would be an unlikely device for preventing hybridization of mixed populations of *H. aurantiaca* and *H. immaculata*, two species which have broadly overlapping ranges in the eastern United States. In addition, this latter species exhibits a temperature modulation of its circadian mating rhythm such that on warm days and nights attraction is initiated at dusk and extends for several hours. On cool days and nights this rhythm is shifted so that attraction occurs during the two hours preceeding sunset (Cardé 1971). Similar temperature shifts have recently been reported for several tortricids (Comeau 1971; Sanders and Lucuik 1972b) and a noctuid (Sower et al. 1971) and indeed this phenomenon may be general among the Lepidoptera.

6.3. Reproductive isolation with multiple compound systems

Structural variations are evident for tortricid attractants, as mentioned above, but they are quite limited, especially for the Tortricinae. In the Lepidoptera, *cis*-11-tetradecenyl acetate (*c*11-14 : Ac) appears to be quite common as an attractant. However, it was discovered that certain chemicals could be evaporated simultaneously with an attractant either to increase (synergize) or decrease (inhibit) male catches (Roelofs and Comeau 1968). With two tortricid species, the redbanded leafroller, *Argyrotaenia velutinana* (Walker), and the obliquebanded leafroller, *Choristoneura rosaceana*, which both use *c*11-14 : Ac as an attractant, the addition of dodecyl acetate greatly increases catches of redbanded males and decreases catches of obliquebanded males (fig. 6.2) (Roelofs and Comeau 1971a). Other preliminary data indicate the use of other secondary chemicals for attractancy of *Argyrotaenia velutinana*. Each secondary chemical could increase the specificity of the pheromone system by synergizing the attractant for the conspecific males and/or reducing attractancy for males of co-occurring species utilizing the same main attractant.

Males of another tortricid species, *Clepsis melaleucana* (Walker), were attracted only when *cis*-11-tetradecen-1-ol (*c*11-14 : OH) was used in conjunction with *c*11-14 : Ac, and not by either compound alone (Roelofs and Comeau 1971b). This 1 : 1 mixture of *c*11-14 : Ac and *c*11-14 : OH is not attractive to redbanded and obliquebanded leafroller males, suggesting that these males would not be attracted to *C. melaleucana* females, and conversely that the *C. melaleucana* males would not be attracted to the leafroller females, which apparently release predominantly *c*11-14 : Ac.

The alcohol, *c*11-14 : OH, is also attractive to males of the tortricid *Choristoneura fractivittana* (Clemens), but these males are not attracted to traps containing both *c*11-14 : OH and *c*11-14 : Ac, and so presumably they would not be attracted to *Clepsis melaleucana* females. In the same way *C. melaleucana* males would not search for *Choristoneura fractivittana* females, which emit predominantly only one of the required chemicals for attraction of *Clepsis melaleucana* males.

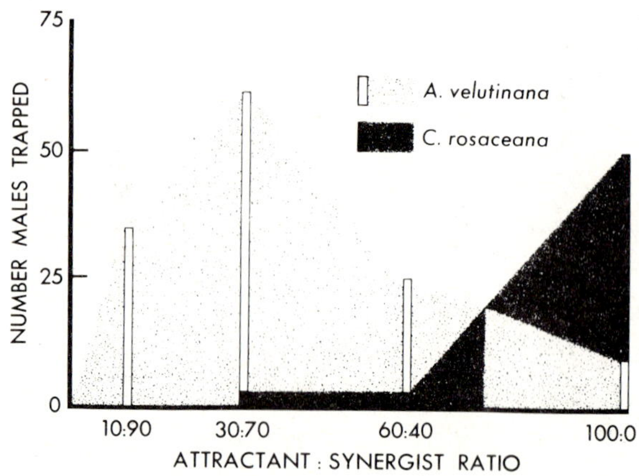

Fig. 6.2. Male catches of two tortricid species with various *c*11-14 : Ac to 12 : Ac ratios (Roelofs and Comeau 1971a).

The synthetic mixtures found by field tests to be the best attractants for some species may not always be the natural pheromone mixture, but they must generally bear close resemblance to it. In the case of *Platynota idaeusalis* (Walker), the tufted apple bud moth, field tests showed that males were attracted to *trans*-11-tetradecen-1-ol (*t*11-14 : OH) (Roelofs and Comeau 1971b), but the addition of the corresponding acetate, *t*11-14 : Ac, greatly increased attractancy (Comeau 1971). Later, analysis of female gland extracts proved that both compounds are indeed produced by the females (Hill et al. 1974).

The evidence is increasing in support of Wright's (1964) prediction that most insects use more than one attractant chemical. Pressures from sympatric species, which utilize a common attractant, could contribute to the importance placed on secondary chemicals as a means of reducing communication interference. Continued selection could result in the evolution of a pheromone system in which the secondary chemical becomes the main component and the original attractant chemical is used as a minor chemical or not at all. An example of species possibly at different stages in this sort of model is that of *Adoxophyes orana* Fischer von Röslerstamm and *Clepsis spectrana* (Treitschke). Although these co-occurring

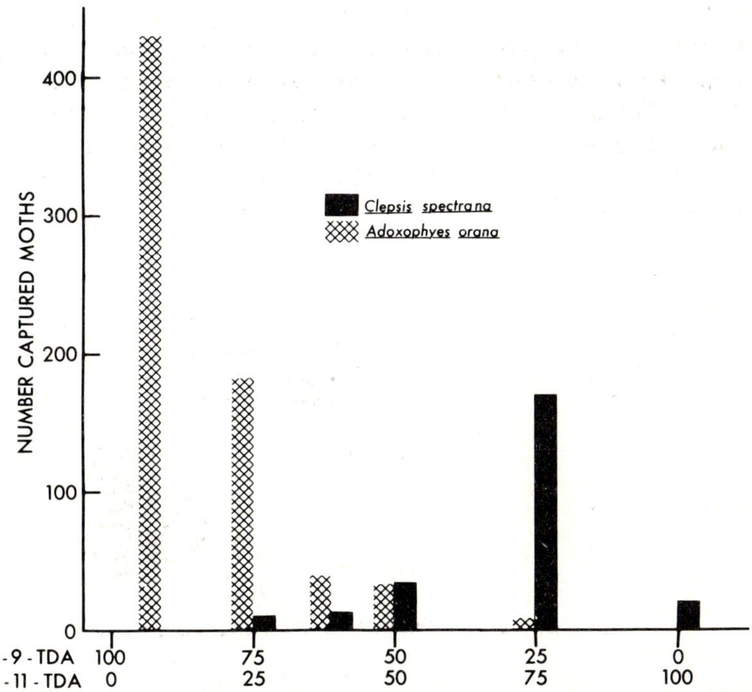

Fig. 6.3. Male catches of two tortricid species with various ratios of *c*9-14 : Ac and *c*11-14 : Ac (Minks et al. 1973).

species have similar diel mating cycles and utilize the same two chemicals for attractants, they are reproductively isolated by discriminating among different ratios of these chemicals (fig. 6.3) (Minks et al. 1973). *C. spectrana* males are attracted by *c*11-14 : Ac alone, but are attracted in much larger numbers when *c*9-14 : Ac is present in a 1 : 3 (*c*9 : *c*11) ratio. Although *c*9 is a synergist at low ratios, it becomes quite inhibitory at ratios above 1 : 1. Males of *Adoxophyes orana* are not attracted until *c*9 is present in high ratios, optimally 9 : 1 (*c*9 : *c*11). Males are not attracted, or even stimulated in laboratory bioassays, by *c*9 alone, so *c*11 is an obligatory secondary compound, which becomes inhibitory in the field when present in too high a ratio to *c*9. It is possible that both species evolved from ancestors which employed *c*11-14 : Ac. One species, then, has evolved a pheromone system with *c*9-14 : Ac as a secondary component and the other species has evolved to the point where *c*9-14 : Ac is no longer a secondary compound, but rather is the main component of the mixture.

It has become impossible to predict which chemicals are going to be inhibitory and which ones synergistic for any given species, although certain generalities can be given for potential synergists and inhibitors. According to the receptor model described by Roelofs and Comeau (1971a), hydrophobic, hydrophilic and electrostatic bonding of the attractant with a flexible membrane protein could cause the conformational change to trigger nerve impulse-producing mechanisms. Three main 'active sites' were described as possibly being important for attractancy. These included the terminal functional group, the area of unsaturation, and the terminal methyl group. Compounds most likely to modulate attractancy are those which interact with at least two of the active sites, for example: 1) geometrical isomers; 2) compounds of the same carbon chain length and position of unsaturation, but different functional groups, such as alcohol, acetate or aldehyde; 3) compounds with one of the mentioned functional groups, but of carbon-chain length terminating at the unsaturated active sites, for example, dodecyl or undecyl acetate interacting with receptors for the attractant *c*11-14 : Ac; 4) compounds with one of the mentioned functional groups, but of carbon-chain length similar to the attractant compound, for example, tetradecyl acetate interacting with receptors for the attractant *c*11-14 : Ac; and 5) compounds with nucleophilic atoms, such as N, O or S interacting with two active sites, for example 10-propoxydecan-1-yl acetate interacting with the receptors for *c*11-14: Ac. As mentioned, compounds fitting the above criteria can be potential synergists or inhibitors or both, depending on which ratio of chemical to attractant is used, even though two or more antennal receptors may be involved in multiple chemical perception. The addition of *t*11-14 : Ac to *c*11-14 : Ac (1 : 1) can procedure an attractive mixture for males of the smartweed borer, *Ostrinia obumbratalis* (Lederer) (Klun and Robinson 1972), but the presence of *t*11-14: Ac at this same ratio causes strong inhibition for males of the redbanded leafroller (Roelofs and Comeau 1971a) and European corn borer (Klun and Robinson 1971). Voerman and Minks (1973) tested the effect of 70 chemicals on the

Adoxophyes orana attractant mixture (*c*9- and *c*11-14 : Ac (9 : 1)). They found that in the series of alcohols and acetates of varying carbon chain lengths and an oxygen atom varying from positions 8 through 12, only 8-butoxyoctan-1-yl, 11-methoxy- and 11-ethoxyundecan-1-yl acetates were strongly inhibitory. In accordance with the model theory discussed above, inhibition was less pronounced 1) with 11-propoxyundecanyl acetate, which extends the chain length beyond that of the 14-carbon chain length of the attractants; and 2) with compounds containing the oxygen atom in positions other than the 9 or the 12. The inhibitory compounds mentioned, with an oxygen atom in position 9 or 12, could conceivably be interacting with receptors for the *c*9 and *c*11 unsaturated sites of the attractants (these sites involve carbons 9 and 10 and carbons 11 and 12, respectively, on the two attractants). It is interesting to find that 11-ethoxyundecanyl acetate is a strong inhibitor in this case, but is strongly synergistic for redbanded leafroller attraction (Roelofs and Comeau 1971a).

Dodecyl acetate synergizes the attractancy of *c*11-14 : Ac for redbanded leafroller, but it is an inhibitor for *Grapholitha molesta* (Busck)(Roelofs et al. 1973). Dodecyl alcohol, on the other hand, is synergistic to the *G. molesta* pheromone (*c*8-12 : Ac). A structurally similar pheromone (*c*7-12 : Ac) of the cabbage looper moth is inhibited by the corresponding alcohol, *c*7-12 : OH (Tumlinson et al. 1972b), whereas the spruce budworm pheromone, *c*11-14 : Ald, is inhibited by the corresponding acetate (Sanders et al. 1972).

A mixture of two related mono- and di-unsaturated compounds (*cis*-9-tetradecenyl acetate (*c*9-14 : Ac) and *cis*-9, *trans*-12-tetradecadienyl acetate (*c*9,*t*12-14: Ac) was identified from females of the southern army worm, *Spodoptera eridania* (Cramer) (Jacobson et al. 1970) and found to stimulate males in laboratory bioassays and attract them in simulated field conditions (Redfern et al. 1971). On the other hand, *c*9-14 : Ac strongly inhibits the activity of female extracts from three species of phycitids that utilize *c*9,*t*12-14 : Ac as an attractant (Brady 1969; see later in chapter).

The pheromone of the European pine shoot moth, *Rhyacionia buoliana* (Schiffermüller), is unidentified, but in field studies with sixteen 12-carbon chain acetates (Daterman et al. 1972; Lange and Hoffman 1972), only the *c*7, *c*8 and *c*9-12 : Ac effectively inhibited attractancy of live females, which suggests that these compounds bear close resemblance to the pheromone structure.

In some cases several receptor sites may be involved in the perception of synergists, inhibitors and attractants. Electrophysiological studies on the antenna of the male redbanded leafroller moth with whole antennal responses (Roelofs and Comeau 1971c), or with single cell recordings (O'Connell 1972), have not resolved the question of the number of receptor sites involved with the attractant, inhibitor and synergist. O'Connell (1972) was able to find one cell (cell-2) for which the inhibitor, *t*11-14 : Ac, elicited large excitatory responses and another cell (cell-1) for which it elicited small inhibitory responses. Both cells responded to the attractant, *c*11-14 : Ac, although the latter cell (cell-1) exhibited the greater increase in response frequency. The synergist, dodecyl acetate, did not stimulate either cell, but a mixture of synergist and attractant elicited a larger response from cell-1 than expected from a sum of individual responses. A mixture of inhibitor and attractant elicited a response less than that elicited by the attractant alone.

Since the behavioral effects can be explained, by considering only cell-1, or can be explained by considering both cells, the question of how many receptor sites are actually involved can not yet be answered. If several receptor sites are involved with pheromone perception in some species, then some natural secondary components could presumably differ radically from the main attractant structure. These would first have to be identified by an analysis of gland extract or female effluent before potential compounds could be field tested. It is important to know that all chemicals isolated from the pheromone glands do not necessarily help attractancy. For example, 2-methyl-*cis*-7-octadecane, indicated to be a precursor of the gypsy moth pheromone (*cis*-7,8-epoxy-2-methyloctadecane) (Bierl et al. 1970), was found to be very inhibitory to male attractancy (Cardé et al. 1973). Sanders and Lucuik (1972a) also found the presence of an inhibitory component in spruce budworm gland extracts. The function of an inhibitor in the gland is not known and these chemicals may not actually be released by the female.

Other recent reports suggest the presence of secondary chemicals. Berisford and Brady (1973) found evidence that two Olethreutinae species, *Rhyacionia frustrana* (Comstock), Nantucket pine tip moth, and *R. rigidana* (Fernald), pitch pine tip moth, may emit several components, some of which are inhibitory to males of the wrong species. The pheromone systems, therefore, appear to be an important mechanism in the reproductive isolation of these two species.

The chemical, *c*9,*t*12-14 : Ac, described above as one component of the southern armyworm pheromone mixture, has also been identified in five phycitid species (Indian meal moth, *Plodia interpunctella* (Hübner); Brady et al. 1971b; Dahm et al. 1971b Kuwahara et al. 1971b); Mediterranean flour moth, *Anagasta kühniella* (Zeller) (Brady et al. 1971a; Kuwahara et al. 1971a); Almond moth, *Cadra cautella* (Walker) (Brady et al. 1971b; Kuwahara et al. 1971b); Tobacco moth, *Ephestia elutella* (Hübner) (Brady and Nordlund 1971); and the Raisin moth, *Cadra figulilella* (Gregson) (Brady and Daley 1972) and one other noctuid species (Beet armyworm, *Spodoptera exigua* (Hübner) (Brady and Ganyard 1972)). Since several of the phycitid species have similar food preferences, broadly overlapping diel mating cycles and geographical distribution, it is not surprising to find evidence for multiple component pheromone systems in these moths. Secondary components have been indicated for *Ephestia elutella* (Brady and Nordlund 1971), *Cadra cautella* (Brady et al. 1971b), and *Plodia interpunctella* (Ganyard and Brady 1971).

In the subfamily Plusiinae (Noctuidae) at least 10 species have been reported to be attracted by *c*7-12 : Ac (Berger 1966; Roelofs and Comeau 1971b; Tumlinson et al. 1972a; Kaae et al. 1973b). Many different premating isolating mechanisms are involved, but there is evidence in one case that females of *Trichoplusia ni* emit a substance which may not be synergistic for its own males, but is inhibitory for males of *Pseudoplusia includens* (Walker) (Mitchell 1972). Both species respond to the same high release rates of *c*7-12 : Ac (Kaae et al. 1973b).

6.4. *Multiple components and sound*

Up to this point we have discussed a pheromone system with a female emitter and a male receiver. However, within the Lepidoptera, some moth species have the reverse interaction. Males of the greater waxmoth, *Galleria mellonella* (L.), release a pheromone with a musklike odor – identified to be undecanal (Röller et al. 1968) – from a pair of wing glands, which attracts females for mating. This same compound was found in lesser waxmoth, *Achroia grisella* (F.), males, but it failed to elicit behavioral responses with the females. Activity was obtained when another component of the male wing extract was identified (*c*11-18 : Ald) and added to undecanal (Dahm et al. 1971a). Although intense excitation was elicited by the mixture, there was no directed response of the females to the odor source until auditory cues of a small stirrer (simulating male wing vibration) were added (Dahm et al. 1971a). In this case, the pheromone system consists of the olfactory stimuli from a multiple component chemical mixture and auditory cues, which could presumably also be varied to help effect reproductive isolation.

6.5. *Variation of pheromone systems within 'species'*

Species are most probably on a continuum of ever-evolving pheromone blends as they respond to changes in their chemical environment that tend to reduce sensitivity and specificity. It would not be surprising, then, to find populations of a species in different geographical areas to be evolving differences in their pheromone blends, as shown among various bark beetles (Lanier et al. 1972). Continued allopatric development of different secondary components, ratios and release rates could gradually produce populations no longer able to communicate with each other for mating if found sympatrically in nature. A possible example of this may be found in the European corn borer, *Ostrinia nubilalis*. In Iowa, the main attractant chemical was identified as *c*11-14 : Ac (Klun and Brindley 1970; Klun and Robinson 1971). In New York, the main attractant chemical was found to be the geometrical isomer, *t*11-14 : Ac, from field trapping studies (Roelofs et al. 1972) and then by chemical identification from female pheromone gland extracts (Kochansky et al. 1974). Preliminary trapping experiments in various parts of Europe, where the various introductions to the United States probably originated, showed that neither the *cis* nor *trans* compound appears to be effective in attracting male corn borers. Differences in the pheromone systems of the introduced corn borers in Iowa and New York have evidently occurred to such an extent that if these populations were sympatric they would now be reproductively isolated by differing chemical communication systems. In this case, they would be classified as different species.

6.6. Conclusion

The complexities of describing species-specific pheromone blends has brought the challenge of pheromone identifications from the chemistry laboratory back to the field. Although chemical characterizations must still be continued to unveil the intriguing sex pheromones used by many other species, especially those in families for which no identification has as yet been made, the final duplication of any natural pheromone blend can only be accomplished by analysis of various ratios and release rates under field conditions. An exact reproduction of the pheromone input should enable man to attract males very efficiently and specifically. On the other hand, one must bear in mind that the long-term use of fairly exact blends could merely serve as an artificial pressure causing the insect to further modify its chemical communication system.

References

Ambros, W. (1940) Einige Beobachtungen und Untersuchungen an der Nonne im Jahre 1938, Zentralbl. Ges. Forstw., 66, 131–147 and 166–169.

Bartell, R. J. and H. H. Shorey (1969) Pheromone concentrations required to elicit successive steps in the mating sequence of males of the light-brown apple moth, *Epiphyas postvittana*. Ann. Entomol. Soc. Am. 62, 1206–1207.

Bierl, B. A., M. Beroza and C. W. Collier (1970) Potent sex attractant of the gypsy moth: its isolation, identification, and synthesis. Science 170, 87–89.

Berger, R. S. (1966) Isolation, identification, and synthesis of the sex attractant of the cabbage looper, *Trichoplusia ni*, Ann. Entomol. Soc. Am. 59, 767–771.

Berisford, C. W. and U. E. Brady (1973) Specificity and inhibition of attraction of male *Rhyacionia frustrana* and *R. rigidana* to their female sex pheromone. Nature (London) 241, 68–69.

Brady, U. E. (1969) Inhibition of the behavioral response of males of Indian-meal moths, *Plodia interpunctella*, and related species to female sex pheromones: exposure to sex pheromones of unrelated species. J. Ga. Entomol. Soc. 4, 41–45.

Brady, U. E. and R. C. Daley (1972) Identification of a sex pheromone from the female raisin moth, *Cadra figulilella*. Ann. Entomol. Soc. Am. 65, 1356–1358.

Brady, U. E. and M. C. Ganyard, Jr. (1972) Identification of a sex pheromone of the female beet armyworm, *Spodoptera exigua*. Ann. Entomol. Soc. Am. 65, 898–899.

Brady, U. E. and D. Nordlund (1971) *cis*-9, *trans*-12-Tetradecadien-1-yl acetate in the female tobacco moth *Ephestia elutella* (Hübner) and evidence for an additional component of the sex pheromone. Life Sci. 10, Part II, 797–801.

Brady, U. E., D. A. Nordlund and R. C. Daley (1971a) The sex stimulant of the Mediterranean flour moth *Anagasta kuehniella*. J. Ga. Entomol. Soc. 6, 215–217.

Brady, U., J. Tumlinson, III, R. Brownlee and R. Silverstein (1971b) Sex stimulant and attractant in the Indian-meal moth and in the almond moth, Science 171, 802–804.

Cardé, R. T. (1971) Aspects of reproductive isolation in the *Holomelina aurantiaca* complex (Lepidoptera: Arctiidae). Ph.D. Thesis, Cornell Univ.

Cardé, R. T., C. C. Doane and W. L. Roelofs (1974) Diel periodicity of male sex pheromone response and female attractiveness in the gypsy moth. Can. Entomol. (in press).

Cardé, R. T., W. L. Roelofs and C. C. Doane (1973) Natural inhibitor of the gypsy moth sex attractant. Nature (London) 241, 474–475.

Chapman, P. J. (1973) Bionomics of the apple-feeding Tortricidae. Ann. Rev. Entomol. 18, 73–96.

Collins, C. W. and S. F. Potts (1932) Attractants for the flying gipsy moths as an aid to locating new infestations. U. S. Dept. Agric. Tech. Bull. 356, 43 p.

Collins, M. M. and R. D. Weast (1961) Wild silk moths of the United States. Saturniinae. (Collins Radio Company, Cedar Rapids, Iowa), 138 pp.

Comeau, A. (1971) Physiology of sex pheromone attraction in Tortricidae and other Lepidoptera (Heterocera). Ph.D. Thesis, Cornell Univ.

Comeau, A. and W. Roelofs (1973) Sex attraction specificity in the Tortricidae. Entomol. Exptl. Appl. 16, 191–200.

Dahm, K., D. Meyer, W. Finn, V. Reinhold and H. Röller (1971a) The olfactory and auditory mediated sex attraction in *Achroia grisella* (Fabr.). Naturwissenschaften 58, 265–266.

Dahm, K. H., I. Richter, D. Meyer and H. Röller (1971b) The sex attractant of the Indian-meal moth, *Plodia interpunctella* (Hübner). Life Sci. 10, Part II, 531–539.

Daterman, G. E., G. D. Davies, Jr. and M. Jacobson (1972) Inhibition of pheromone perception in European pine shoot moth by synthetic acetates. Envir. Entomol. 1, 382–383.

Ferguson, D. C. (1953) On the identity and status of *Eubaphe lamae* Freeman (Lepidoptera, Arctiidae). Can. Entomol. 85, 371–373.

Ferguson, D. C. (1971–72) Bombycoidea (Saturniidae) *In*: Dominick et al., The moths of America north of Mexico. fasc. 20.2, 275 pp.

Forbush, E. H. and C. H. Fernald (1896) The Gypsy Moth (Wright and Potter Printing Company, Boston) 495 pp.

Freeman, T. N. (1953) The spruce budworm, *Choristoneura fumiferana* (Clem.), and an allied new species on pine. (Lepidoptera: Tortricidae). Can. Entomol. 85, 121–127.

Freeman, T. N. (1967) On coniferophagous species of *Choristoneura* (Lepidoptera: Tortricidae) in North America. I: Some new forms of *Choristoneura* allied to *C. fumiferana*. Can. Entomol. 99, 449–455.

Ganyard, M. C., Jr. and U. E. Brady (1971) Inhibition of attraction and cross-attraction by interspecific sex pheromone communication in Lepidoptera. Nature (London) 234, 415–416.

Granges, J. and M. Baggiolini (1971) Une phéromone sexuelle synthétique attractive pour le carpocapse des prunes (*Grapholitha funebrana* Tr. (Lep. Tortricidae)). Rev. Suisse Vitic. Arboric. 3, 93–94.

Henderson, H. E. and F. L. Warren (1972) Sex pheromones. *cis*-Dec-5-en-1-yl 3-methyl butanoate as the pheromone from the pine emperor moth (*Nudaurelia cytherea cytherea* Fabr.). Chem. Comm. 686–687.

Hill, A., A. Comeau, R. Cardé, W. Bode and W. Roelofs (1974) Sex pheromones of the tufted apple bud moth (*Platynota idaeusalis*) (in press).

Jacobson M., R. E. Redfern, W. A. Jones and M. H. Aldridge (1970) Sex pheromones of the southern armyworm moth: isolation, identification and synthesis. Science 170, 542–544.

Jacentovský, D. (1932) Nový způsob kontroly mnišky. Les. Pr. 11, 149–152.

Jacentkovský, D. (1934) Výskyt bekyně velkohlavé (*Liparis dispar* L.) v polesí Rafajna (Podk. Rus.). Les. Pr. 13, 27–36.

Kaae, R. S., H. H. Shorey and L. K. Gaston (1973a) Pheromone concentration as a mechanism for reproductive isolation between two lepidopterous species. Science 179, 487–48.

Kaae, R. S., H. H. Shorey, S. U. McFarland and L. K. Gaston (1973b) Sex pheromones of Lepidoptera. XXXVII. Role of sex pheromones and other factors in reproductive isolation among ten species of Noctuidae. Ann. Entomol. Soc. Am. 6, 444–448.

Kochansky, J., R. T. Cardé and W. L. Roelofs (1974) Sex pheromone of the European corn borer (New York) (in preparation).

Klun, J. A. and T. A. Brindley (1970) *Cis*-11-Tetradecenyl acetate, a sex stimulant of the European corn borer. J. Econ. Entomol. 63, 779–780.

Klun, J. A. and J. F. Robinson (1971) European corn borer moth: sex attractant and sex attraction inhibitors. Ann. Entomol. Soc. Am. 64, 1083–1086.

Klun, J. A. and J. F. Robinson (1972) Olfactory discrimination in the European corn borer and several pheromonally analogous moths. Ann. Entomol. Soc. Am. 65, 1337–1340.

Kuwahara, Y., H. Hara, S. Ishii and H. Fukami (1971a) The sex pheromone of the Mediterranean flour moth. Agr. Biol. Chem. 35, 447–448.

Kuwahara, Y., C. Kitamura, S. Takahashi, H. Hara, S. Ishii and H. Fukami (1971b) Sex pheromone of the almond moth and the Indian-meal moth: *cis*-9, *trans*-12-tetradecadienyl acetate. Science 171, 801–802.

Lange, R. and D. Hoffman (1972) Essigsaure-*cis*-dodecen-(9)-yl-ester, ein Inhibitor des Sexualpheromons des Kiefernknospertriebwicklers. Naturwissenschaften 59, 217.

Lanier, G. N., M. C. Birch, R. F. Schmitz and M. M. Furniss (1972) Pheromones of *Ips pini* (Coleoptera: Scolytidae): variation in response among three populations. Can. Entomol. 104, 1917–1923.

Meijer, G. M., F. J. Ritter, C. J. Persoons, A. K. Minks and S. Voerman (1972) Sex pheromones of summer fruit tortrix moth *Adoxophyes orana*: two synergistic isomers. Science 175, 1469–1470.

Minks, A. K., W. L. Roelofs, F. J. Ritter and C. J. Persoons (1973) Reproductive isolation of two tortricid moth species by different ratios of a two-component sex attractant. Science 180, 1073–1074.

Mitchell, E. R. (1972) Female cabbage loopers inhibit attraction of male soybean loopers. Envir. Entomol. 1, 444–446.

O'Connell, R. J. (1972) Responses of olfactory receptors to the sex attractant, its synergist and inhibitor in the red-banded leaf roller, *Argyrotaenia velutinana. In*: Olfaction and Taste IV; ed.: D. Schneider (Wissenschaftliche Verlagsgesellschaft MBH, Stuttgart). pp. 180–186.

Powell, J. A. (1964) Biological and taxonomic studies on Tortricinae moths, with reference to the species in California. Univ. Calif. Publ. Entomol. 32, 1–317.

Rau, P. and N. L. Rau (1929) The sex attraction and rhythmic periodicity in the giant saturniid moths. Trans. Acad. Sci. St. Louis 26, 83–221.

Read, J. S., F. L. Warren and P. H. Hewitt (1968) Identification of the sex pheromone of the false codling moth. Chem. Commun. 792–793.

Redfern, R. E., E. Cantu, W. A. Jones and M. Jacobson (1971) Response of the male southern armyworm in a field cage to prodenialure A and prodenialure B. J. Econ. Entomol. 64, 1570–1571.

Roelofs, W. and H. Arn (1968) Sex attractant of the red-banded leafroller moth, Nature (London) 219, 513.

Roelofs, W. and R. Cardé (1971) Hydrocarbon sex pheromone in tiger moths (Arctiidae). Science 171, 684–686.

Roelofs, W. and A. Comeau (1968) Sex pheromone perception. Nature (London) 220, 600–601.

Roelofs, W. and A. Comeau (1969) Sex pheromone specificity: Taxonomic and evolutionary aspects in Lepidoptera. Science 165, 398–400.

Roelofs, W. and A. Comeau (1970) Lepidopterous sex attractants discovered by field screening tests. J. Econ. Entomol. 63, 969–974.

Roelofs, W. and A. Comeau (1971a) Sex pheromone perception: synergists and inhibitors for the redbanded leafroller attractant. J. Insect Physiol. 17, 435–449.

Roelofs, W. L. and A. Comeau (1971b) Sex attractants in Lepidoptera. *In*: Chemical Releasers in Insects, vol. III; ed.: A. Tahori, (Gordon and Breach, New York) pp. 91–114.

Roelofs, W. and A. Comeau (1971c) Sex attractant perception: electroantennogram responses of the red-banded leafroller moth. J. Insect Physiol. 17, 1969–1982.

Roelofs, W. and K. C. Feng (1968) Sex pheromone specificity tests in the Tortricidae – an introductory report. Ann. Entomol. Soc. Am. 61, 312–316.

Roelofs, W. and J. Tette (1970) Sex pheromone of the oblique-banded leaf roller. Nature (London) 226, 1172.

Roelofs, W., R. Cardé, R. Bartell and P. Tierney (1972) Sex attractant trapping of the European corn borer in New York. Envir. Entomol. 1, 606–608.

Roelofs, W., R. Cardé, G. Benz and G. Von Salis (1971a) Sex attractant of the larch bud moth found by electroantennogram method. Experientia 27, 1438–1439.

Roelofs, W. L., R. T. Cardé and E. F. Taschenberg (1974) Sex pheromone of the grape berry moth: release rate and trap design (in preparation).

Roelofs, W., R. Cardé and J. Tette (1973) Oriental fruit moth attractant synergists. Envir. Entomol. 2, 252–254.

Roelofs, W., A. Comeau, A. Hill, and G. Milicevic (1971b) Sex attractant of the codling moth: characterization with electroantennogram technique. Science 174, 297–299.

Roelofs, W., A. Comeau and R. Selle (1969) Sex pheromone of the oriental fruit moth. Nature (London) 224. 723.

Roelofs, W., J. Tette, E. F. Taschenberg and A. Comeau (1971c) Sex pheromone of the grape berry moth: identification by classical and electroantennogram methods, and field tests. J. Insect Physiol. 17, 2235–224.

Röller, H., K. Biemann, J. S. Bjerke, D. W. Norgard and W. H. McShan (1968) Sex pheromones of pyralid moths. I. Isolation and identification of the sex attractant of *Galleria mellonella* (greater waxmoth). Acta Entomol. Bohemoslov. 65, 208–211.

Sanders, C. J. (1971a) Daily activity patterns and sex pheromone specificity as sexual isolating mechanisms in two species of *Choristoneura* (Lepidoptera: Tortricidae). Can. Entomol. 103, 498–502.

Sanders, C. J. (1971b) Sex pheromone specificity and taxonomy of budworm moths (*Choristoneura*). Science 171, 911–913.

Sanders, C., R. Bartell and W. Roelofs (1972) Field trials for synergism and inhibition of *trans*-11-tetradecenal, the sex pheromone of the eastern spruce budworm. Can. Dept. Envir. Bi-mon. Res. Notes 28, 10.

Sanders, C. J., G. E. Daterman, R. F. Sheppard and H. Cerezke (1973) Sex attractants for two western spruce budworms, *Choristoneura biennis* and *C. viridis* (Lepidoptera: Tortricidae) (manuscript).

Sanders, C. J. and G. S. Lucuik (1972a) Masking of female sex pheromone of the eastern spruce budworm by excised female abdomen tips. Can. Dept. Envir. Bi-mon. Res. Notes 28, 10–11.

Sanders, C. J. and G. S. Lucuik (1972b) Factors affecting calling by female eastern spruce budworm, *Choristoneura fumiferana* (Lepidoptera: Tortricidae). Can. Entomol. 104, 1751–1762.

Schönherr, V. J. (1972) Die Wirkung von Disparlure auf die Nonne, *Lymantria monacha* L. Z. Angew. Entomol. 71, 260–263.

Schwinck, I. (1955) Weitere Untersuchungen zur Frage Geruchsorientierung der Nachtschmetterlinge: Partielle Fühleramputation bei Spinnermännchen, insbesondere am Seidenspinner *Bombyx mori* L. Z. Vergl. Physiol. 37, 439–458.

Smith, S. G. (1954) A partial breakdown of temporal and ecological isolation between *Choristoneura* species (Lepidoptera: Tortricidae). Evolution 8, 206–224.

Sower, L. L., H. H. Shorey and L. K. Gaston (1971) Sex pheromones of noctuid moths. XXV. Effects of temperature and photoperiod on circadian rhythms of sex pheromone release by females of *Trichoplusia ni*. Ann. Entomol. Soc. Am. 64, 488–492.

Stehr, G. W. (1967) On coniferophagous species of *Choristoneura* (Lepidoptera: Tortricidae) in North America. II. Geographic distribution in accordance with forest regions. Can. Entomol. 99, 456–463.

Tamaki, Y., H. Noguchi, T. Yushima and C. Hirano (1971a) Two sex pheromones of the smaller tea tortrix: isolation, identification, and synthesis. Appl. Entomol. Zool. 6, 139–141.

Tamaki, Y., H. Noguchi, T. Yushima, C. Hirano, K. Honma and H. Sugawara (1971b) Sex pheromone of the summerfruit tortrix: isolation and identification. Konchu 39, 338–340.

Traynier, R. M. M. (1968) Sex attraction in the Mediterranean flour moth, *Anagasta kühniella*: location of the female by the male. Can. Entomol. 100, 5–10.

Tumlinson, J. H., E. R. Mitchell, S. M. Browner and D. A. Lindquist (1972a) A sex pheromone for the soybean looper. Envir. Entomol. 1, 466–468.

Tumlinson, J. H., E. R. Mitchell, S. M. Browner, M. S. Mayer, N. Green, R. Hines and D. A. Lindquist (1972b) *cis*-7-dodecen-1-ol, a potent inhibitor of the cabbage looper sex pheromone. Envir. Entomol. 1, 354–358.

Voerman, S. and A. K. Minks (1973) Sex pheromones of summerfruit tortrix moth *Adoxophyes orana*. II. Compounds influencing their attractant activity. Envir. Entomol. 2, 751–756.

Weatherston, J., W. Roelofs, A. Comeau and C. Sanders (1971) Studies of physiologically active arthropod secretions. X. Sex pheromone of the eastern spruce budworm, *Choristoneura fumiferana* (Lepidoptera: Tortricidae). Can. Entomol. 103, 1741–1747.

Wright, R. H. (1964) After pesticides – what? Nature (London) 204, 121–125.

CHAPTER 7

Aphrodisiac pheromones in insects

Martin BIRCH

7.1. Introduction

Aphrodisiac is a popular term loosely applied to many pheromones which are thought to play an important role in the successful achievement of copulation through their use in courtship behavior. The standard pheromone model for bringing sexual partners together is that one sex, usually the female, releases a pheromone into the atmosphere often only under prescribed environmental and physiological conditions (Shorey ch. 4). The opposite sex, usually male, is stimulated by this pheromone to approach the source. At close range, other stimuli (visual, auditory or tactile) alone or in conjunction with the pheromone may stimulate him to continue courtship and to copulate. The higher concentration of the female sex pheromone near the source may be enough on its own to release courtship and copulatory behavior (sect. 7.2) and, in that case, would be utilized as both an attractant and a courtship or copulatory pheromone in the two different contexts. However, other pheromones may be released specifically during courtship and at no other time. Examples are the pheromones disseminated by the hairpencils of danaiine butterflies during courtship flight which induce the female to alight (sect. 7.4.1) or the male cockroach secretion (sect. 7.3) which induces the female to mount the male and thus attain the correct copulatory stance.

The term aphrodisiac pheromone has become widely used since Butler (1967a) introduced it into the current literature on pheromones and defined it as a 'substance produced by one or other sex, usually by the male and often as only a part of a complex pattern of courtship behavior, preparing the opposite sex for copulation *after* the pair has been brought together by olfactory sex attractants and other means'. The emphasis is mine since it clearly differentiates between sex pheromones that act as aphrodisiacs and those that attract the opposite sex over a distance. Materials which may act as aphrodisiacs by inducing courtship or other sexual behavior, but which come from the environment (e.g. Riddiford 1967) are eliminated from our discussion since they are not pheromones. Shorey (1973) has recently taken up the term aphrodisiac, but with reservations. He contends that a true aphrodisiac should directly affect that part of the nervous system in the female that controls her mating behavior, increasing the chance that she will accept the male in copulation (it could equally well be a female to male effect), whereas many of the pheromones described as aphrodisiacs exert their effect on other parts of the nervous system, such as inhibiting flight or stimulating feeding behavior. Such criticism, however, appears to be somewhat teleological in attempting to avoid the rigor of behavioral experiment and critical observation by cloaking it with terminology. Nor is the neurophysiological basis for behavior well enough defined to know, morphologically or neurologically, what part of the nervous system, if it is a specific part, controls mating behavior. It is also easy to confuse the function of a behavior pattern with its mechanism. The mechanisms of behavior involved in feeding or in the inhibition of locomotion may be involved in an identical way as part of food searching, escape from predation or sexual behavior, but this in no way lessens their function in releasing specific parts of precopulatory behavior and directly promoting successful copulation, even if this is not clear at first glance.

The use of a label, such as aphrodisiac, can nevertheless be criticized as can the labels attached to many pheromones, since it derives from the final result of the behavior and thus assumes that the behavior was aimed toward that goal (Kennedy 1972). Part of the problem is clearly the heavy anthropomorphic overtones carried by the word (Comfort ch. 20) and in the assumption that an aphrodisiac is always 'successful'. Courtship pheromone might avoid this problem since it specifies only when the pheromone is used and does not speculate on the outcome. However, aphrodisiac is now an established word and if the dangers in its use are borne in mind it does usefully describe a functionally distinct group of pheromones. It is used here according to Butler's definition and thus only three criteria are required: the substance must be a pheromone; it must be released after the insects have come together; and it must, as far as is known, clearly facilitate courtship and/or copulation.

7.2. Some candidate pheromones

Most insect species probably employ sex pheromones which act as stimulants when the sexes come into near or direct contact (Jacobson 1972; Shorey 1973). The literature abounds with references to such effects, but most are anecdotal or circumstantial and only the few which have been experimentally analyzed in any detail will be discussed here.

Honey bee queen substance: One of the most versatile pheromones known is the queen substance of the honey bee, *Apis mellifera* L. This substance, 9-oxodec-*trans*-2-enoic acid, is produced by the mandibular glands of the queen but not the workers. Depending on the context, it can function as an attractant for workers in colony cohesion and swarming, as an inhibitor of queen cell construction and of ovary development in workers, and as a sex attractant and a mating stimulant for drones (Butler 1967a; Gary 1970, and ch. 11).

Drone bees attracted by the queen substance to an experimental area, closely examined queens, worker bees and models of queen bees as long as they were suspended eight m above ground (Butler 1967b). The drones confined their mounting almost entirely to queens, workers, or models which had open sting-chambers. However, the drones did not attempt to grasp a model even with an open sting chamber unless 9-oxodec-*trans*-2-enoic acid was present. Then they would seize and attempt to copulate with it. Butler concluded that both open sting-chamber and odor of queen substance are required stimuli to induce a drone to mount a queen in flight and that the queen substance functions as an aphrodisiac. Clearly this short-range effect of the queen substance in releasing drone sexual behavior is highly dependent on the context of perception.

However, the behavior pattern may not be quite as straightforward as this (Gary ch. 11). Mandibular glands producing the queen substance can be excised from virgin queens, before the glands become functional, but this procedure does not inhibit all queens from mating successfully (Morse et al. 1962). The mandibular glands of queen bees also produce a series of ten-carbon acids (Callow et al. 1964). Their function, if any, is unknown although they are apparently not active individually in sex attraction (Butler and Fairey 1964). Butler (1971) has since suggested that a further unidentified pheromone from the abdominal tergites may stimulate mounting and copulation. The indications are that there is a lot more to discover about honey bee behavior supposedly mediated by queen substance alone. It seems highly likely that chemical modifiers, such as synergists and inhibitors, will be found here too as in other insect orders.

Close-range role of female sex pheromones: A hierarchy of behavior in response to stimulation by female sex pheromone has been demonstrated for a large number of insects from several orders (Shorey 1973, for references). In *Trichoplusia ni* (Hübner), for example, a quantitative increase in concentration of female sex pheromone alone is sufficient for the initiation of each successive step in the response sequence including the release of male copulatory behavior (Shorey and Gaston 1970). This phenomenon also occurs in species from other families of Lepidoptera, e.g. *Porthetria dispar* (L.) (Lymantriidae) (Doane 1968) and *Anagasta kühniella* (Zeller) (Phycitidae) (Traynier 1968). Some authors have claimed to have identified sex attractant pheromones of Lepidoptera from assays which by design could only identify a stimulatory role of the pheromone. However, although the same stimulus in different concentrations may elicit all responses through attraction and copulation, it is possible that the compounds isolated may evoke copulatory attempts or stimulation, but not attraction. The difference between attractant and stimulant is very real (Brady et al. 1971), but unfortunately frequently ignored. In *Cadra cautella* (Walker) one pheromone (*cis*-9, *trans*-12-tetradecadien-1-yl-acetate) produced by the female will elicit a stimulation response in the males but does not release orientation to the source by itself (Brady et al. 1971). In fact, increased concentration may inhibit male activity. At least one other sex pheromone is required to elicit the whole response in *C. cautella* up to and including copulatory behavior. With the related *Plodia interpunctella* (Hübner) the same compound is sufficient to stimulate and attract.

The behavior released by female sex pheromones in initiating copulatory attempts after the sexes have been brought together might include them in our definition of aphrodisiacs. However, at least in the Lepidoptera, the female sex attractants are released continuously and may not be involved in a courtship sequence at all – the male may arrive and copulate at once, without preliminaries. Thus it seems more logical to restrict the term aphrodisiac to those pheromones produced *only* after the sexes have come together (see sect. 7.1) and to continue to use the terms sex attractant and sex stimulant as proposed by Dethier et al. (1960) for the female sex pheromones.

Other possible aphrodisiacs: Mating behavior in both Diptera and Hymenoptera is apparently initiated in response to fairly non-specific visual stimuli (Shorey 1973), but the threshold for releasing sexual behavior may be lowered by the odor of food or of aggregation sites. In *Lucilia cuprina* (Wied.) contact with the partner dramatically increases the mating potential if the partner is female, possibly due to a contact pheromone (Bartell et al. 1969). Similarly, when a male *Drosophila melanogaster* (Meigen) has oriented towards another fly, additional stimuli, probably gustatory or other contact pheromones, assist in determining whether courtship is broken off or continues through to copulation (Shorey and Bartell 1970). Courtship in *Rhodnius prolixus* (Stal.) is already initiated before the female releases her pheromone, although its production is essential for releasing successful male copulatory behavior (Baldwin et al. 1970). Pantle (1971) showed that a compound from the male milkweed bug, *Oncopeltus fasciatus* (Dallas), can be perceived by both sexes and suggests that if, as indicated, there is an effect at close range then the compound has the characteristics of an aphrodisiac. Mating behavior of the hen flea, *Ceratophyllus gallinae* (Schrank), is only initiated if the male comes into direct contact with the female and receives some specific stimulus from her abdomen through his maxillary palps (Humphries 1967). These few examples clearly show the potential existence of aphrodisiac pheromones, but a lot of detailed experimental work is required to analyze the complex interactions of intimate behavior.

Happ (1969) coined the term 'anti-aphrodisiac' for a pheromone which inhibits the response of other males to the female scent of *Tenebrio molitor* L. This clearly represents a broader usage of the word since its opposite would apply aphrodisiac to a pheromone produced by males to enhance the response of other males to a female. As, however, August (1971) finds no effect of male pheromone on other males in this species, the term may be short-lived. Burkholder (in ch. 22) describes the aphrodisiac effect of high concentrations of the female pheromone of *Attagenus megatoma* (F.) (Dermestidae) in releasing male copulatory behavior.

7.3. *Gustatory aphrodisiacs*

Sex pheromones acting through the gustatory sense require that the male and female make contact and are thus likely to have an aphrodisiac function.

In many species of Orthoptera the virgin female produces a sex pheromone which attracts males. Courting males of some species will themselves produce a pheromone which stimulates the female to mount, feed on the secretion and thus attain the correct position for copulation. Such male pheromones have been described for *Blatella germanica* (L.) and *Supella supellectilicum* Serville (Roth 1962); *Blatta orientalis* L. (Roth and Willis 1952); *Nauphoeta cinerea* (Olivier) (Roth 1962); *Byrsotria fumigata* (Guerin) (Roth and Barth 1964); *Leucophaea maderae* (Fab.) (Roth 1965) and *Periplaneta americana* (L.) (Barth 1970). The female feeding response is known from at least 25 species (Roth and Dateo 1966), in all of which courtship behavior is essentially similar. The male first makes antennal contact with the body of the female, orienting the exposed abdominal tergites towards her. She straddles his abdomen and the male assists this behavior by moving back under her. The female is observed to 'feed' on the exposed tergal surface. This behavior allows the male to contact the female genitalia and to copulate. As soon as the connection is made the pair adopts an opposed position for the duration of copulation.

As the wings are raised to the vertical position the terminal abdominal sternites are pressed to the substrate so that the upper surface of the abdomen becomes somewhat concave. Female feeding behavior may involve actual ingestion or palpation of the dorsal surface, chemical or tactile stimuli from which stimulates the male to engage the genitalia. Because the role of the female can be duplicated in *Byrsotria fumigata* by stroking the exposed male tergites with a fine brush (Roth and Barth 1964) the stimulus imparted by the female of this species is apparently largely tactile.

There is no obvious discrete gland in *Periplaneta americana* (Barth 1970), but Roth (1952) described a very distinct gland on the seventh abdominal tergite of *Supella supellectilicum*, consisting of a circular depressed area with a mound at its center. Setae arising from the mound have a glossy appearance due to secretion from cells at their bases. In *Blatella germanica* (L.) (Roth 1952) there are double pouches on the seventh and eighth tergites with glandular cells leading via a tubule to the lumen of each pouch. Roth and Dateo (1966) isolated a pheromone from males of *Nauphoeta cinerea* which elicits the typical behavior of females attracted to a courting male's tergum. Females were highly attracted to dummies containing the active extract and rushed up to them, placing their mouthparts on the filter paper source. The pheromone is a polar neutral lipid of low volatility. It was named *seducin* for its role in releasing female sexual feeding behavior which directly permits copulation to take place.

Gabbutt (1954) describes a similar, somewhat more involved courtship behavior in the cricket, *Nemobius sylvestris* (Bosc.). The female may mount a receptive male and 'feed' by running her labial palps over the surface of the male's right tegmen, while the male introduces a spermatophore. However, no morphological evidence of glandular structures could be found. The female eats the first spermatophore, but a second bigger spermatophore is formed which is inserted when the female mounts a second time. Gurney (1947) suggested that the function of the female's feeding behavior may be to distract her attention away from the second spermatophore until the sperm have passed into the spermatheca. Male *Rioxa pernia* (Walker) (Diptera, Tephritidae) produce a fluid from the proboscis, apparently secreted by the salivary glands, which creates a white foam when it is mixed with air. Receptive females actually consume the foam while the male mounts (Pritchard 1967).

There are undoubtedly many other species in which sex pheromones released on the surface of the body or over a very short distance act as stimulants for the copulatory act. For example, Mathes' (1962) observations of the courtship of many species of malachiid beetles indicated that glands over the body surface of males produce a gustatory pheromone during courtship.

These gustatory secretions fit our definition of aphrodisiac in that they prepare the opposite sex for copulation after the sexes have been brought together. Feeding behavior is a very specific and ritualized part of copulatory behavior. It immobilizes the female and allows the male to make his copulatory attempt. Such an immobilization response is more dramatic in the Lepidoptera.

7.4. *Olfactory aphrodisiacs in Lepidoptera*

The principal female response to male-produced aphrodisiac pheromones appears to be either inhibition of the female's natural tendency to fly or cessation of flight. In day-flying butterflies males are initially attracted to a female flying overhead. They fly up to and overtake the female, distributing scent over her in an attempt to induce her to land. In nocturnal species (moths) the initial attraction of males to a receptive female is usually olfactory. The male pheromone appears to function in preventing the female from taking flight as the male makes contact, or in some cases inducing the female to take an acceptance posture.

Taking the Lepidoptera as a whole, the range in structure and position of male scent-disseminating structures is tremendous (fig. 7.2). They are found on the legs, thorax or abdomen and vary from simple tufts of hair to complex eversible organs displaying elaborate methods for secretion, storage and release of scent. Müller's remarkable series of observations (1874, 1877, 1878) described the great variety of male scales in detail and deduced their function with great accuracy. By the late nineteenth century enough literature had accumulated on the male scent-organs in

Lepidoptera to warrant a review (Dalla-Torre 1885). However, the only definite information acquired until very recently was that the organs were male specific, had glandular structures associated with them, were odoriferous to man, were eversible, and probably played some role in the sexual life of the insects. An indication of the historical background can be gained from Brower et al. (1965), Jacobson (1972) and Varley (1962). Numerous early references were 'anecdotal', describing dancing butterflies and brush displays during courtship (see Brower et al. 1965 for references), but there was no attempt at critical observation or analysis of the behavior. Still less was known about nocturnal species. As Varley (1962) points out, the problem was not so much the nocturnal habits of the insects but more one of attitude: any 'behavior' that the insect was permitted resulted in measurable damage to a potential cabinet specimen!

A land mark study of courtship behavior was the work of Tinbergen et al. (1942; also in Tinbergen 1951) on the grayling butterfly, *Eumenis semele* (L.) (Satyridae). During courtship, males touch the scent scales on their forewings to the antennae of the female before walking behind her and attempting to copulate. Brower et al. (1965) have since analyzed the courtship behavior of the queen butterfly (Nymphalidae: Danaiinae) in detail.

7.4.1. Danaiinae

In the queen butterfly, *Danaus gilippus berenice* (Cramer), the male flies after the female, overtakes her and induces her to alight by rapidly extruding two hair-pencils from the posterior of his abdomen which release the male pheromone near the female antennae (fig. 7.1) (Brower et al. 1965). A receptive female will alight and fold her wings. The male may hover and continue his hair-pencilling before alighting and attempting to copulate. When coupled, the male flies with the female to a quiet area where copulation lasts for several hours. Males may initiate the entire sequence again if the alighted female is unresponsive. The presence of hair-pencils is essential for successful courtship. Excision of the hair-pencils from males drastically reduces their mating success (Pliske and Eisner 1969) since males without hair-pencils readily court females but cannot induce them to remain on the ground long enough to copulate.

The hair-pencils are covered with cuticular particles which are transferred to the surface of the female, including the surface of the sensory pegs on the antennae, during the hair-pencilling activity. Two components have been isolated from the hair-pencils – a volatile ketone and a viscous terpenoid alcohol. The ketone is the essential aphrodisiac pheromone and the terpene alcohol functions as a glue to stick the cuticular particles to the female antennae and possibly to carry more pheromone. Laboratory-reared males fed on a ketone deficient natural food plant, *Asclepias tuberosa rolfsii*, are relatively unsuccessful sexually, but their mating competence can be restored by adding the ketone to the hair-pencils (Pliske and Eisner

1969). Schneider and Seibt (1969) confirmed the activity of the ketone electrophysiologically. Receptor responses of male and female antennae were equally strong when stimulated with either crude hair-pencil odor or ketone alone, but were only weakly responsive to the terpene alcohol. Myers and Brower (1969) demonstrated by behavioral means that only the short, thin-walled sensillae perceive the male pheromone. Schneider and Seibt's (1969) work also showed that hair-pencils of another danaiine butterfly, *Lycorea ceres ceres* (Cramer), are as effective as queen hair-pencils in eliciting an electrophysiological response from the queen antennae, but that the hair-pencils of the monarch, *Danaus plexippus* (L.), are not.

The ketone in *D. gilippus* has been identified as a crystalline pyrrolizidinone (1) (fig. 7.1) and the viscous compound as a terpenoid diol (2) (Meinwald et al. 1969). The ketone is also found in *Lycorea ceres*, explaining the electrophysiological cross activity. However, in *Lycorea* the diol is replaced by two aliphatic acetate esters (6 and 7) (Meinwald et al. 1966) which may possibly fulfil the same biological role as the diol. The monarch, *Danaus plexippus*, does not produce either the ketone or the diol so that its sensitivity to the ketone remains unexplained. Curiously, Schneider and Seibt (1969) could not obtain any electrophysiological response from the laboratory-reared monarchs in response to their own hair-pencils. The major components isolated from the hair-pencils of *D. plexippus* are two aliphatic acids (4 and 5) (Meinwald et al. 1968; Meinwald et al. 1969) present in neither of the other species, which may explain why the monarch hair-pencils were unable to elicit responses from the queen antennae. Meinwald et al. (1971) have also examined an African danaiine, *D. chrysippus* L., and find that it contains the same ketone as does *D. gilippus*, together with an alcohol (3) similar in structure to the queen diol. It is not surprising then that taxonomically the old world *D. chrysippus* and the new world *D. gilippus* are thought to be more closely related to each other than either is to *D. plexippus*. The indistinguishable electrophysiological response to females of *D. gilippus*, *Lycorea ceres* and *Danaus plexippus* appears to conflict with the hypothesis that male aphrodisiac pheromones are a mechanism for discrimination between species following the rather non-discriminatory initial attraction. Further behavioral and physiological work is clearly indicated.

7.4.2. Noctuidae and other nocturnal families

Müller's (1877) speculation that volatile secretions from the male scent brushes of moths were used in courtship has recently been proven correct (Birch 1970a; Grant 1970, 1972). Noctuid males commonly have brushes either on the ventral surface of the eighth abdominal segment, e.g. *Plusia gamma* (L.) (fig. 7.2) and *Trichoplusia ni*, or a pair of brush-organs at the anterior end of the abdomen, e.g. *Apamea monoglypha* (Huf.) (fig. 7.2) and *Phlogophora meticulosa* (L.).

In *P. meticulosa* (Birch 1970b) two brush-organs arising from each side of the second abdominal sternite are mounted at the tip of a sclerotised arm and everted by a

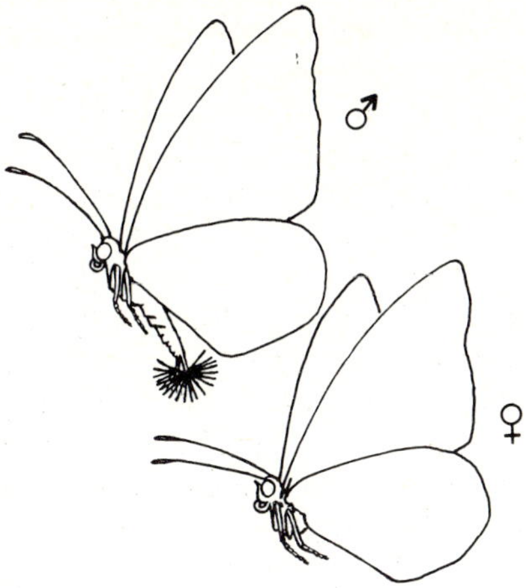

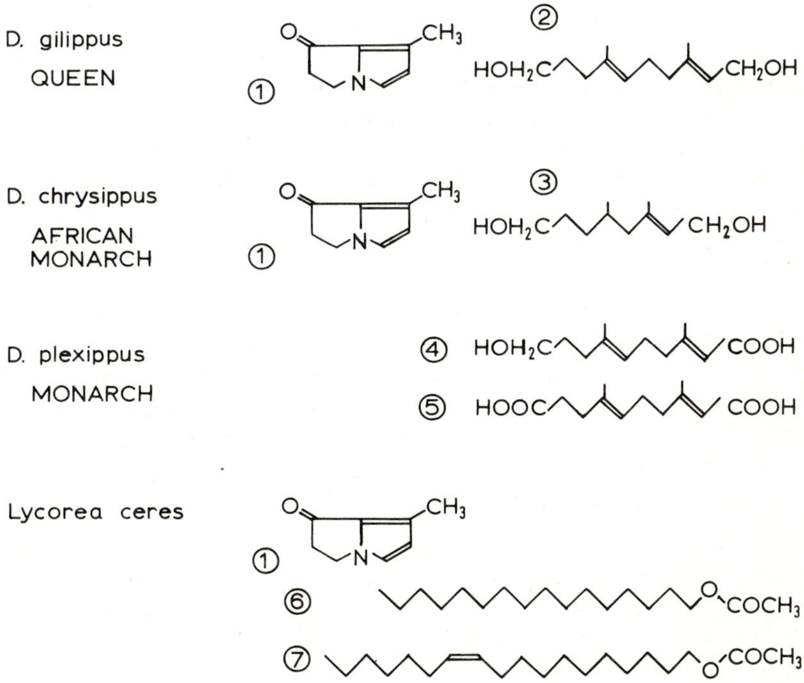

Fig. 7.1. (upper) *Danaus gilippus.* Male hair-pencilling female in courtship flight (from Brower et al. 1965). (lower) Compounds identified from the hair-pencils of four species of Danainae. 1) 2,3-dihydro- 7-methyl-l *H*-pyrrolizin-l-one; 2) *trans, trans*-3,7-dimethyl-deca-2, 6-dien-1,10-diol; 3) 3,7-dimenthyloct-2-en-1,8-diol; 4) *trans*, *trans*-10-hydroxy-3,7-dimenthyl-2,6-decadienoic acid; 5) *trans*, *trans*-3,7-dimethyl-2,6-decadien-l,10-dioic acid; 6) *n*-hexadecyl acetate; 7) *cis*-vaccenyl acetate (from Meinwald et al. 1971).

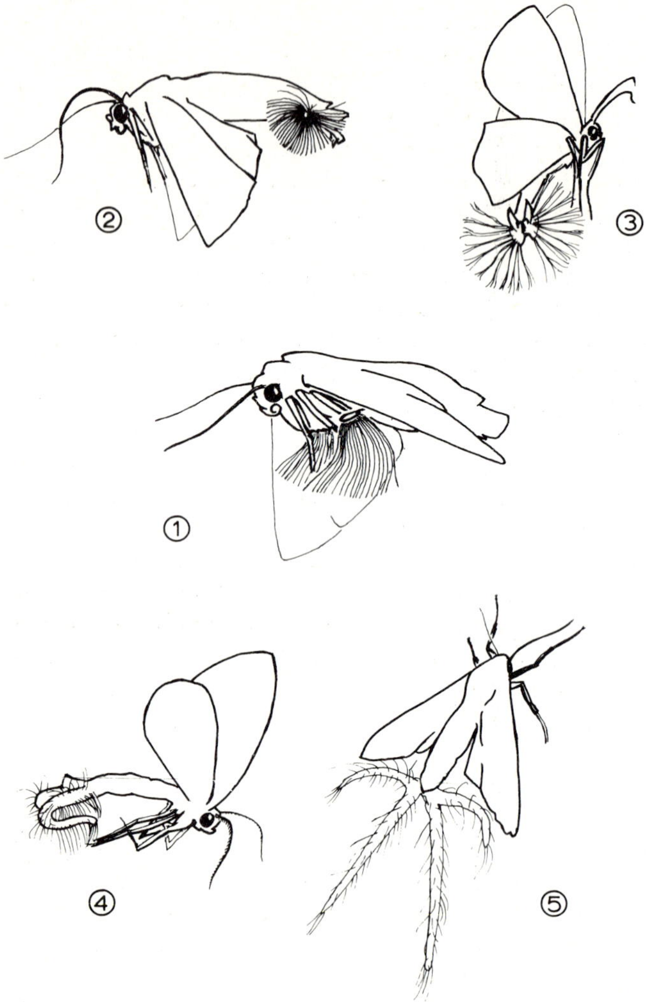

Fig. 7.2. Some of the variety of male brush-organs and coremata in the Lepidoptera. 1) Noctuidae, *Apamea monoglypha* – anterior abdominal brushes on either side of the abdomen, expanded just before copulation. In this species the main component on the brushes is pinocarvone. 2) Noctuidae, *Plusia gamma* – paired brushes on the 8th abdominal segment; very similar to those of *Trichoplusia ni.* 3) Geometridae, *Bapta temerata* (Denis and Schiff) – tufts of hair arise from inflatable sacs at the base of the genitalia. In this species *n*-butyric acid is the principal component secreted. 4) Geometridae, *Xanthorhoe ferrugata* – long air-filled tubes or coremata are inflated in flight just before genital contact is attempted. 5) (after Pagden 1957) Arctiidae, *Creatonotus gangis* (L.) – huge air-filled coremata are inflated as some part of courtship behavior.

complex of antagonistic muscles and a lever arrangement. Normally the brushes are concealed in abdominal folds or pockets. A secretion is accumulated on the brushes while they are in the pockets from a pair of glands in the second abdominal segment, first described by Stobbe (1912) and now known as Stobbe's glands (Varley 1962). Each gland is a group of hairs whose secretory bases are deeply invaginated within the second segment. Their secretion passes along the hairs onto the brush. The glands are active in the pharate adult, but the enormously hypertrophied cells collapse and discharge their entire contents when the moth emerges from the pupa. They then atrophy and are no longer functional (Birch 1970b). (Clearwater and Sarafis (1973) have now shown a similar state in *Pseudaletia separata* (Walker).) Thus the entire secretion for a male moth is stored on the brushes or in the scales lining the pocket until required for use.

Males exposed to receptive females in the laboratory (Birch 1970a) are stimulated to perform a sequence of responses. The antennae swing forward, wings are vibrated rapidly, genitalia extruded and flexed, and the males fly upwind to the vicinity of the female, appearing to find her precise location by tactile sense or vision. Once contact is established courtship is rapid indeed. The male curls his genitalia towards the female and simultaneously everts both brushes. The brushes remain exposed for only one or two seconds and almost immediately the male attempts to engage the genitalia. There is no overt female response. No male ever attempted copulation in the laboratory without everting the brushes, nor were males from which the brushes had been removed capable of mating. Their courting behavior suggested that general viability was not decreased. Since the brushes do not touch the female when everted, it is assumed that lack of success in this case was due to lack of an olfactory rather than a tactile stimulation. Further laboratory experiments showed that the males can 'charge' the brushes with secretion already in the pockets between two and three times during their adult life (Birch 1970a).

Grant (1970) demonstrated that the male 'genital' brushes of *Trichoplusia ni* are used in essentially the same way. Just before the male attempts to engage the genitalia, the paired scent-brushes are extruded and spread briefly without touching the female. The structure of these brushes and their related gland cells is complicated, but one striking parallel with the structures in *Phlogophora meticulosa* is that the gland cells are completely atrophied within one or two days after emergence (Grant 1971a).

Compounds identified from the male brushes are all simple terpenoids, aromatics and carboxylic acids (Aplin and Birch 1968, 1970; Birch 1972; Clearwater 1972; Grant et al. 1972) (fig. 7.3). Such low molecular weight, volatile compounds would probably be very inefficient in distance communication. However, the quantities produced are relatively large; >5 μg of benzaldehyde per brush in *Leucania impura* (Hübner) (Aplin and Birch 1968); over 10 μg benzaldehyde and 0.04 μg benzyl alcohol per brush in *Pseudaletia unipuncta* (Haworth) (Grant et al. 1972). Lack of any overt behavioral response in the female and the nocturnal courtship in these species has made it difficult to determine which or all of the components affect the female's responsiveness. In *Phlogophora meticulosa* for example, we know that the total secretion is essential for successful courtship since males without the hair-pencils or with discharged hair-pencils are unable to succeed in copulating. However, if the secretion is to be described as a pheromone, a specific effect on the female must be demonstrated either by stimulating adoption of a specific acceptance posture or by inhibiting movement.

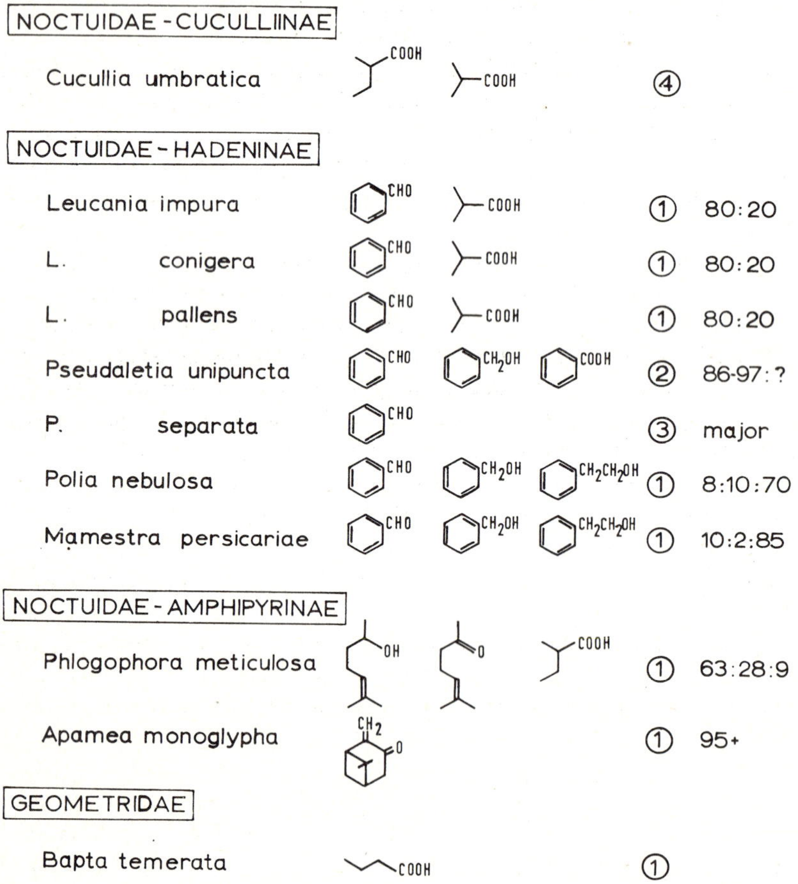

Fig. 7.3. Compounds identified from the male brushes of Lepidoptera (Noctuidae and Geometridae) Left to right: species, compounds, references to published identification, percentages of each of the components as isolated. References – 1) Aplin and Birch 1970; 2) Grant et al 1972; 3) Clearwater 1972; 4) Birch 1972. Benzaldehyde, alone or with other minor components, has since been identified from five more species of Hadeninae and *iso*-valeric acid from a *Cucullia* species (J. R. Clearwater unpublished data).

Although no noctuid females have shown any specific acceptance response, such a posture has been observed in the phycitid moth, *Plodia interpunctella* (Grant 1972 and personal communication). The male everts brushes on the costal margin of the forewings as he approaches and comes to face the female. The female's antennae come close to the wing brushes. If she is receptive, she raises the tip of her abdomen up between her wings in an acceptance posture. However, if she lacks antennae or the male lacks brushes she will not adopt this posture and copulation does not occur. In the Noctuidae, receptive females of *Phlogophora meticulosa* fly or move away when males without brushes attempt to copulate, or after antennectomy when any object approaches very close or touches them. Clearwater (1972) attempted to clarify and quantify the female response by introducing benzaldehyde, isolated from the male brushes, into an olfactometer containing virgin female *Pseudaletia separata*. Although his results were not conclusive he did find that females were less active in the presence of benzaldehyde than under control conditions, supporting ideas that the effect of the secretion on the female is to inhibit movement.

Electrophysiological studies have been made (Grant 1970, 1971b; Birch 1971; Grant et al. 1972) in an attempt to circumvent this behavioral block. The results of these investigations indicate that male scent brushes or even compounds identified from the scent brushes do not elicit antennal responses that are specific either with respect to sex tested or to chemical compounds employed; nor in general is there any difference between male and female responsiveness. It seems that no consistent distinction can be drawn between electroantennograms (EAGs) produced by scent-brush compounds and related chemicals (Birch 1971; Grant et al. 1972). In contrast, the female sex pheromones in Lepidoptera usually have lower threshold values than any other chemicals related or not, and produce larger EAGs than other compounds at concentrations within the normal physiological range (Grant et al. 1972).

The conclusion must be that the ability to perceive an odor stimulus is not necessarily correlated with naturally intraspecific biologically active compounds. Further behavioral evidence is needed to determine which component(s) are actually the pheromones.

7.4.3. Evolution of male aphrodisiacs in Lepidoptera

The immediate function of the male pheromones from both the hair-pencils of the Daniinae and the brush-organs of the Noctuidae is to cause inhibition of locomotion in the female, promoting successful mating by blocking her normal escape-flight response to a strange object. In addition to this immediate effect there is also the possibility that the pheromone may also function in a number of other ways: (1) as a species-specific signal to prevent cross breeding; (2) as a primer pheromone to initiate oogenesis; (3) to deter other males; (4) to repel predators.

(1) One immediately attractive theory is that the male pheromones provide a species-specific signal preventing cross-mating, particularly since now we know that considerable cross-attraction occurs to synthetic pheromones and to some extent naturally (Jacobson 1972). However, several species of Noctuidae appear to have similar or identical male pheromones (fig. 7.3). In particular, three species of *Leucania* all produce a mixture of benzaldehyde and *iso*-butyric acid in the same ratio (80/20). All these species can occur in the same locality in England. All have larvae which apparently feed on the same variety of common grasses and all emerge at the same time of year. It is possible that the female sex pheromones are different, but the male antennae of each species respond equally (EAG) to the female pheromones of the other two. The only obvious difference is that each species flies at a different though overlapping time of the night (Birch unpublished). EAG recordings from several noctuid species indicate that the male scent brushes and compounds isolated from them are very unspecific. So far no threshold differences have been found for substances from one species as opposed to another. For example, Grant (1971b) found that eight noctuid species all responded similarly to the hair-pencils of *Trichoplusia ni*. Working with *Pseudaletia unipuncta* Grant et al. (1972) also found that both male and female antennae responded equally well to each chemical extracted from the brushes (fig. 7.3) and that scent brush compounds were no more stimulating than other compounds. Any specificity in the Noctuidae remains to be found.

There is little more evidence for specificity in the Danaiinae. Chemicals are different for each of the species identified (fig. 7.1), although only one, the ketone, has been shown to have biological activity. Antennae of the monarch (which lacks the ketone) respond equally to hair-pencils of the queen, to *Lycorea ceres*, and to the pure ketone.

(2) Pliske and Eisner (1969) suggested that, since the diol from the hair-pencils of *Danaus gilippus* has some chemical similarities to farnesol – a juvenile hormone mimic, it might stimulate yolk deposition during oogenesis. Topical administration during courtship would be perfect timing for a hormone acting in this way. However, this exciting possibility seems at most to be a very minor effect, if it occurs at all. Virgin females hand-paired to males lacking the hair-pencils produced normal numbers of viable offspring, nor did the diol later show any juvenile hormone activity when tested in *Pyrrhocoris*.

(3) Several males may compete to copulate with a receptive female possibly resulting in delayed copulation, no copulation, or attraction of predators to the scene. If so, it would be an advantage to the female or to the first male to be able to shut off female pheromone production or to deter males from approaching. It is conceivable, though quite hypothetical at this time, that the male pheromone could act in these ways in addition to inhibiting female locomotion. We only know that males of several Noctuidae (Grant 1971b; Grant et al. 1972) and Danaiinae (Schneider and Seibt 1969) are capable of perceiving their own pheromone.

(4) The last function postulated is that of deterrence to predators. One reason why this is likely is that the compounds so far identified from the male brushes are similar to defensive secretions. Benzaldehyde has been implicated as a possible antibacterial agent in aquatic Dytiscidae (Gilmour 1965), and as a defensive compound of an ant (Blum et al. 1969) and of numerous Diplopoda (Weatherston and Percy 1970). *Iso*-butyric acid is also a defensive compound in a wide range of insects (e.g. Schildknecht et al. 1968; Eisner et al. 1970; Pattendon and Staddon 1972). The second reason is that the copulation period in moths may last from a few minutes to several hours, either immobile on the ground or in clumsy flight, and is undoubtedly a very vulnerable period in the life of moths. There would be a considerable selective advantage to predators able to key in to the sex pheromones of their prey. This is well documented in other orders (e.g. Borden ch. 8 sect. 5). A predator could also respond to the site of increased activity when several males are attracted to a female, bats to moths, for example; production of a deterrent would then be selected for and if used only when male and female are in proximity, might also explain why a defensive substance should be found only in one sex.

The extreme range of male scent structures in Lepidoptera indicates considerable parallel evolution and convergence. Male structures may take the form of brush-organs, as in the Noctuidae (Birch 1970b); brushes associated with the genitalia, as in *Trichoplusia ni* (Grant 1971a); coremata, the eversible tubes inflated with air found in numerous Arctiidae, Geometridae, and some Noctuidae (Varley 1962); or small tufts of hair or brushes on almost any part of the body. In spite of this variety, there are basic requirements common to all – a glandular source of secretion, storage area and modified scales for distribution. The eversible tubes (coremata) or the lever arrangement of the Noctuidae are both mechanisms for opening their brushes rapidly and thus disseminating the scent material with considerable force, a factor apparently common to brush-organs wherever they are located. Observations of the mating behavior of other moths indicates that coremata and other male brushes are used in a similar way to the Danaiinae (Brower et al. 1965) and Noctuidae (Birch 1970a; Grant 1970). The brushes of *Plusia gamma* and *P. chrysitis* (L.) and the coremata of *Xanthorhoe ferrugata* (Clerck.) (fig. 7.2) and *X. fluctuata* (L.) (Geometridae) are everted by the males just before attempting to engage the genitalia (Birch 1970a). However, some species with well developed organs, such as *Spilosoma lubricipeda* (L.) (Arctiidae) will copulate readily in the laboratory without using them (Birch 1969, 1970a).

Just as the range of structures throughout the Lepidoptera indicates powerful evolutionary pressures to develop male scent disseminating organs, the number with partial organs indicates that it has just as clearly been advantageous for many species to lose the structures again. Deployment of a male pheromone is evidently a fundamental phenomenon, 'relatively ancient and invariable in principle, but deployed by mechanisms which are highly specialized and adapted to the individual requirements of each species' (McColl 1969). The question remains as to how the male brush-organs, hair-pencils and coremata originally evolved. Miriam Rothschild proposed the idea (quoted in Birch 1970c) that insect attractants and courtship pheromones evolved in connection with food plant odors. A character fulfilling the double function of linking flowers and pollinators in time and space would have a much better chance of selection than one with a single beneficial attribute. Their role as courtship pheromones would have subsequently diverged and developed from this and the odors strengthened to function both as courtship pheromones and possibly as deterrents to other species.

Brower (1963) suggested that a complex male scent apparatus was more likely to develop in those species or groups where visual signals are reduced or confusing, such as Müllerian mimics, in order to overcome the potential difficulty of visual recognition between species. This may be one way in which selective pressures would encourage the development of scent-organs. However, Vane-Wright (1972) points out that many Müllerian groups lack a complex scent apparatus whereas several sex-limited mimics do have scent-organs. There is clearly no universal evolutionary route towards scent-organs and no simple connection between their presence or absence and the ability to become sexually dimorphic, polymorphic or mimetic in any particular fashion. Visual information might indeed be confused or minimal in the nocturnal Lepidoptera, though, as noted, scent-organs are certainly not universal for these families nor are they known to be involved in species recognition. It seems equally feasible that they should have been selected for as deterrents.

The brush-organs of the Sphingidae may now be at this stage of development. Many sphingid species have complex male abdominal brush-organs (Birch 1969; Grant and Eaton 1973), which are everted as part of a warning/defensive display when handled or disturbed. This may be the primitive function of male scent organs in general (Birch 1970c), but it is difficult to see how only one sex could develop such a defensive mechanism unless the defensive function arose secondarily (Grant and Eaton 1973) or coincidentally with a sexual function. There is virtually no evidence as to the real function of the sphingid brushes.

A different line of development could have been by specializing from a more generalized male sex pheromone. For example, males of *Achroia grisella* (Fabr.), the lesser waxmoth, produce an attractant pheromone: the female, as far as is known, produces no sex pheromone. The male pheromone attracts females and, together with auditory stimuli, facilitates copulation (Dahm et al. 1971). This may have been the primitive role of male aphrodisiac pheromones with the attractant function being later taken over by the female.

All we can say at present is that the male pheromones and their organs of production have evolved by some means, that they have evolved independently many times, and also have been lost very many times. The selection pressures behind their evolution (and subsequent loss) may be one or many, probably the latter. However, where they exist, the male pheromones are used in courtship behavior in such a way that they are clearly within the category – aphrodisiac pheromones.

7.5. Conclusion

There is a distinct group of pheromones which mediate behavior patterns immediately prior to copulation. They are sex pheromones, i.e., produced by either the male or the female, but in contrast to the female sex attractant pheromones, they are employed after the sexes have been brought together. Such close-range pheromones may evoke a direct copulatory attempt or they may initiate a different behavioral response, such as feeding or inhibition of locomotion, which itself facilitates copulation. The term aphrodisiac is widely used to describe this phenomenon, but care should be exercised in its use because of anthropomorphism, the tendency of anecdotal observations to be given more credence than they deserve, and the assumption that an aphrodisiac is always successful. Male aphrodisiacs are widespread and most well known from the Lepidoptera, but even in this group we know little about the initimate behavioral interactions, the role of these pheromones in the population biology of the insects, or their significance in evolution.

Acknowledgments

Many thanks are especially due to J. R. Clearwater and G. G. Grant for making unpublished material available and to U. E. Brady, G. G. Grant and C. R. Pantle for their generous help in reviewing the chapter.

References

Aplin, R. T. and M. C. Birch (1968) Pheromones from the abdominal brushes of male noctuid Lepidoptera. Nature (London) 217, 1127–1128.

Aplin, R. T. and M. C. Birch (1970) Identification of odorous compounds from male Lepidoptera. Experientia 26, 1193–1194.

August, C. J. (1971) The role of male and female pheromones in the mating behaviour of *Tenebrio molitor*. J. Insect Physiol. 17, 739–751.

Baldwin, W. F., A. G. Knight and K. R. Lynn (1970) A sex pheromone in the insect *Rhodnius prolixus*. Can. Entomol. 103, 18–22.

Bartell, R. J., H. H. Shorey and L. Barton-Browne (1969) Pheromonal stimulation of the sexual activity of the males of the sheep blowfly *Lucilia cuprina* (Calliphoridae) by the female. Anim Behav. 17, 576–585.

Barth, R. H., Jr. (1964) The mating behavior of *Byrsotria fumigata* (Guerin) (Blattidae, Blaberinae) Behaviour 23, 1–30.

Barth, R. H. (1970) The mating behaviour of *Periplaneta americana* (Linnaeus) and *Blatta orientalis* Linnaeus (Blattaria, Blattinae) with notes on three additional species of *Periplaneta* and interspecific action of female sex pheromones. Z. Tierpsychol. 27, 722–748.

Birch, M. C. (1969) Scent organs in male Lepidoptera. D. Phil. thesis (University of Oxford) 178 pp.

Birch, M. C. (1970a) Pre-courtship use of abdominal brushes by the nocturnal moth, *Phlogophora meticulosa* (L.) (Lepidoptera: Noctuidae). Anim. Behav. 18, 310–316.

Birch, M. C. (1970b) Structure and function of the pheromone-producing brush-organs in males of *Phlogophora meticulosa* (L.) (Lepidoptera: Noctuidae). Trans. Roy. Entomol. Soc. (London) 122, 277–292.

Birch, M. C. (1970c) Persuasive scents in moth sex life. Nat. Hist. 79, 34–39, 72.

Birch, M. C. (1971) Intrinsic limitations in the use of electroantennograms to bioassay male pheromones in Lepidoptera. Nature (London) 233, 57–58.

Birch, M. C. (1972) Male abdominal brush-organs in British noctuid moths and their value as a taxonomic character. (Part I) Entomologist 105, 185–205. (Part II) Entomologist 105, 233–244.

Blum, M. S., F. Padovani, A. Curley and R. E. Hawk (1969) Benzaldehyde: a defensive secretion of a harvester ant. Comp. Biochem. Physiol. 29, 461–465.

Brady, U. E., J. H. Tumlinson, R. G. Brownlee and R. M. Silverstein (1971) Sex stimulant and attractant in the indian meal moth and in the almond moth. Science 171, 802–804.

Brower, L. P. (1963) Evolution of sex-limited mimicry in butterflies. Proc. XVIth Int. Congr. Zool. 4, 173–179.

Brower, L. P., J. v. Z. Brower and F. P. Cranston (1965) Courtship behaviour of the queen butterfly, *Danaus gilippus berenice* (Cramer). Zoologica (New York) 50, 1–39.

Butler, C. G. (1967a) Insect pheromones. Biol. Rev. Cambridge Phil. Soc. 42, 42–87.

Butler, C. G. (1967b) A sex attractant acting as an aphrodisiac in the honey bee (*Apis mellifera* L.) Proc. Roy. Entomol. Soc. London Ser. A, 42, 71–76.

Butler, C. G. (1971) The mating behaviour of the honey bee (*Apis mellifera* L.). J. Entomol. 46, 1–11.

Butler, C. G. and E. M. Fairey (1964) Pheromones of the honey bee: biological studies of the mandibular secretion of the queen. J. Apicult. Res. 3, 65–76.

Callow, R. K., J. R. Chapman and P. N. Paton (1964) Pheromones of the honey bee: chemical studies of the mandibular gland secretion of the queen. J. Apicult. Res. 3, 77–89.

Clearwater, J. R. (1972) Chemistry and function of a pheromone produced by the male of the southern armyworm *Pseudaletia separata*. J. Insect Physiol. 18, 781–789.

Clearwater, J. R. and V. Sarafis (1973) The secretory cycle of a gland involved in pheromone production in the noctuid moth, *Pseudaletia separata*. J. Insect Physiol. 19, 19–28.

Dahm, K. D., D. Meyer, W. E. Finn, V. Reinhold and H. Röller (1971) The olfactory and auditory mediated sex attraction in *Achroia grisella* (Fabr.). Naturwissenschaften 58, 265–266.

Dalla-Torre, K. W. v. (1885) Die Duftapparate der Schmetterlinge. Kosmos (Stuttgart) 2, 354–423.

Dethier, V. G., L. Barton-Browne and C. N. Smith (1960) The designation of chemicals in terms of the responses they elicit from insects. J. Econ. Entomol. 53, 134–136.

Doane, C. C. (1968) Aspects of mating behavior of the gypsy moth. Ann. Entomol. Soc. Am. 61, 768–773.

Eisner, T., T. E. Pliske, M. Ikeda, D. F. Owen, L. Vásquez, H. Pérez, J. G. Franclemont and J. Meinwald (1970) Defense mechanisms of arthropods. XXVII. Osmeterial secretions of papilionid caterpillars (*Baronia, Papilio, Eurytides*). Ann. Entomol. Soc. Am. 63, 914–915.

Gabbutt, P. D. (1954) Notes on the mating behaviour of *Nemobius sylvestris* (Bosc.) (Orth., Gryllidae). Brit. J. Animal Behav. 2, 84–88.

Gary, N. E. (1970) Pheromones of the honeybee, *Apis mellifera* L. *In*: Control of Insect Behavior by Natural Products; eds.: D. L. Wood, R. M. Silverstein and M. Nakajima (Academic Press; N. Y.) pp. 29–54.

Gilmour, D. (1965) The Metabolism of Insects (Oliver and Boyd, Edinburgh.) pp. 343.

Grant, G. G. (1970) Evidence for a male sex pheromone in the noctuid *Trichoplusia ni*. Nature (London) 227, 1345–1346.

Grant, G. G. (1971a) Scent apparatus of the male cabbage looper, *Trichoplusia ni*. Ann. Entomol. Soc. Am. 64, 347–352.

Grant, G. G. (1971b) Electroantennogram responses to the scent brush secretions of several male moths. Ann. Entomol. Soc. Am. 64, 1428–1431.

Grant, G. G. (1972) Courtship behaviour of phycitid moths. Section C. Joint meeting of the Entomological Societies of America, Canada and Quebec, Montreal, Nov. 26–30, 1972.

Grant, G. G. and J. L. Eaton (1973) Scent brushes of the male tobacco hornworm *Manduca sexta* (Lepidoptera, Sphingidae). Ann. Entomol. Soc. Am. (in press).

Grant, G. G., U. E. Brady and J. M. Brand (1972) Male armyworm scent brush secretion: identification and electroantennogram study of major components. Ann. Entomol. Soc. Am. 65, 1224–1227.

Gurney, A. B. (1947) A new species of *Pristoceuthopilus* from Oregon and remarks on certain special glands of Orthoptera. J. Wash. Acad. Sci. 37, 430–435.

Happ, G. M. (1969) Multiple sex pheromones of the mealworm beetle, *Tenebrio molitor* L. Nature (London) 222, 80–81.

Humphries, D. A. (1967) The mating behaviour of the hen flea *Ceratophyllus gallinae* (Schrank) (Siphonaptera: Insecta). Anim. Behav. 15, 82–90.

Jacobson, M. (1972) Insect Sex Pheromones (Academic Press, New York) 392 pp.

Kennedy, J. S. (1972) The emergence of behaviour. J. Aust. Entomol. Soc. 11, 168–176.

Matthes, D. (1962) Excitatoren und Paarungsverhalten mitteleuropäischer Malachiiden. Z. Morphol. Oekol. Tiere 51, 375–546.

McColl, H. P. (1969) The sexual scent organs of male Lepidoptera. M. Sc. Thesis (University College of Swansea, Wales) 214 pp.

Meinwald, J., A. M. Chalmers, T. E. Pliske and T. Eisner (1968) Pheromones. III. Identification of *trans, trans*-10-hydroxy-3, 7-dimethyl-2, 6-decadienoic acid as a major component in 'hair-pencilling' secretion of the male monarch butterfly. Tetrahedron Lett. 47, 4893–4896.

Meinwald, J., A. M. Chalmers, T. E. Pliske and T. Eisner (1969a) Identification and synthesis of *trans, trans*-3,7-dimethyl-2,6-decadien-1,10-dioic acid, a component of the pheromonal secretion of the male monarch butterfly. Chem. Commun. 1969, 86–87.

Meinwald, J., Y. C. Meinwald and P. H. Mazzocchi (1969b) Sex pheromone of the queen butterfly: chemistry. Science 164, 1174–1175.

Meinwald, J., Y. C. Meinwald, J. M. Wheeler, T. Eisner and L. P. Brower (1966) Major components in the exocrine secretion of a male butterfly (*Lycorea*). Science 151, 583–585.

Meinwald, J., W. R. Thompson, T. Eisner and D. F. Owen (1971) Pheromones. VII. African monarch: major components of the hair-pencil secretion. Tetrahedron Lett. 38, 3485–3488.

Morse, R. A., N. E. Gary and T. S. Johansson (1962) Mating of virgin queen honey bees (*Apis mellifera* L.) following mandibular gland extirpation. Nature (London) 194, 605.

Müller, F. (1874) The habits of various insects. Nature (London) 10, 102–103.

Müller, F. (1877) Über Haarpinzel, Filzfleche und ähnliche Gebilde auf den Flügeln männlicher Schmetterlinge. Jena Z. Naturw. 9, 99.

Müller, F. (1878) Scent organs in butterflies. Trans. Entomol. Soc. (London) 1878, 211–221.

Myers, J. and L. P. Brower (1969) A behavioural analysis of the courtship pheromone receptors of the queen butterfly, *Danaus gilippus berenice*. J. Insect Physiol. 15, 2117–2130.

Pagden, H. T. (1957) The presence of coremata in *Creatonotus gangis* (L.) (Lepidoptera: Arctiidae) Proc. Roy. Entomol. Soc. London Ser. A, 32, 90–94.

Pantle, C. (1971) The use of electroantennograms to study olfactory responses of the milkweed bug, *Oncopeltus fasciatus*. Ph. D. Thesis (St. Louis University).

Pattenden, G. and B. W. Staddon (1972) Identification of *iso*-butyric acid in secretion from Brindley's scent glands in *Rhodnius prolixis* (Heteroptera: Reduviidae). Ann. Entomol. Soc. Am. 65, 1240–1241.

Pliske, T. E. and T. Eisner (1969) Sex pheromone of the queen butterfly: biology. Science 164, 1170–1172.

Pritchard, G. (1967) Laboratory observations on the mating behaviour of the island fruit fly, *Rioxa pornia* (Diptera: Tephritidae). J. Aust. Entomol. Soc. 6, 127–132.

Riddiford, L. M. (1967) Trans-2-hexenal: mating stimulant for polyphemus moths. Science 158, 139–141.

Roth, L. M. (1952) The tergal gland of the male cockroach *Supella supellectilicum*. J. Morphol. 91, 469–477.

Roth, L. M. (1962) Hypersexual activity induced in females of the cockroach *Nauphoeta cinerea*. Science 138, 1267–1269.

Roth, L. M. (1965) Loci of sensory end-organs used by cockroaches in mating behavior. Proc. 12th Int. Congr. Entomol., London 1964, 305.

Roth, L. M. and R. H. Barth, Jr. (1964) The control of sexual receptivity in female cockroaches. J. Insect Physiol. 10, 965–975.

Roth, L. M. and G. P. Dateo (1966) A sex pheromone produced by males of the cockroach *Nauphoeta cinerea*, J. Insect Physiol. 12, 255-265.

Roth, L. M. and E. R. Willis (1952) A study of cockroach behavior. Am. Midland Naturalist 47, 66–129.

Schildknecht, H., H. Winkler and U. Maschwitz (1968) Vergleichend chemische Untersuchungen der Inhaltsstoffe der Pygidialwehrblasen von Carabiden. Z. Naturforsch. 236, 637–644.

Schneider, D. and V. Seibt (1969) Sex pheromone of the queen butterfly: electroantennogram responses. Science 164, 1173–1174.

Shorey, H. H. (1973) Behavioral responses to insect pheromones. Ann. Rev. Entomol. 18, 349–380.

Shorey, H. H. and R. J. Bartell (1970) Role of a volatile female sex pheromone in stimulating male courtship behaviour in *Drosophila melanogaster*. Anim. Behav. 18, 159–164.

Shorey, H. H. and L. K. Gaston (1970) Sex pheromones of noctuid moths. XX. Short-range visual orientation by pheromone-stimulated males of *Trichoplusia ni*. Ann. Entomol. Soc. Am. 63, 829–832.

Stobbe, R. H. (1912) Die abdominalen Duftorgane der männlichen Sphingiden und Noctuiden. Zool. Jb. 32, 493–632.

Tinbergen, N. (1951) The Study of Instinct (Oxford Univ. Press) 228 pp.

Tinbergen, N., B. J. D. Meeuse, L. K. Boerema and W. W. Varossieau (1942) Die Balz des Samtfalters, *Eumenis* (=*Satyrus*) *semele* (L.). Z. Tierspychol. 5, 182–226.

Traynier, R. M. M. (1968) Sex attraction in the Mediterranean flour moth, *Anagasta kühniella*; location of the female by the male. Can. Entomol. 100, 5–10.

Vane-Wright, R. I. (1972) Pre-courtship activity and a new scent organ in butterflies. Nature (London) 239, 338–340.

Varley, G. C. (1962) A plea for a new look at Lepidoptera with special reference to the scent distributing organs of male moths. Trans. Soc. Brit. Entomol. 15, 3–40.

Weatherston, J. and J. E. Percy (1970) Arthropod defensive secretion. *In*: Chemicals Controlling Insect Behavior; ed.: M. Beroza (Academic Press, New York) pp. 95–144.

CHAPTER 8

Aggregation pheromones in the Scolytidae

John H. BORDEN

8.1. Introduction

Insect aggregation pheromones cause 'other members of the same species to aggregate in a particular area' (Shorey 1973). With a few possible exceptions, they occur throughout the family Scolytidae (Coleoptera) (Borden and Stokkink 1971), in which large numbers of beetles of both sexes are characteristically attracted. Thus, the pheromones serve as population aggregation pheromones. In the majority of scolytid species, the beetles construct galleries in living or recently felled trees – bark beetles in the phloem tissue, and ambrosia (timber) beetles in the xylem tissue. These habits render scolytid beetles extremely important pests of forests and timber, particularly in North America (Davidson and Prentice 1967). It is well known that scolytids aggregate in great numbers in a mass attack on selected hosts. This mass attack (aggregation) is considered essential to overcome the resistance of a living host tree (Anderson 1948) or to utilize temporary habitats to their fullest extent (Atkins 1966a).

The possibility that scolytids use odor to help them find their host was investigated as early as 1916 (Miller and Keen 1960). However, Anderson (1948) produced the first evidence for population aggregation pheromones. Male *Ips pini* (Say) boring in pine logs produced an odor which attracted large numbers of beetles from the surrounding forest. Since that time, pheromones which promote population aggregation have been demonstrated in over 30 species (Borden and Stokkink 1971). Chemical identifications and/or structures have been described for the pheromones of several species (see table 8.1). A considerable body of data has also accumulated on behavior and ecology related to pheromone production and response in scolytid beetles and their insect associates (Borden and Stokkink 1971).

It is generally agreed that the processes of host selection and mass attack take place in a sequence of genetically controlled, behavioral events. Wood (1972) groups the behavioral events into three phases for the western pine beetle, *Dendroctonus brevicomis* LeConte: dispersal and selection, concentration (aggregation), and establishment. My interpretation of how each phase applies to the individual behavioral components of a scolytid population can be seen in fig. 8.1. A fundamental basis of such a behavioral sequence must be that the insect encounters a 'series of take-it-or-leave-it situations' as described by Thorsteinson (1960) for food-plant selection. An insect will proceed from one type of behavior to another, only when its internal physiological condition, and the external environment are favorable (a 'take-it' situation), i.e. when the environment *permits* a given type of behavior to occur.

If one generalizes sufficiently, the sequence of behavioral steps turns out to be relatively simple (fig. 8.1). The complexity lies in the multitude of different beetle and host species, environmental stimuli and interaction between them, a multiplicity of pheromone compounds produced by either or both sexes, and various perception and response mechanisms which may vary according to the genetic constitution and physiological state of the insect.

It is the intent of this chapter to describe the essential biological role of aggregation pheromones in the processes of scolytid host selection and mass attack as outlined in fig. 8.1. In addition, the role of scolytid pheromones in guiding associated insects to scolytid-attacked hosts will be examined as outlined in fig. 8.2. Specific examples are taken from well researched species to illustrate each step. It is not the intent of this chapter to explore the chemical nature of aggregating pheromones, chemical methodology or the practical use of pheromones.

8.2. *Dispersal*

The conditions under which beetles emerge and take flight determine the availability of insects, the occurrence of the first attack on a new host, and the environment in which beetles must produce and respond to aggregating pheromones, ultimately leading to a mass attack. Emergence and flight are apparently very similar for scolytids of both sexes.

8.2.1. *Emergence*

Most bark and timber beetles emerge from the host in which they have matured, either directly following maturation, or after an overwintering period. Some species emerge from a second (overwintering) host to which they migrated following maturation in the brood host. A third group emerges after spending the winter in a non-host substrate such as litter and duff on the forest floor. Precise seasonal timing is important. The beetles must emerge into a hospitable environment. Generally, temperature must be favorable and rainfall absent so that flight may occur. The new host must be in an acceptable state. For example, new cones must be available for *Conophthorus* spp., winter snow-break and wind-throw trees must be available for ambrosia beetles, or host tree carbohydrate content and composition must be optimal (Pitman 1966). Diel timing is also important, e.g. a crepuscular emergence

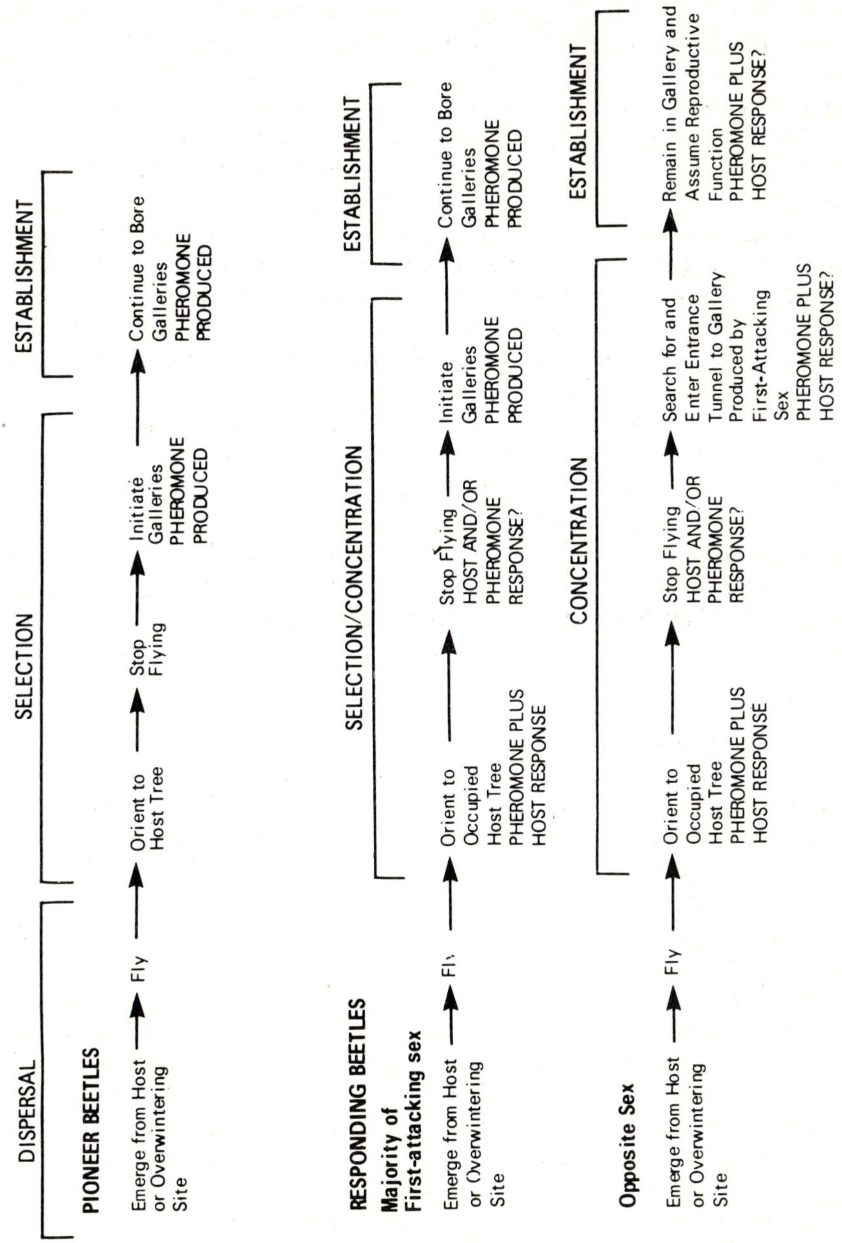

Fig. 8.1. Generalized behavioral sequence in host selection and mass attack by scolytid beetles. Key steps in which aggregation pheromones are known or suspected to play a part are identified.

may serve to avoid adversely high mid-day temperature, or may coincide with maximum activity and pheromone production by prospective mates (Borden 1967).

There are two important internal factors which influence emergence: general physiological readiness and biological rhythms. Physiological readiness may require a maturation feeding. For example, development of flight muscles in *Ips paraconfusus* Lanier* must occur prior to emergence (Borden and Slater 1969a). Diapause must also be terminated, enabling beetles to respond to environmental stimuli. Flight muscles of *Dendroctonus pseudotsugae* Hopkins do not mature while the insect is in diapause (Ryan 1959) and *Trypodendron lineatum* (Olivier), while appearing normal, will not mate while in a winter reproductive diapause (Fockler and Borden 1972). Only for *Xyleborus ferrugineus* (F.) is there extensive evidence that emergence and subsequent flight are under control of a true circadian rhythm (Saunders 1967). However, emergence and flight rhythms often show distinct, predictable diel periodicity (Gara and Vité 1962; Cameron and Borden 1967; Daterman et al. 1965), which may, in fact, reflect endogenous circadian rhythms.

A beetle which has received all the necessary internal feedback information is ready to emerge. Its flight muscles are functional, energy reserves adequate, sensory systems operational, and the alarm bell is ringing on its internal clock. Temperature is apparently the most important environmental factor regulating emergence, possibly because the majority of sites from which the beetles emerge are continually dark and humid. If all internal and external conditions are favorable the beetle will emerge by chewing and/or crawling its way to the surface of a given substrate.

8.2.2. Flight

The emergent beetle is exposed to new environmental conditions such as sunlight, fluctuating relative humidity, wind and heat. At this point in their life cycle, scolytids are characteristically flight positive. Many of the physiological criteria governing emergence must also govern readiness to fly. In addition, emergence periodicity is apparently reflected in the diel flight rhythms of many scolytids (Daterman et al. 1965; Gara 1963; Vité et al. 1964). The environmental conditions most known to determine flight initiation are temperature, light and humidity (Henson 1962; Perttunen and Boman 1965; Borden 1967). For *Conophthorus coniperda* (Schwarz) Henson (1962) observed that '. . .the preflight conditions which lead to the most extensive flight are high humidity in the period between emergence and flight. Maximum flight will take place between 27 and 35 °C and after about 9 hr of light'. He concluded that' . . .the peak of flight may be expected in the early afternoon on bright, dry days following a period of weather which would permit drying of the litter'. Thus, the beetle is under quite precise control by

* Prior to Lanier (1970), referred to in literature as *Ips confusus* (LeConte).

its external environment and can presumably most readily initiate flight in environmental conditions favoring dispersal, host selection and response to pheromones.

8.3. *Pioneer beetles*

8.3.1. *Selection and concentration*

Orientation to host: As a general rule, if the scolytid species is monogamous, as in the genus *Dendroctonus*, females are the first-attacking sex. In polygamous genera such as *Ips*, males initiate the attack. There are some exceptions. For example, *Gnathotrichus sulcatus* (LeConte) is monogamous, but males initiate the attack. Characteristically, a very few beetles of the first-attacking sex make the initial attack on a new host. These are commonly referred to as 'pioneer' beetles. The remaining beetles of the first-attacking sex face a different behavioral task since they orient to a host already attacked by pioneer beetles, which by then may possibly have been joined by their prospective mates. However, for such phenomena as physiological release of host-positive response, cessation of flight, initiation and establishment of galleries, and pheromone production, all beetles of the first-attacking sex are apparently similar.

Early research, primarily on the western pine beetle, *Dendroctonus brevicomis*, resulted in considerable (still unresolved) controversy as to whether the pioneer beetle attack is directed to selected hosts due to a primary (host) attraction, or occurs at random. The various arguments have recently been reviewed by Wood (1972). The *D. brevicomis* controversy has stimulated research on many other scolytids and for the majority of species investigated, primary attraction is a fact. The ambrosia beetles, *Trypodendron lineatum* (Moeck 1970, 1971) and *Gnathotrichus sulcatus* (Cade et al. 1970; Moeck 1971) are attracted to ethanol, apparently produced by anaerobic metabolism in potential hosts (Graham 1968), very much in line with Person's (1931) hypothesis for *Dendroctonus brevicomis.* Species such as *Ips paraconfusus* (Wood 1963), *Dendroctonus pseudotsugae* (Chapman 1963), and *Scolytus ventralis* LeConte (Ferrell 1971) are attracted to uninfested natural hosts. Other studies (Rudinsky 1966b; Perttunen et al. 1970; Oksanen et al. 1970) indicate that host volatiles such as monoterpenes and terpene alcohols serve as primary olfactory attractants. Visual cues may also be important in host selection. For example, *Conophthorus coniperda* orients to silhouettes following an initial photopositive flight (Henson 1962) and *Dendroctonus ponderosae* Hopkins orients most readily to horizontally placed 'log' configuration olfactometers (Pitman and Vité 1969).

Orientation to a host (or to aggregation pheromones) must inevitably be in opposition to dispersal behavior. The behavioral transition involved has been investigated for aphids (Kennedy and Booth 1963a, b) and can be explained in terms of shifting stimulus threshold levels (Johnson 1969). At the beginning of the dispersal phase, the insect has a very low threshold for dispersal stimuli, but a very high threshold for host-positive stimuli. In other words, it would require an extremely intense host stimulus to divert it from dispersal to host orientation. However, after a given flight period, the insect becomes able to respond to a normal stimulus from its host.

Such a flight-dependent, behavioral reversal was discovered by Graham (1959, 1962) for *Trypodendron lineatum.* Subsequently, other researchers unsuccessfully searched for similar mechanisms in other scolytids, e.g. *Ips paraconfusus* (Gara 1963; Borden 1967). However, Graham's (1959, 1962) hypothesis of release from photopositive domination by flight has recently been verified in the laboratory for two scolytids. Female *Dendroctonus pseudotsugae* which were host-negative became host-positive after varying amounts of flight exercise (Atkins 1966b). In addition, Bennett and Borden (1971) found that only after 30 and 90 min of flight on a flight mill would *Trypodendron lineatum* and *Dendroctonus pseudotsugae*, respectively, respond to the odor of pheromone-laden frass by ceasing flight. Graham (1961) hypothesized that *Trypodendron lineatum* swallowed air in flight and developed a large ventricular air bubble, which could provide an internal feedback indication of flight duration. However, ventricular air bubbles have been found in *T. lineatum* which were denied flight (C. E. Fockler and J. H. Borden unpublished results), and stationary *Dendroctonus pseudotsugae* were observed to swallow air on exposure to temperatures conducive to flight (Bennett and Borden 1971).

An alternative threshold determination system may occur in the lipid metabolism of scolytid beetles. Atkins (1966b) found that *D. pseudotsugae* with more than 20% total lipid (per dry weight) were flight-positive and host-negative. Beetles with less than 20% lipid could still fly, but were host-positive if given the appropriate stimuli. Thus, beetles with great energy reserves could afford the luxury of extended dispersal, while beetles with minimal reserves would respond to the first new host and/or pheromone encountered and would conserve their energy reserves for reproduction. In support of the lipid metabolism hypothesis Thompson and Bennett (1971) showed that there was selective oxidation of mono-unsaturated fatty acids (C 16:1 and C 18:1) by male *D. pseudotsugae* in flight. Thus Atkins' (1969) hypothesis that behavioral changes may be stimulated through the accumulation of selective metabolic by-products may be correct.

Cessation of flight: Once a beetle is in the proximity of a host, flight must be inhibited. There is evidence that cessation of flight occurs in response to olfactory stimuli (Borden and Bennett 1969; Bennett and Borden 1971). Preflown *D. pseudotsugae* females (the first-attacking sex) on flight mills ceased flight on exposure to the odor of Douglas-fir phloem tissue, but not to the odor of pheromone-laden frass. Such a selective response could inhibit female beetles from landing on heavily attacked hosts, thus avoiding overcrowding and partially explaining the 'switching phenomenon' by which the center of *Dendroctonus frontalis* Zimmerman aggregation is shifted to unattacked trees (Gara and Coster 1968).

Initiation of galleries: The next key behavior performed by pioneer beetles is to begin to bore into the potential host on which they have alighted. Although the initiation of feeding by scolytids is not extensively researched, in *Scolytus multistriatus* (Marsham) chemical stimuli are known to be predominant. Feeding is deterred by juglone (5-hydroxy-1,4-naphthoquinone) from the bark of the non-host, *Carya ovata* (Mill) K. Koch which must be distinguished from host elms (Gilbert et al. 1967). On *Ulmus americana* L. the beetle is stimulated to feed by the bark tissue chemicals (+)-catechin-5-β-D-xylopyranoside and lupeyl cerotate (Doskotch et al. 1970).

Also significant is the recent report that female *Dendroctonus* stridulate when initiating an attack (Rudinsky and Michael 1973). Thus, female *Dendroctonus* (and other scolytids of the first-attacking sex) might communicate by means of both pheromones and sound, a communication system which could partially explain the non-random (evenly spaced) distribution of galleries observed in *D. ponderosae* (Shepherd 1965) and *Scolytus ventralis* (Berryman 1968). Such spacing would serve to minimize intraspecific competition in scolytid broods.

Pheromone production: At some point before, during or following the initiation of boring activity, pioneer beetles (and others of the first-attacking sex) begin to produce significant amounts of aggregation pheromones. For the majority of species, these pheromones form the basis of secondary attraction, i.e., the attraction emanating from an attacked host, as opposed to primary attraction produced by an unattacked host. Some exceptions to the existence of aggregation pheromones may occur. For example, both laboratory (Oksanen et al. 1970) and field tests (Perttunen et al. 1970) indicate that *Blastophagus piniperda* L. females do not produce a pheromone. There are also some anomalous or unusual phenomena. *Leperisinus fraxini* Pz. females are the first-attacking sex, but the males produce the aggregation pheromone (Schönherr 1970). In *Dendroctonus brevicomis*, both sexes contribute to the aggregation pheromone (table 8.1) (See sect. 8.4).

In every case investigated the site of pheromone production has proven to involve the hindgut (Borden and Stokkink 1971), but the Malpighian tubules also appear to play a part. In laboratory tests, Zenther-Møller and Rudinsky (1967) found that males of *D. pseudotsugae* were arrested by ethanol extracts of the posterior portion of female hindguts. However, if two drops of Douglas-fir phloem extract were added, extracts of the anterior hindgut or Malpighian tubules caused arrestment as well. The Malpighian tubules of *Ips paraconfusus* have also been implicated in pheromone production (Pitman et al. 1965).

There is increasing information available on the mechanisms by which pheromone production and/or release is stimulated. Timing is undoubtedly of vital importance in controlling the events in mass attack by each species. For example, *Dendroctonus* species may require a rapidly released pheromone which would attract the large populations necessary to overcome resistant trees, whereas *Ips* species which attack less vigorous hosts may be better served by a pheromone released after a requisite feeding or excavation period which could indicate the suitability of a given host (Vité and Pitman 1968).

Females of *Dendroctonus frontalis* contain and may be able to release pheromone immediately on arrival at a fresh host tree. Flying *D. frontalis* in the field responded to crushed emergent females (Renwick and Vité 1968; Vité and Renwick 1968), supporting gas chromatographic and mass spectrometric studies that pheromone is produced in the female hindgut prior to attack on a new host (Renwick and Vité 1968; Coster and Vité 1972). Extensive feeding by *D. frontalis* soon inhibits the production and release of pheromones (Vité and Pitman 1968; Coster and Vité 1972).

In other species, there appears to be a requisite excavation period in the new host before pheromone is produced. Hindguts of emergent *Trypodendron lineatum* were only marginally attractive to males (Borden and Slater 1969b) and pheromone was not released until after females initiated boring activity on a new host (Chapman 1966; Borden and Slater 1969b). The question of whether feeding is necessary for *T. lineatum* to produce pheromone is the subject of conflicting reports. In dissections of over 100 female beetles excised from host logs, J. A. Chapman (personal communication) found essentially empty guts and Borden and Slater (1969b) noted that females boring in dye-impregnated wood during the pheromone-producing period did not ingest host material. However, Schneider and Rudinsky (1969) report that pheromone is produced only when bark and wood particles are present in the hindgut site of pheromone production.

In *Ips paraconfusus*, males do not produce attractive frass or develop attraction in the hindgut until feeding has occurred and food material has passed through the gut (Wood and Bushing 1963; Pitman et al. 1965). Such data led to the hypothesis that '. . . . either a precursor is ingested and metabolized to the attractant or the metabolism of food material causes secretory activity in specialized cells' (Wood et al. 1966). However, recent studies indicate that there are two mechanisms of pheromone production in the genus *Ips* and that both mechanisms can occur in the same beetle (Vité et al. 1972). Simple exposure to pine oleoresin vapors for a few hours stimulated males of 12 *Ips* species to produce the pheromone compounds *cis*- and *trans*-verbenol, as identified by gas chromatography of excised guts. Accordingly, Vité et al. (1972) classify verbenol as a 'contact' pheromone. Such pheromones would be found in aggressive scolytid species which require rapid aggregation of large numbers of beetles to overcome host-tree resistance. The pheromone compounds, ipsenol and ipsdienol, were produced only after the male beetles had fed, and are, therefore, termed 'frass' pheromones (Vité et al. 1972).

Elucidation of pheromone biogenesis may be furthered by studies involving juvenile hormone. Treatment of *I. paraconfusus* males with large amounts (at least 25μg) of a juvenile hormone analogue (10,11-epoxyfarnesenic acid methyl ester) (EFA) caused their hindguts to become attractive to females within 18 hr (Borden et al. 1969). Therefore, a host stimulus may be mediated by the hormonal system which then induces pheromone production. Alternatively, the large amount of EFA necessary and the long time before pheromone activity appeared, suggest that EFA may have been metabolically altered by the treated beetles, possibly mimicking the metabolic alteration of similar host compounds, e.g. juvabione-like materials.

More than one pheromone compound is produced in most beetles for which the pheromone chemistry is at least partially known (table 8.1), and there is frequent synergism with compounds from the host. The roles of various pheromone compounds are discussed mainly in sect. 8.4.

8.3.2. Establishment

The final behavioral step in attack by pioneer beetles is to maintain gallery construction, i.e. for the beetles to establish themselves in a new host. On numerous occasions, one can find galleries which have been abandoned early in the initial stages of attack. Often in bark beetles this is due to the physical resistance of the tree. The beetles, at the mercy of their environment, are simply pitched out by the force of oleoresin exudation pressure (Vité and Wood 1961; Wood 1962a). However, other environmental cues such as host moisture content may be screened and assessed by the beetles, which may then vacate unsuitable hosts (Rudinsky 1962).

8.4. Responding beetles

8.4.1. Concentration

Chemical communication and orientation to host: A major and crucial event in the life of most scolytids is to orient successfully to a host containing pheromone-producing members of the first-attacking sex (fig. 8.1). This phenomenon has been both elucidated and rendered increasingly mystifying by chemical studies. When entomologists and chemists originally collaborated to tackle the problem of isolating the aggregation pheromones, they assumed that they were searching for a single compound for each species. How wrong they were! The first successful identification of scolytid pheromones in *I. paraconfusus* disclosed not one but three compounds (Silverstein et al. 1966) which act together to attract both sexes to a newly attacked host (Wood et al. 1968) (table 8.1). Moreover, it is now apparent that some pheromone compounds are shared by more than one species (table 8.1). Another exciting and fundamental discovery was that female *Dendroctonus brevicomis* produce primarily one pheromone compound, brevicomin* (Silverstein et al. 1968), while the responding males produce another, frontalin (Kinzer et al. 1969), both of which are active in the aggregation process (Vité and Pitman 1969). Finally, it was discovered that the host tree may also contribute volatile components to the chemical message (Bedard et al. 1969; Pitman 1969; Bedard et al. 1970). Thus, rather than to refer just to aggregating pheromones, it is more appropriate to speak

* Exo-brevicomin is referred to brevicomin troughout this chapter.

TABLE 8.1

Pheromones and other chemicals isolated and/or identified in the Scolytidae by May, 1973: their source and biological activity.

Species	Pheromone or other chemical[a]	Source and biological activity
Ips paraconfusus	ipsenol *cis*-verbenol ipsdienol linalool	Ipsenol, *cis*-verbenol and ipsdienol isolated and identified from male frass (Silverstein et al. 1966). In the field, all 3 synthetic compounds combined competitive with male-infested logs and attracted beetles in the same sex ratio (Wood et al. 1968). *Ips latidens* (LeConte) attracted to a mixture of ipsenol and *cis*-verbenol (Wood et al. 1967). Linalool isolated from cold-trapped volatiles, function unknown (J. C. Young, personal communication)[b].
Ips grandicollis	ipsenol	Differential diagnosis (Vité and Renwick 1970) used to identify ipsenol from male hindguts. Attractive to both sexes in the field; sex ratio more natural when deployed with *trans*-verbenol (Vité and Renwick 1971a).
Ips calligraphus	ipsdienol *cis*-verbenol *trans*-verbenol	Identified from male hindguts. Ipsdienol attractive in the field in combination with either *trans*- or (primarily) *cis*-verbenol. Addition of host volatiles produced comparable attraction to male-infested log (Renwick and Vité 1972).
Ips pini	linalool	Isolated from male frass, function unknown (J. C. Young, personal communication)[b].
Gnathotrichus sulcatus	6-methyl-5-hepten-2-ol (sulcatol)	Isolated and identified from boring dust, male hindguts and volatiles from infested logs. Synthetic compound attractive in laboratory and field[c].
Dendroctonus brevicomis	brevicomin frontalin verbenone *trans*-verbenol *endo*-brevicomin	Brevicomin isolated and identified from female frass (Silverstein et al. 1968), frontalin from male hindguts (Kinzer et al. 1969). Both pheromones, synergized principally by host terpene myrcene (Bedard et al. 1969), attractive in the field, brevicomin mainly to males and frontalin to females (Vité and Pitman 1969). Verbenone and *trans*-verbenol identified from hindguts of males and females, respectively (Renwick 1967). *Trans*-verbenol and verbenone inhibit response (Wood 1972). Verbenone proposed as attack termination factor (Renwick and Vité 1970). *Endo*-brevicomin found in females, and suggested as species-specificity-regulating pheromone in frontalin-responding *Dendroctonus* (Vité and Renwick 1971b).

Table 8.1 (continued)

Species	Pheromone or other chemical[a]	Source and biological activity
Dendroctonus frontalis	frontalin *trans*-verbenol verbenone *endo*-brevicomin	Frontalin identified in minute quantities in female hindguts (Kinzer et al. 1969). Attractive to both sexes in the field in combination with host volatiles, particularly α-pinene (Renwick and Vité 1969). *Trans*-verbenol and verbenone identified from hindguts of males and females, respectively (Renwick 1967). *Trans*-verbenol synergistic with frontalin; verbenone proposed as attack termination factor (Renwick and Vité 1970). *Endo*-brevicomin found in trace amounts in some male hindguts (Vité and Renwick 1971b). (See *D. brevicomis* for suggested function.)
Dendroctonus ponderosae	*trans*-verbenol brevicomin	*Trans*-verbenol isolated and identified from female hindguts (Pitman et al. 1968); attractive to both sexes in the field in combination with host volatiles, particularly α-pinene (Pitman 1969). Brevicomin identified from hindguts of both sexes (Pitman et al. 1969); function unknown (Renwick and Vité 1970).
Dendroctonus jeffreyi Hopkins	*trans*-verbenol brevicomin	*Trans*-verbenol identified from female hindguts, brevicomin from both sexes (Pitman et al. 1969). Function not investigated.
Dendroctonus pseudotsugae	frontalin *trans*-verbenol 3-methyl-2-cyclohexen-1-one (MCH) 3-methyl-2-cyclohexen-1-ol (seudenol)	Frontalin (Pitman and Vité 1970), *trans*-verbenol (Rudinsky et al. 1972b), MCH (Kinzer et al. 1971) and seudenol (Vité and Pitman 1972) all isolated or identified from female hindguts. Frontalin and seudenol (G. B. Pitman, personal communication)[d] in combination with host volatiles, principally camphene or α-pinene (Pitman and Vité 1970; Furniss and Schmitz 1971) attractive to both sexes in the field. *Trans*-verbenol synergistic with frontalin (Rudinsky et al. 1972b), but role unclear in other tests (Rudinsky et al. 1972a; Furniss et al. 1972). Attraction nullified by addition of MCH to an attractive mixture (Rudinsky et al. 1972a; Furniss et al. 1972).

[a] Accepted trivial names used in all possible cases. See references cited for chemical names and structures. Only compounds with demonstrated biological activity or identified by 2 or more methods, e.g. by gas-liquid chromatography and verified by mass spectrometry, are listed.

[b] Canada Agriculture, Chemistry and Biology Research Institute, Ottawa, Ontario, Canada.

[c] K. J. Byrne, A. Swigar, R. M. Silverstein, J. H. Borden and E. Stokkink. Manuscript in preparation.

[d] BTI Forest Research Laboratory, P.O. Box 1119, Grass Valley, California, 95945, U.S.A.

of secondary attraction, i.e. the complex of beetle-produced pheromones and host compounds responsible for population aggregation of a species and mass attack of the host.

Although early studies demonstrated that both sexes aggregate on or in the same host (Anderson 1948; Miller and Keen 1960), it was not at first clear that members of the first-attacking sex (with the exception of the pioneer beetles) responded to aggregation pheromones. However, the demonstration that male *Ips paraconfusus* respond to their own aggregation pheromone (Wood and Vité 1961; Wood 1962b) led to the eventual discovery that the first-attacking sex responds similarly in almost all species investigated.

The response of members of the first-attacking sex to secondary attraction is characteristically lower than that of the opposite sex (Wood and Bushing 1963; Chapman 1966; Rudinsky 1966a). In the genus *Ips*, typical response sex ratios have been obtained in field tests in which known pheromone and/or host compounds have been deployed in mixtures which attempt to mimic the odors of naturally-infested hosts (Wood et al. 1968; Vité and Renwick 1971a; Renwick and Vité 1972). However, in *Dendroctonus brevicomis*, the sex ratio of responding beetles is apparently regulated by the changing concentration of particular pheromone and host compounds (Vité and Pitman 1969, 1970; Renwick and Vité 1970). Comparative response behavior of *Ips paraconfusus* has been studied in the laboratory (Wood and Bushing 1963). Females respond in a " 'point' or 'straight line' orientation", while the response of males, the first-attacking sex, was characterized as an " 'area' orientation".

It is possible that some species employ only one pheromone compound in population aggregation. For example, ipsenol alone has been identified as a pheromone from *I. grandicollis* (Eichhoff) (Table 8.1). However, Vité and Renwick (1971a) report the presence of at least 'two additional, apparently insect-produced components' in the male hindgut. Systems of chemical communication, involving a sequential release of various compounds, have been proposed for *Dendroctonus ponderosae*, *D. brevicomis* and *D. frontalis* (Renwick and Vité 1970). For example, the postulated attack mechanism for *D. brevicomis* is as follows (Renwick and Vité 1970). 'Attacking females release small amounts of frontalin and brevicomin, and their boring activity causes resin exudation, with the resultant evaporation of terpenes. Both males and females are attracted to this mixture, although it is likely that more frontalin is produced during the beetles' struggle against the resin flow. An excess of frontalin would then draw more females to the tree, thus accelerating the mass attack and rapidly weakening the tree. As soon as the females are able to feed, brevicomin production increases to a high level so that more males are attracted. The concentration of verbenone released by aggregating males then builds up to inhibit further response to a tree or that portion of a tree which has been successfully colonized. At the same time, the terpene concentration drops as resin exudation ceases. However, the relatively large amount of frontalin released by the male beetles assures simultaneously continued response of female beetles to the area of pheromone release. The combination of response eliciting and inhibiting factors, then, triggers the shifting of attack to unoccupied host material within the sphere of the population attractant.'

Of considerable interest is the ubiquitous presence of *cis*- or *trans*-verbenol (table 8.1). Either or both isomers may serve as contact pheromones in *Ips* species (Vité et al. 1972), but although *trans*-verbenol is present in at least five *Dendroctonus* species, it apparently serves as a major aggregating pheromone compound only in *D. ponderosae* (Pitman et al. 1968).

The definitive role of host-tree monoterpenes as synergistic components of an aggregating pheromone complex was elucidated by the isolation of myrcene from the frass of female *D. brevicomis* (Silverstein, 1970) and the subsequent demonstration that in field tests the pure compound was synergistic with the pheromone compound, brevicomin (Bedard et al. 1969). Other terpenes also have a synergistic role with beetle-produced pheromones: e.g. 3-carene in *D. brevicomis* (Pitman 1969), although it is not as effective as myrcene (Bedard et al. 1970); α-pinene in *D. frontalis* (Renwick and Vité 1969) and *D. ponderosae* (Pitman 1969); and camphene in *D. pseudotsugae* (Pitman and Vité 1970), although it may not be as effective as α-pinene (Furniss and Schmitz 1971), or differ significantly from other host volatiles (Rudinsky et al. 1972a).

Assuming that all external and internal environmental factors are favorable, flying beetles of both sexes orient to a host occupied by aggregation pheromone-producing beetles of the first-attacking sex. The threshold for pheromone response stimuli must be low and for dispersal stimuli, high. The physical environment must permit flight and the appropriate blend of host and beetle-produced volatiles must be present on the wind. The responding beetles perceive the odor with their antennae (Borden and Wood 1966; Payne 1970, 1971) and, as established for *Ips paraconfusus* (Gara 1963; Wood and Bushing 1963; Borden and Wood 1966), orient upwind in what can be described as an 'anemo-chemo-klinotaxis'.

Cessation of flight: If the orientation process is successful, a responding beetle arrives in the immediate proximity of an infested host. Just as with pioneer beetles, cessation of flight is a key step in the concentration phase. It commits the responding beetles to make contact with the host in or on which they may find others of the first-attacking sex or prospective mates, as the case may be. Again duration of flight (Bennett and Borden 1971) and concurrent lipid metabolism (Atkins 1969; Thompson and Bennett 1971) apparently predispose beetles to respond. It is not established whether responding beetles cease flight in response to pheromones. For example, males of *Dendroctonus pseudotsugae* ceased flight in response to either odor of host phloem tissue or attractive female frass (Bennett and Borden 1971). Once it has alighted, a responding beetle may be inhibited from further flight by the presence of volatile pheromones. Contact with or presence of the odor of attractive frass almost completely inhibited take-offs in both sexes of *Ips paraconfusus* (Borden 1967). Thus inhibited from response to dispersal stimuli, the responding beetle is free to perform a new series of behavioral tasks.

Orientation to prospective mates: Both odor and sound are used in the short-range communication involved in location and recognition of a mate. Contact with male frass is sufficient to induce female *Ips calligraphus* (Germar) to search for and find the entrance to a male nuptial chamber (Wilkinson et al. 1967). Physical presence of a male is not necessary in *I. paraconfusus.* When females encountered male frass around artificial entrance holes, they searched for and entered the holes just as they would the normal entrance to a nuptial chamber (Barr 1969). Stridulation by female *Ips* occurs when they encounter the entrance to a nuptial chamber, apparently in response to male-produced pheromones. In response, the male admits the female into the nuptial chamber (Wilkinson et al. 1967; Barr 1969).

Verification of the interaction of aggregation pheromones and stridulation has been shown for *Dendroctonus pseudotsugae* (Rudinsky and Michael 1972). Males stridulate at or near the entrance to a female-occupied gallery to produce a recognizable 'courtship' sound, distinguishable in oscilloscope traces from distress sounds. An identical sound is produced on exposure to frontalin, 3-methyl-2-cyclohexen-1-one (MCH) and *trans*-verbenol, all female-produced pheromones (table 8.1). A *D. pseudotsugae* female is able to mask her aggregation pheromone in response to the male's stridulation, or to a non-stridulating male placed in her gallery (Rudinsky 1968, 1969, 1970; Rudinsky and Michael 1972). The pheromone mask stops within 9 to 14 min after males are removed from galleries (Rudinsky 1968) or after the stridulation sound is stopped (Rudinsky and Michael 1972). It does not mask the primary response to host volatiles and is limited to a small area around a gallery entrance. Thus, flying females can still respond to volatiles from unattacked regions of a host tree and males can respond to nearby unmated females (Rudinsky 1970).

Attack termination: It has recently been demonstrated that MCH is, in fact, the natural pheromone mask released by female *D. pseudotsugae* (Rudinsky et al. 1973). Since MCH inhibits the response of beetles in the field to aggregation pheromones (Rudinsky et al. 1972a), it is probably the attack termination factor responsible for inhibiting response to saturated hosts. Pheromone masks or response inhibitors may occur in species other than *D. pseudotsugae*. Solitary virgin or mated *Trypodendron lineatum* produce secondary attraction, but the presence of males in the galleries greatly reduces the attraction, possibly because they can mask the aggregating pheromone (Nijholt 1970). Verbenone inhibits pheromone response in *Dendroctonus frontalis* (Renwick and Vité 1969) and *D. brevicomis* (Renwick and Vité 1970; Wood 1972).

In part, termination of mass attack may be in response to decreasing production of aggregation pheromone. For example, frass expelled from the galleries, and male *Ips paraconfusus* guts lose attraction in proportion to the number of females in the gallery, with attraction being completely lost after three or four females are present (Borden 1967). In support of this result, Vité et al. (1972) found that male *I. calligraphus* joined by three or more females quickly cease to synthesize the frass pheromone ipsdienol.

8.4.2. Establishment

In order for reproduction to occur in most scolytid species, both sexes remain in the host and participate in a fairly intricate type of reproductive behavior (Swaine 1918; Reid 1958b; Wilkinson et al. 1967; Barr 1969; Borden 1969; Schmitz 1972). Although there is little or no experimental evidence, the environmental cues for establishment must include various host factors such as taste, smell, moisture and temperature, and must also include the presence of the opposite sex. This last factor is also little understood, but recognition probably occurs through chemical, acoustic and tactile communication, particularly in the dark reaches of a cryptic gallery. Whether or not various aggregation pheromones or other compounds serve as close-range recognition factors has not been investigated. Finally, if all factors are acceptable, the beetles of both sexes become physiologically tied to their hosts through degeneration of their flight muscles and consequent temporary inability to leave the host (Chapman 1957; Reid 1958a; Hensen 1961; Atkins and Farris 1962; Bhakthan et al. 1970).

Thus, the sequence is complete.* Beetles have emerged from their previous host or overwintering site and through a sequence of genetically controlled, behavioral events have successfully colonized a new host in which they will reproduce. Without the employment of aggregation pheromones in host selection and concentration of the population, successful large scale colonization of this type would be improbable.

8.5. Associated insects

In addition to scolytid beetles, which are the principal colonists in most of their hosts, a large complex of other species may join them. Some of these may compete for host tissue, or utilize areas of the host not inhabited by the scolytid species in question. Among such insects are other scolytid species, cerambycid and buprestid beetles and siricid woodwasps. In addition to other host feeders, there are many insect associates which are commensals, parasites (parasitoids) or predators of scolytids.

* For simplicity, re-emergence and re-attack by parent beetles have not been included in the foregoing discussion.

One might hypothesize that the parasitic, predaceous or commensal associates would follow a similar generalized sequential type of behavior (fig. 8.2) to the scolytids themselves (fig. 8.1)*. One may note that two of the accepted phases of host selection for parasitoids, host habitat finding and host finding (Doutt 1965) are borrowed and extended to apply to predators and commensals. Literally speaking, host finding need not be practiced by commensals which live in the gallery of scolytids, but in actual fact most species are so closely associated with the scolytids that actual contact would appear inevitable. One might expect that associated insects would utilize bark beetle pheromones in the orientation process. However, there are several means by which they could find the host tree. If they arrive early in the phase of scolytid colonization they could rely on the same primary attraction mechanisms as the scolytids themselves. Included in this group would be most of the insects which compete for or share host tissue.

If the associates arrive after the scolytids are established in the new host, they could also respond to stimuli from the host plant in its altered state following scolytid attack. For example, Fitzgerald and Nagel (1972) doubt that the common dipteran predator of scolytid larvae, *Medetera aldrichii* Wh., responds to bark beetle pheromones 'since ovipositing *M. aldrichii* are present in the field after prey species have ceased pheromone production'. Similarly, *Heydenia unica* Cook and Davis, a pteromalid parasite of *Dendroctonus frontalis* respond in the field to α-pinene, and response was not significantly increased by combining known bark beetle pheromones with α-pinene (Camors and Payne 1972). Berisford and Franklin (1971) noted that three hymenopteran parasites of southern *Ips* species, *Coeloides pissodes* (Ashmead), *Heydenia unica* and *Roptocerus eccoptogastri* (Ratz.), oriented to infested trees in peak numbers 7 to 10 days after the peak *Ips* response, 'suggesting a response to something other than aggregating pheromone . . .'.

Finally, if the associated insects arrive during the period of aggregation pheromone production, they could utilize them as kairomones (ch. 1). Brown et al. (1970) proposed the term kairomone and defined it as 'a transpecific chemical messenger, the adaptive benefit of which falls on the recipient rather than on the emitter'. Thus, an associated predator, parasite or commensal of scolytid beetles which utilizes scolytid pheromones to locate a suitable host tree or beetle is, in fact, using them as kairomones. In host habitat finding a relatively small number of insect scolytid associates have definitely been shown to exhibit a kairomone response to scolytid pheromones (table 8.2). However, virtually nothing is known about the possible use of kairomones in host finding. All kairomone-responding species begin to arrive at, or very shortly after, the initial attack of the host and are thus present and flying in an environment permeated by scolytid aggregation pheromones. Significantly, all are entomophagous insects which are intimately associated with bark beetles and depend on them as larval and/or adult food. The four beetles

* Phoretic mites are excluded from this discussion.

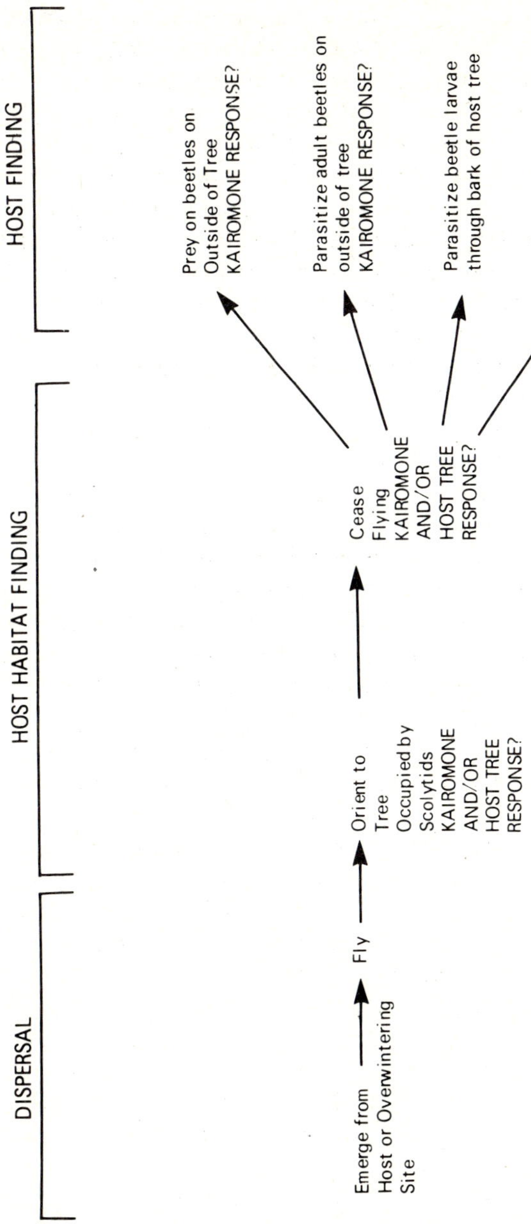

Fig. 8.2. Generalized behavioral sequence in host selection followed by predaceous, parasitic or commensal insect associates of scolytid beetles. Key steps in which kairomones are known or could possibly play a part are identified.

are predators which attack and consume adult beetles on a new host as well as ovipositing on the bark of infested trees so that their larvae will be near their prey, the developing bark beetle brood. Although Furniss and Schmitz (1971) did not demonstrate that *Dendroctonus pseudotsugae* pheromones attracted any more clerids or ostomids than host terpenes, subsequent studies resulted in large catches of the clerid *Thanasimus undatulus* Wolc. to frontalin (table 8.2). In fact, the high response rates to frontalin by *Trypodendron undatulus* and *Thanasimus dubius* (Fab.) and by *Temnochila chlorodia* (Mann.) to *exo*-brevicomin (table 8.2), have provoked questioning of proposed aggregation pheromone control programs since they could remove large numbers of predators from the forest.

The parasitic wasp, *Tomicobia tibialis* Ashmead, is nearly specific to *Ips* species (Bedard 1965) and must locate incoming beetles on the bark surface so it can mount the beetles and oviposit through the pronotum or elytra. Lastly, the fly, *Medetera bistriata* Parent, oviposits on the bark around newly formed *Dendroctonus frontalis* or *Ips avulsus* Eichhoff galleries and young larvae enter the galleries to feed on scolytid larvae (Thatcher 1960).

Curiously, Pitman and Vité (1971) recorded only a marginal response of *Enoclerus lecontei* (Wolcott) to the aggregating pheromones frontalin and *exo*-brevicomin (fewer than to myrcene), despite their coincident arrival with their prey, *Dendroctonus brevicomis*, on a host tree under mass attack (Berryman 1970). Moreover, *Temnochila chlorodia* preys on a large number of scolytid species as well as on buprestids and cerambycids, despite the apparent lack of brevicomin in the pheromone complex of such genera as *Ips*. Clearly we have yet much to learn about the precise kairomone orientation mechanisms for most early arriving parasites and predators. Such knowledge must probably await our complete understanding of scolytid aggregation pheromones.

TABLE 8.2

Kairomone response of entomophagous insect associates of scolytids. Only well documented cases in which associates use scolytid aggregating pheromones as kairomones are included.

Associated insect	Natural source of kairomone, or active kairomone compounds, if known	Response information
COLEOPTERA		
Temnochila chlorodia (Trogositidae)	brevicomin	Response in large numbers occurs to brevicomin alone (Bedard et al. 1969; Pitman and Vité 1971). Many references indicate low level response to other scolytid and host volatiles.

Table 8.2 (continued)

Enoclerus lecontei (Cleridae)	ipsenol *cis*-verbenol ipsdienol *Pinus ponderosa* logs infested with male *Ips pini*	Wood et al. (1968) trapped numerous *E. lecontei* responding to a mixture of all 3 compounds in field tests of *Ips paraconfusus* synthetic pheromones. In field tests in California and Idaho, more strongly attracted to odor produced by boring *Ips pini* males from New York than from California or Idaho (Lanier et al. 1972).
Thanasimus dubius (Cleridae)	frontalin *trans*-verbenol verbenone	Response occurs in same diel rhythm as its prey, *Dendroctonus frontalis*, to frontalin alone or in combination with oleoresin or *trans*-verbenol (Vité and Williamson 1970). Verbenone raised ratio of male response, but lowered overall response level.
Thanasimus undatulus (Cleridae)	frontalin	Attracted in large numbers to frontalin in field tests (E. D. A. Dyer[a] and R. F. Schmitz[b], personal communication).
HYMENOPTERA		
Tomicobia tibialis (Pteromalidae)	*Pinus ponderosa* logs infested with male *Ips paraconfusus* or male *Ips pini*	Both sexes attracted to odor produced by boring male *Ips paraconfusus* (Bedard 1965; Rice 1969). Responded in greater numbers to *Ips pini* than to *Ips paraconfusus. Ips pini* from California or Idaho more attractive than those from New York (Lanier et al. 1972). Not attracted to *Dendroctonus*-infested *Pinus ponderosa* (Rice 1968).
DIPTERA		
Medetera bistriata	frontalin *trans*-verbenol verbenone *Pinus taeda* logs infested with *Ips grandicollis* males	Frontalin or α-pinene alone not attractive. Mixtures of frontalin with α-pinene, *trans*-verbenol plus α-pinene, or verbenone plus α-pinene all attractive (Williamson 1971). Verbenone caused change in sex ratio in favor of females. Attraction of logs infested with *Ips grandicollis* males equal to that from logs infested with *Dendroctonus frontalis* females.

[a] Pacific Forest Research Centre, Canadian Forestry Service, Victoria, B. C., Canada.

[b] USDA, Forest Service, Forestry Sciences Laboratory, Moscow, Idaho, U.S.A.

Acknowledgments

I thank G. B. Pitman, J. A. Rudinsky, R. F. Schmitz, J. P. Vité and J. C. Young for providing information on recent data not available in published form at the time of writing, and B. A. Barr, M. C. Birch, M. M. Furniss, R. F. Schmitz and J. C. Young for critical review of the manuscript.

Note added in proof

Recent studies have elucidated the production of 'contact' pheromones in the genus *Dendroctonus* in response to monoterpenes or host tree volatiles (Hughes, P. R., Z. angew. Entomol. 73, 294–312 (1973); Hughes, P. R., Naturwissenschaften 60, 261–262 (1973); Renwick, J. A. A., P. R. Hughes and DeJ. T. Tanletin, J. Insect Physiol. 19, 1735–1740 (1973)) (see p. 143).

Laboratory tests have confirmed that verbenone in high concentrations acts as an inhibitor of pheromone response in *D. frontalis*. However, in lower concentrations and when combined with other pheromones and host volatiles, verbenone and MCH act as attraction, arrestment and stridulation inducing factors in *D. frontalis* and *D. pseudotsugae*, respectively (Rudinsky, J. A., Environ. Entomol. 2, 511–514 (1973); Rudinsky, J. A., Environ. Entomol. 2, 579–585 (1973)). Studies in the field (Nijholt, W. W., Can. Entomol. 105, 583–590 (1973)) and laboratory (J. H. Borden, unpublished results) have provided conclusive evidence that male *T. lineatum* are able to mask the female pheromone. (See pp. 148–149).

References

Anderson R. F. (1948) Host selection by the pine engraver. J. Econ. Entomol. 41, 596–602.

Atkins, M. D. (1966a) Behavioral variation among scolytids in relation to their habitat. Can. Entomol. 98, 285–288.

Atkins, M. D. (1966b) Laboratory studies on the behavior of the Douglas-fir beetle, *Dendroctonus pseudotsugae* Hopkins. Can. Entomol. 98, 953–991.

Atkins, M. D. (1969) Lipid loss with flight in the Douglas-fir beetle. Can. Entomol. 101, 164–165.

Atkins, M. D. and S. H. Farris (1962) A contribution to the knowledge of flight muscle changes in the Scolytidae (Coleoptera). Can. Entomol. 94, 25–32.

Barr, B. A. (1969) Sound production in the Scolytidae (Coleoptera) with emphasis on the genus *Ips*. Can. Entomol. 101, 636–672.

Bedard, W. D. (1965) The biology of *Tomicobia tibialis* (Hymenoptera: Pteromalidae) parasitizing *Ips confusus* (Coleoptera: Scolytidae) in California. Contrib. Boyce Thompson Inst. 23, 77–81.

Bedard, W. D., R. M. Silverstein and D. L. Wood (1970) Bark beetle pheromones. Science 167, 1638–1639.

Bedard, W. D., P. E. Tilden, D. L. Wood, R. M. Silverstein, R. G. Brownlee and J. O. Rodin (1969) Western pine beetle: field response to its sex pheromone and a synergistic host terpene, myrcene. Science 164, 1284–1285.

Bennett, R. B. and J. H. Borden (1971) Flight arrestment of tethered *Dendroctonus pseudotsugae* and *Trypodendron lineatum* (Coleoptera: Scolytidae) in response to olfactory stimuli. Ann. Entomol. Soc. Am. 64, 1273–1286.

Berisford, C. W. and R. T. Franklin (1971) Attack patterns of *Ips avulsus* and *I. grandicollis* (Coleoptera: Scolytidae) on four species of southern pines. Ann. Entomol. Soc. Am. 64, 894–897.

Berryman, A. A. (1968) Distribution of *Scolytus ventralis* attacks, emergence, and parasites in grand fir. Can. Entomol. 100, 57–68.

Berryman, A. A. (1970) Evaluation of insect predators of the western pine beetle. *In*: Studies on the population dynamics of the western pine beetle, *Dendroctonus brevicomis* Le Conte (Coleoptera: Scolytidae); eds.: R. W. Stark and D. L. Dahlsten (Univ. Calif. Div. Agric. Sci., Berkeley) pp. 102-112.

Bhakthan, N. M. G., J. H. Borden and K. K. Nair (1970) Fine structure of degenerating and regenerating flight muscles in a bark beetle, *Ips confusus*. I. Degeneration. J. Cell Sci. 6, 807–820.

Borden, J. H. (1967) Factors influencing the response of *Ips confusus* (Coleoptera: Scolytidae) to male attractant. Can. Entomol. 99, 1164–1193.

Borden, J. H. (1969) Observations on the life history and habits of *Alniphagus aspericollis* (Coleoptera: Scolytidae) in southwestern British Columbia. Can. Entomol. 101, 870–878.

Borden, J. H. and R. B. Bennett (1969) A continuously recording flight mill for investigating the effect of volatile substances on the flight of tethered insects. J. Econ. Entomol. 62, 782–785.

Borden, J. H. and C. E. Slater (1969a) Flight muscle volume change in *Ips confusus* (Coleoptera: Scolytidae). Can. J. Zool. 47, 29–32.

Borden, J. H. and C. E. Slater (1969b) Sex pheromone of *Trypodendron lineatum*: production in the hindgut – Malpighian tubule region. Ann. Entomol. Soc. Am. 62, 454-455.

Borden, J. H. and E. Stokkink (1971) Secondary attraction in the Scolytidae. Canada Dept. Fish. and For. Inf. Rept. BC-X-57, 77 pp.

Borden, J. H. and D. L. Wood (1966) The antennal receptors and olfactory response of *Ips confusus* (Coleoptera: Scolytidae) to male sex attractant in the laboratory. Ann. Entomol. Soc. Am. 59, 253–261.

Borden, J. H., K. K. Nair and C. E. Slater (1969) Synthetic juvenile hormone: induction of sex pheromone production in *Ips confusus*. Science 166, 1626–1627.

Brown, W. L., Jr., T. E. Eisner and R. H. Whittaker (1970) Allomones and kairomones: transspecific chemical messengers. BioScience 20, 21–22.

Cade, S. C., B. F. Hrutfiord and R. I. Gara (1970) Identification of a primary attractant for *Gnathotrichus sulcatus* isolated from western hemlock logs. J. Econ. Entomol. 63, 1014–1015.

Cameron E. A. and J. H. Borden (1967) Emergence patterns of *Ips confusus* (Coleoptera: Scolytidae) from ponderosa pine. Can. Entomol. 99, 236–244.

Camors, F. B., Jr. and T. L. Payne (1972) Response of *Heydenia unica* (Hymenoptera: Pteromalidae) to *Dendroctonus frontalis* pheromones and a host-tree terpene. Ann. Entomol. Soc. Am. 65, 31–33.

Chapman, J. A. (1957) Flight muscle change during adult life in the Scolytidae. Can. Dept. Forestry Bi-Mon. Progr. Rept. 13(1), 3–4.

Chapman, J. A. (1963) Field selection of different log odors by scolytid beetles. Can. Entomol. 95, 673–676.

Chapman, J. A. (1966) The effect of attack by the ambrosia beetle *Trypodendron lineatum* (Olivier) on log attractiveness. Can. Entomol. 98, 50–59.

Coster, J. E. and J. P. Vité (1972) Effects of feeding and mating on pheromone release in the southern pine beetle. Ann. Entomol. Soc. Am. 65, 263–266.

Daterman, G. E., J. A. Rudinsky and W. P. Nagel (1965) Flight patterns of bark and timber beetles associated with coniferous forests of western Oregon. Ore. State Univ. Agric. Exptl. Sta. Tech. Bull. 87, 46 pp.

Davidson, A. G. and R. M. Prentice, eds. (1967) Important forest insects and diseases of mutual concern to Canada, the United States and Mexico. Canada Dept. For. and Rural Dev., Ottawa, 248 pp.

Doskotch, R. W., S. K. Chatterji and J. W. Peacock (1970) Elm bark derived feeding stimulants for the smaller European elm bark beetle. Science 167, 380–382.

Doutt, R. L. (1965) Biological characteristics of entomophagous adults. *In*: Biological Control of Insect Pests and Weeds; ed.: P. De Bach (Reinhold Pub. Co.) pp. 145–167.

Ferrell, G. T. (1971) Host selection by the fir engraver, *Scolytus ventralis* (Coleoptera: Scolytidae): preliminary field studies. Can. Entomol. 103, 1717–1725.

Fitzgerald, T. D. and W. P. Nagel (1972) Oviposition and larval bark-surface orientation of *Medetera aldrichii* (Diptera: Dolichopodidae): response to a prey-liberated plant terpene. Ann. Entomol. Soc. Am. 65, 328–330.

Fockler, C. E. and J. H. Borden (1972) Sexual behavior and seasonal mating activity of *Trypodendron lineatum* (Coleoptera: Scolytidae). Can. Entomol. 104, 1841–1853.

Furniss, M. M. and R. F. Schmitz (1971) Comparative attraction of Douglas-fir beetles to frontalin and tree volatiles. U.S.D.A. Forest Service Res. Pap. INT.-96, 16 pp.

Furniss, M. M., L. N. Kline, R. F. Schmitz and J. A. Rudinsky (1972) Tests of three pheromones to induce or disrupt aggregation of Douglas-fir beetles (Coleoptera: Scolytidae) on live trees. Ann. Entomol. Soc. Am. 65, 1227–1232.

Gara, R. I. (1963) Studies on the flight behavior of *Ips confusus* (LeC.) (Coleoptera: Scolytidae) in response to attractive material. Contrib. Boyce Thompson Inst. 22, 51–66.

Gara, R. I. and J. E. Coster (1968) Studies on the attack behavior of the southern pine beetle. III. Sequence of tree infestation within stands. Contrib. Boyce Thompson Inst. 24, 77–85.

Gara, R. I. and J. P. Vité (1962) Studies on the flight patterns of bark beetles (Coleoptera: Scolytidae) in second growth ponderosa pine forests. Contrib. Boyce Thompson Inst. 21, 275–289.

Gilbert, B. L., J. E. Baker and D. M. Norris (1967) Juglone (5-hydroxy-1,4-naphthoquinone) from *Carya ovata*, a deterrent to feeding by *Scolytus multistriatus*. J. Insect Physiol. 13, 1453–1459.

Graham, K. (1959) Release by flight exercise of a chemotropic response from photopositive domination in a scolytid beetle. Nature (London) 184, 283–284.

Graham, K. (1961) Air swallowing: a mechanism in photic reversal of the beetle *Trypodendron*. Nature (London) 191, 519–520.

Graham, K. (1962) Photic behavior in the ecology of the ambrosia beetle *Trypodendron lineatum*. Proc. Int. Congr. Entomol. 11th. (1960) 2, 226.

Graham, K. (1968) Anaerobic induction of primary chemical attractancy for ambrosia beetles. Can. J. Zool. 46, 905–908.

Henson, W. R. (1961) Laboratory studies on the adult behavior of *Conophthorus coniperda* (Schwarz) (Coleoptera: Scolytidae). I. Seasonal changes in the internal anatomy of the adult. Ann. Entomol. Soc. Am. 54, 698-701.

Henson, W. R. (1962) Laboratory studies on the adult behavior of *Conophthorus coniperda* (Coleoptera: Scolytidae). III. Flight. Ann. Entomol. Soc. Am. 55, 524–530.

Johnson, C. G. (1969) Migration and Dispersal of Insects by Flight. (Methuen, London) 763 pp.

Kennedy, J. S. and C. O. Booth (1963a) Free flight of aphids in the laboratory. J. Exptl. Biol. 40, 67–85.

Kennedy, J. S. and C. O. Booth (1963b) Co-ordination of successive activities in an aphid. The effect of flight on the settling responses. J. Exptl. Biol. 40, 351–369.

Kinzer, G. W., A. F. Fentiman, Jr., R. L. Foltz and J. A. Rudinsky (1971) Bark beetle attractant: 3-methyl-2-cyclohexen-1-one isolated from *Dendroctonus pseudotsugae*. J. Econ. Entomol. 64, 970–971.

Kinzer, G. W., A. F. Fentiman, Jr., T. F. Page, Jr., R. L. Foltz, J. P. Vité and G. B. Pitman (1969) Bark beetle attractants: identification, synthesis and field bioassay of a new compound isolated from *Dendroctonus*. Nature (London) 221, 477–478.

Lanier, G. N. (1970) Biosystematics of North American *Ips* (Coleoptera: Scolytidae). Hopping's group IX. Can. Entomol. 102, 1139–1163.

Lanier, G. N., M. C. Birch, R. F. Schmitz and M. M. Furniss (1972) Pheromones of *Ips pini* (Coleoptera: Scolytidae): variation in response among three populations. Can. Entomol. 104, 1917–1923.

Miller, J. M. and F. P. Keen (1960) Biology and control of the western pine beetle. U. S. Dept. Agric. Misc. Publ. 800, 381 pp.

Moeck, H. A. (1970) Ethanol as the primary attractant for the ambrosia beetle *Trypodendron lineatum* (Coleoptera: Scolytidae). Can. Entomol. 102, 985–995.

Moeck, H. A. (1971) Field test of ethanol as a scolytid attractant. Bio-Mon. Res. Notes, Canada Dept. Fisheries and Forestry, Ottawa, 27(2), 11–12.

Nijholt, W. W. (1970) The effect of mating and the presence of the male ambrosia beetle, *Trypodendron lineatum*, on 'secondary' attraction. Can. Entomol. 102, 894–897.

Oksanen, H., V. Perttunen and E. Kangas (1970) Studies on the chemical factors involved in the olfactory orientation of *Blastophagus piniperda* (Coleoptera: Scolytidae). Contrib. Boyce Thompson Inst. 24, 299–304.

Payne, T. L. (1970) Electrophysiological investigations on response to pheromone in bark beetles. Contrib. Boyce Thompson Inst. 24, 275–282.

Payne, T. L. (1971) Bark beetle olfaction. I. Electroantennogram responses of the southern pine beetle (Coleoptera: Scolytidae) to its aggregation pheromone frontalin. Ann. Entomol. Soc. Am. 64, 266–268.

Person, H. L. (1931) Theory in explanation of the selection of certain trees by the western pine beetle. J. Forest. 31, 696–699.

Perttunen, V. and T. Boman (1965) Laboratory experiments on the spontaneous take-off activity of *Blastophagus piniperda* (Col., Scolytidae) in relation to temperature and light intensity at different seasons of the year. Proc. 12th Int. Congr. Entomol. (1964) 5, 344–345.

Perttunen, V., H. Oksanen and E. Kangas (1970) Aspects of the external and internal factors affecting orientation of *Blastophagus piniperda* (Coleoptera: Scolytidae). Contrib. Boyce Thompson Inst. 24, 293–297.

Pitman, G. B. (1966) Studies on the pheromone of *Ips confusus* (LeConte). III. The influence of host material on pheromone production. Contrib. Boyce Thompson Inst. 23, 147–158.

Pitman, G. B. (1969) Pheromone response in pine bark beetles: influence of host volatiles. Science 166, 905–906.

Pitman, G. B. and J. P. Vité (1969) Aggregation behavior of *Dendroctonus ponderosae* (Coleoptera: Scolytidae) in response to chemical messengers. Can. Entomol. 101, 143–149.

Pitman, G. B. and J. P. Vité (1970) Field responses of *Dendroctonus pseudotsugae* (Coleoptera: Scolytidae) to synthetic frontalin. Ann. Entomol. Soc. Am. 63, 661–664.

Pitman, G. B. and J. P. Vité (1971) Predator-prey response to western pine beetle attractants. J. Econ. Entomol. 64, 402–404.

Pitman, G. B., R. A. Kliefoth and J. P. Vité (1965) Studies on the pheromone of *Ips confusus* (LeConte). II. Further observations on the site of production. Contrib. Boyce Thompson Inst. 23, 13–18.

Pitman, G. B., J. P. Vité, G. W. Kinzer and A. F. Fentiman, Jr. (1968) Bark beetle attractants: *trans*-verbenol isolated from *Dendroctonus*. Nature (London) 218, 168–169.

Pitman, G. B., J. P. Vité, G. W. Kinzer and A. F. Fentiman, Jr. (1969) Specificity of population-aggregating pheromones in *Dendroctonus*. J. Insect Physiol. 15, 363–366.

Reid, R. W. (1958a) Internal changes in the female mountain pine beetle, *Dendroctonus monticolae* Hopk., associated with egg laying and flight. Can. Entomol. 90, 464–468.

Reid, R. W. (1958b) The behavior of the mountain pine beetle, *Dendroctonus monticolae* Hopk., during mating, egg laying, and gallery construction. Can. Entomol. 90, 505–509.

Renwick, J. A. A. (1967) Identification of two oxygenated terpenes from the bark beetles *Dendroctonus frontalis* and *Dendroctonus brevicomis*. Contrib. Boyce Thompson Inst. 23, 355–360.

Renwick, J. A. A. and J. P. Vité (1968) Isolation of the population aggregating pheromone of the southern pine beetle. Contrib. Boyce Thompson Inst. 24, 65–68.

Renwick, J. A. A. and J. P. Vité (1969) Bark beetle attractants: mechanism of colonization by *Dendroctonus frontalis*. Nature (London) 224, 1222–1223.

Renwick, J. A. A. and J. P. Vité (1970) Systems of chemical communication in *Dendroctonus*. Contrib. Boyce Thompson Inst. 24, 283–292.

Renwick, J. A. A. and J. P. Vité (1972) Pheromones and host volatiles that govern aggregation of the six-spined engraver beetle, *Ips calligraphus*. J. Insect Physiol. 18, 1215–1219.

Rice, R. E. (1968) Observations on host selection by *Tomicobia tibialis* Ashmead (Hymenoptera: Pteromalidae). Contrib. Boyce Thompson Inst. 24, 53–56.

Rice, R. E. (1969) Response of some predators and parasites of *Ips confusus* (LeC.) (Coleoptera: Scolytidae) to olfactory attractants. Contrib. Boyce Thompson Inst. 24, 189–194.

Rudinsky, J. A. (1962) Ecology of Scolytidae. Ann. Rev. Entomol. 7, 327–348.

Rudinsky, J. A. (1966a) Host selection and invasion by the Douglas-fir beetle, *Dendroctonus pseudotsugae* Hopkins, in coastal Douglas-fir forests. Can. Entomol. 98, 98–111.

Rudinsky, J. A. (1966b) Scolytid beetles associated with Douglas-fir: response to terpenes. Science 152, 218–219.

Rudinsky, J. A. (1968) Pheromone-mask by the female *Dendroctonus pseudotsugae* Hopk., an attraction regulator. Pan-Pac. Entomol. 44, 248–250.

Rudinsky, J. A. (1969) Masking of the aggregating pheromone in *Dendroctonus pseudotsugae* Hopk. Science 166, 884–885.

Rudinsky, J. A. (1970) Sequence of Douglas-fir beetle attraction and its ecological significance. Contrib. Boyce Thompson Inst. 24, 311–314.

Rudinsky, J. A. and R. R. Michael (1972) Sound production in the Scolytidae: chemostimulus of sonic signal by the Douglas-fir beetle. Science 175, 1386–1390.

Rudinsky, J. A. and R. R. Michael (1973) Sound production in Scolytidae: stridulation by female *Dendroctonus* beetles. J. Insect Physiol. 19, 689–705.

Rudinsky, J. A., M. M. Furniss, L. N. Kline and R. F. Schmitz (1972a) Attraction and repression of *Dendroctonus pseudotsugae* (Coleoptera: Scolytidae) by three synthetic pheromones in traps in Oregon and Idaho. Can. Entomol. 104, 815–822.

Rudinsky, J. A., G. W. Kinzer, A. F. Fentiman, Jr., and R. L. Foltz (1972b) *Trans*-verbenol isolated from Douglas-fir beetle: laboratory and field bioassays in Oregon. Environ. Entomol. 1, 485–488.

Rudinsky, J. A., M. Morgan, L. M. Libbey and R. R. Michael (1973) Sound production in Scolytidae: 3-methyl-2-cyclohexen-1-one released by female Douglas-fir beetle in response to male sonic signal. Environ. Entomol. 2, 505–509.

Ryan, R. B. (1959) Termination of diapause in the Douglas-fir beetle, *Dendroctonus pseudotsugae* Hopkins (Coleoptera: Scolytidae), as an aid to continuous laboratory rearing. Can. Entomol. 91, 520–525.

Saunders, J. L. (1967) Diurnal emergence of *Xyleborus ferrugineus* (Coleoptera: Scolytidae) from cacao trunks in Ecuador and Costa Rica. Ann. Entomol. Soc. Am. 60, 1094–1096.

Schmitz, R. F. (1972) Behavior of *Ips pini* during mating, oviposition, and larval development (Coleoptera: Scolytidae). Can. Entomol. 104, 1723–1728.

Schneider, I. and J. A. Rudinsky (1969) The site of pheromone production in *Trypodendron lineatum* (Coleoptera: Scolytidae): bioassay and histological studies of the hindgut. Can. Entomol. 101, 1181–1186.

Schönherr, J. (1970) Evidence of an aggregating pheromone in the ash-bark beetle, *Leperisinus fraxini* (Coleoptera: Scolytidae). Contrib. Boyce Thompson Inst. 24, 305–307.

Shepherd, R. F. (1965) Distribution of attacks by *Dendroctonus ponderosae* Hopk. on *Pinus contorta* Dougl.var. *latifolia* Engelm. Can. Entomol. 97, 207–215.

Shorey, H. H. (1973) Behavioral responses to insect pheromones. Ann. Rev. Entomol. 18, 349–380.

Silverstein, R. M. (1970) Methodology for isolation and identification of insect pheromones – examples from Coleoptera. *In*: Control of Insect Behavior by Natural Products; eds.: D. L. Wood, R. M. Silverstein and M. Nakajima (Academic Press, N. Y.) pp. 285–299.

Silverstein, R. M., R. G. Brownlee, T. E. Bellas, D. L. Wood and L. E. Browne (1968) Brevicomin: principal sex attractant in the frass of the female western pine beetle. Science 159, 889–890.

Silverstein, R. M., J. O. Rodin and D. L. Wood (1966) Sex attractants in frass produced by male *Ips confusus* in ponderosa pine. Science 154, 509–510.

Swaine, J. M. (1918) Canadian bark beetles, II. A preliminary classification with an account of the habits and means of control. Can. Dept. Agric. Entomol. Br. Bull. 14, 143 pp.

Thatcher, R. C. (1960) Bark beetles affecting southern pines: a review of current knowledge. U. S. Forest Serv. S. Forest Exptl. Sta. Occas. Paper 180, 25 pp.

Thompson, S. N. and R. B. Bennett (1971) Oxidation of fat during flight of male Douglas-fir beetles, *Dendroctonus pseudotsugae*. J. Insect Physiol. 17, 1555–1563.

Thorsteinson, A. J. (1960) Host selection in phytophagous insects. Ann. Rev. Entomol. 5, 193–218.

Vité, J. P. and G. B. Pitman (1968) Bark beetle aggregation: effects of feeding on the release of pheromones in *Dendroctonus* and *Ips*. Nature (London) 218, 169–170.

Vité, J. P. and G. B. Pitman (1969) Aggregation behavior of *Dendroctonus brevicomis* in response to synthetic pheromones. J. Insect Physiol. 15, 1617–1622.

Vité, J. P. and G. B. Pitman (1970) Management of western pine beetle populations: use of chemical messengers. J. Econ. Entomol. 63, 1132–1135.

Vité, J. P., G. B. Pitman, A. F. Fentiman, Jr. and G. W. Kinzer (1972) 3-methyl-2-cyclohexen-1-ol isolated from *Dendroctonus*. Naturwissenschaften, 59, 469.

Vité, J. P. and J. A. A. Renwick (1968) Insect and host factors in the aggregation of the southern pine beetle. Contrib. Boyce Thompson Inst. 24, 61–63.

Vité, J. P. and J. A. A. Renwick (1970) Differential diagnosis and isolation of population attractants. Contrib. Boyce Thompson Inst. 24, 323–328.

Vité, J. P. and J. A. A. Renwick (1971a) Population aggregating pheromone in the bark beetle, *Ips grandicollis*. J. Insect Physiol. 17, 1699–1704.

Vité, J. P. and J. A. A. Renwick (1971b) Inhibition of *Dendroctonus frontalis* response to frontalin by isomers of brevicomin. Naturwissenschaften 58, 418.

Vité, J. P. and D. L. Williamson (1970) *Thanasimus dubius*: prey perception. J. Insect Physiol. 16, 233–239.

Vité, J. P. and D. L. Wood (1961) A study on the applicability of the measurement of oleoresin exudation pressure in determining susceptibility of second growth ponderosa pine to bark beetle infestation. Contrib. Boyce Thompson Inst. 21, 67–78.

Vité, J. P., A. Bakke and J. A. A. Renwick (1972) Pheromones in *Ips* (Coleoptera: Scolytidae): occurrence and production. Can. Entomol. 104, 1967–1975.

Vité, J. P., R. I. Gara and H. D. Von Scheller (1964) Field observations on the response to attractants of bark beetles infesting southern pines. Contrib. Boyce Thompson Inst. 22, 461–470.

Wilkinson, R. C., W. T. McClelland, R. M. Murillo and E. O. Ostmark (1967) Stridulation and behavior in two southeastern *Ips* bark beetles (Coleoptera: Scolytidae). Florida Entomol. 50, 185–195.

Williamson, D. L. (1971) Olfactory discernment of prey by *Medetera bistriata* (Diptera: Dolichopodidae). Ann. Entomol. Soc. Am. 64, 586–589.

Wood, D. L. (1962a) Experiments on the interrelationship between oleoresin exudation pressure in *Pinus ponderosa* and attack by *Ips confusus* (LeC.) (Coleoptera: Scolytidae). Can. Entomol. 94, 473–477.

Wood, D. L. (1962b) The attraction created by males of a bark beetle *Ips confusus* (LeConte) attacking ponderosa pine. Pan-Pac. Entomol. 38, 141–145.

Wood, D. L. (1963) Studies on host selection by *Ips confusus* (LeConte) (Coleoptera: Scolytidae) with special reference to Hopkins' host selection principle. Univ. Calif. Publ. Entomol. 27, 241–282.

Wood, D. L. (1972) Selection and colonisation of ponderosa pine by bark beetles. *In*: Insect/Plant Relationships; ed.: H. F. van Emden. Symp. Roy. Entomol. Soc. (London) 6, 101–117.

Wood, D. L. and R. W. Bushing (1963) The olfactory response of *Ips confusus* (LeConte) (Coleoptera: Scolytidae) to the secondary attraction in the laboratory. Can. Entomol. 95, 1066–1078.

Wood, D. L. and J. P. Vité (1961) Studies on the host selection behavior of *Ips confusus* (LeConte) (Coleoptera: Scolytidae) attacking *Pinus ponderosa*. Contrib. Boyce Thompson Inst. 21, 79–95.

Wood, D. L., L. E. Browne, W. D. Bedard, P. E. Tilden, R. M. Silverstein and J. O. Rodin (1968) Response of *Ips confusus* to synthetic sex pheromones in nature. Science 159, 1373–1374.

Wood, D. L., L. E. Browne, R. M. Silverstein and J. O. Rodin (1966) Sex pheromones of bark beetles – I. Mass production, bio-assay, source, and isolation of the sex pheromone of *Ips confusus* (LeC.). J. Insect Physiol. 12, 523–536.

Wood, D. L., R. W. Stark, R. M. Silverstein and J. O. Rodin (1967) Unique synergistic effects produced by the principal sex attractant compounds of *Ips confusus* (LeConte) (Coleoptera: Scolytidae). Nature (London) 215, 206.

Zenther-Møller, O. and J. A. Rudinsky (1967) Studies on the site of sex pheromone production in *Dendroctonus pseudotsugae* (Coleoptera: Scolytidae). Ann. Entomol. Soc. Am. 60, 575–582.

CHAPTER 9

Pheromones in speciation of Coleoptera

Gerald N. LANIER and Wendell E. BURKHOLDER

9.1. *Introduction*

The current emphasis on development of ecologically acceptable means of manipulating and monitoring economic pests, together with recent advances in chemical technology, have resulted in an explosion of information on attractant pheromones. Since attractant pheromones can enforce premating isolation between related sympatric species (Mayr 1963), considerable interest has been aroused in pheromones as taxonomic indicators and in the role of pheromones in speciation. Shorey et al. (1968) pointed out that 'contrary to the general popular impression, insect sex pheromones are not necessarily species-specific – sometimes not even genus-specific or family-specific.' Wood (1970) stated that 'sex pheromones are an important isolating mechanism and a study of their specificity should contribute to a more enlightened view of insect biosystematics and evolution'. Roelofs and Comeau (1969, 1970) proposed that mutations in pheromone systems might result in speciation without the necessity of geographic isolation and genetic selection. Conversely, Shorey (1970) expressed the opinion that pheromone changes follow speciation because sex pheromone specificity is a premating isolating mechanism which can prevent gamete wastage and therefore is subject to considerable selection pressure. This chapter will examine in depth the subject of species-specificity of attractant pheromones in Coleoptera, the evolution of pheromone differences and the role of pheromones in speciation.

Attractant pheromones in Coleoptera are generally classed as sex pheromones or aggregating pheromones (reviews by Silverstein 1970 and Jacobson 1972). Sex pheromones are usually released by one sex and attract the other. The release of sex pheromone may occur irrespective of habitat whenever the releasing individual is ready to mate, as is apparently the case in some Scarabidae (Ladd 1970; Hoyt et al. 1971). Aggregating pheromones are usually released by either or both sexes when a suitable breeding habitat is located (see Borden, ch. 8). Typically, the sex which initiates feeding in the habitat releases a pheromone which is attractive to both sexes, as in the boll weevil, *Anthonomus grandis* Boheman (Tumlinson et al. 1970; Hardee 1970) and most bark beetles (Silverstein 1970). *Leperisinus varius fraxini* Pz.) appears to be exceptional because the female initiates feeding and gallery construction in ash logs but the male releases the aggregating pheromone (Schönherr 1970).

Both habitat cues and pheromones are operative in the aggregation of many beetles, but they vary in the order of precedence. The dermestid beetles apparently seek the habitat first, then locate mates within the habitat by using short range pheromones. In contrast, many Scolytidae will virtually ignore uninfested host material in the presence of other host material which has been marked for colonization by pheromones. Habitat odors and beetle pheromones may produce an integrated aggregating attractant such as that of the western pine beetle, *Dendroctonus brevicomis* LeConte, in which a pheromone from each sex plus a host terpene are necessary for optimum attraction (Wood 1972). Habitat cues seem to be of little importance to mating in beetles which release a sex attractant, mate and then seek a suitable oviposition site. In the other extreme, habitat or host odors, per se, may bring the sexes together (Oksanen et al. 1970). For example, both sexes of the cerambycid genus *Monochamus* are strongly attracted to injured or cut conifers upon which they encounter and mate without any apparent pheromonal signal.

9.2. *Specificity of pheromone systems in Coleoptera*

9.2.1. *Components of pheromone systems*

Chemical communication involves emission and perception of volatile compounds. Either or both of these components may convey *response specificity* among two or more species. Similarity or dissimilarity of the emission products, i.e., *pheromone specificity*, may be inferred from the results of bioassays or by comparisons of the putative active compounds present in different species. Similarity in capacity to receive chemical messages, i.e., *receptor specificity*, may be inferred from behavioral tests or directly assessed by an electroantennogram (EAG). An EAG is made by inserting micro-electrodes into the nerve of the living antenna and recording the magnitude of the change in electrical potential when the antenna is presented with olfactory stimuli (see Payne, ch. 3). The two criteria, production and response, must be met before a compound can be classified as a pheromone.

Although pheromonal attraction is known to occur in several coleopteran families, the pheromone systems of only the dermestid genus, *Trogoderma*, and the scolytid genera, *Ips* and *Dendroctonus*, are sufficiently known to warrant discussion of pheromone specificity. Because direct information on pheromone and receptor specificity is extremely limited much of the discussion in this section is based upon inferences. This procedure seems valid because, whenever available, direct information is usually compatible with the results of behavioral tests.

9.2.2. *Specificity of pheromones in Trogoderma*

Species of *Trogoderma* are distributed rather evenly among different faunal zones, on every continent and in every climate from subarctic to tropical (Beal 1954). The world-wide distribution of *Trogoderma* reflects an ancient origin of this genus as well as its recent distribution by commerce. Three of the 14 species occurring in North America were introduced and two of these, *T. glabrum* (Herbst) and *T. variabile* Ballion (=*parabile* Beal), are among the most damaging and widely spread pests of stored products. The infamous Khapra beetle, *T. granarium* Everts, was once introduced but subsequently eradicated from the United States. Hinton (1945) identified several elytral and antennal variations in Eurasian *T. glabrum.* Beal (1954) found only one of these varieties in North America and speculated that the Nearctic populations resulted from a single introduction and perhaps a single gravid female. Similarly, *T. variabile* is morphologically extremely uniform in North America. In contrast to the exotic species, the *Trogoderma* native to North America are rather variable, often rare, and usually of minor economic significance.

Although *Trogoderma* species are broadly sympatric, cohabitation of two or more species is rare. The various species have different ecological and food preferences in their natural habitats (Strong et al. 1959; Partida and Strong 1970) but this is not sufficiently strict to account for the lack of mixed species colonies in stored products. When *T. granarium* and *T. variabile* were initially established in the same experimental grain bin *T. variabile* became extinct (Nutting 1959). It is interesting that the introduced *T. glabrum* and *T. variabile* are among the most damaging and widespread species. In the central and northern parts of the United States these are by far the most important *Trogoderma.* A three year survey by Kantack and Staples (1969) reveales that infestations of *T. glabrum* were well established in grain storages in 43 Nebraska counties. These species are the most important *Trogoderma* in Wisconsin and P. K. Harein* (personal communication) reported that ca. 95% of the *Trogoderma* sp. identified at the University of Minnesota are either *T. glabrum* or *T. variabile.*

Beal (1954) reported that males of *T. sternale maderae* Beal, *T. grassmani* Beal, *T. simplex* Jayne and *T. variabile* were sexually stimulated by contact with the dorsum of a female of any of these species. Males of five species of *Trogoderma* showed considerable interspecific response to crude extracts of attractants from seven species (Vick et al. 1970). The same five species, plus a sixth, were attracted to the synthetic pheromone of *T. inclusum* (14-methyl-*cis*-8-hexadecen-1-ol) (Rodin et al. 1969) although *T. glabrum* was much more sensitive to its own pheromone (14-methyl-*trans*-8-hexadecen-1-ol) (Burkholder et al. 1973). *T. sternale* showed relatively low cross attractiveness to any species and relatively high threshold response to either the *cis* or *trans* alcohol (table 9.1).

* University of Minnesota, Dept. of Entomol. Fisheries and Wildlife, St. Paul, Minnesota 55101, U.S.A.

TABLE 9.1

Interspecific response by *Trogoderma* males in the laboratory.

Attractant	Species of males tested					
Female extract[a]	*inclusum*	*simplex*	*variabile*	*grassmani*	*glabrum*	*sternale*
		Index of response[b]				
inclusum	100 α	111 α	109α	–	20 α	0 α
simplex	98 α	100 α	109 α	–	6 α	0 α
variabile	85 α	89 α	100 α	–	0 α	0 α
granarium	70 αβ	84 α	93 α	–	11 α	0 α
grassmani	98 α	91 α	109 α	–	20 α	55 αβ
glabrum	42 β	27 β	2 β	–	100 β	58 αβ
sternale	80 α	31 β	6 β	–	13 α	100 β
Synthetic pheromone[c]	Concentration (μg) of compound required for 50% male response					
inclusum (*cis*-alcohol)	0.0011	0.1219	0.0017	0.0001	0.4745	0.2930
glabrum (*trans-alcohol*)	0.1143	1.7043	0.2036	0.0300[d]	0.0036	10,0000[d]

[a] 0.01 Female equivalent; Vick et al. (1970).

[b] Index of response = interspecific response (%)/conspecific response (%) x 100. Indices followed by the same letter (α or β) in vertical columns are not significantly different at the 5% level, as determined by Duncan's multiple range test.

[c] Burkholder et al. (1973).

[d] Nonsignificant linear regression.

Although they are apparently not species-specific, *Trogoderma* pheromones seem to be genus-specific. Male *T. granarium* responded to extracts of female *T. inclusum* and *T. glabrum*, but not to those of *Anthrenus flavipes* LeConte (=*vorax* Waterhouse), *Attagenus megatoma* (Fab.) or *Dermestes maculatus* DeGeer (Levinson and Bar Ilan 1970). Similarly, *Attagenus megatoma* did not respond to extracts of *Trogoderma inclusum* or *T. glabrum*, and none of the *Trogoderma* species responded to *Attagenus megatoma* (Burkholder 1970).

9.2.3. Specificity of pheromone systems in Ips

The North American *Ips* have been divided into ten groups of closely related species (Hopping 1963). The species concepts have been subjected to some revision but the groups have survived considerable taxonomic scrutiny (Lindquist 1969; Lanier 1966, 1970b, 1970c, 1972, 1974). Typically several species of *Ips* occur in a given geographic area and some of them may compete for the same host material. However, these sympatric species belong to different groups. For example, *Ips calligraphus calligraphus* (Germar) (Group X), *I. grandicollis* (Eichhoff) (Group IX) and *I. avulsus* (Eichhoff) (Group IV) are respectively frequently found in the lower, middle and upper portions of the same pine tree in the southeastern states. The widely distributed *I. pini* (Say) (Group IV) is usually found with *I. integer* (Eichhoff) (Group III) or *I. calligraphus ponderosae* Swaine (Group X) in the Rocky Mountain states and with *I. paraconfusus* Lanier (Group IX) or *I. plastographus* (LeConte) (Group III) on the western slope of the Sierra Nevada.

Laboratory and field bioassays have invariably demonstrated a high degree of response specificity in *Ips* species of different groups (Vité and Gara 1962; Vité et al. 1964; Lanier and Wood 1973). In most tests, interspecific responses were not significantly above the background levels and, even when significant responses were observed in the laboratory, cross attractiveness was much lower or nil in the field. For example, the highest attraction indices* observed in the laboratory between *Ips* of different groups were 38 and 30 for reciprocal tests of females of *I. pini* and *I. paraconfusus* respectively (table 9.2). However, none of the aggregate of nearly 2000 *I. pini* and *I. paraconfusus* trapped in a field test responded to the 'wrong' species (Lanier et al. 1972).

In contrast to the sympatry of *Ips* of different species groups, species of the same group are generally allopatric or parapatric. In Group IX, for example, *I. para-*

TABLE 9.2

Indices of attraction[a] between *Ips* species of different groups in the laboratory.

Group	Species exposed (♀♀)	Air only	*plast.*	*pini*	*para.*	*callig.*	Other species
III	*plastographus*	9	100	24	16	22	–
IV	*pini*	13	14	100	38	16	–
IX	*paraconfusus*	9	16	30	100	27	0 – 13[b]
X	*calligraphus*	–	18	19	14	100	–

[a] Index of attraction = interspecific attraction (%)/conspecific attraction (=) x 100 (Lanier 1970a). Data from Lanier and Wood (1973).

[b] Indices of attraction of *paraconfusus* to other species are as follows: *latidens* – 11, *sabininae* – *13* (both group 0); *concinnus* – 9, *mexicanus* – 9 (both group I); *pilifrons* – 0, *woodi* – 0 (both Group VI); *tridens* – 3 (Group VIII).

* The attraction index is an expression of response to a different species or population, relative to the level of response to the same species or population (Lanier 1970a).

confusus is contiguously allopatric with *I. montanus* (Eichhoff) in Oregon and northern California and with *I. confusus* (LeConte) in southern California. *I. confusus* meets *I. hoppingi* Lanier near the border of the U.S.A. and Mexico. *I. cribricollis* (Eichhoff) overlaps the geographical distribution of *I. hoppingi* but occurs at higher elevations and in different hosts. *I. lecontei* Swaine is the exceptional species in this group because it is partially sympatric with and occasionally infests the same host material as *I. cribricollis*, *I. confusus* and *I. hoppingi* (Lanier 1970b).

Also in contrast to the situation among *Ips* of different groups, species of the same group are usually cross attractive (Vité et al. 1964; Wood 1970; Vité and Renwick 1971b; Lanier and Wood 1973). In laboratory bioassays of individual samples of attractant frass, response to species of the same group was usually as strong as conspecific response (table 9.3). *I. lecontei* was again exceptional among Group IX-species owing to its moderate response and attractiveness to other species. When two attractant samples were presented simultaneously, *I. paraconfusus* demonstrated a clear preference for conspecific attractant while *I. montanus* and *I. confusus* discriminated against only the *I. lecontei* attractant (Wood 1970; Lanier and Wood 1973). In the field *I. paraconfusus*, *I. montanus* and *I. confusus* were strongly cross attractive. In addition, female *I. paraconfusus* mated with males of *I.*

TABLE 9.3

Indices of attraction[a, b] between *Ips* species of Group IX when samples are presented individually (I) and simultaneously (S) in the laboratory.

Species exposed ♀♀		Species producing frass ♂♂ *para.*	*conf.*	*hopp.*	*mont.*	*lec.*	*crib.*
paraconfusus	I	100	97	–	86	76*	–
	S	100	55***	63**	35***	59***	114
confusus	I	99	100	–	111	64	–
	S	111	100	–	–	78	–
montanus	I	122	125	–	100	25***	–
	S	83	119	–	100	–	–
lecontei	I	63*	65**	–	65*	100	–
	S	51***	47**	39***	45***	100	16***
hoppingi	S	144	–	100	–	–	–
cribricollis	S	–	–	–	–	113	100

[a] Index of attraction = interspecific attraction (%) / conspecific attraction (%) × 100 (Lanier 1970a). Data from Lanier and Wood (1973).

[b] Differences in raw data significant at 0.05 – *; 0.01 – ** and 0.001 – *** levels of confidence (Chi-square test).

montanus and *I. confusus* boring in uncaged bolts placed in an area where only *I. paraconfusus* occurred (Lanier and Wood 1973). Vité and Renwick (1971b) reported 'interspecific attraction' among *I. confusus*, *I. paraconfusus*, *I. montanus*, *I. cribricollis* and *I. grandicollis* but they did not state which combinations were tested and what level of attraction was observed. In one experiment (Vité et al. 1964), *I. grandicollis* seemed to favor the frass of *I. paraconfusus* over its own attractant, but this test cannot be considered definitive because the sources used were not equivalent.

The index of response for females of *I. tridens* (Mannerheim) to males of *I. pilifrons* Swaine (both Group VIII) was 37 in the laboratory but 16 and 0 in two field tests (Lanier 1970a). It seems probable that whenever attraction is less than the base 100 in the laboratory, attraction will be still lower in the field, but when a species does not show preference for its own attractant in the laboratory, it may not discriminate in the field.

Three pheromones – ipsenol, *cis*-verbenol and ipsdienol* – are known in *Ips*; all of them were originally identified from frass of *Ips paraconfusus* (Silverstein et al. 1966). Each of the three pheromones elicited some response from *I. paraconfusus* in laboratory bioassays, but a mixture of all three compounds was necessary for effective attraction in the field (Wood et al. 1967). The same compounds are produced by *I. confusus* but only ipsenol is attractive to this species (Young et al. 1973). Ipsenol was reported to act alone as the pheromone of *I. grandicollis* (Vité and Renwick 1971b), which also produces *cis*-verbenol (Vité et al. 1972), and ipsdienol plus *cis*-verbenol have been reported to be pheromones of *I. calligraphus* (Renwick and Vité 1972). Compounds which, on the basis of gas chromatographs, are believed to be the three pheromones appear in the hindguts of males of several additional species (Vité et al. 1972) (table 9.4). However, the structure of these compounds have not been verified, their optical rotation is unknown and their role in attraction of the species involved has not been determined.

The verified pheromones are consistent with response behavior of *Ips*. Strong attraction of *I. grandicollis* and *I. paraconfusus* is explained by the relatively large amount of ipsenol produced by the latter species. Lack of cross attraction between *I. grandicollis* and *I. calligraphus* is expected owing to their clear pheromonal differences. That *I. calligraphus* is not attracted to *I. paraconfusus*, which produces all three pheromones, indicates that reponse is blocked, possibly by ipsenol. *I. latidens* is attracted to a mixture of ipsenol and *cis*-verbenol but ipsdienol blocks response (Wood et al. 1967; Wood 1970).

Vité and Renwick (1971b) noted that behavioral tests indicated that ipsenol was also produced by *I. montanus* and *I. cribricollis*. Since the attractants of *I. monta-*

* The trivial names, ipsenol and ipsdienol were suggested by Silverstein (personal communication) and used by Renwick and Vité (1972) for 2-methyl-6-methylene-7-octen-4-ol and 2-methyl-6-methylene-2,7-octadien-4-ol, respectively.

TABLE 9.4

Attractant pheromones in *Ips*.

Group	Species	Ipsenol	*cis*-verbenol	Ipsdienol
0	*latidens*[b,1,2]	?Rs[a]	?Rs	?B
II	*knausi*[3]	O?	P?	P?
III	*integer*[3]	O?	P?	P?
IV	*avulsus*[3]	O?	P?	P?
	pini[3]	O?	P?	P?
	bonanseai[3]	O?	P?	P?
VI	*typographus*[c,3]	P?	P?	P?
IX	*paraconfusus*[1,2,4]	PRs	PRs	PRs
	confusus[5]	PR	PO	PO
	grandicollis[6]	PR	P?	O?
	cribricollis[3]	P?	P?	O?
	montanus[2]	?r	?r	?r
X	*calligraphus*[7]	O?	PRs	PRs
–	*accuminatus*[c,3]	P?	P?	P?
–	*sexdentatus*[c,3]	P?	P?	P?

[a] P = produced, B = blocking, R = response, Rs = response synergized, r = response in the laboratory, O = not produced or no response, ? = unknown production (if in front of letter) or unknown response (if behind).

[b] References are keyed to numbers as follows: 1. Wood et al. (1967); 2. Wood (1970); 3. Vité et al. (1972a); 4. Silverstein et al. (1966); 5. Young et al. (1973); 6. Vité and Renwick (1971b); 7. Renwick and Vité (1972).

[c] European species: contrary to Hopping (1965) and Vité et al. (1972a), *I. sexdentatus* is not closely related to *calligraphus* (Lanier 1972).

nus and *I. confusus* appeared to be interchangeable with respect to *I. paraconfusus* and to each other, it seems probable that *I. montanus* also used only ipsenol as its pheromone. On the other hand, the semi-specificity of *I. lecontei* indicated that this species used at least one compound not shared by the other species of Group IX.

The gas chromatograms of Vité et al. (1972a) are consistent with the observed cross attraction between *I. pini* and *I. bonanseai* (Hopkins) and between *I. cribricollis* and *I. paraconfusus*. *I. pini* and *I. avulsus* appear to be biochemically similar to *I. calligraphus* but these species are not cross attractive. Renwick and Vité (1972) stated that the mutual production of ipsdienol 'may be responsible for the cross attraction between *I. avulsus* and *I. calligraphus*, which frequently co-inhabit the same tree'. However, the only published data (Vité et al. 1964) give an index of

14 for the attraction of *I. calligraphus* to *I. avulsus* and an index of 0.2 for the reciprocal. In the same test the index of attraction of *I. calligraphus* to *I. grandicollis* (which produces no ipsdienol) was 12. This behavioral evidence and the cohabitation of these species clearly does not 'corroborate to some extent' (Vité et al. 1972) the biochemical similarity of *I. calligraphus* and *I. avulsus*. Either the identification of the pheromone of *I. avulsus* is incorrect or additional compounds confer specificity between this species and *I. calligraphus*. Behavioral specificity among European *Ips* and among *I. knausi* Swaine, *I. integer* and *I. bonanseai* of the southwestern U.S.A. is not known, but it seems safe to predict that these species will not be strongly cross attractive. Unidentified compounds will probably be decisive in the specificity of their pheromone bouquets.

9.2.4. *Specificity of pheromone systems in Dendroctonus*

Unlike the situation in the genus *Ips*, generalities about the geographic distribution of *Dendroctonus* species relative to their phylogenetic relationship are not readily apparent. Certain closely related species such as *D. simplex* LeConte and *D. pseudotsugae* Hopkins or *D. valens* LeConte and *D. terabrans* (Olivier) are allopatric (Wood 1963). However, other very closely related species, such as *D. ponderosae* Hopkins and *D. jeffreyi* Hopkins and *D. rufipennis* Kirby (=*obesus* Mannerheim) and *D. murrayanae* Hopkins, are broadly sympatric but they attack different hosts (Wood 1963; Lanier and Wood 1968). *D. brevicomis* LeConte and *D. frontalis* Zimmerman are largely allopatric but they overlap geographically and overlap in host preference in parts of the southwestern U.S.A. and Mexico, where they may compete for the same host material with *D. approximatus* Dietz, *D. adjunctus* Blandford and *D. ponderosae* (Wood 1963). In contrast, *D. valens* avoids serious competition with its more distant relatives by concentrating its attacks on the root collar of pines. Most of the species discussed here feed in pines, but the normal host of *D. simplex* is larch, *D. rufipennis* attacks spruces and the usual host of *D. pseudotsugae* is Douglas-fir.

Also in contrast to the genus *Ips*, more is known about the chemistry of the *Dendroctonus* pheromones and response to attractive compounds than about response specificity in the natural system (i.e., beetles boring in trees). The only controlled experiment on response specificity of *Dendroctonus* yet published revealed that *D. rufipennis* boring in white spruce and *D. pseudotsugae* boring in either white spruce or Douglas-fir were strongly cross attractive (Chapman and Dyer 1969). *D. rufipennis* refused to bore in Douglas-fir, so that treatment could not be assessed. From these results Chapman and Dyer (1969) concluded that the pheromones of *D. rufipennis* and D. *pseudotsugae* are very similar or identical.

Three attractive compounds, brevicomin, frontalin and *trans*-verbenol have been reported in five of the 16 *Dendroctonus* species and a fourth attractant, 3-methyl-2-cyclohexen-1-ol, has recently been identified from *D. pseudotsugae* (Vité et

TABLE 9.5

Attractant pheromones in *Dendroctonus*.

Species	Attractants			Inhibitors		Optimum attractant
	t-verbenol	brevicomin	frontalin	verbenone	MCH[a]	
frontalis 1,2,3,4,5,6,7						
♂♂	ps[c]	pi	0R	Pi	--	F + α-pinene[4]
♀♀	Ps	0I	pR	pi	--	
brevicomis 1,2,6,7,8,9,10,11,12						
♂♂	pi	0R	PR	Pi	--	B + F + myrcene >[11]
♀♀	Pi	Pr	0R	pi	--	3-carene[10,11]
ponderosae 6,7,13						
♂♂	0R	P0	00	o?	--	*t*-V + α-pinene[5]
♀♀	PR	p0	00	p?	--	
jeffreyi 7						
♂♂	p?	P?	0?	o?	--	Unknown
♀♀	P?	p?	0?	p?	--	
pseudotsugae 14,15,16,17						
♂♂	?0	??	?R	??	?I	F + camphene,[17]
♀♀	P0	??	PR	??	pI	α-pinene[17]
adjunctus 18						
♂♂	??	??	?R	??	--	Unknown
♀♀	??	??	?R	??	--	

[a] MCH = 3-methyl-2-cyclohexene-1-one; the corresponding alcohol, 3-methyl-2-cyclohexene-1-ol, is produced by the female *D. pseudotsugae* (and probably by female *D. rufipennis*) and is thought to be an attractant (Vité et al. 1972b).

[b] References are indicated by numbers as follows: 1. Renwick (1967); 2. Kinzer et al. (1969); 3. Vité and Renwick (1968); 4. ibid (1971a) 5. Renwick and Vité (1969); 6. ibid (1970); 7. Pitman et al. (1969); 8. Silverstein et al. (1968); 9. Bedard et al. (1969); 10. Vité and Pitman (1969b); 11. Bedard et al. (1970); 12. Wood (1973); 13. Pitman and Vité (1969); 14. Renwick and Vité (1968); 15. Pitman and Vité (1970); 16. Kinzer et al. (1971); 17. Rudinsky et al. (1972a, b); 18. Vité and Renwick (1970).

[c] P = Produced; p = produced in trace quantities; R = response; I = strong inhibitor; i = weak inhibitor; 0 = not produced or not attractive; F =

1972b) (table 9.5). At least two of these compounds appear in each sex of each species, but the combinations present differ between sexes and species. An additional two compounds, 3-methyl-2-cyclohexen-1-one (MCH) (Rudinsky et al. 1972a) and verbenone (Renwick and Vité 1970), appear to play a role in 'turning off' the attraction in some species. Some of the compounds may have multiple roles; brevicomin and *trans*-verbenol are attractants to some species and inhibitors of response in others (Vité and Renwick 1971a; Vité and Islas 1973; Wood 1973).

Host terpenes synergize the attraction to pheromones of *Dendroctonus* species. For example, *D. ponderosae* showed almost no attraction to *trans*-verbenol until this pheromone was combined with host odors (Pitman and Vité 1969). However, the response of *D. pseudotsugae* to frontalin *per se* compared favorably to the response to females boring in logs (Rudinsky et al. 1972b).

The only direct study of olfactory reception in beetles is the EAG work on *Dendroctonus brevicomis* and *D. frontalis* by Payne (1970, 1971). Antennal receptors of these two species were not specific to the pheromones frontalin and brevicomin or to various terpenes on a response–no response basis. However, the relative amplitude of the EAG in response to various stimuli was consistent with the behavioral response of the beetles. For example, EAGs of antennae of female *D. brevicomis* showed greater response to frontalin than to brevicomin although the reverse was true of the males. This mirrors the relative attractiveness of the two pheromones to the sexes in the field (Bedard et al. 1969; Vité and Pitman 1969b). The EAGs represent the aggregate response of the stimulated receptors; it is not possible to determine whether the same receptors or different receptors, as suggested by Renwick (1970), are responding to the pheromones and host terpenes.

Reports of interspecific response in the field tend to corroborate the chemical evidence presented in the above discussion (table 9.6). *D. frontalis* responded strongly to frass (Vité et al. 1964) and crushed, mixed sexes (Vité and Renwick 1968) of *D. brevicomis*. Vité and Renwick (1968) stated that males of *D. brevicomis*, which contained large amounts of frontalin, were strongly attractive to *D. frontalis* whereas females, which produced mostly brevicomin, were only slightly attractive (no data supporting this statement have been published). *D. frontalis* was also strongly attracted to crushed *D. pseudotsugae* females, which produce frontalin, but not to crushed males or to either sex of *D. ponderosae*, which do not produce frontalin (Renwick and Vité 1968). Similarly, crushed females of *D. brevicomis* and *D. frontalis*, which produce substantially more *trans*-verbenol than do males, were 'strongly' attractive to *D. ponderosae* (Pitman and Vité 1969). Finally, *D. brevicomis* males and females were attracted to crushed males of *D. ponderosae* which produce substantial amounts of brevicomin (Vité and Pitman 1969a).

Pitman et al. (1969) hypothesized that since the pheromones in *Dendroctonus* are shared by several species, the pheromone receptors convey response specificity. The mechanism proposed is that the combination of the pheromone and a host terpene convey a species specific message. For example, specificity between

TABLE 9.6

Interspecific response by *Dendroctonus* in the field.

Species responding		Material tested	Attraction index
frontalis	*brevicomis*	frass extract[a,1]	400[6]
frontalis	*brevicomis*	mixed sexes, crushed[2]	306
frontalis	*brevicomis*	males, crushed[2,3]	high
frontalis	*brevicomis*	females, crushed[3]	slight
frontalis	*pseudotsugae*	males, crushed[2]	0[6]
frontalis	*pseudotsugae*	females, crushed[2]	91[b]
frontalis	*ponderosae*	males, crushed[3]	nil
frontalis	*ponderosae*	females, crushed[3]	nil
brevicomis	*ponderosae*	males, crushed[4]	53[b]
ponderosae	*brevicomis*	females, crushed + oleoresin[5]	high
ponderosae	*brevicomis*	males, crushed + oleoresin[5]	slight
ponderosae	*brevicomis*	infested material[6]	'respond readily'
ponderosae	*frontalis*	females, crushed + oleoresin[5]	high
ponderosae	*frontalis*	males, crushed + oleoresin[5]	slight
pseudotsugae	*rufipennis*	boring in white spruce[7]	73
rufipennis	*pseudotsugae*	boring in white spruce[7]	27
rufipennis	*pseudotsugae*	boring in Douglas-fir[7]	52

[a] References are keyed to numbers as follows: 1. Vité et al. (1964); 2. Renwick and Vité (1968); 3. Vité and Renwick (1970); 4. Vité and Pitman (1969a); 5. Pitman and Vité (1969); 6. Pitman et al. (1968); 7. Chapman and Dyer (1969).

[b] Attraction indices based on data from tests which were not exactly equivalent.

D. brevicomis and *D. pseudotsugae*, both of which are attracted to frontalin, could be maintained by the terpenes 3-carene and camphene in the respective host species (Pitman and Vité 1970). Subsequently it was found that α-pinene is interchangeable with camphene in the *D. pseudotsugae* attractant (Rudinsky et al. 1972a) and that myrcene is a superior terpene synergist for the *D. brevicomis* attractant (Bedard et al. 1969). Detailed examination of terpene composition in the host species of the different beetles revealed a number of specific criticisms to the situation hypothesized above. However, the most important criticism of this work is that pheromone specificity was assumed without being tested. It is not known, for example, that *D. brevicomis* and *D. pseudotsugae* are *not* cross attractive.

In every published case in which cross attractiveness of *Dendroctonus* species has been tested, beetles responded in a number that would have been predicted by the bouquet of compounds they are known to produce. *D. pseudotsugae* forced to bore in several factitious or occasional hosts were attractive to the flying population (Jantz and Rudinsky 1965; Chapman and Dyer 1969). *D. ponderosae* reportedly responds to *D. brevicomis* boring in ponderosa pine (Pitman et al. 1968). There is no reason to believe that *D. brevicomis* would not be attracted to *D. ponderosae* boring in ponderosa pine or in another host even though *D. brevicomis* cannot successfully attack certain species (Smith 1961, 1963, 1965). It seems clear that neither production nor reception of attractant compounds from both the beetle and the tree is sufficient to enforce reproductive isolation among many of the species of sympatric *Dendroctonus*.

9.3. *Pheromone systems and reproductive isolation*

9.3.1. *Role of pheromones*

Our knowledge of behavioral specificity in *Trogoderma* and *Ips* exceeds our understanding of pheromone specificity. The reverse is true in *Dendroctonus*. The role of pheromone systems in maintaining reproductive isolation appears, at this early stage of the field, to be quite different in these genera. Pheromone systems effectively prevent interspecific insemination in *Ips* because sympatric species are not (or only minimally) cross attractive. These species may share some attractive compounds, as do *I. paraconfusus* and *I. calligraphus*, but the bouquet is unique, and blocking or some other mechanism mediates against cross attractiveness (Wood et al. 1967; Renwick and Vité 1972). Pheromone systems per se appear not to isolate most *Trogoderma* and certain sympatric *Dendroctonus* such as *D. brevicomis* and *D. ponderosae* or *D. rufipennis* and *D. pseudotsugae*. Synergism by specific terpenes may play a role in minimizing attraction between two *Dendroctonus* species which produce some of the same pheromones, but infest different hosts (as theorized by Pitman et al. 1969), although this hypothesis has never been tested. To the contrary, conspecific and interspecific attraction between *D. pseudotsugae* and *D. rufipennis* (Jantz and Rudinsky 1965; Chapman and Dyer 1969) prove that, in some cases, host species is of little consequence to pheromone attractiveness.

9.3.2. *Consequence of interspecific attraction*

Breeding experiments demonstrated reproductive isolation among all combinations of the *Trogoderma* species listed in table 9.1 (Beal and Spitler 1959; Strong and Arndt 1962). Only the reciprocal combination of *T. granarium* and *T. glabrum* produced brood, but these were totally sterile. These studies did not report whether mating occurred in interspecific pairings other than *T. glabrum* x *T. granarium*. Beal (1954) stated that females of several *Trogoderma* species refused interspecific insemination. After initial mating *Trogoderma* females typically refuse further copulation for a period ranging from two hours to the remainder of their lives (Vick et al. 1972); possibly, the females that Beal (1954) observed had already mated. Vick (1973) found that *T. inclusum* and *T. glabrum* readily intermated but the *T. inclusum* female rejected the foreign spermatophore and mated again. The *T. glabrum* female accepted the *T. inclusum* spermatophore and was refractory to further mating. Thus, an interspecifically mated *T. glabrum* would be effectively sterilized while the reciprocal cross would be of little consequence if *T. inclusum* males were available for subsequent mating.

Among the *Ips*, the propensity for interspecific mating was closely correlated with cross attraction. Females readily entered the nuptial chambers of males of cross attractive species, mated, and laid eggs, but hatchability of these eggs was in the inverse order of the attractiveness (Lanier 1966, 1970b, c, 1972). Interspecific insemination among the highly cross attractive species within Groups IV, IX and X resulted in no fertile progeny. *I. plastographus* and *I. integer* of Group III showed low cross attraction and produced a low number of semifertile hybrids. *I. borealis* and *I. tridens* were minimally cross attractive and difficult to breed, but the few resulting hybrids were fertile, intermediate in attractiveness, and readily crossed back to either parent species (Lanier 1970a).

Less is known about the propensity and the consequences of *Dendroctonus* species to intermate. *D. ponderosae* and *D. jeffreyi* were compatible as mates but the single hybrid resulting from 1250 eggs was sterile (Lanier and Wood 1968). *D. pseudotsugae* and *D. simplex* readily intermated and produced fertile hybrids when the latter was the female (Furniss 1973) but eggs laid by interspecifically mated *D. pseudotsugae* failed to hatch. Nothing is known about the response specificity between these pairs of species, although the former pair produce similar bouquets of compounds known to be attractants (Pitman et al. 1969).

9.3.3. *Isolating mechanisms*

Specificity of pheromone systems is clearly not the principal mechanism enforcing reproductive isolation in *Trogoderma* and *Dendroctonus*. Hybridization among any of the currently recognized species of *Dendroctonus* is probably rare in nature even if interspecific mating is not. Attraction in *Dendroctonus* probably does not result in mating although this is generally the case in *Ips* and possibly *Trogoderma*. Pheromone systems are probably only one of a number of isolating mechanisms which function in various combinations between different species. Detailed discussion of these is beyond the scope of this chapter, but they are outlined and exemplified in table 9.7.

9.4. *Geographic variation in pheromone systems*

The assumption that the pheromone system of a species is uniform throughout its geographic range has been discounted by the discovery of dramatic differences between pheromone systems of eastern and western *Ips pini* (Lanier 1972; Lanier et al. 1972) and between proximal populations of *I. tridens* (table 9.8). Other tests have revealed probable intraspecific pheromonal differences in *I. calligraphus calli-*

TABLE 9.7

Mechanisms which may affect reproductive isolation among sympatric species of *Trogoderma* and *Dendroctonus*.

Premating isolation
1. Ecological stratification of the habitat and hosts within generally overlapping ranges. *Dendroctonus pseudotsugae* and *D. rufipennis* are cross attractive but inhabit distinct forest types (Chapman and Dyer 1969). Various *Trogoderma* show distinct climate associations in California (Partida and Strong 1970).
2. Differences in flight periods or diel activity. *Trogoderma* show differences in diel patterns of activity although this may be insufficient to enforce reproductive isolation. Most *Dendroctonus* have different peak flight periods in the first spring flight but later flight is concurrent.
3. Pheromones
4. Differences in the host compounds which are optimum pheromone synergists. Myrcene is the most potent synergist of attraction of *D. brevicomis* to frontalin and brevicomin. This terpene is characteristic of ponderosa pine but absent or only minimally present in most non-host species (Bedard et al. 1969, 1970).
5. Food preference and antiattraction effects (i.e., repellency) *D. rufipennis* refused to establish galleries in Douglas-fir even though it was attracted to *D. pseudotsugae* boring in that host (Chapman and Dyer 1969).
6. Toxic effects of the "wrong" host *D. ponderosae, D. brevicomis* and *D. jeffreyi* are less sensitive to the fumigant and contact toxic effects of terpenes of host species than to those non-host species (Smith 1961, 1963, 1965).
7. Specificity of stridulation or other courtship rituals The stridulating organs of six species of *Dendroctonus* showed marked differences. A detailed analysis revealed that sonic patterns produced by *D. ponderosae* and *D. pseudotsugae* were very distinct (Michael and Rudinsky 1972).
8. Genital mismatch The male genitalia of *Dendroctonus* and *Trogoderma* are distinct (Wood 1963; Beal 1954, 1964). However, these differences did not prevent insemination in laboratory pairings of closely related species (Lanier and Wood 1968; Furniss 1973; Beal and Spitler 1959; Strong and Arndt 1962; Vick 1973).

Postmating isolation
1. Spermatophore rejection The female *Trogoderma inclusum* will reject a *T. glabrum* spermatophore and be receptive to reinsemination (Vick 1973).
2. Nonfertility Eggs resulting from matings between *D. ponderosae* and *D. jeffreyi* (Lanier and D. L. Wood 1968) generally failed to hatch.
3. Sterility of hybrids The hybrids of *T. glabrum* and *T. granarium* are sterile (Beal and Spitler 1959; Strong and Arndt 1962) as was the only F_1 individual resulting from pairings of *D. jeffreyi* and *D. ponderosae* (Lanier and D. L. Wood 1968).

graphus and *I. calligraphus ponderosae* (Lanier 1972). The response of *Dendroctonus frontalis* to frontalin was inhibited by endo-brevicomin in the southwestern U.S.A. (Vité and Renwick 1971a) but in Mexico *D. frontalis* was attracted to endo-brevicomin (Vité and Islas 1973). As pheromones become more widely tested additional reports of geographic variation are certain to follow. In some instances the entities revealed by pheromonal differences will prove to be sibling species. Sympatric sibling species of moths have already been discovered by their differential response to attractant compounds (Roelofs and Comeau 1969, 1970).

Reproductive isolation, and hence the species status according to the definition of the biological species by Mayr (1969), is not proven by the demonstration of different pheromonal preferences among geographical isolates. It is unwarranted to assume that, since pheromones are important in mate-finding, differences in pheromone systems per se constitute reproductive isolation. Eastern and western *Ips pini* are less cross attractive than are a number of 'good' species – i.e., *I. paraconfusus*, *I. confusus* and *I. montanus* (Wood 1970; Lanier and Wood 1973). Nevertheless, cross attraction is sufficient to insure cross insemination between individuals of eastern and western *I. pini* if they were present together in the field. Interpopulational hybrids of *I. pini* are highly fertile and hybrid males are intermediate in attractiveness at least to the eastern population (Piston and Lanier 1973). The pheromonal differences, like the slight morphological differences in both the insect (Hopping 1964) and its parasitic mites (Lindquist 1969), probably intergrade in the Rocky Mountains of the northern U.S.A. and Canada.

The most complex intrapopulational variation in pheromone systems discovered to date is exhibited in *I. tridens* and *I. borealis* Swaine. The concepts of these species were revised considerably following the discovery that seven names (considered synonyms here) were based on different forms of polymorphic females (Lanier 1973). The two remaining species are basically western and eastern in their respect-

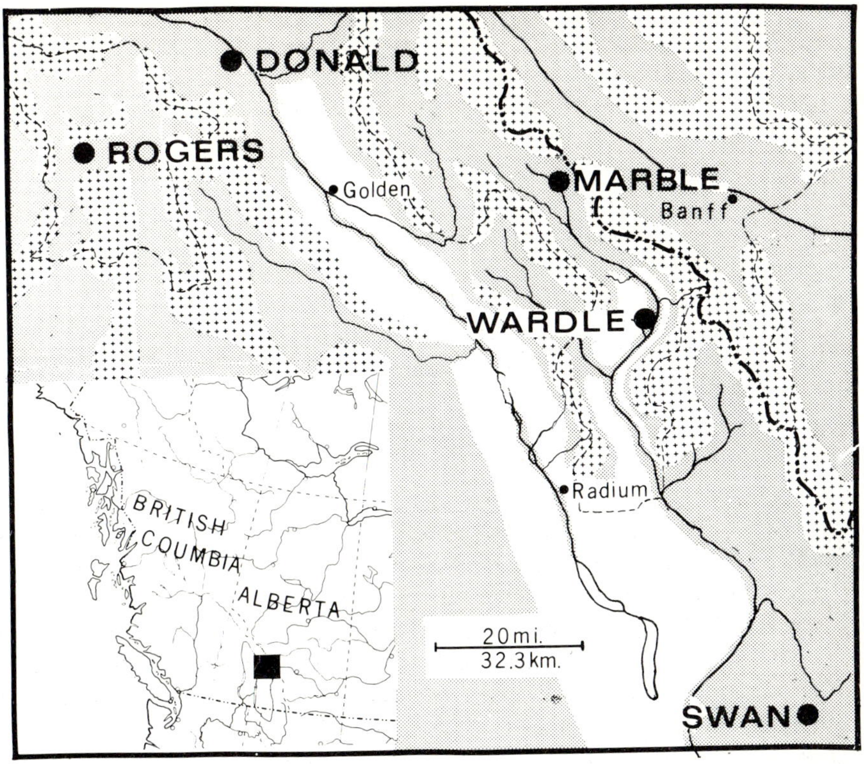

Fig. 9.1. Pheromonally variable populations of *Ips tridens* in the Rocky Mountain National Parks region of Canada. Large dots represent the collection localities (with elevations) as follows: 'Rodgers' – Rodgers Pass (4300 ft.); 'Marble' – Marble Canyon (5000 ft); 'Wardle' – Wardle Creek (4200 ft); 'Swan' – White Swan Lake (3800 ft.) 'Donald' – Donald Station (2800 ft.). The area with crosses represents barrier mountains, the shaded area represents the distribution of spruce and the unshaded area represents area occupied by other conifers. The black rectangle on the insert map indicates the area detailed.

ive distributions, but they exist sympatrically along the eastern ranges of the Canadian Rocky Mountains. Near Banff, Alberta, the two species were found in discrete gallery systems in the same spruce trees; reproductive isolation was enforced by specificity of attractant pheromones (Lanier 1970a). Field and laboratory bioassays of seven populations of each species demonstrated high degrees of pheromone specificity between sympatric populations of the two species. The same tests revealed a startling variability in pheromone systems among populations of the same species. The following discussion illustrates this variability among five populations of *I. tridens* from the Rocky Mountain National Parks region of British Columbia (fig. 9.1). A detailed description of methods and results is published elsewhere (Lanier 1974).

Males of *I. tridens* from Marble Canyon (Marble), Wardle Creek (Wardle), and Donald Station (Donald) were tested concurrently in each of these three areas and at White Swan Lake (Swan) and Rodgers Pass (Rodgers) (fig. 9.1). In all cases males used in the tests were reared in the laboratory in bolts of the same spruce tree and introduced into fresh bolts cut from another tree.

In most tests, females responded preferentially to males of the same population. Exceptions to this generality are that Marble females showed no clear preference for Marble males over Wardle males in two field tests and Donald females did not discriminate between Wardle and Donald males in four laboratory tests (table 9.8). Even slight differentiation between the respective pheromones by Marble and Wardle females was surprising because these populations are separated by a distance of only 20 miles over which *I. tridens* is continuously distributed. The extremely strong discrimination between Marble and Wardle males by females of Swan and Rodgers indicated that the volatiles produced by males of the two populations were even more different than could have been suspected from the reciprocal tests. This discrimination may have resulted from differences in pheromone bouquets which were of little consequence to the Marble and Wardle populations, but important for response by Swan and Rodgers. The same phenomenon may explain the relatively high response of *Trogoderma sternale* males to *T. grassmani* females despite its zero response to four other species, which, on the basis of reciprocal attraction, appear to be pheromonally identical to *T. grassmani* (table 9.1).

9.5. *Genetic control of pheromone systems*

No direct information on the genetics of pheromone specificity has been published. However, insight into genetic control of pheromones and pheromone receptors can be gleaned from bioassays of hybrids of species in the following three groups of *Ips*: (1) hybrids of *I. tridens* (=amiskwiensis Hopping) with *I. borealis* and *I. pilifrons* (Lanier 1970a); (2) *I. plastographus* and *I. integer* (Lanier 1970b); (3) *I. pini* from Idaho and New York (Piston and Lanier 1973).

In all cases, hybrid males were intermediate in attractiveness to the parental types. When males of the backcross generations (B_1) were included in the bioassays, levels of response by the parent population were again in direct order of 'blood' relationship. For example, the indices of response of female *I. pilifrons* to male *I. pilifrons*, B_1 *P* (*t–p**, F_1 *t–p*, B_1 *t* (*p–t*) and *I. tridens* were 100, 35, 27, 13, and 11, respectively (Lanier 1970a). The only exception was that the ability of *I. tridens* to discriminate among its backcrosses broke down in the presence of the F_1 *t–p*. The only hybrid females bioassayed were those of the spruce *Ips*. F_1 *t–p* females were slightly more attracted to males of their own kind than to those of the

* *I. tridens* = *t*; *I. pilifrons* = *p*; B_1 *p* (*t–p*) symbolizes the progeny resulting from backcrosses of the F_1 to *pilifrons*.

two parent species. Backcross females were generally most attracted to pure males of the backcross species. For example, B_1 $p(t-p)$ females had indices of response of 143, 100 and 30 to males of *I. pilifrons*, the B_1, and *I. tridens*, respectively. All of the F_1 and B_1 individuals tested appeared to be influenced by genotypes of their parents in both their attractant and response behavior. This clearly showed that genes controlling pheromone production and reception were not sex-linked.

It seems unlikely that hybrids produce 'new' compounds which evoke intermediate response in receptors of the parent species or that hybrids have 'new' receptors which are sensitive to both parental pheromones. It is especially unlikely that 'new' hybrid receptors are automatically 'keyed' to new hybrid pheromones – as would be necessary to explain the preference of F_1 $t-p$ females for their brother's pheromone. The simplest explanation for the observed results is that hybrids have pheromones and pheromone receptors of both parental types. Thus, the hybrid $t-p$ was most responsive to hybrid males because the mixture of pheromones would excite the maximum number of pheromone receptors. The least complex genetic situation possible is single loci for pheromone and pheromone receptor type. Thus, the genotype for receptors of the F_1 *tridens–pilifrons* would be *TP* and those of

TABLE 9.8

Geographic variation in pheromone response in *Ips tridens*[a].

Responding females		*Index of response*[c] *to male attractant*		
Population[b]	Test	Marble	Wardle	Donald
Marble	lab	100	60*	75
	field	100	100	35***
Wardle	lab	76	100	32***
	field	71*	100	19***
Donald	lab	74	107	100
	field	45**	48*	100
Swan	lab	27***	100	68
	field	0***	100	74
Rodgers	field	100	17***	29***

[a] See Lanier (1974) for complete explanation of methods and additional data.

[b] Localities of populations are indicated in fig. 1.

[c] Index of response expresses the relative attraction between populations with the response to males of the same population (or in the case of Swan and Rodgers, the most attractive population) as base 100. Differences in raw data significant to 0.05*, 0.01**, and 0.001*** percent confidence levels, respectively (Chi-square test).

the backcross to *pilifrons* would be ½TP and ½PP. The response of backcross females with the TP genotype is expected to be similar to that of the F_1 female. Those with the PP genotype should respond in a manner similar to *I. pilifrons*. If the response levels of the two genotypes predicted by the attraction indices are summed, it is clear that the *I. pilifrons* pheromone will provide the greatest aggregate attraction to backcross females. If more than one locus is responsible for determining receptor type, this preference of the B_1 to the backcross species should be accentuated.

9.6. *Mechanisms for pheromone system shift*

9.6.1. *Sympatric changes*

In the process of field-screening a number of synthetic candidate compounds, three cases were discovered in which pairs of sympatric species of moths were attracted to geometric isomers (Roelofs and Comeau 1969, 1970). In each case the isomers can technically be classed as sex attractants but they cannot be termed pheromones because it has not been shown that they are actually produced by the moths. The geometric isomer of the attractant was not attractive and a mixture of both isomers inhibited response in the two cases tested. This is similar to the earlier discovery that the response of the red-banded leaf roller (*Argyrotarnia velutinana* Walker) to its sex pheromone (*cis*-11-tetradecenyl acetate) was inhibited by the *trans* isomer (Roelofs and Comeau 1968). Roelofs and Comeau (1969) proposed that these pairs of sibling species may have developed sympatrically by mutation of a gene to produce the geometric isomer of the pheromone. This would not be attractive to males of the parent population, but a simultaneous mutation of a gene controlling the perception of the 'new' compound could result in a strain which is reproductively isolated from the other members of the population. Thus the two entities would pursue separate courses of evolution.

There are at least three major problems confronting this 'instant species' hypothesis. One is that the resultant two entities would be competing for exactly the same niche, unless mutations for niche accompanied mutations for pheromone system. A second problem is that the mutant types would have vastly fewer potential mates than normal individuals. If the chance of mutant individuals finding mates is lower than that of the normal individuals, the percentage of mutant alleles in the population will decrease in each succeeding generation; in order for the mutant pheromone system to become established, it must convey more efficiency in mate-finding or be linked with genes for superior survival. The third problem is the difficulty of insuring the inbreeding necessary to consolidate the mutant alleles. One of the mutant alleles – either for pheromone production or reception – must occur on the Y chromosome in order that the progeny of a mutant mating have more than 50% chance of inbreeding. A mutaticn for pheromone production on the

Y chromosome of a lepidopteran female would be passed on to all of her daughters; an equivalent mutation on the Y chromosome of a male *Ips* would be inherited by all of his sons. However, the Y chromosome is practically devoid of genes in those systems known genetically and in *Ips*, the genes controlling the pheromone system are not sex-linked.

In *Ips* the alleles which control both production and reception of pheromones are codominant and autosomal. If a male *Ips* which is heterozygous for a mutant pheromone allele breeds a female which is heterozygous for a receptor allele keyed to the mutant pheromone, 1/4 of the progeny will be doubly heterozygous, 1/2 will carry one mutant allele, and 1/4 will carry no mutant alleles. If it is assumed that each female mates with the male which is theoretically the most attractive to her, 1/96 of the following generation would be expected to be homozygous for both of the mutant alleles. If the mutation were between *cis* and *trans* isomers of the pheromone and if a mixture of the pheromones is inhibitory, as suggested by Roelofs and Comeau (1969), the pheromone mixture produced by the heterozygous genotype would be totally unattractive. Hence, the criteria necessary for mate-finding among mutant types would be lost in the first generation. The hypothesis of Roelofs and Comeau (1969) requires totally dominant mutations or simultaneous mutation of both pheromone alleles. However, females homozygous for mutant pheromone alleles would produce unattractive heterozygous daughters after mating with a male having receptor mutations but normal alleles for pheromone production.

9.6.2. *Allopatric changes*

Transition in pheromone systems in geographic isolation encounters some of the difficulties in shift of pheromone systems outlined above, but it does not require that entities with identical genomes (except for pheromone systems) compete for the same niche. Changing of the geographic range of a species by immigration or by disruption (as by glaciation, etc.) results in intensive selection for genotypes suited for the new situation. New combinations of genes which convey superior survival are continually disrupted by panmictic mating in the general population and between adjacent populations. Any gene which helps to prevent outmating of highly adapted genotypes would itself have survival value. Hence, a change in the pheromone system could be co-adaptive with genes which convey high survival value in the modified environment. This mechanism could result in a shift in pheromone systems without direct pressure on the pheromone system itself.

It is probable that evolution of the pheromone system is usually accomplished by direct selection pressure. The force involved could be selection for pheromone bouquets least attractive to natural enemies and/or disruptive selection for reproductive isolation of species using the same pheromones. Predators and parasites have broken the chemical code of bark beetles and capitalized upon pheromone systems to locate their host or prey (Rice 1969, inter alia). These natural enemies could exert considerable selection pressure on the pheromone system of bark beetles by their differential response to various components of a pheromone bouquet (Vite and Williamson 1970; Pitman and Vité 1971). Variations in the pheromone system of a widely distributed species may result from selection pressure to minimize mortality to the natural enemies which occur in different parts of its range. In Idaho and California *I. pini* from New York were four times more attractive to the black-bellied clerid, *Enoclerus lecontei* (Wolcott) than were the western *I. pini* (Lanier et al. 1972). However, the eastern clerid species, *Enoclerus nigripes* (Say) and *Thanasimus dubius* (F.), did not distinguish between the eastern and western *Ips pini* males (Piston and Lanier 1973). Clearly, selection pressure against the eastern pheromone could be considerable in the west.

Disruptive selection against the pheromone system could accommodate the coexistence of two species which use the same pheromones but occupy different niches. Cross attraction could result in interspecific mating or, in the case of bark beetles, increased cohabitation and mutually disadvantageous competition for the same host material. Perhaps pheromone variability between eastern and western *I. pini* (Lanier et al. 1972) resulted from disruptive selection for pheromone specificity with respect to different sets of sympatric *Ips*.

The existence of sympatric sibling species with different pheromone systems could also be explained by disruptive selection. The sibling species may have pursued courses in evolution in the traditional allopatric manner. If the species reconverge, their ecological requirements (different hosts, etc.) may be sufficiently different to permit their coexistence. Not having been under evolutionary pressure, the pheromone systems may have remained unchanged during geographic isolation. Mating between the two entities will result and they may hybridize introgressively. However, if sufficient genetic and/or chromosomal changes accumulated to cause subnormal zygote viability or hybrid sterility, or if disruption of the adapted genotype was sufficient to mediate against survival of hybrids, the entities could not exist sympatrically until premating isolating mechanisms developed. Thus, *Trogoderma* species, may not be able to persist on the same food source because indiscriminate mating resulting from cross attraction produces no brood. The species which is least abundant on the food source probably will disappear (as observed by Nutting 1959) because of failure to reproduce. Lanier (1970a) suggested that the cross attractiveness of *Ips paraconfusus, I. montanus* and *I. confusus* enforced their contiguously allopatric distribution. Intrusion of individuals of one of these species into the range of another would probably result in inviable interspecific mating and the genetic death of the individuals involved. On the other hand, *I. lecontei* can coexist with *I. confusus* owing to differences in pheromone systems (Lanier and Wood 1973) and, probably, stridulating mechanisms (Lanier 1970b). Michael and Rudinsky (1972) found major differences among *Dendroctonus* species in stridulating organs and their sounds. It is possible that stridulation as well as differences in host preference, etc. (table 9.7) act as premating isolating mechanisms in cases where pheromone systems fail.

The response of *Ips grandicollis* to host terpenes is inhibited by the *Dendroctonus* pheromone, frontalin (Werner 1972). This intergeneric inhibition could be mutually advantageous owing to the consequent decrease in competition. However, it seems unlikely that intergeneric inhibition could result in a shift of the pheromones produced by closely related species.

A shift in the pheromone system need not require de novo appearance of a new compound or new receptors. Schneider (1969) hypothesized that most insect species possess olfactory receptors which are specialists and others which are generalists. The specialists could be cued to pheromones and occur in great redundancy while the generalists might be of several types and have overlapping response spectra. Pheromone specificity could evolve by promotion of a 'secondary' compound to pheromone status and selection for redundancy of receptors already responsive to the compound. For example, both *D. brevicomis* and *D. ponderosae* produce brevicomin and *trans*-verbenol and each of these compounds is an attractant of the respective species. However, brevicomin does not appear to have a role in the pheromone system of *D. ponderosae* and *trans*-verbenol is not attractive to *D. brevicomis*. It is possible that each species perceives the pheromone of the other even though no behavioral response is elicited (Payne 1970). Hence, differences in minor secondary compounds may be accentuated by disruptive selection until one or both species is (are) committed to secondary compounds, either as principal pheromones or as synergists or antiattractants.

9.6.3. *Pheromone systems and speciation*

The three beetle genera discussed here appear to be conservative in speciation. Species such as *Trogoderma glabrum, Dendroctonus ponderosae* and *Ips pini* are widely distributed and show geographic variation, but intensive investigations (Beal 1954; Hay 1956; Lanier and Wood 1968; Lanier 1972) have shown them to have continuity of reproduction. There is no evidence that pheromone systems precipitated speciation; rather, pheromone systems in these genera probably tended to maintain reproductive ties among populations which were temporarily isolated.

There is little (if any) factual support and scant theoretical basis for sympatric speciation of Coleoptera resulting from spontaneous changes in the pheromone system. Conversely, changes in pheromone systems probably followed allopatric evolution and resulted from selection for premating isolation to prevent inviable interspecific mating and disruption of highly adapted genotypes.

9.7. *Suggestions for research*

A number of gaps in available information became readily apparent during the writing of this chapter. Research in the areas outlined below could contribute to the usefulness of existing data toward clarifying the role of pheromones in the evolution of Coleoptera.

1) Data on pheromone systems of beetles have accrued rapidly during the past decade. However, the contribution of these data in advancing our knowledge of the role of pheromones in speciation is limited by the unevenness of the progress within the various groups of beetles. Additional data on pheromones and response specificity are needed. Putative pheromones which have been tentatively identified by gas chromatography in *Dendroctonus* and *Ips* require confirmation by spectrometric techniques and bioassays. The apparent similarity in the pheromone systems in *Trogoderma* based on beetle response (table 9.1) needs confirmation by indentification of pheromones in additional species. Rigorous chemical identification of pheromones is a costly process which can usually be justified only for species of considerable economic importance. On the other hand, modest expenditures for bioassays of behavioral specificity and of compounds known to be pheromones of related species can make substantial contributions to the subject of this chapter. Particularly in need of clarification is the cross attractiveness of various *Dendroctonus* species and the propensity for and the consequence of interspecific insemination.

2) Circumstantial evidence implies the existence of compounds which inhibit interspecific response between species using the same (or similar) attractant. Information on these blocking compounds would be a major contribution to the study of pheromone specificity.

3) The role of optical rotation in pheromone specificity should be investigated. Riley et al. (1973) found that the (–) enantiomer of the alarm pheromone (+)-4-methyl-3-heptanone, was inactive in the ant, *Atta texana* (Buckley). This suggests that optical activity could be a mechanism conveying specificity to pheromones which are otherwise identical. For example, *Ips avulsus* and *I. calligraphus* are not cross attractive even though they appear to produce the same compounds (Vité et al. 1972a). To date, the only bark beetle pheromones for which the optical enantiomers have been determined are those of *I. paraconfusus* (Silverstein et al. 1966).

4) Analysis of variation in pheromone systems within and between populations of the same species would constitute a considerable contribution to the understanding of the role of pheromones in reproductive isolation. Breeding experiments which test the assortment of different types of pheromones and receptors could be especially useful.

5) The hypothesis presented in this chapter that differences in pheromone systems of closely related species may result from disruptive selection could be tested by monitoring mixed colonies of cross attractive species for changes in the propensity for interspecific mating. It would also be interesting to monitor popula-

tion levels in mixed colonies to determine whether inviable interspecific mating can result in the extinction of one or both of the species.

Acknowledgments

We acknowledge with deep appreciation the constructive reviews of the manuscript by Richard S. Beal, Graduate Dean at the University of Northern Arizona, Flagstaff; Theodore T. Kozlowski, Professor of Forestry at the University of Wisconsin, Madison; and Robert M. Silverstein, Professor of Ecological Chemistry at the College of Environmental Science and Forestry, Syracuse, N. Y. We are also grateful to numerous additional colleagues for their contribution to the conceptual framework of this chapter and for their permission to cite unpublished reports or manuscripts in press.

References

Beal, R. S., Jr. (1954) Biology and taxonomy of the nearctic species of *Trogoderma*. Univ. Calif. Publ. Entomol. 10, 35–102.

Beal, R. S., Jr. (1964) A new superficially cryptic species of *Trogoderma* from the southwestern United States. Proc. Entomol. Soc. Wash. 66, 79–84.

Beal, R. S., Jr. and G. H. Spitler (1959) Report on crossbreeding experiments in *Trogoderma*. Proc. Entomol. Soc. Wash. 61, 1–6.

Bedard, W. D., P. E. Tilden, D. L. Wood, R. M. Silverstein, R. M. Brownlee and J. O. Rodin (1969) Western pine beetle: field response to its sex pheromone and a synergistic host terpene, myrcene. Science 164, 1284–1285.

Bedard, W. D., R. W. Silverstein and D. L. Wood (1970) Bark beetle pheromones. Science 167, 1638–1639.

Burkholder, W. E. (1970) Pheromone research with stored product Coleoptera. *In*: Control of Insect Behavior by Natural Products; eds.: D. L. Wood, R. M. Silverstein and M. Nakajima (Academic Press, N. Y.) pp. 1–20.

Burkholder, W. E., J. E. Gorman, J. Coffelt and D. G. H. Halstead (1973) Interspecific response to the synthetic pheromones of *Trogoderma* inclusum *(Coleoptera: Dermestidae). Ann. Entomol. Soc. Am. (In press).*

Chapman, J. A. and E. D. A. Dyer (1969) Cross attraction between the Douglas-fir beetle (*Dendroctonus pseudotsugae* Hopk.) and the spruce beetle (*D. obesus* (Mann.)). Bi-Mon. Res. Notes Canada Dep. Fish. and Forest 25, 31.

Furniss, M. M. (1973) Controlled breeding, comparative anatomy and bionomics of *Dendroctonus simplex* LeConte and *Dendroctonus pseudotsugae* Hopkins. Univ. Idaho Publ. Entomol (in press).

Hardee, D. D. (1970) Pheromone production by male boll weevils as affected by food and host factors. Contrib. Boyce Thompson. Inst. 24, 315–321.

Hay, C. J. (1956) Experimental crossing of mountain pine beetle with Black Hills beetle. Ann. Entomol. Soc. Am. 49, 567–671.

Hinton, H. E. (1945) A Monograph of the Beetles Associated with Stored Products (British Museum, London).

Hopping, G. R. (1963) The natural groups of species in the genus *Ips* De Geer (Coleoptera: Scolytidae) in North America. Can. Entomol. 95, 508–516.

Hopping, G. R. (1964) The North American species in groups IV and V of *Ips* De Geer (Coleoptera: Scolytidae). Can. Entomol. 96. 970–978.

Hopping, G. R. (1965) The North American species in group X of *Ips* De Geer (Coleoptera: Scolytidae). Can. Entomol. 97, 803–809.

Hoyt, C. P., G. O. Osborne and A. P. Mulcock (1971) Production of an insect sex attractant by symbiotic bacteria. Nature (London) 230, 472–473.

Jacobson, M. (1972) Insect Sex Pheromones (Academic Press, N. Y.) 382 pp.

Jantz, O. K. and J. A. Rudinsky (1965) Laboratory and field methods for assaying olfactory responses of the Douglas-fir beetle, *Dendroctonus pseudotsugae* Hopkins. Can. Entomol. 97, 935–941.

Kantack, B. H. and R. Staples (1969) The biology and ecology of *Trogoderma glabrum* (Herbst) in stored grains. Res. Bull. Univ. Nebr. 232, 1–24.

Kinzer, G. W., A. F. Fentiman, T. F. Page, R. L. Foltz, J. P. Vité and G. B. Pitman (1969) Bark beetle attractants: identification, synthesis and field bioassay of a new compound isolated from *Dendroctonus*. Nature (London) 222, 477–478.

Kinzer, G. W., A. F. Fentiman, R. L. Foltz and J. A. Rudinsky (1971) Bark beetle attractants: 3-methyl-2-cyclohexene-1-one isolated from *Dendroctonus pseudotsugae*. J. Econ. Entomol. 64, 970–971.

Ladd, T. L. (1970) Sex attraction in the Japanese beetle. J. Econ. Entomol. 63, 905–908.

Lanier, G. N. (1966) Interspecific mating and cytological studies of closely related species of *Ips* De Geer and *Orthotomicus* Ferrari (Coleoptera: Scolytidae). Can. Entomol. 98, 175–188.

Lanier, G. N. (1970a) Sex pheromones: abolition of specificity in hybrid bark beetles. Science 169, 71–72.

Lanier, G. N. (1970b) Biosystematics of North American *Ips* (Coleoptera: Scolytidae) Hopping's Group IX. Can. Entomol. 102, 1139–1163.

Lanier, G. N. (1970c) Biosystematics of the genus *Ips* (Coleoptera: Scolytidae) in North America. Hopping's Group III. Can. Entomol. 102, 1404–1423.

Lanier, G. N. (1972) Biosystematics of the genus *Ips* (Coleoptera: Scolytidae) in North America. Hopping's Groups IV and X. Can. Entomol. 104, 361–388.

Lanier, G. N. (1974) Biosystematics of the genus *Ips* (Coleoptera: Scolytidae) in North America. Hopping's Groups VI, VII and VIII (in preparation).

Lanier, G. N. and D. L. Wood (1968) Controlled mating, karyology, morphology, and sex ratio in the *Dendroctonus ponderosae* complex. Ann. Entomol. Soc. Am. 61, 517–526.

Lanier, G. N. and D. L. Wood (1973) Specificity of population aggregating pheromones in the genus *Ips* (Coleoptera: Scolytidae) (unpublished manuscript).

Lanier, G. N., M. C. Birch, R. F. Schmitz and M. M. Furniss (1972) Pheromones of *Ips pini* (Coleoptera: Scolytidae): variation in response among three populations. Can. Entomol. 104, 1917–1923.

Levinson, H. Z. and A. R. Bar Ilan (1970) Lack of an interspecific attractant in male *Trogoderma granarium*. Riv. Parasitol. 31, 70–72.

Lindquist, E. E. (1969) Review of holarctic tarsenemid mites (Acarina: Prostigmata) parasitizing eggs of Ipine bark beetles. Mem. Entomol. Soc. Can., No. 60.

Mayr, E. (1963) Animal Species and Evolution (The Belknap Press, Harvard University Press, Cambridge, Mass.).

Mayr, E. (1969) Principles of Systematic Zoology (McGraw-Hill, New York) pp. 24–27.

Michael, R. R. and J. A. Rudinsky (1972) Sound production in Scolytidae: specificity in male *Dendroctonus* beetles. J. Insect Physiol. 18, 2189–2201.

Nutting, W. L. (1959) A study of the food habits of the Khapra beetle in natural environments. Final Report for the period 1 July 1955 to 30 June 1958. Univ. Ariz. Agr. Exptl. Sta., Dept. of Entomology. 12pp.+ 2 figs.

Oksanen, H., V. Pertunnen and E. Kangas (1970) Studies on the chemical factors involved in the olfactory orientation of *Blastophagus piniperda* (Coleoptera: Scolytidae). Contrib. Boyce Thompson Inst. 24, 299–304.

Partida, G. L. and R. G. Strong (1970) Distribution and relative abundance of *Trogoderma* spp. in relation to climate zones of California. J. Econ. Entomol. 63, 1553–1560.

Payne, T. L. (1970) Electrophysiological investigations on response to pheromones in bark beetles. Contrib. Boyce Thompson Inst. 24, 275–282.

Payne, T. L. (1971) Bark beetle olfaction. 1. Electroantennogram responses of the southern pine beetle (Coleoptera: Scolytidae) to its aggregating pheromone frontalin. Ann. Entomol. Soc. Am. 64, 266–268.

Piston, J. J. and G. N. Lanier (1973) Pheromones of *Ips pini* (Coleoptera: Scolytidae): relative attractiveness of interpopulational hybrids and interpopulational response to males boring in two host species (in preparation).

Pitman, G. B. and J. P. Vité (1969) Aggregation behavior of *Dendroctonus ponderosae* (Coleoptera: Scolytidae) in response to chemical messengers. Can. Entomol. 101, 143–149.

Pitman, G. B. and J. P. Vité (1970) Field response of *Dendroctonus pseudotsugae* (Coleoptera: Scolytidae) to synthetic frontalin. Ann. Entomol. Soc. Am. 63, 661–664.

Pitman, G. B. and J. P. Vité (1971) Predator-prey response to western pine beetle attractants. J. Econ. Entomol. 64, 402–404.

Pitman, G. B. J. P. Vité, G. W. Kinzer and A. F. Fentiman, Jr. (1968) Bark beetle attractants: *trans*-verbenol isolated from *Dendroctonus*. Nature (London) 218. 168–169.

Pitman, G. B. J. P. Vité, G. W. Kinzer and A. F. Fentiman (1969) Specificity of population-aggregating pheromones in *Dendroctonus*. J. Insect Physiol. 15, 363–366.

Renwick, J. A. A. (1967) Identification of two oxygenated terpenes from the bark beetles *Dendroctonus frontalis* and *Dendroctonus brevicomis*. Contrib. Boyce Thompson Inst. 23, 255–260.

Renwick, J. A. A. (1970) Chemical aspects of bark beetle aggregation. Contrib. Boyce Thompson Inst. 24, 337–341.

Renwick, J. A. A. and J. P. Vité (1968) Isolation of the population aggregating pheromone of the southern pine beetle. Contrib. Boyce Thompson Inst. 24, 65–68.

Renwick, J. A. A. and J. P. Vité (1969) Bark beetle attractants: mechanism of colonization by *Dendroctonus frontalis*. Nature (London) 224, 1222–1223.

Renwick, J. A. A. and J. P. Vité (1970) Systems of chemical communication in *Dendroctonus*. Contrib. Boyce Thompson Inst. 24, 283–292.

Renwick, J. A. A. and J. P. Vité (1972) Pheromones and host volatiles that govern aggregation of the six-spined engraver beetle, *Ips calligraphus*. J. Insect Physiol. 18, 1215–1219.

Rice, R. E. (1969) Response of some predators and parasites of *Ips confusus* (LeC.) (Coleoptera: Scolytidae) to olfactory attractants. Contrib. Boyce Thompson Inst. 24, 189–194.

Riley, R. G., R. M. Silverstein and J. C. Moser (1973) Biological response of the alarm pheromone of *Atta texana* and the enantiomer thereof (in preparation).

Rodin, J. O., R. M. Silverstein, W. E. Burkholder and J. E. Gorman (1969) Sex attractant of female dermestid beetle *Trogoderma inclusum* LeConte. Science 165, 904–906.

Roelofs, W. L. and A. Comeau (1968) Sex pheromone perception. Nature (London) 220, 600–601.

Roelofs, W. L. and A. Comeau (1969) Sex pheromone specificity: taxonomic and evolutionary aspects in Lepidoptera. Science 165, 398–400.

Roelofs, W. L. and A. Comeau (1970) Lepidopterous sex attractants discovered by field screening tests. J. Econ. Entomol. 63, 969–974.

Rudinsky, J. A., M. M. Furniss, L. N. Kline and R. F. Schmitz (1972a) Attraction and repression of *Dendroctonus pseudotsugae* (Coleoptera: Scolytidae) by three synthetic pheromones in traps in Oregon and Idaho. Can. Entomol. 104, 815–822.

Rudinsky, J. A., G. W. Kinzer, A. W. Fentiman, Jr. and R. L. Foltz (1972b) *Trans*-verbenol from Douglas-fir beetle: laboratory and field bioassay in Oregon. Environ. Entomol. 1, 485–488.

Schneider, D. (1969) Insect olfaction: deciphering system for chemical messages. Science 163, 1031–1037.

Schönherr, J. (1970) Evidence of an aggregating pheromone in the ash-bark beetle, *Leperisinus fraxini* (Coleoptera: Scolytidae). Contrib. Boyce Thompson Inst. 24, 305–307.

Shorey, H. H. (1970) Sex pheromones of Lepidoptera. *In*: Control of Insect Behavior by Natural Products: eds.: D. L. Wood, R. M. Silverstein and M. Nakajima (Academic Press, N. Y.) pp. 249–281.

Shorey, H. H., L. K. Gaston and R. N. Jefferson (1968) Insect sex pheromones. *In*: Advances in Pest Control Research; ed.: R. L. Metcalf (Interscience Publishing, N. Y. and London) pp. 57–126.

Silverstein, R. M. (1970) Attractant pheromones of Coleoptera. *In*: Chemicals Controlling Insect Behavior; ed.: M. Beroza (Academic Press, N. Y.) pp. 21–40.

Silverstein, R. M., R. G. Brownlee, T. E. Bellas, D. L. Wood and L. E. Browne (1968) Brevicomin: principal sex attractant in the frass of the female western pine beetle. Science 159, 889–891.

Silverstein, R. M., J. O. Rodin and D. L. Wood (1966) Sex attractants in frass produced by male *Ips confusus* in ponderosa pine. Science 154. 509–510.

Smith, R. H. (1961) The fumigant toxicity of three pine resins to *Dendroctonus brevicomis* and *D. jeffreyi*. J. Econ. Entomol. 54, 365–369.

Smith, R. H. (1963) Toxicity of pine resin vapors to three species of *Dendroctonus* bark beetles. J. Econ. Entomol. 56, 827–831.

Smith, R. H. (1965) A physiological difference among beetles of *Dendroctonus ponderosae* (=D. monticolae) and *D. ponderosae* (=*D. jeffreyi*). Ann. Entomol. Soc. Am. 58, 440–442.

Strong, R. G. and R. G. Arndt (1962) Crossbreeding studies with seven species of *Trogoderma*. J. Econ. Entomol. 55, 445–448.

Strong, R. G., G. T. Okumura and D. E. Sbur (1959) Distribution and host range of eight species of *Trogoderma* in California. J. Econ. Entomol. 52, 830–836.

Tumlinson, J. H., R. C. Gueldner, D. D. Hardee, A. C. Thompson, P. A. Hedin and J. P. Minyard (1970) The boll weevil sex attractant. *In*: Chemicals Controlling Insect Behavior; ed.: M. Beroza (Academic Press, N. Y.) pp. 41–59.

Vick, K. W. (1973) Effect of interspecific mating of *Trogoderma glabrum* and *T. inclusum* on oviposition and remating. Ann. Entomol. Soc. Am. 66, 237–239.

Vick, K. W., W. E. Burkholder and J. E. Gorman (1970) Interspecific response to sex pheromones of *Trogoderma* species (Coleoptera: Dermestidae). Ann. Entomol. Soc.Am. 63, 379–381.

Vick, K. W., W. E. Burkholder and B. J. Smittle (1972) Duration of mating refractory period and frequency of second matings in female *Trogoderma inclusum* (Coleoptera: Dermestidae). Ann. Entomol. Soc. Am. 65, 790–793.

Vité, J. P. and R. I. Gara (1962) Volatile attractants from ponderosa pine attacked by bark beetles (Coleoptera: Scolytidae). Contrib. Boyce Thompson Inst. 21, 251–273.

Vité, J. P. and F. Islas (1973) Biochemical separation of *Dendroctonus* populations from east Texas and central Mexico, (unpublished manuscript).

Vité. J. P. and G. B. Pitman (1969a) Insect and host odors in the aggregation of the western pine beetle. Can. Entomol. 101, 113–117.

Vité, J. P. and G. B. Pitman (1969b) Aggregation behavior of *Dendroctonus brevicomis* in response to synthetic pheromones. J. Insect Physiol. 15, 1617–1622.

Vité, J. P. and J. A. A. Renwick (1968) Insect and host factors in the aggregation of the southern pine beetle. Contrib. Boyce Thompson Inst. 24, 61–63.

Vité, J. P. and J. A. A. Renwick (1970) Differential diagnosis and isolation of population attractants. Contrib. Boyce Thompson Inst. 24, 323–328.

Vité, J. P. and J. A. A. Renwick (1971a) Inhibition of *Dendroctonus frontalis* response to frontalin by isomers of brevicomin. Naturwissenschaften 58, 418.

Vité, J. P. and J. A. A. Renwick (1971b) Population aggregating pheromone in the bark beetle, *Ips grandicollis*. J. Insect Physiol. 17, 1699–1704.

Vité, J. P. and D. L. Williamson (1970) *Thanasimus dubius*: prey perception. J. Insect Physiol. 16, 233–239.

Vité, J. P., A. Bakke and J. A. A. Renwick (1972a) Pheromones in *Ips* (Coleoptera: Scolytidae): occurrence and production. Can. Entomol. 104, 1967–1975.

Vité, J. P., R. I. Gara and H. D. Von Scheller (1964) Field observations on the response to attractants of bark beetles infesting southern pines. Contrib. Boyce Thompson Inst. 22, 461–470.

Vité, J. P., G. B. Pitman, A. F. Fentiman and G. W. Kinzer (1972b) 3-methyl-2-cyclohexene-1-ol isolated from *Dendroctonus*. Naturwissenschaften 59, 469.

Werner, R. A. (1972) Response of the beetle, *Ips grandicollis*, to combinations of host and insect produced attractants. J. Insect Physiol. 18, 1403–1412.

Wood, D. L. (1970) Pheromones of bark beetles. *In*: Control of Insect Behavior by Natural Products; eds.: D. L. Wood, R. M. Silverstein and M. Nakajima (Academic Press, N. Y.) pp. 301-316.

Wood, D. L. (1972) Selection and colonization of ponderosa pine by bark beetles. *In*: Insect/Plant Relationships; ed.: H. F. van Emden. Symp. Roy. Entomol. Soc. (London) 6, 101–117.

Wood, D. L., R. W. Stark, R. M. Silverstein and J. O. Rodin (1967) Unique synergistic effects produced by the principal sex attractant compounds of *Ips confusus* (LeConte) (Coleoptera: Scolytidae). Nature (London) 215, 206.

Wood, S. L. (1963) A revision of the bark beetle genus *Dendroctonus* Erichson (Coleoptera: Scolytidae). Great Basin Natur. 23, 1–117.

Young, J. C., R. M. Silverstein and M. C. Birch (1973) Aggregation pheromone of the bark beetle *Ips confusus*: Isolation and identification. J. Insect Physiol. 19, 2273–2277.

CHAPTER 10

Pheromonal bases of social manifestations in insects

Murray S. BLUM

10.1. Introduction

Presocial insects, which display varying degrees of non-sexual interactive behavior, have a widespread distribution in the Insecta (Wheeler 1928), and the number recognized is increasing steadily. Presociality has developed eclectically in the Insecta and is present in all stages leading to the truly social or eusocial insects – the ants, termites and highly organized wasps and bees. Michener (1969) classified the major steps in the establishment of insect sociality and it is important to recognize that all developmental stages leading to the verge of eusociality have been achieved by presocial insects. In essence, adult and adult-immature interactions of increasing temporal and spatial complexity characterize the evolutionary stages of the social imperative as expressed by various insect phyletic lines.

Subsocial behavior, in which the adults care for their young, is well developed in many groups of Hemiptera (Bequaert 1935), Coleoptera (Hinton 1944), Dermaptera (Fulton 1924), Orthoptera (West and Alexander 1963), wasps (Evans 1958), bees (Michener 1969), and species in several other orders. Among the bees, the complete evolutionary progression from subsocial to eusocial is well established, and includes communal, quasisocial, and semisocial stages, in which members of the same generation share a nest either with (quasisocial) or without (communal) cooperation in brood care. In the semisocial stage, reproductive division of labor occurs and the immature reproductives are cared for by adult workers (Michener 1969). Eusociality reflects active cooperation of offspring and parents, so that the semisocial stage is surpassed as a consequence of the presence of cooperating individuals of more than one generation. Most of the female offspring are relatively sterile sisters, a fact which focuses on the genetic bases of eusociality, most recently analyzed by Hamilton (1972).

In light of our present knowledge of the pheromonal basis of eusociality, it seems almost certain that chemical releasers are foundational to many of the observed intra specific interactions of presocial insects. Unfortunately, presociality has been described mostly in anecdotal terms and the precise behavioral stimuli have been illuminated for only a few of the species that have evolved a presocial *modus vivendi*. Conceivably, the developmental steps which have culminated in an elegant eusociality, may also be amenable to analysis in terms of a greater dependence of the species on diverse pheromonal stimuli to regulate the increasingly complex interactions that are manifested as societies become more highly organized. At this juncture, there is an obvious and compelling need to establish whether an increasing emphasis on chemical releasers and primers of social behavior is correlated with the upward thrust toward eusociality that characterizes the sequential steps along the presocial road.

The widespread occurrence of sex pheromones in arthropods clearly demonstrates that the prerequisites for successful chemical communication have evolved in numerous non-social as well as social species. The ability of an insect to produce a chemical messenger that encodes information and to discharge the compound into the external environment where it can be perceived and ultimately translated into specific behavior by another individual of the same species, presupposes that several exacting conditions have been fulfilled. These are: (1) the presence of enzymatic pathways for the synthesis of the pheromone(s); (2) glandular tissue in which the pheromone or its precursor are synthesized; (3) a reservoir associated with the biosynthetic organ; (4) a duct system (or its equivalent) for discharging the pheromone to the exterior; (5) specific olfactory chemoreceptors for rapid perception of the pheromone, usually in trace quantities; (6) rapid decoding in the central nervous sytem; and (7) the ability of the receiver to respond in a rather stereotyped manner.

The presence of chemical releasers of sexual behavior in primitive insects demonstrates that these biochemical, physiological, and behavioral criteria have been satisfactorily met and suggests that, in theory, presocial insects could possess the capacity to utilize other types of pheromones as well. Indeed, numerous investigations of presocial insects indicate that a variety of behavioral interactions may be based primarily on the availability of chemical stimuli and it seems alsmost certain that chemical releasers and primers will be frequently implicated in many more aspects of presocial insect behavior when these phenomena are subjected to detailed analyses. Functionally, the stimulus-response effect of releasers, mediated exclusively by the central nervous system, contrasts with primer stimuli which cause an alteration of rèproductive or endocrinological systems.

10.2. Chemical stimuli of aggregative behavior

Although gregarious behaviour is characteristic of presocial insects, it also occurs in some species in which adults do not care for the young, or, for that matter, adults are excluded entirely. Thus, aggregative propensities are exhibited by many orthopterous, heteropterous, and lepidopterous species and in some cases, it has been established that pheromonal stimuli are key elements in triggering this gregariousness. In addition, it has been demonstrated that pheromones can regulate some facets of either the behavior or development of individuals in these assemblages. Pheromonal initiation of these intraspecific interactions can be of manifest selective advantage, especially if chemical releaser or primer stimuli can affect the population distribution so as to reduce crowding or to promote reproductive synchrony of developing adults (Chauvin and Noirot 1968). Group effects are probably much more widespread among gregarious species than has been suspected and pheromones may ultimately be demonstrated to be the primary driving force in initiating these interactive phenomena.

Pheromonally-induced group oviposition may be widespread in the Insecta. This phenomenon has been observed in females of the blowfly *Lucilia cuprina* (Wied.) (Barton Browne et al. 1969) and the mosquito *Culex tarsalis* Coquillet (Hudson and McLintock 1967). Gregariousness in females of the desert locust *Schistocerca gregaria* (Forskal) is promoted by pheromonal stimuli and results in adults ovipositing in close proximity to each other (Norris 1963). Indeed, the presence of chemical stimuli which promote the formation of assemblages has been well established for several species of crickets and grasshoppers. Sexton and Hess (1968) reported that the European house cricket, *Acheta domesticus* (L.), produces an aggregation pheromone to which both sexes respond; it is relatively non-volatile and is produced by both sexes. However, it is chiefly in the Blattaria, an order which is characterized by the presence of numerous gregarious species (Roth and Willis 1960), that both the source and specificity of some of these aggregative pheromones have been determined. These chemical releasers are widespread among cockroaches and appear to be the primary *raison d'être* for assemblages of these insects.

Ishii and Kuwahara (1967, 1968) reported that nymphs of the German cockroach, *Blattella germanica* (L.), aggregated in response to a pheromone present in the feces and presumably originating from rectal pad cells. The aggregation pheromone of *B. germanica* is not species specific and its presence results in the formation of nymphal assemblages of *Periplaneta americana* (L.), *P. fuliginosa* (Serville), and *P. japonica* Karny, and vice versa. However, species appear to be more responsive to their own pheromones than those produced by other species (Ishii 1970).

Recently, Bell et al. (1972) demonstrated the presence of aggregation pheromones in nymphs representing five species in two families of cockroaches. The blattids *Blatta orientalis* (L.) and *Periplaneta americana*, as well as the blaberids *Eublaberus posticus* (Erichson), *Byrsotria fumigata* (Guerin) and *Blaberus discoidalis* (Serville) exhibited varying degrees of intra- and interspecific attraction to the chemical releasers of aggregative behavior. On the other hand, nymphs of the blattellid *Parcoblatta pennsylvanicus* (De G.) did not aggregate on either their own conditioned papers or those conditioned by the other species. In general, the blaberid species showed much more family specificity than the blattids. It may be significant that whereas the blattid and blattellid pheromones are reported to be derived from rectal secretions in admixture with feces, those of the blaberid *Blabe-*

rus craniifer Burmeister have been localized in the secretion of the mandibular glands (Brossut 1970).

Species in a wide variety of coleopterous families form aggregations, and in several cases it has been established that these beetle assemblages result from pheromonal cues. Secretions from both male and female Khapra beetles, *Trogoderma granarium* Everts, function as local assembling agents (Finger et al. 1965; Yinon and Shulov 1967) in the stored grains on which these insects feed. The 'assembling scent' of *T. granarium* is comprised primarily of the ethyl esters of palmitic, stearic, oleic, and linoleic acids. The esters are of equivalent attractiveness and no synergistic effects are evident (Ikan et al. 1969).

Pheromones released by males of the lycid, *Lycus loripes* (Chevrolat), attract both males and females of this species (Eisner and Kafotos 1962) and the resulting aggregations of these distasteful beetles produce a conspicuous collective display of aposematism. Similarly, males of some scolytid beetles, after attacking a suitable tree, act as pheromonal beacons for individuals of both sexes (Wood 1962). The large hibernative aggregations of the coccinellid *Semiadalia undecimnotata* Schneid. are induced by pheromones (Hodek 1960) and these bisexual assemblages, like those of other coleopterous species, are admirably suited to promote reproduction. The aerial swarms of some Diptera, Ephemeroptera, Trichoptera, and Lepidoptera are also probably pheromonally mediated and the integrity of these temporary aggregations may be maintained by chemical releasers.

10.3. Chemical stimuli of dispersive behavior

Since aggregations of insects represent a real bonanza for effective predators, it would be of great selective value for the clustered individuals to disperse in the presence of a voracious intruder. Alarm pheromones would seem to constitute ideal despersive agents and, in fact, have recently been demonstrated to be highly functional releasers of escape behavior for several gregarious species in the order Hemiptera. Kislow and Edwards (1972) reported that the aphid *Myzus persicae* (Sulzer) as well as species in four other genera, discharged secretions from their abdominal cornicles which acted as a powerful chemical stimulus for dispersion of nearby aphids. In some species, escape behavior resulted in individuals dropping from the plant. This alarm pheromone has been identified as *trans*-β-farnesene (Bowers et al. 1972) and has been isolated from species in three different genera. Furthermore, since three other species in two additional genera display alarm behavior in the presence of this compound, it must be regarded as one of the most non-specific pheromones identified to date.

Nymphs of the pyrrhocorid *Dysdercus intermedius* Distant are typical of many hemipterous species in forming rather compact aggregations. When a nymph is disturbed, the secretions from its third dorsal scent gland are utilized for defense while simultaneously releasing alarm behavior in adjacent individuals (Calam and

Youdeowei 1968). The primary alarm pheromone has been identified as 2-hexenal, a compound also serving as an alarm releaser for the ant *Crematogaster africana* Mayr (Bevan et al. 1961; Blum et al. 1969). On the other hand, the secretion of the two anterior scent glands differs from that of the third gland and it has been demonstrated that the products from these two glands function as aggregation pheromones (Youdeowei and Calam 1969). Such specialization in the roles of exocrine glands may be widespread in gregarious insects and would be of great adaptive significance in exploiting the environment with a finite number of exocrine products.

10.4. Primer pheromones

Reproductive synchrony in certain coleopterous and orthopterous species is mediated by primer pheromones and it is very likely that this phenomenon will be found to occur commonly in insect species which possess aggregative propensities. Developmental synchrony maximizes the number of sexually mature adults that are simultaneously available and as a consequence, promotes the reproductive potential of the local population. Norris (1954) observed that the presence of mature males of the locust *Schistocerca gregaria* hastens the maturation of immatures of both sexes. In addition, mature females accelerate the development of immature males but this effect is much weaker than that produced by mature males and only occurs when males are crowded with the females. Norris (1968) has also demonstrated that young adults or last-instar nymphs of both sexes, retard the maturation of males, a phenomenon presumably associated with primer pheromones different from those which expedite development.

Group effects attributable to the presence of chemical primers have been demonstrated for the mealworm beetle *Tenebrio molitor* L. Both oocyte development and rate of sex pheromone emission are increased if isolated adult females are exposed to airstreams containing the scents of either mature males or females (Happ et al. 1970). The male scent accelerates both oocyte growth and the rate of sex attraction liberation at the end of three days, whereas the female scent affects egg development only after seven days. These results demonstrate that beetles, like locusts, temporally regulate reproduction in local populations by utilizing primer pheromones elaborated by both sexes.

In an elegant series of experiments, McFarlane (1964) reported that the cricket *Acheta domesticus* (L.) would inhibit the growth of another cricket, *Gryllodes sigillatus* (Walk.); however, extracts of *Acheta domesticus* inhibited the growth of *both* species. Subsequently, McFarlane and Henneberry (1965) observed that the methyl esters of C_{12}–C_{18} fatty acids inhibited the growth of *Gryllodes sigillatus* nymphs, presumably after entry through the external body wall. Group-reared nymphs of *G. sigillatus* exhibit reduced survival in the presence of methyl palmitate but this ester does not affect the survival of singly-reared individuals (McFarlane

1966a). On the other hand, methyl laurate increased the body weight of both group-reared and singly-reared males of *Acheta domesticus* but this effect is concentration dependent so that higher dosages of the ester had no effect on group-reared individuals (McFarlane 1966b). Significantly, the effects of a free fatty acid and a methyl ester on *Gryllodes sigillatus* nymphs appear to result from different inhibitory mechanisms and to affect different developmental systems during sensitive growth periods (McFarlane 1968). The results of these investigations emphasize the possible primer effect which compounds may mediate as cuticular penetrants and indicate that this phenomenon should be considered when nutritional studies are undertaken.

10.5. Eusociality: the social imperative

The various phylogenetic lines of Hymenoptera that have become eusocial have done so through the evolution of a variegated series of communicative stimuli to which they are programmed to respond adaptively. These insect societies exhibit a complex of behavioral interactions which, in their totality, surpass those that are encountered in any of the species of presocial insects. The very nature of the eusocial state dictates that a high degree of organization be maintained in order to optimally integrate the activities of the colonial members. Different degrees of eusociality are present among the Hymenoptera and Isoptera but in all cases, they possess three fundamental qualities in common: 1) individuals of the same species cooperate in caring for the young; 2) a reproductive division of labor which includes more or less sterile adults caring for reproductives; and 3) overlapping generations resulting in offspring functioning alongside their parents in colonial maintenance. This trio of conditions set the stage for a multitude of interactions between immatures, adult workers and reproductives, which are fundamental to the maintenance of a viable eusociality. Significantly, it now seems evident that chemical signals are the principal vehicles governing specific behavioral interactions between individuals. Therefore, eusociality became possible only after a finite number of adaptively favorable patterns of interaction, initiated chiefly by chemical stimuli, had been established by natural selection in the colonial milieu.

A potpourri of behavioral reactions induced by pheromones is included in table 10.1.

This list is by no means intended to be inclusive, since pheromones may also constitute the interactive stimuli for many additional social responses, both recognized and cryptic. Also, no strict terminological exactitude is meant to be implied by either the described reactions or their chemical stimulators since the former may actually represent the behavioral end products of a series of overlapping responses, and the latter may constitute the same pheromone being utilized for more than one function. It is also striking that, in spite of the vastly different evolutionary pathways by which they became eusocial, the termites and highly organized hymenop-

TABLE 10.1

Varied expressions of exocrine communication in the main groups of eusocial insects*.

Reaction	Type of chemical stimulus	Group
Primers		
Caste determination	Reproductive-caste inhibitory pheromone	Bees, wasps, termites
Ovarian inhibition	Queen substance	Ants, bees, termites
Inhibition or stimulation of queen-cell construction	Queen substance	Ants, bees, termites
Releasers		
Regurgitation and solid food exchange	Solicitation pheromone	Ants, bees, wasps, termites
Alarm behavior	Alarm pheromone; trail pheromone	Ants, bees, wasps, termites
Recruitment and emigration	Trail pheromone; alarm pheromone; specialized attractant pheromones	Ants, bees, termites
Oral grooming	Surface pheromone	Ants, bees, wasps, termites
Aggregative (=clustering) behavior	Aggregation pheromone	Ants, bees, termites
Attraction of alate reproductives	Territorial pheromone; sex attractant	Ants, bees, wasps, termites
Queen identification by workers	Queen-recognition pheromone; queen substance	Ants, bees, wasps, termites
Flight induction of sexual alates	Flight induction pheromone	Ants
Repellency	Alarm (?) pheromone	Ants, bees
Abdominal pumping by adults	Thermoregulatory pheromone	Wasps

*Colony odor has not been demonstrated to be of exocrine origin and is not included in this list.

terans utilize a repertoire of chemically homologous pheromones as key regulatory stimuli. Thus, although the particulars of the hymenopterous and isopterous eusocialities are widely divergent, their chief types of integrative nexuses, the pheromones, are remarkably similar. Since nearly all of the pheromonal regulators listed in table 10.1 may be common to isopterous and highly organized hymenopterous species, it appears that both groups of insects arrived at the eusocial state through utilization of strikingly comparable chemical stimuli as the behavioral integrators of a complex societal structure.

The functions of pheromones in the colonial milieu may be contextually variable, as is evident from table 10.1. Alarm behavior may be triggered by both trail and alarm pheromones but, on the other hand, the same two pheromones may be utilized simultaneously to function as powerful stimuli for recruitment. Functional eusociality is also reflected in the presence of pheromones for regulating liquid food exchange (trophallaxis) between adults and immatures. Food exchange constitutes an excellent mechanism for distributing relatively non-volatile pheromones throughout the colony and the 'communal stomach' thus constitutes an ideal social organ. Queen substances, key chemical stimuli which generate a steady state cohesiveness among workers, are, to a large extent, trophallactically distributed as an effective device that demonstrates the colonial omnipresence of the reproductive female. Grooming pheromones (table 10.1) promote frequent interactions at the level of individual pairs and these apparent surface stimuli serve admirably to establish a tightly knit 'family' unit at the colonial level. In all probability, aggregation or clustering pheromones are of similar adaptive significance in that these releasers favor social interactions among the individuals forming the assemblages.

At a glance, the pheromones underlying the eusocial state would appear to constitute a veritable omnium-gatherum, but if these chemical stimuli are viewed strictly as societal integrators, they can actually be classified as members of a few functional categories. Thus, the hallmark of eusocial insects, the group response, is initiated by pheromones identified with alarm, trail following, attraction and even alate flight behavior. On the other hand, colonial cohesiveness is guaranteed by a group of chemical stimuli which result in such diverse responses as food exchange, queen recognition, grooming, and control of production of reproductives through effects on both the behavior and physiology of workers. Therefore, the viable eusocial state represents the subtle interplay of chemical stimuli required: 1) to maintain colony homeostasis through the utilization of pheromones engineered; 2) to produce limited behavioral and physiological interactions chiefly in the milieu of the nest; and 3) to stimulate mass responses which rapidly utilize the collective resources of a programmed society.

10.6. Conclusions

The road to insect sociality was paved with pheromones. The pheromonal leitmotif characterizing the eusocial state provides the primary means of regulating the dazzling variety of behavioral interactions identified within the true insect societies. However, many of the chemical stimuli which have been blended into a viable eusociality arose from those associated with presocial species belonging to a wide range of insect orders. Indeed, some of the subsocial insects possess certain communicative systems as elaborate as those exhibited by eusocial species, and as a consequence, the latter societies must be regarded as the end product of a multitude of presocial evolutionary 'experiments'. Certainly, the eusocial genesis occurred in a society which already possessed complex behavioral patterns and a rich chemical 'language', legacies derived from subsocial species evolving along the path toward the ultimate social imperative.

References

Barton Browne, L., R. J. Bartell and H. H. Shorey (1969) Pheromone-mediated behavior leading to group oviposition in the blowfly *Lucilia cuprina*. J. Insect Physiol. 15, 1003–1014.

Bell, W. J. , C. Parsons and E. A. Martinko (1972) Cockroach aggregation pheromones: Analysis of aggregation tendency and species specificity (Orthoptera: Blattidae). J. Kansas Entomol. Soc. 45, 414–421.

Bequaert, J. (1935) Presocial behavior among the Hemiptera. Bull. Brooklyn Entomol. Soc. 30, 177–191.

Bevans, C. W. L., A. J. Birch and H. Caswell (1961) An insect repellent from black cocktail ants. J. Chem. Soc. p. 488.

Blum, M. S. , R. M. Crewe, J. H. Sudd and A. W. Garrison (1969) 2-Hexenal: Isolation and function in a *Crematogaster* (*Atopogyne*) sp. J. Ga. Entomol. Soc. 4, 145–148.

Bowers, W. S. , L. R. Nault, R. E. Webb and S. R. Dutky (1972) Aphid alarm pheromone: isolation, identification, synthesis. Science, 177, 1121–1122.

Brossut, R. (1970) L'interattraction chez *Blabera craniifer* Burm. (Insecta, Dictyoptera): sécrétion d'une phéromone par les glandes mandibulaires. C. R. Acad. Sci . 270D, 714–716.

Calam, D. H. and A. Youdeowei (1968) Identification and functions of secretion from the posterior scent gland of fifth instar larvae of the bug *Dysdercus intermedius*. J. Insect Physiol. 14, 1147–1158.

Chauvin, R. and C. Noiret, eds. (1968) L'effet de groupe chez les animaux. Colloques Internationaux du Centre National de la Recherche Scientifique, Paris, 1967, No. 173, 390 pp.

Eisner, T. and F. C. Kafotos (1962) Defense mechanisms of arthropods.X A pheromone promoting aggregation in an aposematic distasteful insect. Psyche 69, 53–61.

Evans, H. E. (1958) The evolution of social life in wasps. Proc. Int. Congr. Entomol. 10th (1956) 2, 449-457.

Finger, A. (Bar Ilan), V. Stanic and A. Shulov (1965) Attracting substance (pheromone) produced by virgin females of *Trogoderma granarium* Everts. (Col., Dermestidae). Riv. Parassitol. 4, 39–58.

Fulton, B. B. (1924) Some habits of earwigs. Ann . Entomol. Soc. A. 17, 357–367.

Hamilton, W. D. (1972) Altruism and related phenomena, mainly in social insects. Ann. Rev. Ecol. Systematics 3, 193–232.

Happ, G. M., M. E. Schroeder and J. C. H. Wang (1970) Effects of male and female scent on reproductive maturation in young female *Tenebrio molitor*. J. Insect Physiol. 16, 1543–1548.

Hinton, H. E. (1944) Some general remarks on sub-social beetles, with notes on the biology of the staphylinid, *Platystethus arenarius* (Fourcroy). Proc. Roy. Entomol. Soc. London Ser. 19, 115–128.

Hodek, J. (1960) Hibernation-bionomics in Coccinellidae. Cas. Csl. Spol. Entomol. 57, 1–20.

Hudson, A and J. McLintock (1967) A chemical factor that stimulates oviposition by *Culex tarsalis* Coquillet (Diptera, Culicidae). Anim. Behav. 15, 336–341.

Ikan, R., E. D. Bergmann, U. Yinon and A. Shulov (1969) Identification, synthesis, and biological activity of an 'Assembling Scent' from the beetle *Trogoderma granarium*. Nature (London) 223, 317.

Ishii, S. (1970) An aggregation pheromone of the German cockroach, *Blattella germanica* (L.). 2. Species specificity of the pheromone. Appl. Entomol. Zool. 5, 33–41.

Ishii, S. and Y. Kuwahara (1967) An aggregation pheromone of the German cockroach *Blattella germanica* L. (Orthoptera: Blattellidae). I. Site of the pheromone production. Appl. Entomol. Zool. 2, 203–217.

Ishii, S. and Y. Kuwahara (1968) Aggregation of German cockroach (*Blattella germanica*) nymphs. Experientia 24, 88–89.

Kislow, C. J. and L. J. Edwards (1972) Repellent odour in aphids. Nature (London) 235, 108–109.

McFarlane, J. E. (1964) Interaction between two species of crickets reared together. Can. J. Zool. 42, 689–691.

McFarlane, J. E. (1966a) Studies on group effects in crickets. III. Wing development of *Gryllodes sigillatus* (Walk.) Can. J. Zool. 44, 1017–1021.

McFarlane, J. E. (1966b) Studies on group effects in crickets. II. A temperature and a concentration effect on *Acheta domesticus* (L). Can. J. Zool. 44, 1013–1016.

McFarlane, J. E. (1968) Fatty acids, methyl esters and insect growth. Com. Biochem. Physiol. 24, 377–384.

McFarlane, J. E. and G. O. Henneberry (1965) Inhibition of the growth of an insect by fatty acids. J. Insect Physiol. 11, 1247–1252.

Michener, C. D. (1969) Comparative social behavior of bees. Ann. Rev. Entomol. 14, 299–342.

Norris, M. J. (1954) Sexual maturation in the desert locust (*Schistocerca gregaria* (Forskål)) with special reference to the effects of grouping. Anti-Locust Bull. No. 18, 44 pp.

Norris, M. J. (1963) Laboratory experiments on gregarious behaviour in ovipositing females of the desert locust (*Schistocerca gregaria* (Forsk.)). Entomol. Exptl. Appl. 6, 279–303.

Norris, M. J. (1968) Further experiments on the effects of social factors on the rate of sexual maturation in the desert locust. Nature (London) 219, 865–866.

Roth, L. M. and E. R. Willis (1960) The biotic associations of cockroaches. Smithson. Misc. Collect. No. 141, 470 pp.

Sexton, O. J. and E. H. Hess (1968) A pheromone-like dispersant affecting the local distribution of the European house cricket *Acheta domestica*. Biol. Bull. 134, 490–502.

West, M. J. and R. D. Alexander (1963) Sub-social behavior in a burrowing cricket (*Anurogryllus muticus* (De Geer)). (Orthoptera: Gryllidae) Ohio J. Sci. 63, 19–24.

Wheeler, W. M. (1928) The Social Insects: Their Origin and Evolution (Kegan Paul, Trench, Trubner Co., Ltd., London) 378 pp.

Wood, D. L. (1962) The attraction created by males of a bark beetle *Ips confusus* (LeConte) attacking ponderosa pine. Pan-Pac. Entomol. 38, 141–145.

Yinon, U. and A. Shulov (1967) New findings concerning pheromones produced by *Trogoderma granarium* (Everts.) (Coleoptera, Dermestidae). J. Stored Prod. Res. 3, 251–254.

Youdeowei, A. and D. H. Calam (1969) The morphology of the scent glands of *Dysdercus intermedius* Distant (Hemiptera: Pyrrhocoridae) and a preliminary analysis of the scent gland secretions of the fifth instar larvae. Proc. Roy. Entomol. Soc. London Ser. A 44, 38–44.

CHAPTER 11

Pheromones that affect the behavior and physiology of honey bees

Norman E. GARY

11.1. Introduction

This chapter is concerned with research on pheromones that influence the behavior and physiology of the honey bee, *Apis mellifera* L. Data and interpretations from many researchers are integrated, and in some cases reconciled, in order to develop a composite view of pheromonal mechanisms in the honey bee colony. Other reviews have been published by Butler (1970), Gary (1970), and Pain (1971, 1973). However, this chapter is intended to be more than a review in the sense that there is free speculation on pheromones and mechanisms yet to be documented. Such speculation, based to some extent on empirical evidence, is intended to suggest new directions for future research and to encourage new interpretations of existing data. The chapter emphasizes the research advantages inherent in a mechanistic approach, as opposed to the subtle barriers to objective thinking inherent in anthropomorphic interpretations of behavior induced by pheromones.

11.2. Barriers to understanding pheromonal mechanisms

The premise that honey bees are reacting *mechanistically* to environmental stimuli is still not universally accepted. Complex and unexplained behavior can be more easily attributed to a degree of intelligence than to fundamental mechanisms, which can be experimentally elucidated. Anthropomorphic and romantic interpretations of bee activities can explain bee behavior without reference to pheromones or other stimuli, but they do not help in understanding the functions of behavioral mechanisms. Some of the major barriers to understanding the function of pheromones of social insects, and honey bees in particular, are as follows:

1) Man's long and close association with honey bees has led to the use of terminology replete with connotations of human values and activities. Bees in the worker caste become guards, nurses, house-bees, field-workers or attendants, all of which subtly and tacitly imply a degree of man's intelligence, an awareness of destiny and a degree of conscious option in exercising alternative behavioral re-

sponses to pheromones. Worker bees are credited with the options of 'refusing' to approach a queen, 'offering' food, 'grooming' the queen and 'attacking' colony 'enemies'. They are able to 'guard' the hive, as if there is an awareness of some imminent danger, a concept that implies an awareness of safety and its implications for the future life of the individual, welfare of the colony and finally the survival of the species. Although more complex behavior is observed in the worker bee, the queen often gets 'credit' for directing the colony activities and somehow judiciously 'dispensing' pheromones for the colony welfare. However, it is possible to view the queen bee as an ordinary female reproductive insect with no more or less 'intelligence' than the worker bee, her genetic equivalent.

All these responses are genetically 'programmed' and their behavioral expression is contingent upon transient factors such as age, physiological condition, previous experiences (learning) and the status of endogenous and exogenous stimuli in the immediate area of each bee. Objective analysis must be based on the assumption that the bee has no awareness of any future event, even during the next millisecond. To concede the existence of any foresight is to obscure and to attenuate a critical analysis of the basic *mechanisms* regulating behavior at that instant. Thus, the assumption that the queen bee is 'searching' for an empty cell in which to lay an egg tends to inhibit critical thinking and the formulation of a hypothesis that the queen may be attracted to cells and compelled to lay eggs in them by pheromones deposited in the cell interior by worker bees. The anthropomorphic notion that nurse bees feed larvae because they are hungry tends to abort critical analysis just short of asking the question, 'Is brood feeding behavior of nurse bees stimulated by pheromones secreted by larvae?'

2) It is often assumed that there is a *purpose* for each observed activity. If bees are responding mechanically to stimuli, it becomes inappropriate to speculate on the purpose. However, it is appropriate to speculate on the function of pheromones as they appear to facilitate colony survival. Objectively, there is no more purpose to a behavioral activity than there is to a stone rolling down a hillside . . . both are a function of transient physical and chemical energy, and both activities are not consciously oriented toward any specific accomplishments or future events, such as survival.

3) Since honey bees are obligate social animals, bioassays to evaluate pheromone activity – qualitatively and quantitatively – must be conducted with groups rather than individuals. This introduces the problem that the observed behavior may be caused by secondary pheromones, released in response to the primary pheromones that are the object of the investigation. The physiological condition and genetic composition of bees used in bioassays are variable and can dramatically affect the results. Use of caged bees for bioassays also imposes a serious stress and increases the risk of observing aberrant responses.

4) The complex composition of honey bee secretions may contain may more pheromones than similar secretions of non-social insects (Gary 1970). Multiple

compounds may differ greatly in physical and chemical properties. The isolation and subsequent assay of the individual components of a bioactive complex may lead to erroneous conclusions. Compounds, which act synergistically in the secretion, may be inactive when tested singly. These problems seem likely to be encountered frequently, owing to the great number of pheromones in the honey bee colony and the selective advantage conferred by an increase in communication potential through the evolution of responses to pheromonal mixtures.

5) The fact that most of the identified honey bee pheromones are relatively stable compounds may be caused primarily by the loss of highly volatile and/or labile pheromones during extracting and processing procedures in the laboratory. There is some empirical evidence that such compounds are utilized as pheromones (Gary unpublished data). Furthermore there is the problem of inadvertently altering the ratios of compounds in the complex, with the attendant risk of changing the nature of the 'information' that is communicated.

6) Bees are extremely sensitive to very small quantities of pheromones that are far beyond the detection range of sophisticated analytical instruments, such as gas chromatography. High sensitivity, combined with persistence of some of the more stable pheromones, has created interesting problems. Residues of the most abundant queen pheromone, 9-oxo-2-decenoic acid, may persist for a period of years after initial contamination. The handling of queen bees is a common activity at apicultural research laboratories and *all* objects contacted by people who handle bees are likely to be contaminated*.

7) Finally there is a tendency to assume subconsciously that bees literally see where they are going inside the hive and can thus anticipate the next activity. Some of this bias arises from the necessity of observing behavior through glass-walled observation hives illuminated by artificial light. Man's intellect and superior visual sense gives him the ability to see and predict activities and some of this capability is often mentally transferred to the bee. Consequently, observers tend to emphasize visual and tactile mechanisms, at the expense of olfactory mechanisms.

11.3. Characteristics of the honey bee colony

A typical colony of honey bees contains three castes: a) Workers (20,000–60,000) – non-reproductive females, which comprise most of the population and perform

* The problem of contamination by pheromones can be dramatic. For example the air circulation system at the Anti-Locust Research Centre in London (now the Centre for Overseas Pest Research) recirculated air from gregarious rearing quarters for the locust, *Schistocerca gregaria* (Forskal), throughout the breeding rooms. The maturation pheromone (W. Loher (1960) Proc. Roy. Soc. V. 153, 380–397) was distributed to such an extent that solitary phase locusts could not be reared in that facility (P. E. Ellis and S. Gillet, (1968) Colloques, Int. Cent. Natn. Rech. Scient. 173, 173–182: S. Gillet (1968) Nature (London) 218, 782–783).

most of the colony activities, such as nest construction, defense, feeding brood and foraging; b) Drones (several hundred) – the males; active primarily outside the hive during mating activities; c) A single queen – the fully developed female that normally lays all of the eggs and hence produces the population of the colony.

Honey bees (at least *Apis mellifera*) live in enclosed nests, such as dark cavities in hollow trees, crevices in rocks, or box-like structures provided by man. In such dark enclosures, the thousands of bees crowd closely together, living in an apparently highly organized society. Regardless of the degree of organization per se, effective communication is the primary means whereby all activities are integrated. Communication is defined as the intra-specific transfer of stimuli that elicit behavioral and/or physiological responses in receptive individuals. Thus, at any given time worker bees are constantly 'sending' and 'receiving' information, primarily through the media of tactile and olfactory senses. The dark nest would seem to prevent communication by visual means and favor the evolution of elaborate mechanisms involving tactile and olfactory communication. A cursory examination of the honey bee nest reveals several attributes that probably facilitate communication by volatile pheromones. First, the enclosed nest offers protection from variable wind currents that could dissipate chemical 'messages'. Nest enclosure, combined with active ventilation behavior, permits some control of pheromone concentration, particularly through exhausting pheromones that could persist beyond the functional period and leave meaningless 'odor messages'. Ventilation is regulated by fanning bees. The air flow is orderly, that is, at the nest entrance one can detect intake and exhaust areas. The same ventilation activity apparently spreads chemical messages very quickly throughout the colony, complementing the mechanism of diffusion. Other nest attributes also favor a degree of stability of pheromone distribution, for example, the relatively constant temperature (35 °C).

All activities within the hive are potentially mediated to some degree by pheromones. The search for such pheromones has been enhanced greatly by transferring colonies from the protected, dark nest cavities into glass-enclosed observation hives. Behavioral activities can be observed easily in these hives, without apparently disturbing the bees inside.

11.4. Queen pheromones

11.4.1. Effects of queen pheromones on worker bees

Queen pheromones greatly influence the physiology and behavior of worker bees. The two identified pheromones are found primarily in the secretion of the mandibular glands (fig. 11.1). The major one, originally named queen substance (Butler 1954a), is 9-oxodec-*trans*-2-enoic acid (hereafter designated, 9-O-2). 9-O-2 was identified by Callow and Johnston (1960) and Barbier and Lederer (1960), and synthesized by Callow and Johnston (1960), Barbier et al. (1960), Barbier and Hügel

(1961) and Butler et al. (1961). The other pheromone is 9-hydroxydec-*trans*-2-enoic acid, isolated by Butler et al. (1964). Evidence for pheromones at other body sites has been presented by many researchers, e.g. Velthuis (1970a), but these pheromones have not been identified. Seasonal variations in pheromone production have been noted in both queens and worker bees (Pain et al. 1972).

Colonies containing healthy queens behave in a characteristic manner in which the various activities of workers proceed somewhat orderly and efficiently. The casual observer is not likely to get the impression that there is a direct influence of queen pheromones on worker activities, except perhaps on the workers immediately surrounding the queen. Nevertheless, the effects of queen pheromones can be demonstrated simply by removing the queen from the colony. Workers soon begin to move around in an 'agitated' or excited state. Fanning activity greatly increases within several minutes of queen removal. The fanning sound is so noticeable that some beekeepers utilize this behavior when searching for the queen bee. They divide the brood combs into two chambers, delay a few minutes, then search for the queen in the quiet brood chamber. Fanning and locomotion both exist at low levels even when the queen is present. Fanning probably facilitates the distribution of queen pheromones throughout the hive and locomotion increases the probability that the 'agitated' bees would encounter the queen. A more popular interpretation is that the 'agitated' bees are *searching* for the queen. This is probably not true in the literal sense (see sect. 11.2). It follows, then, that queen pheromones possibly

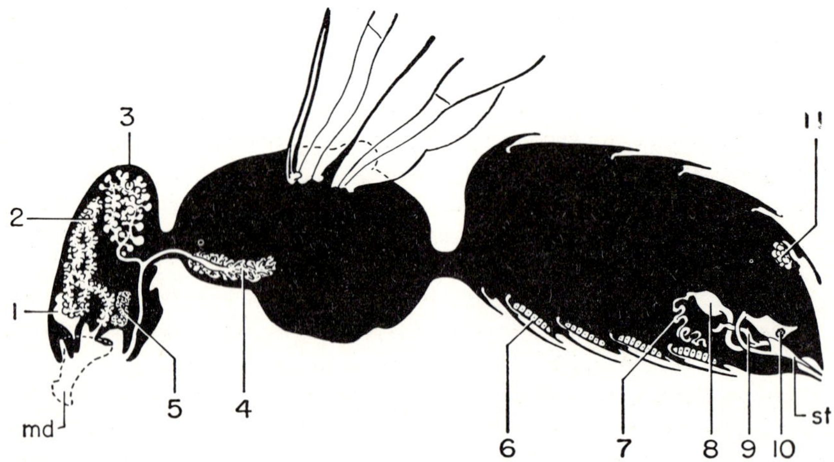

Fig. 11.1. Exocrine glands of the honey bee worker indicated as sources or potential sources of pheromones: 1) mandibular gland; 2) hypopharyngeal gland; 3) head labial gland; 4) thorax labial gland; 5) postgenal gland; 6) wax glands; 7) poison gland; 8) vesicle of poison gland 9) Dufour's gland; 10) Koschewnikow gland; 11) Nassanoff gland. (md, mandible; st, sting) (Adapted from Wilson, copyright (3 Sept. 1965) by the American Association for the Advancement of Science.)

inhibit locomotion and fanning behavior in a portion of the worker population: the frequency and intensity of locomotion and fanning by this particular population is perhaps in equilibrium with the pheromone concentration at any given time within the colony. Complete removal of the queen would remove the inhibitory pheromones, leading to maximal fanning and locomotion responses.

Another colony response to the loss of queen pheromones is the construction of queen cells, in which ordinary worker cells containing larvae less than three days old are shaped into queen cells and provisioned lavishly with food, ultimately leading to the production of a new queen. Queen cell construction is usually begun within 48 hr after the queen is lost or removed from the colony. Such behavior indicates that queen pheromones inhibit queen cell construction. This hypothesis has been validated in various bioassays by many researchers, for example, Butler and Callow (1968) and reviewed by Butler (1970) and Gary (1970).

Queen pheromones possibly affect the behavior of nurse bees in provisioning queen cells with brood food (royal jelly). In commercial rearing of queens, approximately 80–90% of introduced queen cells containing one-day old larvae are 'accepted' and provisioned throughout larval life when the cells are placed in colonies without queens. However, only approximately 40% of such cells placed in the brood chamber of colonies containing normal queens are accepted and provisioned (Gary 1959). Queen cell destruction appears to be stimulated by queen pheromones. In colonies without queens, introduced queen cells normally remain until queen emergence. However, approximately 50% of mature cells (within 24 hr before emergence) are destroyed before queen emergence when such cells are placed in the brood chambers of colonies containing normal queens (Gary 1959). There is some evidence (Gary and Morse 1962) that some worker bees destroy queen cells at the same time other bees are engaged in cell construction and provisioning. Differences in physiological state may partially account for the opposing responses to identical pheromonal stimuli.

The construction and provisioning of cells occur during the presence of the queen (and presumably her pheromones) prior to swarming and prior to supersedure of the old queen. It is possible that the pheromone production of queens changes qualitatively and quantitatively during such cell construction, perhaps in combination with physiological changes in workers, which might temporarily change their behavior regarding cell construction and provisioning.

Significant changes in worker bee physiology are related to queen pheromones. Gast (1967) found that the *corpora allata* undergo two growth phases, a first phase which is inhibited by 9-O-2 and a second phase in which development occurs only when a queen is present. Inhibition of oogenesis in workers has been reported by many researchers (e.g., Voogd, 1955; Butler 1957; Verheijen-Voogd 1959; Pain 1961; Velthuis 1970b, 1972) and has been demonstrated by confining worker bees in cages without queens or queen extracts. When such bees are properly nourished, the normally diminutive ovaries enlarge. In advanced stages, a few eggs may be produced. When these workers are in colonies, some lay unfertilized eggs in worker cells. Apparently, the presence of the queen (and her pheromones) generally tends to inhibit female attributes related to reproduction, leading to a degree of regulation of worker bee activities which some authors interpret as a kind of 'dominance'. Workers with enlarged ovaries apparently mimic queen pheromones to some degree. Velthuis et al. (1965) found that laying workers (advanced stage of oogenesis) and/or extracts of laying workers elicited retinue behavior and inhibited oogenesis in young workers under experimental conditions. Pain et al. (1967) did not detect 9-O-2 in laying workers.

11.4.2. Distribution of queen pheromones

The distribution of queen pheromones within the colony probably involves several mechanisms, one of which is clearly dissipation in the air currents within the hive. Butler (1954b, 1956) suggested that distribution is primarily by frequent food transfer between workers, in which 'queen substance' (9-O-2) is mechanically distributed, after being obtained initially by licking the queen's body. The food transfer mechanism is theoretically possible. Nixon and Ribbands (1952) demonstrated that sugar syrup containing P_{32} rapidly was distributed to most workers within a few hours of feeding small quantities to a few workers in a colony. Loss of inhibitory effects (oogenesis and queen cell building) was observed when queen extracts were mixed with sugar syrup higher than 5–10% (Verheijen-Voogd 1959; Erp 1960; Pain 1961), although Butler (1956) and Butler and Gibbons (1958) did not detect any influence of sugar concentration on worker response. Johnston et al. (1965) fed radioactive 9-O-2 to workers in order to study the rate of metabolism and the nature of metabolites produced within the worker bee gut. They found that 9-O-2 was quickly metabolized to 9-ketodecanoic acid, 9-hydroxydecanoic acid, and 9-hydroxydec-2-enoic acid, and suggested that the speed of conversion into these compounds was sufficiently rapid to account for the rapid onset of queenless behavior following the separation of the queen from the workers. Consequently, transmission of pheromones in transferred food is possible, but the efficiency of this mechanism is very difficult to evaluate. Velthuis (1972) suggested that queen pheromones are more likely to be disseminated by those worker bees which contact the queen during retinue behavior. The pheromones 'adhere' to the other workers where the materials express effects through the mechanism of olfactory perception – primarily antennal. This mechanism was suggested earlier by Verheijen-Voogd (1959) who proposed that olfactory perception alone is sufficient to elicit worker responses. Further support for the olfactory perception mechanism was found by Erp (1960), Butler (1961), Butler and Fairey (1963), and others.

Butler, Callow, Greenway and Simpson (personal communication) followed the distribution of tritiated 9-O-2 applied to thoraces of isolated queens and workers, which were prevented from grooming by removal of wings and the use of leg constraints. Subsequent analyses of heads and abdomens from these bees revealed tritiated 9-O-2, thus indicating absorption and translocation within the body. More tritiated 9-O-2 was found inside the body than on the surface, suggesting that 9-O-2 may be transported in the circulatory system. Butler and Fairly (1963) reported that the injection of worker bees with 9-O-2 partially inhibited oogenesis, but did not inhibit queen rearing.

11.5. Worker–queen behavioral interactions

The most obvious and perhaps most significant effects of queen pheromones are found in the behavioral interactions between queens and workers in the immediate vicinity of the queen. As queens move near the workers, they are usually encircled by worker bees. Such retinue behavior is apparently stimulated primarily by pheromones. Similar behavior can be induced by queen extracts placed on dummy queens. Several kinds of behavioral responses are stimulated, presumably influenced by the physiological state of the workers and the pheromone concentration, most likely a function of pheromone dilution in space as the distance between workers and queen increases. There is also the possibility that different worker responses are stimulated by different pheromones localized on various parts of the queen. The most frequently observed responses of workers to queens are as follows:

1) Turning toward the queen
2) Walking toward the queen
3) Arrested (short duration) locomotion a few millimeters from the queen's body
4) Backward locomotion, as if repelled by high pheromone concentration
5) Advancing close to the queen's body and initiation of antennal tapping, proboscis extension and licking of cuticular surfaces, particularly the abdomen
6) Advancing to the head region, spreading the mandibles and releasing a glandular secretion which is received by the queen
7) Grasping the queen's body parts with the mandibles
8) Stinging behavior – curling of the abdomen and sting protrusion
9) 'Crowding' near the queen and arrested (prolonged) locomotion.

Unfortunately, virtually all of these behavioral responses have been interpreted anthropomorphically by most observers. Instead of proposing meaningful hypotheses they conclude that such bees are simply 'caring for their queen'. However, although further documentation is required, most of the observed worker behavior near the queen can be explained theoretically as mechanistic responses to changes in the quality and quantity of pheromones emanating from the queen. The distance between the queen and workers especially affects the response. This concept is shown diagramatically in fig. 11.2. Thus, worker bees in zone A constantly perceive a very low 'background' concentration which facilitates continuation of normal activities, such as foraging. Workers in zone B turn and approach the queen. As they approach, the pheromone concentration increases sharply in zone C, thus momentarily arresting further locomotion toward the queen. If the queen is moving steadily few workers advance beyond zone C. Stationary workers in the path of the queen are frequently exposed to zone C by virtue of the queen's movements. These bees are very effectively repelled by the approaching queen and respond by backward locomotion, thus clearing the area and facilitating queen movement. If the queen is stationary, some workers behave as if they have undergone physiological adaptation, to the extent that they are no longer repelled by pheromones in zone C. These workers then move into zone D, where the antennae contact the queen. Extension of the proboscis may be stimulated by antennal contact and there is an opportunity for contact detection of essentially non-volatile pheromones in the cuticle waxes. It is also interesting to speculate that workers may possibly be depositing pheromones on the queen's cuticle while licking the queen's body. Bees that happen to be in the head region (zone E) may possibly receive different pheromones that specifically elicit a feeding response. If this postulate is valid, the same food-offering behavior would be expected to occur at other areas of the queen's body if such a pheromone could be transferred there experimentally.

Although sound and tactile stimuli from queens may also affect worker behavior, pheromones are probably the primary stimuli accounting for queen-oriented worker behavior. For example, the extirpation of mandibular glands (the primary source of queen pheromones) from living queens causes approximately 85% loss of attraction of workers to the queen (Gary 1961a; Morse and Gary 1963; Zmarlicki and Morse 1964) and reduced aggressive responses (Yadava and Smith 1971a).

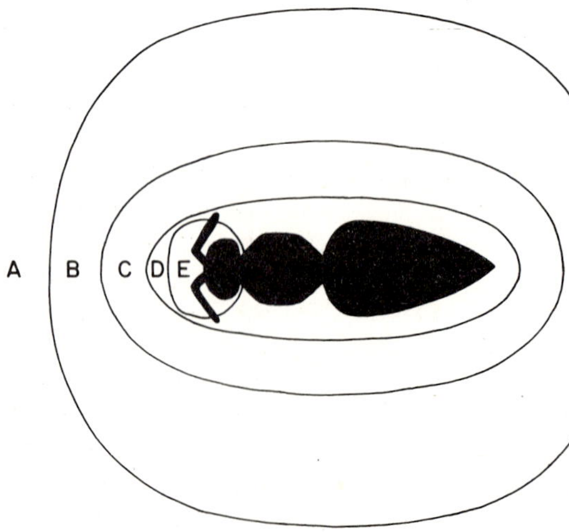

Fig. 11.2. Zones near queen where differential 'retinue' behavior of worker bees is apparently stimulated by variable pheromone quality and concentration (diagrammatic).

Attraction to the queen is the common first step in the 'chains' of worker behavior which concern feeding, 'grooming', receiving queen pheromones that are distributed to other workers, or even 'attacking' the queen.

Under some conditions, worker bees will respond aggressively to queen pheromones, sometimes killing the queen, through starvation or stinging. This occurs especially when: (a) a normal, mated queen is placed in a different colony; (b) a queen is removed from her colony for several hours, then replaced; (c) a second queen is released into a colony containing an established primary queen; and (d) the colony is disturbed excessively by manipulation. During this behavior workers crowd tightly around the queen, forming a compact cluster or 'ball' (hence termed 'balling' by beekeepers). This response may start initially as a kind of hyper-attraction of workers and can be induced experimentally by impregnating objects, such as filter paper, or coating worker bees with queen mandibular gland secretion (Gary 1961b; Yadava and Smith 1971a). Pheromonal mechanisms are involved in this behavior, but the precise mechanisms are somewhat obscure. Gary (1961b, 1970) proposed that: (a) high concentration of queen mandibular gland pheromones may elicit antagonistic, stinging behavior whereas low concentrations elicit attraction and licking behavior; (b) a concentration above a critical threshold level may stimulate the release of alarm pheromones by nearby workers, which in turn stimulates the 'balling' response; (c) the sudden changes in the microenvironment of the queen, e.g., high temperature, caused by hyper-attraction and intensive clustering, may place great 'stress' on some workers and the queen in the interior of the cluster, causing the release of alarm and/or other pheromones.

The above mechanisms seem likely if one assumes that a normal queen produces a relatively constant flow of mandibular gland secretion released at short intervals from the base of the mandible in response to frequent stimulation by workers feeding her. Disruption of this behavior for a significant time may cause an abnormal accumulation of the secretion. At such a time the 'excitation state' or threshold level of workers deprived of the queen pheromones changes greatly. When the queen and workers are placed together again, the hyperstimulated queen releases an abnormally large quantity of secretion. This presents a super-stimulus to which the workers respond maximally, causing the 'balling' responses. Gary (1970) postulated that the worker–queen 'balling' behavior may facilitate the rejection of abnormal queens, i.e., those producing and/or releasing pheromones erratically or somehow out of phase with colony requirements. Yadava and Smith (1971b) postulated the existence of a highly volatile 'stress' pheromone released by the queen when 'attacked' by worker bees. They also demonstrated that the 'balling' behavior stimulated by virgin queens could be eliminated by extirpating the mandibular glands (Yadava and Smith 1971a). Worker bees behaved more aggressively toward queens as the attractiveness of queens increased (Yadava and Smith 1971c).

The 'balling' response, which develops when a queen is placed in another hive, with or without an established queen, is probably caused in part by 'foreign' colony odors on the queen. In this context 'balling' may be stimulated initially by worker pheromones. 'Balling' behavior is likely to involve both worker and queen pheromones, functioning in concert.

11.6. Mating pheromones

Mating pheromones in the honey bee were first determined by Gary (1962), who developed a drone attraction bioassay in which multiple tethered queens were suspended approximately 10–20 m high by helium-filled weather blimps or stationary towers. Elevated queens were found to be highly attractive to drones on mating flights and a series of experiments led to the conclusion that the primary source of pheromones is the oily secretion from the large mandibular glands of the queen. When the mandibular gland secretion of virgin queens was fractionated chemically, at least two compounds were attractive to flying drones. The primary active compound was identified as 9-O-2 (Gary 1962) and Butler and Fairey (1964) identified 9-hydroxydec-2-enoic acid as a secondary component attractive to flying drones. The total lipid complex of the mandibular glands is more attractive to drones than pure 9-O-2 (Gary 1962; Pain and Ruttner 1963). However, Butler and Fairey (1964) reported that 100 μg of synthetic 9-O-2 was as attractive to drones as an alcohol extract of the single virgin queen they used in the experiment. Virgin queens contain only about 108 μg (Pain et al. 1967) to 130 μg (Butler and Paton 1962) of 9-O-2, but there is no information on how much is actually exposed on the surface of the body or released at any given moment from living queens.

Butler (1967) proposed that 9-O-2 also functions as an aphrodisiac in stimulating the mounting of queens by drones. He also suggested that there is an additional, as yet unidentified, pheromone associated with the abdominal tergites, that stimulates mounting and copulation (Butler 1971). This suggestion was based in part on the report of Renner and Baumann (1964) who noticed that unicellular glands on abdominal tergites II, III and IV produce a fragrant, volatile secretion, especially noticeable in virgin queens of the age for mating. They postulated that the secretion may function as a sex attractant.

There may be additional pheromones associated with the sting chamber. For example, pheromones from the Koschewnikow glands (Butler and Simpson 1965) possibly may be released when the sting chamber is opened. Regardless of the intensity of the pheromone stimuli from all sources, mating does not occur unless there is an open sting chamber, or its equivalent (Gary 1963; Butler 1967). The physical requirements for mating, i.e., the diameter and depth of the sting chamber, were documented by Gary and Marston (1971). Drones mated with wooden queen models, which were coated with mandibular gland secretion to enhance attraction. It was found that the wooden queen models treated with queen pheromones were comparable to living queens in attraction, an observation that was also confirmed by Gerig (1971).

The perception of queen odors and synthetic 9-O-2 has been studied by Beetsma and Schoonhoven (1966), Boeckh et al (1966), Beetsma (1967), Kaissling and Renner (1968) and Ruttner and Kaissling (1968). Sense organs, e.g., *sensilla placodea*, are located primarily on the antennae. Drones do not respond to queen pheromones released inside the hive (Pain 1973), but will respond during mating flights, which occur on warm, sunny afternoons when the wind is less than approximately 20 km/hr.

Drones on mating flights tend to assemble in large numbers at 'congregation' areas. There is no evidence that pheromones are involved in the formation of drone congregations, although the possibility has been suggested by Gerig (1972) and others.

Mating pheromones in *Apis* are active interspecifically. Drones of *Apis mellifera* are attracted to the queen pheromones of *A. florea* (Fab.) and *A. cerana* (Fab.) (Butler et al. 1967). Shearer et al. (1970) determined that 9-O-2 produced by *A. dorsata* (Fab.) and *A. cerana* is identical to 9-O-2 produced by queens of *A. mellifera*; Sannasi et al. (1971) confirmed this.

In some insect species, congeners of sex attractant pheromones function as masking agents or synergists with respect to the primary attractant pheromone. This possibility was tested in the honey bee by Blum et al. (1971) who prepared an extensive series of analogues and homologues of 9-O-2 and analyzed the compounds for drone attraction. All structural modifications caused complete loss of attractiveness to drones. Included in the series of 19 alkenoic acids was 9-hydroxy-*trans*-2-enoic acid, found earlier to be attractive to drones by Butler and Fairly (1964). Doolittle et al. (1970) also compared drone attraction to the *cis* and *trans* isomers of 9-O-2, and found that the *cis* isomer was not attractive. However, the *cis* isomer was photoisomerized to the *trans* isomer after prolonged exposure to sunlight, and attraction was restored. The *cis* isomer had no masking activity when tested in combination with the *trans* isomer in a 1:1 ratio.

The number of variables involved in evaluating drone attraction under field conditions is not sufficiently emphasized in published papers. Drone behavior varies greatly according to the population density and the uncontrolled weather variables. The difficulties of conducting mating pheromone bioassays under field conditions are also frequently underestimated. If bioassays are to be conducted under natural conditions as much as possible, they should be conducted in natural drone congregation areas where there are usually large populations (hundreds) of drones. Small numbers of drones may be attracted to queen pheromones in many locations, but these locations should not be regarded as true congregation areas. The population density is an important variable because drones seem to become more excited and active as the population increases. Thus, it appears more likely that drones will approach and mount queens and queen models, or approach displayed pheromone samples, when the population is high. One problem with high populations is recording drone visitation accurately. For example, the sudden, erratic arrivals and departures of up to 100 drones around each source of pheromone will challenge any recording system. When marginally attractive pheromone sources are tested, few drones may be attracted to the immediate vicinity of the candidate pheromones, and weakly attractive compounds may not be detected. In order to ensure large, active drone populations throughout the tests, living queens can be displayed downwind within a few meters from the candidate materials. If drones are sufficiently sparse to permit visual counting of individual drones, the investigator should eliminate each drone by some means after recording each visitation. Otherwise, multiple observations may be made inadvertently on only a few drones, thus possibly introducing bias as a consequence of the uncontrolled genetic and learning variables. In bioassays intended to evaluate relative attraction, multiple samples should be displayed simultaneously in the same immediate area to minimize the variables of time, attractiveness of area, and observer bias inherent when multiple observers operate independently at different observation stations.

Although queen mating pheromones from the mandibular gland secretion are certainly a major communication mechanism which functions during orientation and mating behavior of drones, these pheromones are not absolutely essential for successful mating. Morse et al. (1962) extirpated the mandibular glands from very young virgin queens, prior to the functioning of these glands, and found that a small percentage mated successfully.

Experimental use of queen mating pheromones has greatly facilitated studies of mating behavior. Drones attracted to the pheromones can be photographed, exposed to many kinds of treatments, and captured, tagged and released for flight range studies. This is particularly so since the development of a magnetic recapture system (Gary 1971), which permits automatic recapture of metal, numbered tags at the hive entrances after drones return to their respective hives.

11.7. Pheromones used in nest defense

Because honey bees have many natural 'enemies', it is not surprising that rather elaborate nest defense mechanisms involving pheromonal communication have evolved. Huber (1814) discovered that freshly excised bee stings elicited stinging behavior when placed near the hive entrance. Apiculturists who are stung while manipulating bee colonies are aware that there is a 'sweet' odor, reminiscent of banana oil, associated with the sting. They also notice that the probability of receiving stings increases greatly after the first sting is received. The detailed behavior elicited by pheromones associated with colony defense has been described by Maschwitz (1966). Many insects have alerting pheromones (Maschwitz 1964a; Blum 1969) termed 'alarm' pheromones by Maschwitz (1964b) and Wilson (1965). In the honey bee these compounds seem to be associated with the glandular cells lying against the inner surface of the quadrate plates at the base of the sting (Ghent and Gary 1962), but the precise secretion site is unknown.

The primary active alarm pheromone is *iso*-pentyl acetate (Boch et al. 1962). *Iso*-pentyl acetate is absent in newly emerged worker bees and found primarily in bees 15–30 days old, at the rate of 1–5 μg/bee (Bosch and Shearer 1966). All four *Apis* species contain *iso*-pentyl acetate (Morse et al. 1967). A secondary alarm pheromone, 2-heptanone, is produced in the worker mandibular glands (Shearer and Boch 1965; Boch and Shearer 1967). The existence of this pheromone was indicated when Maschwitz (1964b) placed mandibular gland secretion at the hive entrance and elicited aggressive responses in guard bees. It is possible that 2-heptanone released at the nest entrance is more effective as a repellent to potential enemies, e.g. robber bees (Simpson 1966) than as a primary alarm stimulus. Simpson (1966) and Butler (1966) noted that worker mandibular gland secretion is strongly repellent to foraging bees. The comparative efficacy of *iso*-pentyl acetate and 2-heptanone was studied by Boch et al. (1970), who determined that 20–70 times more 2-heptanone was required to elicit comparable reactions by guard bees at the hive entrance. They concluded that the potency of alarm pheromone is primarily, but not entirely, a function of *iso*-pentyl acetate. Morse et al. (1967) assayed *Apis* species for 2-heptanone and found this compound only in *A. mellifera*, although it elicits alarm in all *Apis* species.

Another possible function of the worker alarm pheromone has been reported by Morse (1972). Alarm odor released near queens in a swarm caused the termination of scenting behavior, stopping the release of the attractive Nassanoff gland pheromone. He suggested that this may be a mechanism by which worker bees identify and join a familiar queen, or reject a 'foreign' queen from another swarm.

Alarm pheromones are released whenever the sting is extruded slightly, but full release probably occurs only when the sting is torn from the bee's body and imbedded in the flesh substrate. Intravenom pheromones would seem to have less adaptive value, inasmuch as the signalling function of the deposited sting would be lost when the sting is inserted into the substrate. Yet, bees disturbed during cold weather elevate the abdomen and release a droplet of venom at the tip of the sting (Morse 1966), suggesting the possibility of an intravenom pheromone release. One alarm pheromone (*iso*-pentyl acetate) has been found in honey bee venom (Gunnison 1966).

Alarm pheromone bioassays have been developed (e.g. Free 1961; Stort, 1972), in which objects and materials simulating the appearance, size, odor, and texture of animals have been displayed near the hive entrance. The assays are usually evaluated by determining the number of deposited stings per unit time. Alarm pheromone bioassays are extremely challenging in that it is difficult or impossible to regulate the quantity and quality of the pheromone owing to rapid dissipation. Additional uncontrolled pheromones may also be released by the first bees stimulated. When sting deposition is used as a criterion of alarm response, the variable size and texture of the substrate present special problems. During maximal response, the substrate is completely covered with bees and the bioassay may measure little more than the number of workers that the substrate can physically accommodate during the exposure period. Ghent and Gary (1962) inserted fresh stings on pieces of filter paper into glass-walled observation hives and noted an 'agitated' response within 15–20 cm from the paper, similar to that described by Butler and Free (1952). The response could not be quantified owing to rapidly changing threshold response levels.

A queen alarm pheromone, referred to as a 'stress' pheromone, has been postulated by Yadava and Smith (1971b) as a mechanism to explain their observations in which queens stimulated massive aggressive behavior by apparently releasing a 'stress' pheromone.

The defensive system of honey bees can be disrupted momentarily by blowing smoke inside the hive, a procedure that is routinely used to prevent stinging behavior when opening and examining colonies. It would be interesting to determine if some components of smoke are causing partial adaptation of the sensilla that are functional in the detection of alarm pheromones.

11.8. Foraging activities

Foraging bees sometimes release pheromones from the Nassanoff gland, also called the scent gland (fig. 11.1). The pheromone secretion originates from a pouch-like, invaginated membrane between the last two abdominal terga. The pheromone is released by raising the abdomen, and partially extruding and exposing the membrane, which is moist with secretion. The volatile secretion is disseminated posteriorly from the bee by wing fanning. Scent fanning is rarely observed when bees forage on natural flora, but it is commonly observed when there is foraging at artificial food sources, usually feeders containing sucrose syrup to which a scent has been added. Von Frisch (1923) reported that the scent was released at food sources when the food supply was rewarding and he suggested that Nassanoff gland pheromone attracted new foragers to the food. Wenner et al. (1969) observed that the frequency of Nassanoff gland exposure at feeding stations increased as the food scent concentration decreased. However, they concluded that the pheromone does not contribute to the recruitment of foragers. Free and Williams (1970) observed a high frequency of scenting behavior during water collection and suggested that scenting behavior during the collection of sugar syrup may be an adaptation of water foraging behavior. There was very little correlation between dancing of foragers returning from a feeding station and release of the pheromone on subsequent foraging trips (Free and Williams 1972).

Nassanoff gland secretion is attractive, as determined by Renner (1960), who collected the secretion by wiping the exposed gland area with filter paper and subsequently tested its activity. Boch and Shearer (1962) identified geraniol as an active ingredient. Foraging bees contain approximately 1.0 μg/bee. However, the whole secretion is more attractive than pure geraniol alone (Free 1962), which indicates that geraniol is only a part of the pheromone complex. Nerolic and geranic acids were identified by Boch and Shearer (1964), who concluded that these two compounds, along with geraniol, accounted for most of the worker attraction. A fourth compound, citral (*trans*-geranial), was identified by Weaver et al. (1964), but they concluded that the geraniol and citral mixture is equivalent bioactively to the natural secretion. Boch and Shearer (1963) found that citral was absent in fresh Nassanoff gland secretion but present (Shearer and Boch 1966) in small quantities in secretion stored for several hours at room temperature. Butler and Calam (1969) found approximately 3% citral in fresh, whole Nassanoff gland secretion. The function of Nassanoff gland secretion during foraging activity is still not clear.

Queen pheromones affect foraging activities of workers. Jaycox (1970a, b) found that foraging is stimulated by the presence of a normal queen, queen extract, or synthetic 9-O-2. There is some evidence indicating that pollen foraging is stimulated by brood pheromones (Free 1967; Jaycox 1970b) and perhaps nectar foraging too. Pheromones may also be released during the dancing behavior of foraging bees, but this intriguing possibility has not been investigated.

11.9. Swarming

Queen pheromones are actively involved during swarming, the reproductive division of the colony in which the established queen and thousands of workers suddenly leave the hive, cluster temporarily on an nearby object and then migrate to a new nest site. Cohesion of the swarm as a group is contingent upon the presence of queen pheromones. When experimentally induced swarms occur without the queen, bees cluster very briefly but then return to the colony. Pheromones stimulating clustering and 'organized migration' were found by Morse (1963) and Simpson (1963) in the mandibular glands of the queen. Simpson (1963) and Velthuis and Van Es (1964) determined that 9-O-2 is attractive to swarming bees. Butler et al. (1964) showed that 9-hydroxydec-2-enoic acid facilitates the maintenance of a stable cluster by swarming bees. Butler and Simpson (1967) concluded that 9-O-2 and 9-hydroxydec-2-enoic acid are complementary in action, i.e., 9-O-2 attracts flying bees to the queen and 9-hydroxydec-2-enoic acid stimulates alighting and clustering. Morse and Boch (1971) questioned that 9-hydroxydec-2-enoic acid stimulates clustering behavior. Instead, they concluded that 9-O-2, in combination with Nassanoff gland pheromones, accounts for attraction and stabilization of the swarm cluster.

Other unknown pheromones may be actively involved in swarming. The sudden and rather spectacular egress of swarming bees from the hive may be stimulated by massive release of pheromones inside the hive. Repellency caused by high concentrations of compounds, otherwise attractive in low concentration, is a very common mechanism in the insect world. A massive release of pheromones, perhaps from the Nassanoff and/or mandibular glands, could logically be made by the worker bees because of their high numbers and large pheromone storage capacity when considered collectively.

11.10. *Trail marking and orientation*

Bees returning to the hive orient to the colony odor effluent (Lecomte 1956; Butler et al. 1970), which probably contains pheromones and other odors from many sources within the hive. If the entrance is disturbed, moved, or blocked for several minutes, and then restored to its original condition, the returning foragers that were initially prevented from entering the hive alight on the entrance and remain stationary for a few minutes while exposing the Nassanoff gland, releasing Nassanoff pheromones and fanning. Other returning foragers orient to the fanning workers, alight, and release additional pheromones.

Honey bees do not have the elaborate trail marking systems of ants, but there is evidence of pheromone trails at the hive entrance. Lecomte (1956) demonstrated a trail marking pheromone by rotating a hive 180 degrees, after which returning foragers alighted at the original entrance location, then walked around the hive to the relocated entrance in response to Nassanoff pheromones released by other foragers. A narrow trail of a stable pheromone was deposited by the tarsi and this trail was followed by other workers. The pheromone is probably produced by the Arnhart's glands located on the tarsal extremities (Chauvin 1962). The existence of a trail-marking pheromone was confirmed by Butler et al. (1969), who called it 'footprint substance'.

11.11. *Other honey bee pheromones*

The potential for utilization of pheromones in the honey bee colony is much greater than the published research indicates, even though Pain (1973) lists 31 pheromones believed to exist, of which 13 have been identified. For example, it is likely that pheromones are involved in brood feeding. Other pheromones produced by developing brood may induce incubation and clustering behavior. Evidence for incubation pheromones has been found for two species of *Bombus* (Heinrich 1973). Drone-produced pheromones may function in caste discrimination within the hive. There may be other worker pheromones involved in communication from worker to worker inside the hive. In summary, our sketchy knowledge of honey bee pheromones, combined with a lack of understanding of the neurophysiology of the sensory system, indicate that that the task of elucidating pheromonal mechanisms has just begun.

References

Barbier, M. and M. Hügel, (1961) Synthèses dans la série de l'acide céto-9 décène-2 *trans* oïque (substance royale). Bull. Soc. Chim. Fr. 202, 951–954.

Barbier, J. and E. Lederer (1960) Structure chimique de la substance royale de la reine d'abeille (*Apis mellifica* L.). C. R. Acad. Sci. (Paris) 250, 4467–4469.

Barbier, M., E. Lederer and T. Nomura (1960) Synthèse de l'acide céto-9 décène-2-*trans* oïque (substance royale) et de l'acide céto-8 nonène-2-*trans* oïque C. R. Acad. Sci. (Paris) 251, 1131–1135.

Beetsma, J. (1967) The transmission of regulating factors between the queen and worker honey bees (*Apis mellifica* L.). Vestn. Cesk. Zemed. Mus. 31, 325–328.

Beetsma, J. and L. M. Schoonhoven (1966) Some chemosensory aspects of the social relations between the queen and the worker in the honey bee (*Apis mellifera* L.). Proc. Kon. Ned. Akad. Wetensch. Ser. 69, 645-647.

Blum, M. S. (1969) Alarm pheromones. Ann. Rev. Entomol. 14, 57–80.

Blum, M. S., R. Boch, R. E. Doolittle, M. T. Tribble and J. G. Traynham (1971) Honey bee sex attractant: conformational analysis, structural specificity, and lack of masking activity of congeners. J. Insect Physiol. 17, 349–364.

Boch, R. and D. A. Shearer (1962) Identification of geraniol as the active component in the Nassanoff pheromone of the honey bee. Nature (London) 194, 704–706.

Boch, R. and D. A. Shearer (1963) Production of geraniol by honey bees of various ages. J. Insect Physiol. 9, 431–434.

Boch, R. and D. A. Shearer (1964) Identification of nerolic and geranic acids in the Nassanoff pheromone of the honey bee. Nature (London) 202, 320–321.

Boch, R. and D. A. Shearer (1966) *Iso*-pentyl acetate in stings of honey bees of different ages. J. Apicult. Res. 5, 65–70.

Boch, R. and D. A. Shearer (1967) 2-Heptanone and 10-hydroxy-*trans* dec-2-enoic acid in the mandibular glands of worker honey bees of different ages. Z. Vergl. Physiol. 54, 1–11.

Boch, R., D. A. Shearer and A. Petrasovits (1970) Efficacies of two alarm substances of the honey bee. J. Insect. Physiol. 16, 17–24.

Boch, R., D. A. Shearer and B. C. Stone (1962) Identification of *iso*-amyl acetate as an active compound in the sting pheromone of the honey bee. Nature (London) 195, 1018–1020.

Boeckh, J., K. E. Kaissling and D. Schneider (1966) Insect olfactory receptors. Cold Spring Harbor Symp. Quant. Biol. 30, 263–280.

Butler, C. G. (1954a) The World of the Honeybee. (Collins, London) pp. 97–110.

Butler, C. G. (1954b) The method and importance of the recognition by a colony of honey bees (*A. mellifera*) of the presence of its queen. Trans. Roy. Entomol. Soc. London 105, 11–29.

Butler, C. G. (1956) Some further observations on the nature of 'Queen substance' and of its role in the organization of a honey-bee (*Apis mellifera*) community. Proc. Roy. Entomol. Soc. London Ser. A 31, 256–257.

Butler, C. G. (1957) The control of ovary development in worker honey bees (*Apis mellifera*). Experientia 13, 256–257.

Butler, C. G. (1961) The scent of queen honey bees (*A. mellifera* L.) that causes partial inhibition of queen rearing. J. Insect Physiol. 7, 258–264.

Butler, C. G. (1966) Mandibular gland pheromone of worker honey bees. Nature (London) 212, 530.

Butler, C. G. (1967) A sex attractant acting as an aphrodisiac in the honey bee (*Apis mellifera* L.). Proc. Roy. Entomol. Soc. London Ser. A 42, 71–76.

Butler, C. G. (1970) Chemical communication in insects: behavioral and ecologic aspects. *In*: Communication by Chemical Signals. Vol. 1 eds.: J. W. Johnston, D. G. Moulton and A. Turk (Appleton-Century-Crofts, New York) pp. 35–78.

Butler, C. G. (1971) The mating behaviour of the honey bee (*Apis millifera* L.). J. Entomol. 46, 1–11.

Butler, C. G. and D. H. Calam (1969) Pheromones of the honey bee – the secretion of the Nassanoff gland of the worker. J. Insect Physiol. 15, 237–244.

Butler, C. G. and R. K. Callow (1968) Pheromones of the honeybee (*Apis mellifera* L.): The 'inhibitory scent' of the queen. Proc. Roy. Entomol. Soc. London Ser. B 43, 62–65.

Butler, C. G. and E. M. Fairey (1963) The role of the queen in preventing oogenesis in worker honeybees. J. Apicult. Res. 2, 14–18.

Butler, C. G. and E. M. Fairey (1964) Pheromones of the honeybee: biological studies of the mandibular gland secretion of the queen. J. Apicult. Res. 3, 65–76.

Butler, C. G. and J. B. Free (1952) The behavior of worker honeybees at the hive entrance. Behaviour 4, 263–292.

Butler, C. G. and D. A. Gibbons (1958) The inhibition of queen rearing by feeding queenless worker honeybees (*A. Mellifera*) with an extract of 'queen substance'. J. Insect Physiol. 2, 61–64.

Butler, C. G. and P. N. Paton (1962) Inhibition of queen rearing by queen honey bees (*Apis mellifera* L.) of different ages. Proc. Roy. Entomol. Soc.London Ser. A 37, 114–116.

Butler, C. G. and J. Simpson (1965) Pheromones of the honey bee (*Apis mellifera* L.). An olfactory pheromone from the Koschewnikow gland of the queen. Scientific Studies, Univ. Libcice, Czechoslovakia 4, 33–36.

Butler, C. G. and J. Simpson (1967) Pheromones of the queen honey bee (*Apis mellifera* L.) which enable her workers to follow her when swarming. Proc. Roy. Entomol. Soc. London Ser. A 42, 149–154.

Butler, C. G., D. H. Calam and R. K. Callow (1967) Attraction of *Apis mellifera* drones by the odours of the queens of two other species of honey bees. Nature (London) 213, 423–424.

Butler, C. G., R. K. Callow and J. R. Chapman (1964) 9-Hydroxydec-*trans*-2-enoic acid, a pheromone stabilizing honey bee swarms. Nature (London) 201, 733.

Butler, C. G., R. K. Callow and N. C. Johnson (1961) The isolation and synthesis of queen substance, 9-oxydec-*trans*-2-enoic acid, a honeybee pheromone. Proc. Roy. Soc. Ser. B 155, 417-432.

Butler, C. G., D. J. C. Fletcher and D. Watler (1969) Nest-entrance marking with pheromones by the honeybee *Apis mellifera* L., and by a wasp, *Vespula vulgaris* L. Anim. Behav. 17, 142–147.

Butler, C. G., D. J. C. Fletcher and D. Watler (1970) Hive entrance finding by honey bee (*Apis mellifera*) foragers. Anim. Behav. 18, 78–91.

Callow, R. K. and N. C. Johnston (1960) The chemical constitution and synthesis of queen substance of honeybees (*Apis mellifera*). Bee World 41, 152–153.

Chauvin, R. (1962) Sur l'epagine ϵ et sur les glandes tarsales d'Arnhart. Insectes Soc. 9, 1–5.

Doolittle, R. E., M. S. Blum and R. Boch (1970) *cis*-9-oxo-2-decenoic acid: synthesis and evaluation as a honey bee pheromone and masking agent. Ann. Entomol. Soc. Am. 63, 1180–1185.

Erp, A. V. (1960) Mode of action of the inhibitory substance of the honey bee queen. Insectes Soc. 7, 207–211.

Free, J. B. (1961) The stimuli releasing the stinging response of honey bees. Anim. Behav. 9, 193–196.

Free, J. B. (1962) The attractiveness of geraniol to foraging honey bees. J. Apicult. Res. 1, 52–54.

Free, J. B. (1967) Factors determining the collection of pollen by honeybee foragers. Anim. Behav. 15, 134–144.

Free, J. B. and I. H. Williams (1970) Exposure of the Nasanov gland by honeybees (*Apis mellifera*) collecting water. Behaviour 37, 286–290.

Free, J. B. and I. H. Williams (1972) The role of the Nasanov gland pheromone in crop communication by honeybees (*Apis mellifera* L.). Behaviour 41, 314–318.

Frisch, K. Von (1923) Über die 'Sprache' der Bienen, eine tier-psychologische Untersuchung. Zool. Jb. (Physiol.) 40, 1–186.

Gary, N. E. (1959) A study of natural and induced supersedure of the queen honey bee (*Apis mellifera* L.). Ph.D. Thesis, Cornell University, Ithaca, New York, 145 pp.

Gary, N. E. (1961a) Queen honey bee attractiveness as related to mandibular gland secretion. Science 133, 1479–1480.

Gary, N. E. (1961b) Antagonistic reactions of worker honeybees to the mandibular gland contents of the queen (*Apis mellifera*). Bee World 42, 14–17.

Gary, N. E. (1962) Chemical mating attractants in the queen honey bee. Science 136, 773–774.

Gary, N. E. (1963) Observations of mating behaviour in the honey bee. J. Apicult. Res. 2, 3–13.

Gary, N. E. (1970) Pheromones of the honey bee, *Apis mellifera* L. *In*: Control of Insect Behavior by Natural Products; eds.: D. L. Wood, R. M. Silverstein and M. Nakajima, (Academic Press, Inc., New York) pp. 29–53.

Gary, N. E. (1971) Magnetic retrieval of ferrous labels in a capture-recapture system for honey bees and other insects. J. Econ. Entomol. 64, 961–965.

Gary, N. E. and J. Marston (1971) Mating behaviour of drone honey bees with queen models (*Apis mellifera* L.). Anim. Behav. 19, 299–304.

Gary, N. E. and R. A. Morse (1962) The events following queen cell construction in honey bee colonies. J. Apic. Res. 1, 3–5.

Gast, R. (1967) Untersuchungen über die Einfluss der Königinnensubstanz auf die Entwicklung der endokrinen Drüsen bei der Arbeiterin der Honigbiene (*Apis mellifica*). Insectes Soc. 14, 1–12.

Gerig, L. (1971) Wie Drohnen auf Königinnen-attrapen reagieren. Schweiz. Bienenztg. 94, 558–562.

Gerig, L. (1972) Ein weiterer Duftstoff zur Anlockung der Drohnen von *Apis mellifica* (L.). Z. Angew. Entomol. 70, 286–289.

Ghent, R. L. and N. E. Gary (1962) A chemical alarm releaser in honey bee stings (*Apis mellifera* L.). Psyche 69, 1–6.

Gunnison, A. F. (1966) The collection and analysis of the volatiles of bee venom, and solubility characteristics of bee venom solids. M. S. Thesis (Cornell University, Ithaca, New York) 55 pp.

Heinrich, B. (1973) A self-stimulating pheromone in bumble bees. (in preparation).

Huber, F. (1814) Nouvelles observations sur les abeilles. 2nd. ed., Transl. 1926 (Dadant, Hamilton, Illinois) p. 205.

Jaycox, E. R. (1970a) Honey bee queen pheromones and worker foraging behavior. Ann. Entomol. Soc. Am. 63, 222–228.

Jaycox, E. R. (1970b) Honey bee foraging behavior: Responses to queens, larvae and extracts of larvae. Ann. Entomol. Soc. Am. 63, 1689–1694.

Johnston, N. C., J. H. Law and N. Weaver (1965) Metabolism of 9-ketodec-2-enoic acid by worker honey bees (*Apis mellifera* L.). Biochemistry 4, 1615–1621.

Kaissling, K. E. and M. Renner (1968) Antennale Rezeptoren für Queen Substance und Sterzelduft bei der Honigbiene. Z. Vergl. Physiol. 59, 357–361.

Lecomte, J. (1956) Über die Bildung von 'Strassen' durch Sammelbienen, deren Stock um 180° gedreht wurde. Z. Bienenforsch. 3, 128–133.

Maschwitz, U. W. (1964a) Gefahrenalarmstoffe und Gefahrenalarmierung bei sozialen Hymenopteren. Z. Vergl. Physiol. 47, 596–655.

Maschwitz, U. W. (1964b) Alarm substances and alarm behaviour in social Hymenoptera. Nature (London) 204, 324–327.

Maschwitz, U. W. (1966) Alarm substances and alarm behavior in social insects. Vitam. Horm. (New York) 24, 267–290.

Morse, R. A. (1963) Swarm orientation in honey bees. Science 141, 357–358.

Morse, R. A. (1966) Honey bee colony defense at low temperatures. J. Econ. Entomol. 59, 1091–1093.

Morse, R. A. (1972) Honey bee alarm pheromone: another function. Ann. Entomol. Soc. Am. 65, 1430.

Morse, R. A. and R. Boch (1971) Pheromone concert in swarming honey bees (Hymenoptera: Apidae). Ann. Entomol. Soc. Am. 64, 1414–1417.

Morse, R. A. and N. E. Gary (1963) Further studies of the responses of honey bee (*Apis mellifera* L.) colonies to queens with extirpated mandibular glands. Ann. Entomol. Soc. Am. 56, 372–374.

Morse, R. A., N. E. Gary and T. S. Johansson (1962) Mating of virgin queen honey bees (*Apis mellifera* L.) following mandibular gland extirpation. Nature (London) 194, 605.

Morse, R. A., D. A. Shearer, R. Boch and A. W. Benton (1967) Observations on alarm substances in the genus *Apis*. J. Apicult. Res. 6, 113–118.

Nixon, H. L. and C. R. Ribbands (1952) Food transmission within the honey bee community. Proc. Roy. Soc. London Ser. B 140, 43–50.

Pain, J. (1961) Sur la phéromone des reines d'abeilles et ses effets physiologiques. Ann. Abeille 4, 73–152.

Pain, J. (1971) Phéromones et comportement chez quelques Hyménoptères. Apidologie 2, 319–334, 351–355.

Pain, J. (1973) Pheromones and Hymenoptera. Bee World 54, 11–24.

Pain, J. and F. Ruttner (1963) Les extraits de glandes mandibulaires des reines d'abeilles attirent les mâles lors du vol nuptial. C. R. Acad. Sci. (Paris) 256, 512–515.

Pain, J., M. Barbier and B. Roger (1967) Dosages individuels des acides céto-9-décène-2-oïque et hydroxy-10-décène-2-oïque dans les têtes des reines et des ouvrières d'abeilles. Ann. Abeille 10, 45–52.

Pain, J., B. Roger and J. Theurkauff (1972) Sur l'existence d'un cycle annuel de la production de phéromone (acide céto-9-décène-2-oïque) chez les reines d'abeilles (*Apis mellifica ligustica* Spinola). C. R. Acad. Sci. (Paris) 275, 2399–2402.

Renner, M. (1960) Das Duftorgan der Honigbiene und die physiologische Bedeutung ihres Lockstoffes. Z. Vergl. Physiol. 43, 411–468.

Renner, M. and M. Baumann (1964) Über Komplexe von subepidermalen Drüsenzellen (Duftdrüsen?) der Bienenkönigin. Naturwissenschaften 51, 68–69.

Ruttner, F. and K.-E. Kaissling (1968) Über die interspezifische Wirkung des Sexuallockstoffes von *Apis mellifica* und *Apis cerena*. Z. Vergl. Physiol. 59, 362–370.

Sannasi, A., G. Rajulu and G. Sundara (1971) 9-oxo-*trans*-2-decenoic acid in the Indian honey bees. Life Sci. 10, 195–201

Shearer, D. A. and R. Boch (1965) 2-heptanone in the mandibular gland secretion of the honeybee. Nature (London) 206, 530.

Shearer, D. A. and R. Boch (1966) Citral in the Nassanoff pheromone of the honey bee. J. Insect Physiol. 12, 1513–1521.

Shearer, D. A., R. Boch, R. A. Morse and F. M. Laigo (1970) Occurrence of 9-oxodec-*trans*-2-enoic acid in queens of *Apis dorsata*, *Apis cerana*, and *Apis mellifera*. J. Insect Physiol. 16, 1437–1441.

Simpson, J. (1963) Queen perception by honey bee swarms. Nature (London) 199, 94–95.

Simpson, J. (1966) Repellency of the mandibular gland scent of worker honey bees. Nature (London) 209, 531–532.

Stort, A. C. G. (1972) Metodologia para o estudo da genetica da agressividade de *Apis mellifera*. Proc. lst Congr. Brasileiro de Apicultura (Florianopolis) pp. 36–50.

Velthuis, H. H. W. (1970a) Queen substances from the abdomen of the honey bee queen. Z. Vergl. Physiol. 70, 210–222.

Velthuis, H. H. W. (1970b) Ovarian development in *Apis mellifera* worker bees. Entomol. Exptl. Appl. 13, 377–394.

Velthuis, H. H. W. (1972) Observations on the transmission of queen substances in the honey bee colony by the attendants of the queen. Behaviour 41, 105–129.

Velthuis, H. H. W. and J. van Es (1964) Some functional aspects of the mandibular glands of the queen honeybee. J. Apicult. Res. 3, 11–16.

Velthuis, H. H. W., F. J. Verheijen and A. J. Gottenbos (1965) Laying worker honey bee: similarities to the queen. Nature (London) 207, 1314.

Verheijen-Voogd, C. (1959) How worker bees perceive the presence of their queen. Z. Vergl. Physiol. 41, 527–582.

Voogd, S. (1955) Inhibition of ovary development in worker bees by extraction fluid of the queen. Experientia 11, 181–182.

Weaver, N., C. C. Weaver and J. H. Law (1964) The attractiveness of citral to foraging honeybees. Progr. Rep. Tex. Agric. Exptl. Stn. No. 2324, 1–7.

Wenner, A. M., P. H. Wells and D. L. Johnson (1969) Honey bee recruitment to food sources: Olfaction or language? Science 164, 84–86.

Wilson, E. O. (1965) Chemical communication in the social insects. Science 149, 1064–1071.

Yadava, R. P. S. and M. V. Smith (1971a) Aggressive behavior of *Apis mellifera* L. workers towards introduced queens. II. Role of the mandibular gland contents of the queen in releasing aggressive behavior. Can. J. Zool. 49, 1179–1183.

Yadava, R. P. S. and M. V. Smith (1971b) Aggressive behaviour of *Apis mellifera* L. workers towards introduced queens. I. Behavioural mechanisms involved in the release of worker aggression. Behaviour 39, 212–236.

Yadava, R. P. S. and M. V. Smith (1971c) Aggressive behavior of *Apis mellifera* L. workers towards introduced queens. III. Relationship between the attractiveness of the queen and worker aggression. Can. J. Zool. 49, 1359–1362.

Zmarlicki, C. and R. A. Morse (1964) The effect of mandibular gland extirpation on the longevity and attractiveness to workers of queen honey bees, *Apis mellifera*. Ann. Entomol. Soc. Am. 57, 73–74.

CHAPTER 12

Pheromonal sociality in the Hymenoptera

Murray S. BLUM

12.1. Introduction

Hymenopterans are richly endowed with exocrine glands and it has become quite apparent that these structures constitute some of the most versatile biosynthetic tissues which are encountered in animals. A dazzling array of pheromones have been identified in the secretions of social insects testifying to the major use of volatile information-bearing agents as behavioral regulators. The widespread utilization of pheromones by these insects reflects their programmed responsiveness to these selective stimuli because of the great acuity and discriminatory elegance of their olfactory chemoreceptors. Rapid processing of information encoded in pheromonal stimuli appears to be a hallmark of social insects which guarantees the viability of a communicative system predicated primarily on olfactory triggers. In a sense, the variegated aspects of chemical communication in the Hymenoptera mirror many of the salient characteristics that have enabled these insects to develop the societal complexity so often identified with species of ants, bees, and wasps.

Although our present knowledge of the chemistry of hymenopterous pheromones is extremely limited, it is nevertheless worthwhile to examine the mainstream of pheromonal sociality as a function of some of the specific chemicals regulating many of the interactions of these insects. In so doing, many of the control systems operating in the social milieu will become comprehensible in terms of precise stimuli whose quintessential roles as pheromones can be probed behaviorally, physiologically, and biochemically. Such a treatment promises to be one viable means of studying the evolution of sociality in the Hymenoptera especially since pheromonal regulators of behavior are by no means restricted in their distribution to the highly organized species. As the same exocrine compounds are often found in both presocial and eusocial species, there are no cogent grounds for concluding that the former do not possess many of the biosynthetic pathways that are expressed in the latter species. Indeed, we shall probably determine that the inability of subsocial hymenopterans to attain a eusocial state is, among other things, not necessarily a reflection of exocrine insufficiency but rather of failure to be genetically programmed to respond adaptively to the variety of natural products in their glandular tissues.

12.2. Trail pheromones

Various types of odor trails are utilized by a wide variety of hymenopterous species (table 12.1) as an effective means of coordinating the movements of groups of individuals. The functions of these trails may be contextually variable and their persistence may reflect such factors as: 1) the number of individuals depositing the pheromone; 2) the nature of the active substances and of the substrate; and 3) the environmental conditions prevailing subsequent to the laying of the trail.

In one of the few investigations made on the stability of trails under field conditions, Torgerson and Akre (1970) determined that those generated in the dry season by Neotropical army ants (*Eciton* spp.) persisted for up to one week whereas trails formed during the rainy season were considerably less stable. Trails established on porous substrates with many absorptive sites, e.g., roots, logs, lianas, were considerably more stable than those laid on soil or leaf litter. Significantly, emigration trails persist longer than raid trails. This observation is reconcilable with the fact that many workers utilize the former and, as a consequence, the concentration of trail pheromone is much higher than it is in trails formed by raiding groups (Torgerson and Akre 1970). It was also determined that trails laid by epigaeic species are more persistent than those produced by hypogaeic forms, and additionally, that well-fed ants generated longer-lasting trails than starved individuals. These sundry observations serve to emphasize some of the multitudinous factors which affect the duration of a trail under natural conditions.

In general, recruitment trails capable of drawing large numbers of workers to food finds constitute the major type of trail generated by hymenopterans. Recruitment trails normally develop from the accretive depositions of trail pheromone paid out by workers returning to the nest from a favorable food source. However, since emigration to a new nest site is also regulated by a recruitment trail, it is obvious that these transient pheromonal pathways can subserve more than one function. In addition, individual ants belonging to legionary ponerine and doryline species lay exploratory trails (Wilson 1963) as they probe the substrate searching for food. These army ants also develop typical emigration trails that are much more persistent that the exploratory ones because the former are reinforced by the pheromonal secretions of many workers whereas the latter are not.

12.2.1. Glandular origins

The protean sources of trail pheromones in the Hymenoptera are evident from table 12.1 in which seven glands have been shown to produce these chemical trail

TABLE 12.1

Glandular sources of trail pheromones in some hymenopterous genera.

Family	Subfamily	Genus	Glandular source	Authority
Vespidae	Vespinae	*Vespula*	Dermal glands (?) (applied with tarsi)	Butler et al. (1969)
Formicidae	Ponerinae	*Termitopone*	Hind gut	Blum (1966a)
		Leptogenys	Poison gland	Fletcher (1971)
	Dorylinae	*Neivamyrmex*	Hind gut	Watkins (1964)
		Eciton	Hind gut	Blum and Portocarrero (1964)
	Myrmicinae	*Atta*	Poison gland	Moser and Blum (1963)
		Monomorium	Poison gland	Blum (1966a)
		Pheidole	Dufour's gland	Wilson (1963)
		Crematogaster	Metathoracic tibial glands (applied with tarsi)	Fletcher and Brand (1968) Leuthold (1968)
	Dolichoderinae	*Monacis*	Pavan's gland	Wilson and Pavan (1959)
	Formicinae	*Myrmelachista*	Hind gut	Blum and Wilson (1964)
		Acanthomyops	Hind gut	Hangartner (1969)
Apidae	Apinae	*Melipona*	Mandibular glands	Lindauer and Kerr (1958)
		Trigona	Mandibular glands	Lindauer and Kerr (1958)
		Apis	Dermal glands (?) (applied with tarsi)	Butler et al. (1969)

stimuli. In almost all cases, a gland normally utilized for other functions has been converted into a social organ, presumably as a consequence of the finite number of exocrine organs available for communicative functions.

Butler et al. (1969) have demonstrated that both honey bees and wasps lay trails with footprints in the vicinity of the hive or nest, and the pheromones appear to be derived from dermal glands. These footprint trails are apparently employed by workers to orient to the nest entrance and it has been suggested that such trails may be present in the vicinity of the nests of other hymenopterans such as ants. Indeed, there is evidence that ants can lay trails with their feet (tarsi) and this phenomenon may be widespread in eusocial insects. Workers of the ant *Eciton hamatum* (Fab.) generate trails with a hind gut secretion (table 12.1) but nevertheless are able to lay weak footprint trails after their abdomens have been removed (Torgerson and Akre 1970). Leuthold (1968) has also reported that, if a well-established trail of the myrmicine *Crematogaster ashmeadi* Mayr is interrupted, the ants will re-establish the trail without exhibiting typical trail-laying behavior involving the hind legs (table 12.1). He interprets this 'passive' trail laying as a function of the deposition of normal footprint material which is less stimulatory than the recruitment pheromone but nevertheless suffices as a low level trail-following stimulus. Although the footprint trails developed by ants, bees, and wasps could not in themselves be completely responsible for the specific odors that the members of each colony possess, they may still serve as an important component of the aromas that accompany the individuals of a nest.

It is only in the stingless bees that the mandibular glands are known to be employed in dispensing trail pheromones (table 12.1). Lindauer and Kerr (1958) demonstrated that these trails are especially distinctive since they actually function as ephemeral aerial flyways accurately followed by airborne bees. These trails develop from a series of droplets deposited at specific intervals from a food source back to the nest. These chemically-developed flyways are particularly well adapted for use in tropical rain forests, and, as they are functional in both the horizontal and vertical component, they can guide bees to the rich flora at the top of the forest canopy.

However, it is among the ants that the independent development of trail organs by different phyletic lines is so clearly expressed (table 12.1). Formicid trail substances are present in glands: 1) secondarily adapted to function as social organs (poison gland and Dufour's gland); 2) extensively hypertrophied to produce trail pheromones (tibial glands); and 3) which arose de novo to play the role as dispensers of chemical releasers of trail following (Pavan's gland). Since members of both the poneroid (Ponerinae and Dorylinae) and myrmecioid (Formicinae) complex (Brown 1954) utilize the hind gut for a source of trail pheromones, the social function of this organ has arisen independently in the two main lines of formicid evolution. In contrast, the poison gland is restricted as a trail organ to species in two subfamilies in the poneroid complex, the Myrmicinae and the Ponerinae. However, in the Myrmicinae, any of three different glands may serve as the source of trail pheromones and one of these cases, the tibial glands of *Crematogaster*, is of special interest because it may constitute a feature unique to this genus.

The unique structure of the abdomen of *Crematogaster* workers militates against using the sting for trail laying, as do the species in other myrmicine genera. The postpetiole is attached to the apparent dorsum of the gaster and can be easily directed dorsally but has little ventral mobility. Independently, Fletcher and Brand (1968) and Leuthold (1968) demonstrated that trails are laid through the tarsi of the metathoracic legs, the trail pheromone originating in the tibial glands. Subsequently, Pasteels et al. (1970) showed that hypertrophied cells surrounding the enlarged unguitractor tendon of the metathoracic legs were the source of the trail pheromone. This pheromone is released from an orifice proximal to the unguitractor plate of the pretarsus while the trail-laying worker executes elaborate 'dance' steps with its hind legs. Neither the prothoracic nor the mesothoracic legs contain a hypertrophied tibial gland and the development of the gland-tendon complex of these legs resembles that of ants in other genera, of termites and of beetles (Pasteels et al. 1970). Thus the trail-laying mechanism of *Crematogaster* seems to represent an extreme elaboration of a system normally underdeveloped in insects.

Pavan's organ is a unique exocrine structure limited in its formicid distribution to species in the subfamilies Dolichoderinae and Aneuretinae. Wilson and Pavan (1959) demonstrated that this gland functions as a generator of chemical trails in certain species but a detailed examination of a large number of species in several dolichoderine genera established that Pavan's organ is not an omnipresent feature of this subfamily (Pavan 1955). As Wilson and Pavan (1959) were able to prepare active trails with tissue from the presumed glandular area of a species (*Liometopum occidentale* Emery) that apparently lacks this organ, it is possible that the trail pheromone is synthesized in poorly differentiated tissues of certain species.

12.2.2. Chemistry and specificity

In spite of relatively little information being available on the chemistry of trail pheromones, it is nevertheless possible to conclude that trails are usually generated with mixtures of compounds, the full significance of which is yet to be determined. Although trail following may be initiated with single compounds isolated from an exocrine gland, the contribution of additional compounds in the glandular exudate will undoubtedly have to be evaluated in order to comprehend the mechanisms responsible for the specificity and persistence of the trails.

Bee trail pheromones: the stingless bee, *Trigona subterranea* Friese, deposits its odor trail from a mandibular gland secretion dominated by neral and geranial, the two stereoisomers of citral (Blum et al. 1970). The potency of these monoterpene aldehydes as attractants for workers is demonstrated by the fact that bees will interrupt a flight pattern between food sources and the nest in order to drop down and investigate citral-treated objects.

Kerr et al. (1963) examined the specificity and persistence of the trails of some *Trigona* species and demonstrated that: 1) more pheromone is deposited at the site farthest from the hive than at closer sites; and 2) the time spent trail marking increases at each successive stop as the bee returns to the nest. These results indicate that the first site is marked with an inordinately large amount of pheromone and it was concluded that consequently, the forager must spend increasingly greater amounts of time attempting to mark sites closer to the nest with the limited amount of trail substance that is still available in the mandibular glands. These results also demonstrate that such trails have great adaptive significance, since the highest concentration of pheromone is registered at the distal end of the trail, a situation which favors the location of the food finds.

Specificity studies with *T. (Scaptotrigona) postica* Latreille, *T. (Scaptotrigona) xanthotricha* Moure, and *T. (Trigona) spinipes* (Fab.) revealed that the trails do not always serve as species-isolating mechanisms. Thus, neither *T. postica* nor *T. spinipes* could follow each other's trails, while *T. xanthotricha* could 'read' the trail of *T. postica* but not vice versa. Analyses of the mandibular gland components of the three species, presented in table 12.2, illuminate the trail 'languages' utilized by these stingless bees.

The mandibular glands of *T. spinipes* are poorly developed (Cruz 1960), and, as trace amounts of only three volatile compounds can be detected, the chemistry of the trail deposited by this species appears to be relatively simple. However, *T. spinipes* has a very effective recruiting system and it seems obvious that the alcohols, especially 2-heptanol, constitute highly effective trail substances. Indeed, by employing 2-heptanol, Kerr, Blum and Fales (unpublished) succeeded, for the first time, in successfully laying an artificial trail for a species of stingless bee. The trail pheromone blend secreted by *T. postica* workers appears to be too complex to be decoded by workers of *T. spinipes*, and presumably the simplicity of the latter's trail pheromone is informationally too inadequate to release trail following in the former.

The pheromonal blends employed by both *T. xanthotricha* and *T. postica* constitute elaborate multicomponent systems (Blum, Fales and Kerr, unpublished) and the ability of the former to follow the latter's trail, but not the reverse, deserves some comment. Although the secretion of *T. postica* contains a few long-chain compounds not detected in that of *T. xanthotricha*, in general, both species produce many of the same methyl ketones and 2-alkanols. The salient difference between these two exudates is large amounts of two isomers of tetradecenyl acetate in the pheromonal blend synthesized by *T. postica* which contrast to a trace of only one isomer of this ester in that of *T. xanthotricha.* Conceivably, the lack of two tetradecenyl acetates in the secretion of *T. xanthotricha* may constitute an informationally-inadequate signal for workers of *T. postica* that are programmed to exhibit trail following to both isomers in the presence of an appropriate pheromonal blend. On the other hand, *T. xanthotricha* workers may derive little information from these esters and as a consequence, the secretion of *T. postica* would prove to be a perfectly suitable stimulant for trail following behavior. Although the bases for the trail specificities of these two species can be determined only after careful experimentation with synthetic mixtures, their complexity underscores the importance of analyzing trail pheromones as pheromonal blends rather than in terms of single compounds.

Ant trail pheromones: methyl 4-methylpyrrole-2-carboxylate, a poison gland product of the myrmicine *Atta texana* (Buckley), is the only ant trail pheromone that has been identified (Tumlinson et al. 1971, 1972). Sonnet and Moser (1972) demonstrated that synthetic analogs in which the 4-methyl group is replaced by either bromine or chlorine atoms are as active as the natural pyrrole. Previously, Moser and Silverstein (1967) observed that the trail pheromone of this species consists of both volatile and relatively non-volatile constituents, and Tumlinson et al. (1972) isolated at least four fractions capable of releasing trail-following behavior. The pyrrole, which is the most volatile and abundant trail pheromone produced

TABLE 12.2

Chemical compositions of the mandibular gland secretions of three *Trigona* species.

Compound	Species		
	T. postica[a]	*T. xanthotricha*[a]	*T. spinipes*[b]
2-Heptanone	++	++	—
2-Heptanol	+++	++	++
2-Nonanone	+	—	—
2-Nonanol	—	+	+
2-Undecanone	+	+	—
2-Undecanol	+	—	—
2-Tridecanone	+++	+++	—
2-Tridecanol	+	++	+
2-Pentadecanone	++	++	—
2-Pentadecanol	+	—	—
2-Heptadecanone	+	—	—
2-Heptadecanol	+	—	—
Tetradecenyl acetate	+++ (2 isomers)	+ (1 isomer)	—
Hexadecenyl acetate	+++ (2 isomers)	+++ (2 isomers)	—
Benzaldehyde	++	++	—

[a] M.S. Blum, H.M. Fales and W.E. Kerr (unpublished)
[b] W.E. Kerr, M.S. Blum and H.M. Fales (unpublished)

in the poison gland, is present at a concentration of about 0.6 ng/worker

Previously, Blum et al. (1964) reported that the poison gland products of species in four genera of fungus-growing ants, representing the broad phylogenetic spectrum of the tribe Attini, completely lacked specificity at the generic level. However, since field observations indicated that well developed attine trails were insulated from violation by species in different genera, it was suggested that the natural trail pheromones were fortified with other compounds that rendered the trails considerably more specific. A veritable plethora of subsequent circumstantial evidence indicates that the hypothesis is correct.

Recently, Robinson, Moser and Blum (unpublished) examined the responsiveness of a wide spectrum of attine species in the genera *Cyphomyrmex, Apterostigma, Trachymyrmex, Acromyrmex*, and *Atta* to methyl4-methylpyrrole-2-carboxylate. Members of all genera were shown to be equally sensitive to this pyrrole when evaluated as a trail pheromone. It was also established that *A. texana* and *A. cephalotes* (L.) would follow trails prepared from poison glands of *Acromyrmex octospinosus* (Reich.) but that *Atta sexdens* (L.) workers would not. It thus appears the secretion of *Acromyrmex octospinosus* lacks the trail pheromone of *Atta sexdens*, notwithstanding the fact that the former species follows trails prepared with the pyrrole. Furthermore, although *A. sexdens* will follow trails prepared from the poison gland of *A. texana*, it will *not* follow a trail generated with methyl 4-methylpyrrole-2-carboxylate, the trail pheromone of the latter species. It is thus clear that *A. sexdens* workers follow a component in the poison gland secretion of *A. texana* which is not identical to the pyrrole and it would be interesting to evaluate the less volatile trail pheromones produced by *texana* in order to ascertain whether any of them functions to release trail following in workers of *sexdens*. It may also be revelant that *A. sexdens* is placed in a different subgenus (*Neoatta*) from those in which *A. cephalotes* (*Atta*) and *A. texana* (*Archeatta*) are classified, but until other species in the subgenus *Neoatta* are challenged with the pyrrole, the significance of the non-responsiveness of *Atta sexdens* to this compound cannot be ascertained.

A. sexdens is not the first species of fungus-growing ant to utilize a trail pheromone which apparently differs from that of species in genera representing the mainstream of attine evolution. Blum and Portocarrero (1966) demonstrated that a species of *Sericomyrmex*, a rather aberrant attine genus, would not follow trails generated from the poison gland secretions of *Atta texana* or *Trachymyrmex septentrionalis* McCook, two species which readily follow trails prepared with the pyrrolic ester. Furthermore, the poison gland products of *Sericomyrmex* elicit either feeble or no trail-following responses in workers of the other two attine species. Clearly, *Sericomyrmex* has diverged from the main line of attine evolution in its utilization of a different natural product(s) as releasers of trail-following behavior.

Although most of the myrmicine trail pheromones are derived from compounds synthesized in the tissues of the poison gland, it should not be concluded that these natural products are identified with the proteinaceous constituents that normally fortify the venoms of ants in this subfamily. Blum and Ross (1965) observed that a trace constituent in the venom of the myrmicine *Tetramorium guineense* (Fab.) was utilized as a trail pheromone, but this compound was clearly different from the proteins and amino acids which thoroughly dominated the venom. Similarly, the pheromone of *T. caespitum* (L.) appeared to be a minor venomous constituent whose distinctness from that produced by *T. guineense* was indicated by the inabilities of the two species to follow each other's trails. However, in spite of the intrageneric specificities of the trail pheromone secretions employed by these two *Tetramorium* species, that of *T. guineense* releases strong trail following in attine species in two unrelated genera, *Atta* and *Trachymyrmex*. On the other hand, the *secretion of Tetramorium caespitum* did not release trail following in the attine species and *T. caespitum* workers did not follow trails generated from the attine secretions. Since the physical properties of the *T. guineense* pheromone demonstrated that it was different from those present in the attine secretions, it is almost certain that although these three species share common natural products, they are not all utilizing the same one as a trail pheromone (Blum and Ross 1965).

In essence, the results obtained in the specificity studies utilizing *Tetramorium* species and the two attines are most compatible with an explanation based on the presence of a pool of trace natural products in the venoms of myrmicine species. Many of these compounds may be common to the venoms of unrelated species, possibly reflecting the presence of similar metabolic pathways ultimately identified with the biosynthesis of macromolecular toxins. Two different species of myrmicines may, by chance, adopt the same trace constituent as a trail pheromone, and in this case their odor trails would not be species-specific if they are sympatric. However, it is equally possible that two species may utilize separate compounds to function as trail pheromones, but, because the two substances are common to both of their poison gland secretions, transposition studies employing their venoms would suggest that the same compound is serving as a pheromone for both species. Indeed, if the adoption of trace concomitants of the main venom constituents to function as trail pheromones has been widely practiced by myrmicine species, then it is possible that the venoms of species that do *not* lay trails may contain trail pheromones for species that do. The results of two investigations demonstrate that this is precisely the case.

The venom of the primitive dacetine, *Daceton armigerum* (Latreille), contains a powerful releaser of trail following for attines in the genera *Trachymyrmex, Acromyrmex*, and *Atta* (Blum and Portocarrero, 1966). Workers of *Daceton armigerum*, which never lay trails, do not follow extracts of their own poison glands, but, for the attine species, these extracts are equivalent in potency as trail pheromone sources to those of their own poison glands. *Sericomyrmex* workers neither follow artificial trails laid with glandular extracts from the other attine species nor do they follow trails generated from *Daceton armigerum* poison glands. These results demonstrate that the venom of *D. armigerum*, a non-trail-laying species, contains a trace constituent which is either identical to, or very similar to, the trail pheromones utilized by ants in a completely unrelated tribe. This lack of responsiveness of *Sericomyrmex* workers would simply reflect the absence of their trail pheromone in the extracts, a fact inferred previously based on the specificity of the *Sericomyrmex* trail pheromone *vis-à-vis* those of the other attines. Similarly, the venom of another myrmicine, *Cardiocondyla nuda* Forel, which does not utilize chemical trails, contains a moderately-active trail pheromone for *Monomorium minimum* (Buckley) (Blum 1966a). Transposition studies on two additional species of *Monomorium, M. pharaonis* (L.) and *M. floricola* (Jerdon), demonstrated the presence of a peculiar pattern of specificities. Neither *M. pharaonis* nor *M. floricola* would follow any trails other than their own, but *M. minimum*, would follow the trail of *M. pharaonis* in addition to its own. It seems most reasonable to assume that neither the trail pheromone of *M. pharaonis* nor that of *M. floricola* are shared with the other two species of *Monomorium*. On the other hand, the venom of *M. pharaonis* must contain the trail pheromone of *M. minimum* in addition to its own (Blum, 1966a), but the secretion of *M. minimum* must lack the chemical stimulus for trail following of *M. pharaonis.*

Wilson (1962) compared the specificities of the trail pheromones of fire ants in the myrmicine genus *Solenopsis* which lay trails with a secretion from Dufour's gland, rather than the poison gland. The secretion of *S. xyloni* McCook releases strong trail following in workers of *S. invicta* (=*saevissima*) Buren and *S. geminata* (Fab.), whereas the Dufour's gland products of *S. geminata* produced virtually no response in workers of the other two species. Similarly, the secretion of *S. invicta* did not initiate a trail-following response in workers of *S. xyloni.* Wilson (1962) concluded that the pheromone of *S. geminata* differed from those of the other two species and that the pheromones of *S. xyloni* and *S. invicta* differed in their effects on *S. geminata* workers.

These results can also be interpreted in terms of the presence of multiple components in the Dufour's gland secretions of these species. The secretion of *xyloni* probably contains the trail pheromones of the other two species in addition to its own, whereas the Dufour's gland pheromone of *geminata* is clearly different from those of *invicta* or *xyloni*. Since the pheromone utilized by *invicta* is different from that of *geminata* it seems certain that these three species of *Solenopsis* utilize different compounds as releasers of trail following but an apparent lack of specificity results because one species (*xyloni*) produces a blend of compounds among which are found the trail pheromones of the other two species.

Investigations involving species in four dolichoderine genera indicate that their trail pheromones are highly specific (Wilson and Pavan 1959). Transposition studies with species of *Tapinoma, Monacis, Liometopum*, and *Iridomyrmex* demonstrated that trail pheromones produced in Pavan's gland were completely species-specific. If such great specificity is characteristic of dolichoderine species in general, it must reflect the presence of very distinctive natural products which are employed as trail pheromones. Such specificity may be possible because Pavan's gland, a unique formicid organ for the synthesis and dispensing of trail pheromones, may have been selected for the production of particular metabolic end products. Presumably, such specificity would be much more difficult to obtain in species utilizing trace constituents of the poison gland as trail pheromones.

Watkins (1964) demonstrated that there is a complete lack of specificity in the odor trails generated by three species of army ants in the genus *Neivamyrmex*. Subsequently, Watkins et al. (1967) reported that the trails laid by four species of *Neivamyrmex* and by *Labidus coecus* (Latreille) were followed by all five species, but, in general, each species preferred its own trail when presented with a choice. However, a fifth species of *Neivamyrmex, N. pilosus* F. Smith, would not follow any trail other than its own, thus demonstrating that within the Dorylinae, not all species display promiscuous trail following behavior.

The results of Torgerson and Akre (1970) also emphasize that the trail pheromones deposited by army ant species may possess an unpredictable element of specificity. Utilizing five species of *Eciton*, two of *Labidus*, and a single species each of *Neivamyrmex* and *Nomamyrmex*, all variations on a specificity theme were encountered. One species of *Eciton, E. burchelli* (Westwood), followed the trails of the other four *Eciton* species as well as those of the *Neivamyrmex* and the *Labidus* species. Although another species of *Eciton* displayed an almost complete specificity in its response to odor trails, the other four species were relatively non-specific. Species in the other genera were indifferent to the *Eciton* trails, and, with few exceptions, non-responsive to all trails except their own. Torgerson and Akre (1970) noted that workers of some doryline species frequently sensed trails generated by foreign species but these alien trails were seldom followed for more than a few centimeters. They interpret this behavior as a response to a general stimulus distinct from that which results in sustained trail following. It is equally possible that the initial probing along a foreign trail may reflect the highly developed propensity of many ants to orient to foreign odors, and as such, may not be related to true trail-following behavior.

Like the army ants, members of the formicine genus *Camponotus* lay chemical trails with a secretion originating in the hind gut. Barlin (personal communication) evaluated the ability of *Camponotus pennsylvanicus* (De G.) to follow trails of seven other species in this genus and determined that their trail pheromones were particularly specific. However, workers of *C. pennsylvanicus* responded strongly to trails prepaired from hind guts of *C. americanus* Mayr, another species in the subgenus *Camponotus*. Since the other six species of *Camponotus* belong to other subgenera, it is possible that closely related species of *Camponotus* may be capable of utilizing each ohter's trails.

Chemical trails may possibly be guaranteed a greater degree of specificity by containing the products of more than one exocrine gland. This is suggested by the results obtained by Hölldobler (1971a) with the harvester ant *Pogonomyrmex badius* (Latreille). This myrmicine lays orientation trails, derived from the Dufour's gland, from points in its foraging field to the nests and this trail pheromone acts to assist the worker in locating the nest, but *does not* function as a recruiting stimulus. In contrast, this species lays powerful recruitment trails to food sources with a poison gland pheromone (Hölldobler and Wilson 1970) and the possibility that the specificity of this trail could be enhanced with a charge from the Dufour's gland cannot be excluded. The utilization of secondary glandular secretions to identify ant trails with an added element of specificity may constitute a widespread phenomenon and the possible existence of this device should be considered when analyzing odor trails under field conditions.

12.2.3. Inter-ordinal trail following

Whereas ants may utilize subtle blends of exocrine products in order to insulate their trails from other species of ants, they have not been able to prevent a multitude of unrelated animals from following these trails. Insects in several orders, as well as certain arthropods in other classes, are able to respond positively to these odor trails. In general, those animals capable of orienting to ant trails have intimate relationships with the ants, and their ability to follow odor trails is of considerable selective advantage since it maintains them in close contact with their hosts. Myrmecophiles do not exhibit a preference for their host colony over colonies of the same species, and they are often not species-specific (Akre and Rettenmeyer 1968).

A multitude of coleopterous species in the families Histeridae, Staphylinidae, and Limulodidae readily follow the trails of army ants in three genera (Akre and Rettenmeyer 1968). All of these beetles appear to be obligatory myrmecophiles and whereas many of them appear to be quite host specific, others are very promiscuous trail followers and may be found following trails of as many as five different species of ants. These beetles are normally encountered on the emigration trails of the dorylines and are seldom found on the exploratory trails generated by raiding ants. The former trails, due to the large number of ants generating them, undoubtedly are enriched with a high concentration of pheromone and are much more attractive to the myrmecophiles than the weaker exploratory trails. Myrmecophiles can certainly utilize emigration trails to locate their hosts and in some cases even larval staphylinids have been observed to follow them (Rettenmeyer 1961). The report that the carabid, *Helluomorphoides texanus* (LeConte) can follow odor trails of a *Neivamyrmex* species (Plsek et al. 1969) demonstrates that this ability is very widespread among beetles.

Rettenmeyer (1961) also observed that some species of Thysanura can follow doryline trails. That this behavior is not limited to myrmecophilous insects is demonstrated by the reports that macrochelid mites (Akre and Rettenmeyer 1968) and millipedes (Rettenmeyer 1962) exhibit trail following when they encounter army ant trails. Indeed, this ability is not limited to invertebrates since blind snakes orient on these trails with a stereotyped anchorconcertina locomotion (Watkins et al. 1967). These snakes feed on ant brood and their capacity to follow army ant trails is decidedly advantageous since it enables them to locate highly mobile food sources. Gehlbach et al. (1971) demonstrated that typhlopid and leptotyphlopid blind snakes followed army ant trails for considerable distances whereas those of non-army ants were decidedly less attractive.

Cockroaches in the genus *Attaphila* constitute the only myrmecophiles known to follow non-army ant trails. Moser (1964) reported that *A. fungicola* W. M. Wheeler, an inquiline of the attine, *Atta texana*, was particularly responsive to the trails of its host although it was not as sensitive to the trail pheromone as the ant workers. Blum and Portocarrero (1966) demonstrated that an *Attaphila* sp. followed the trail of its host, *Acromyrmex coronatus* (Fab.), and indeed, clung more tenaciously to the odor trails than the ants themselves. Since these cockroaches have been observed on the foraging trails of attines, it is probable that the flightless attaphilids utilize these trails for dispersal.

12.2.4. Informational content of trails

Wilson (1962) examined the ability of the fire ant *Solenopsis invicta* to utilize its odor trail to transmit information pertaining to both distance and direction from a point in its trophic field to the nest. It develops that the trail is highly functional in characterizing these two spatial components. Wilson and Bossert (1963) have described an active odor trail as a semiellipsoidal tunnel, to which the ant orients osmotropotactically as long as the concentration of pheromone is great enough to constitute an active space. This space represents a concentration of pheromone molecules great enough to be stimulatory at a threshold value which releases trail following.

In analyzing the odor trail, it also seems appropriate to consider the nature of the constituents that govern the olfactory signal perceived by worker fire ants. Brand, Blum and Barlin (unpublished) have noted that workers of the fire ant *S. richteri* Forel demonstrated passive trail following after a well established trail is directed to a food source. Trail laying is no longer exhibited and the ants do not manifest the 'excited' trail movements which characterize their following during the initial recruitment phase. Indeed, ants can be drawn easily from an old trail with a trail generated from a Dufour's gland. Thus it seems certain that a fresh trail contains more volatile pheromones that are highly stimulatory, and, as a consequence, are very effective recruitment stimuli. Presumably, after these volatile components evaporate, the ants 'settle down' to restrained (=passive) trail following which is both adequate for food retrieval, and, at the same time, is selectively advantageous, since it results in conserving the available trail pheromone.

Thus, it appears that the functionality of such a system is dependent on the availability of chemical blends which are enriched with more than one chemical stimulus of trail following. Brand, Blum, and Barlin (unpublished) demonstrated that the Dufour's gland secretion of *S. richteri* contained more than 30 compounds, some of which were hydrocarbons with considerably lower vapor pressures than that of the trail pheromone. Quite possibly, stimulatory compounds possessing highly different vapor pressures may provide a simple means of encoding both short term and long term information in a chemical trail. The most volatile compounds may function as potent stimuli of recruitment, whereas the less volatile chemostimulants may operate as 'keepers' to maintain the integrity of the chemical trail over a sustained period of time. This explanation is consistent with the observation by Barlin (personal communication) that in addition to the main trail pheromone, the Dufour's gland secretion of *S. richteri* also contains another chemical stimulus of trail following. Gas-chromatographic analyses have demonstrated that this second trail pheromone is present in trace quantities relative to the main chemical releaser of trail following. In addition, this minor exocrine compound is considerably less volatile than the recruitment trail pheromone, and could presumably function as an ideal long-term trail stimulus.

Thus, the informational content of chemical trails must be ultimately viewed in terms of multiple chemical releasers of trail following, the individual and collective properties of which will affect both the spatial and temporal qualities of the trail. Such factors as: (1) physical properties (e.g., vapor pressure); (2) stability; (3) concentration; and (4) chemostimulatory efficiency will have to be determined for the individual components of a pheromonal blend before the functional *raison d'être* of a chemical trail can be comprehended.

Moser and Silverstein (1967) emphasized that workers of *Atta texana* respond to both volatile and relatively non-volatile trail pheromones and Tumlinson et al. (1972) demonstrated that at least four different fractions are identified with trail-following activity. Worker ants are extraordinarily sensitive to the most volatile pheromone, methyl 4-methylpyrrole-2-carboxylate, and can follow 0.08 pg/cm, but it remains to be seen how sensitive they are to the minor components that are present. Indeed, these unidentified compounds could constitute the keepers for the long-lived trails that are characteristic of *Atta* species.

Brand, Blum and Barlin (unpublished) have determined that a worker of the fire ant, *Solenopsis richteri*, contains about one nanogram of the main trail pheromone per Dufour's gland. However, workers can detect about 0.02 pg/cm of this compound, and Barlin (personal communication) has calculated that a trail containing 3×10^{7} moles/cm will be readily perceived by workers. Since a worker contains about 3×10^{12} molecules of this pheromone in its Dufour's gland, it is evident that the generation of a successful trail is effected with no more than a trace of the pheromone present in its glandular reservoir. Whether workers can obtain detectable information from the minor trail pheromones during the initial deposition of a trail can only be ascertained after these compounds are identified and behaviorally evaluated.

12.3. Alarm pheromones

Hymenopterans employ a large variety of compounds as releasers of alarm behavior (table 12.3) and this number will undoubtedly be expanded as the alarm pheromones of species in other genera are chemically analyzed. The majority of compounds listed in table 12.3 are derived from ants as they have been the most successfully investigated family. Although some species of eusocial wasps possess alarm pheromones (Maschwitz 1964), none has been assigned a structure and only a handful of these releasers have been characterized in bees. Therefore, at this juncture, any comparative exocrinology of these pheromones is largely limited to members of the family Formicidae.

12.3.1. Glandular sources

The mandibular glands of meliponine bees are the source of all alarm pheromones so far characterized in this subfamily (Blum et al. 1970; Blum, Fales and Kerr, unpublished). Since many of the same compounds are also used to lay chemical trails, the functions of these substances can be contextually variable, a phenomenon that has been referred to as pheromonal parsimony (Blum 1969). Similarly, Maschwitz (1964) demonstrated that the alarm pheromones of wasps are derived from a secretion also having an entirely unrelated function, e.g., the poison gland secretion of *Vespa* species releases alarm behavior and is also a source of toxic defensive compounds.

In the Formicidae, species in the main subfamilies generally synthesize their alarm pheromones in the mandibular glands. Alarm pheromones are produced in the mandibular glands of species in the subfamilies Ponerinae, Dorylinae, Myrmicinae, and Formicinae. Maschwitz (1964) demonstrated that, in addition to the mandibular glands, certain formicine species can generate alarm signals with secretions from the poison and Dufour's glands. However, dolichoderine species generate an alarm signal with the products of their anal glands (Wilson and Pavan 1959), a structure that appears to have been developed to function as both a social and a defensive organ.

12.3.2. Chemistry of alarm pheromones

Many species of ants and bees signal alarm with a large variety of ketones, a class of compounds particularly emphasized as chemical releasers in the Hymenoptera. Twelve ketones have been identified in hymenopterous species (table 12.1) and it is obvious that an extensive variation on a ketonic theme has occurred in the exocrine glands of these insects. In the ants, these carbonyl compounds have a virtual mono-

TABLE 12.3

Typical alarm pheromones utilized by hymenopterous genera.

Compound	Family	Subfamily	Genus	Authority
Ketones				
2-Heptanone	Formicidae	Dolichoderinae	*Iridomyrmex*	Blum et al. (1963)
	Apidae	Meliponinae	*Trigona*	Blum et al. [b]
4-Methyl-2-hexanone	Formicidae	Dolichoderinae	*Dolichoderus*	Cavill and Hinterberger (1962)
4-Methyl-3-hexanone	Formicidae	Myrmicinae	*Manica*	Fales et al. (1972)
6-Methyl-5-hepten-2-one	Formicidae	Dolichoderinae	*Tapinoma*	Trave and Pavan (1956)
3-Octanone	Formicidae	Myrmicinae	*Myrmica*	Crewe and Blum (1970a)
4-Methyl-3-heptanone	Formicidae	Myrmicinae	*Pogonomyrmex*	McGurk et al. (1966)
2-Methyl-4-heptanone	Formicidae	Dolichoderinae	*Tapinoma*	Trave and Pavan (1956)
2-Nonanone	Apidae	Meliponinae	*Trigona*	Blum et al.[b]
3-Nonanone	Formicidae	Myrmicinae	*Myrmica*	Crewe and Blum (1970b)
6-Methyl-3-octanone	Formicidae	Myrmicinae	*Crematogaster*	Crewe et al. (1972)
3-Decanone	Formicidae	Myrmicinae	*Manica*	Fales et al. (1972)
4, 6-Dimethyl-4-octen-3-one	Formicidae	Myrmicinae	*Manica*	Fales et al. (1972)
Aldehydes				
2-Hexenal	Formicidae	Myrmicinae	*Crematogaster*	Bevan et al. (1961)
Citronellal	Formicidae	Formicinae	*Acanthomyops*	Ghent (1961)
Citral (both isomers)	Formicidae	Formicinae	*Acanthomyops*	Ghent (1961)
	Apidae	Apinae	*Trigona*	Blum et al. (1970)

Table 12.3 (continued)

Acids				
Formic	Formicidae	Formicinae	*Formica*	Maschwitz (1964)
Hydrocarbons				
p-Xylene	Formicidae	Myrmicinae	*Messor*	Blum et al.[c]
n-Decane	Formicidae	Formicinae	*Camponotus*	Bergström and Löfqvist (1971)
n-Undecane	Formicidae	Formicinae	*Acanthomyops*	Regnier and Wilson (1968)
n-Dodecane	Formicidae	Formicinae	*Camponotus*	Bergström and Löfqvist (1971)
Miscellaneous				
o-Aminoacetophenone	Formicidae	Myrmicinae	*Mycocepurus*	Blum et al.[a]
Dimethyldisulfide	Formicidae	Ponerinae	*Paltothyreus*	Casnati et al. (1967)
Dimethyltrisulfide	Formicidae	Ponerinae	*Paltothyreus*	Casnati et al. (1967)
2, 5-Dimethyl-3-isopentylpyrazine	Formicidae	Ponerinae	*Odontomachus*	Wheeler and Blum[d]
2, 6-Dimethyl-3-*n*-pentylpyrazine	Formicidae	Ponerinae	*Odontomachus*	Wheeler and Blum[d]
2, 6-Dimethyl-3-*n*-butylpyrazine	Formicidae	Ponerinae	*Odontomachus*	Wheeler and Blum[d]

[a] M.S. Blum, J.M. Brand and E. Amante (unpublished)
[b] M.S. Blum, H.M. Fales and W.E. Kerr (unpublished)
[c] M.S. Blum, G.W.A. Milne and M. Costa (unpublished)
[d] J. W. Wheeler and M. S. Blum (unpublished)

poly among species in the Myrmicinae and Dolichoderinae. Myrmicine species stress the production of ethyl ketones, five of these compounds having been identified among their mandibular gland products. Species in the Dolichoderinae stress methyl ketones, but one of these compounds, 2-heptanone, is also produced by members of the myrmicine genus *Atta* (Blum et al. 1968; Moser et al. 1968). The recent identification of a typical dolichoderine compound, 6-methyl-5-hepten-2-one, in the mandibular glands of a *Lasius* species (Bergström and Löfqvist 1970), demonstrates that the Formicinae share at least one ketonic product with the Dolichoderinae.

Monoterpene aldehydes probably have a widespread occurrence in the Hymenoptera, especially among bees (Kullenberg 1953); and the isomers of citral have recently been identified in the colletid *Hylaeus cressoni* (Cockerell) (Blum and Bohart 1972). The isomers of citral are also characteristic mandibular gland products of certain formicine ants and function as alarm releasers (Chadha et al. 1962; Bergström and Löfqvist 1970). Both isomers of citral have also been identified in the mandibular gland secretion of the myrmicine *Atta sexdens* (Butenandt et al. 1959) but these monoterpenes do not function as alarm releasers for this species but rather, are utilized as defensive compounds (Blum et al. 1968). 2-Hexenal, a common defensive product of cockroaches and many true bugs, appears to be an aberrant alarm pheromone produced by ants in the genus *Crematogaster*, (Bevan et al. 1961), but it has now been demonstrated that this enal is accompanied by the ethyl ketones which are characteristic alarm pheromones of species in this genus (Crewe et al. 1972).

The glands associated with the sting of formicine species are an extraordinarily rich source of alarm pheromones and other natural products. Formic acid, a ubiquitous poison gland product in the Formicinae, is employed by species of *Formica* (Maschwitz 1964) and *Camponotus* (Ayre and Blum 1971) to generate an alarm signal, but species in certain other genera do not display alarm behavior in the presence of this compound. Short-chain hydrocarbons synthesized in the Dufour's gland of a wide variety of formicines, serve as potent releasers of alarm and are discharged in admixture with the formic acid-rich venom. Species of *Acanthomyops* (Regnier and Wilson 1968), *Formica* (Bergström and Löfqvist 1968), *Lasius* (Bergström and Löfqvist 1970), *Camponotus* (Ayre and Blum 1971; Bergström and Löfqvist 1971) signal alarm with these simple alkanes which dominate the glandular constituents. Besides the dominant alkanes, these secretions are abundantly fortified with alkanes, alcohols, acetates, and sesquiterpenes, often in excess of a total of 40 compounds, and the alarm signals of these ants thus also reflect the presence of a multitude of minor but *not* necessarily inconsequential constituents (Bergström and Löfqvist 1971, 1972).

The occurrence of the aromatic compound, *o*-aminoacetophenone, in the mandibular glands of the attine *Mycocepurus goeldii* Forel (Blum, Brand and Amante, unpublished) deserves some comment. This genus appears to constitute an aberrant taxon in the tribe *Attini*, the evolution of which is well documented (Weber 1958). Crewe and Blum (1972) have demonstrated that the alarm pheromones utilized by genera in the mainstream of attine evolution are generally ethyl ketones, often accompanied by their corresponding carbinols. Thus, the synthesis of *o*-aminoacetophenone by workers of *Mycocepurus goeldii* provides strong biochemical evidence for the suggestion that this genus has disgressed considerably from the main attine genera which are not known to produce aromatic compounds in their mandibular glands.

The Ponerinae may constitute an excellent source of novel natural products serving as alarm pheromones. Only a few species in this primitive subfamily have been investigated, but it is already evident that the ponerines exhibit extraordinary biosynthetic capabilities. Dimethyldisulfide and dimethyltrisulfide are known as animal natural products only because of their occurrence in *Paltothyreus tarsatus* (Fa.) (Casnati et al. 1967) and the same can be said for the pyrazines generated by *Odontomachus* species (Wheeler and Blum unpublished). Whereas workers of *O. hastatus* (Fab.) produce only 2,5-dimethyl-3-isopentylpyrazine in their mandibular glands, those of *O. haematodus* L. convey alarm with a mixture of 2,6-dimethyl-3-alkylpyrazines in which the alkyl group is represented by *n*-pentyl, *n*-butyl, *n*-propyl, and ethyl chains. Suffice it to say, the alarm pheromones of the Ponerinae would appear to constitute an exciting formicid *terra incognita*.

12.3.3. The multiple roles of alarm pheromones

In contrast to the other classes of pheromones, the alarm releasers are generally produced in relatively large quantities. This fact reflects the particular ability of exocrine glands to biosynthesize these compounds while at the same time storing them in rather capacious reservoirs. It would seem, a priori, that these abundant pheromones must play an especially critical social role in order to justify the metabolic stress which is placed on the organism by their biogenesis. As certain social insects are particularly sensitive to these compounds (Moser et al. 1968; Regnier and Wilson 1968), there are no grounds for concluding that high concentrations of these pheromones are required to stimulate their olfactory chemoreceptors. Indeed, although this class of pheromones is not characterized by great structural specificity, it is nevertheless true that the discriminatory properties of the antennal receptors are eminently capable of differentiating a natural alarm pheromone from many closely related compounds (Blum et al. 1971). Furthermore, there are additional grounds for concluding that the chemoreceptors accommodating alarm pheromones are capable of discriminating between nearly identical compounds.

Riley, Silverstein and Moser (personal communication) determined that the alarm pheromone produced by workers of *Atta texana* and *A. cephalotes*, 4-methyl-3-heptanone, was present only as the (+)-isomer. Thus, this ketone, which contains an asymmetric carbon atom adjacent to the carbonyl group, is biosynthesized with such exactitude that only one of the two possible optical isomers is produced. In addition to this enzymatic specificity, it has been demonstrated that workers of *A. texana* display a remarkable ability to distinguish the natural (+)-isomer from the (–)-isomer. It will be interesting to determine if both enzymatic specificity and olfactory acuity demonstrated by *Atta* workers is also present in any other formicids which synthesize alarm pheromones containing asymmetric carbon atoms. Such alarm pheromones as 4-methyl-3-hexanone, 4-methyl-2-hexanone, and 6-methyl-3-octanone represent ideal candidates for similar investigations.

It has now been established that among the workers of social insects, the alarm pheromones constitute the most versatile class of releasers available in the social milieu. These pheromones possess several functions clearly separate from that of merely causing alarm in workers, and it is probable that others will eventually be illuminated.

Defensive secretions: Alarm pheromones in large amounts would seem to constitute ideal defensive compounds, and indeed they do. The main alarm pheromone of *Crematogaster* (*Atopogyne*) spp., 2-hexenal (Bevan et al. 1961; Blum et al. 1969), is employed as a defensive product by many non-social insects and there is no reason why these formicids cannot utilize this compound in a similar manner. The same hydrocarbons that dominate the defensive exudates of hemipterans function as alarm releasers for certain formicine species, and these compounds should also serve admirably as defensive substances when the ants spray them on predators. Formic acid is both major defensive product and alarm pheromone for *Formica* spp. (Maschwitz 1964), an adaptation which emphasizes the selective value of utilizing an exocrine product for both alarm and defense. Indeed, since so many of the alarm pheromones of social insects are identical to the defensive compounds of non-social arthropods, it seems certain that the hymenopterans have adapted defensive compounds to subserve secondarily the function of chemical releasers of alarm.

Recruitment stimuli: Wilson (1958) noted that high concentrations of the alarm pheromone of *Pogonomyrmex badius* released strong alarm behavior, whereas low concentrations acted as excellent attractants. Ayre (1968) demonstrated that alarm pheromones are employed by workers of three species of ants to attract workers to prey encountered in their foraging fields. Recently, Hölldobler (1971b) demonstrated that workers of the formicine *Camponotus socius* Roger fortify their recruitment trails with an alarm pheromone, formic acid, and these trails are highly effective in attracting excited recruits. Because of their capacity to function as low level attractants, alarm pheromones have probably been frequently utilized to increase the stimulatory efficiency of a recruitment signal.

Recognition markers: Bergström and Löfqvist (1971) have emphasized that the complex mixtures produced in the Dufour's glands of formicine ants may serve as a specific marker when sprayed on other ants. The blends of alarm pheromones synthesized in the Dufour's glands of formicines appear to be highly species specific (Bergström and Löfqvist 1968, 1970, 1971) and are made up both of relatively volatile and of persistent compounds. These secretions may be employed to mark intruders, which, after the low boiling compounds volatilize, will be 'tagged' with the higher boiling compounds plus their own characteristic volatiles. This combination may enable a social insect to facilely recognize a marked intruder and this recognition–alarm–defense device (Bergström and Löfqvist 1971) may constitute a key survival mechanism evolved by social insect species.

Chemical disarming stimuli: Species of both bees and ants raid other colonies of social insects in order to obtain either food or immature workers that can be utilized as slaves. It has now been established that one of the key developments which made this raiding *modus vivendi* possible was the employment of alarm pheromones to destroy the colonial cohesiveness of the host species.

Blum et al. (1970) demonstrated that citral, the alarm pheromone of the meliponine bee *Lestrimelitta limao* (F. Smith) (Blum 1969b), acted as an elegant disarming agent for raid-susceptible species of stingless bees. When citral is introduced into colonies of *Trigona* or *Melipona* species which are normally raided by *Lestrimelitta limao*, the behavior of the host workers becomes so disrupted that any possible resistance to intruding raiders becomes impossible. *L. limao* has converted an alarm pheromone into a diabolical instrument of temporary subjugation for raid-susceptible workers and in so doing, has developed a means of achieving non-pyrrhic victories. Similarly, Regnier and Wilson (1971) reported that slave-raiding species of *Formica* subdue their hosts by disarming them with the stimulatory alarm pheromones ejected from their Dufour's glands. These pheromones, which are alkyl acetates, are produced in inordinately large amounts, thus providing a powerful disarming tool for the slave-raiding species.

12.4. Territorial pheromones

Males of many species of social insects form assemblages and this aggregative propensity may represent an important device for promoting reproduction. Bees in the genus *Trigona* form large clusters on the outside of the nest and it has been recently reported that wasp males in the genus *Polistes* form large aggregations which are believed to increase mating efficiency (Lin 1972). While it has not been demonstrated that these aggregations are pheromonally-induced, it would appear that such chemical releasers would be ideally suited for this purpose. The territorial sites frequented by male *Bombus* species are marked with mandibular gland secretions and these exocrine products function to attract individuals of both sexes thereby increasing the probability that mating will occur.

Calam (1969) and Kullenberg et al. (1970) have analyzed the mandibular gland products of a large humber of *Bombus* spp. and demonstrated that these secretions are very species-specific and can thus serve as excellent isolating agents for sympatric species of bumblebees. Kullenberg et al. (1970) reported that among the mandibular gland exudates of 13 species of *Bombus* and six species of *Psithyrus* there are certain compounds that are common, but significantly, no two species produce the same qualitative blend of pheromones. These bees produce a rich variety of terpenes as well as aliphatic acetates, alcohols, and ethyl esters, but the mixture possessed by any one species is sufficiently distinctive to be regarded as a highly specific sex attractant. The ability of hymenopterous males to produce species-specific pheromonal blends may represent one aspect of a common reproductive device for insulating a communicative channel from decoding by foreign species.

12.5. Aggregation pheromones

Workers of many social insects form compact clusters within the nest which may persist for sustained periods. These colonial aggregations are induced by pheromones in at least one case, and it is probable that chemical releasers are responsible for most of these assemblages. Ayre and Blum (1971) observed that workers of *Camponotus pennsylvanicus* generate an unoriented alarm signal with formic acid, while the addition of a product from the Dufour's gland, *n*-undecane, results in an oriented reaction by the workers. This synergism between formic acid and *n*-undecane may be representative of the widespread use of the products of two exocrine glands to modulate a signal. In the case of *C. pennsylvanicus*, the alkane alone does not act as an alarm stimulus but may function to produce worker aggregations that persist for up to 12 hours. Thus, the aggregative behavior of this species is governed by an exocrine product that also functions as a key orienting agent when alarm behavior is released. It is attractive to speculate that the colonial aggregations formed by many other hymenopterans are similary induced by comparable pheromones.

12.6. Flight initiation pheromones

The behavioral peculiarities of eusocial hymenopterans may result in the expression of some novel manifestations of chemical sociality. This is certainly the case for the sexual forms of many species in the large formicine genus *Camponotus*. Hölldobler and Maschwitz (1965) observed that the pre-flight activity of females of this genus is initiated by the mandibular gland secretions of the males. Just prior to becoming airborne, the males label the area around the nest with these glandular products which entice the females from the nest and prime them for flight activity. The utilization of male pheromones to incite the females to flight constitutes an apparently unique function for releaser pheromones that has not been detected in any other genera of social insects.

Brand et al. (1973) analyzed the flight initiation pheromones of five species of *Camponotus* and identified several new animal natural products. Species in the subgenus *Myrmentoma* produce methyl anthranilate, the novel acid, 2,4-dimethyl-

2-hexenoic acid, and in one case, methyl 6-methylsalicylate. On the other hand, males of species in the subgenus *Camponotus* synthesize large quantities of methyl 6-methylsalicylate but do not produce detectable quantities of the acid.

Recently, Brand, Fales, Sokoloski, MacConnel, Blum and Duffield (unpublished) examined the chemistry of the mandibular gland secretions of *C. herculeanus* (L.) and *C. ligniperda* (Latreille), the two species studied by Hölldobler and Maschwitz (1965). These species, which are both members of the subgenus *Camponotus*, synthesize large quantities of methyl 6-methylsalicylate, but in addition, they produce a novel lactone, 3,4-dihydro-8-hydroxy-2-methylisocoumarin (mellein), in their hypertrophied mandibular glands. This lactone, which is known as a fungal metabolite, is a major component along with the salicylate ester, and is also present in the glandular exudates of males of several North American species of *Camponotus* (*Camponotus*). The identification of these caste-specific compounds should make it possible to study the initiation of flight behavior in female alates of *Camponotus* in terms of defined chemical releasers.

12.7. *The increasing scope of chemical sociality*

The means by which pheromones regulate the behavioral interactions of hymenopterans are remarkably diverse, and our functional classification of these compounds is being frequently enlarged as new types of releasers and primers are demonstrated. Recently, Ishay (1972) demonstrated that adult wasps in three genera respond to pupal pheromones by a series of abdominal pumping movements which result in warming the developing wasp. These thermoregulatory pheromones represent an elegant device for insuring that pupal development will proceed at an optimal temperature. The existence of such elaborate control mechanisms, which are governed by pheromonal stimuli, is undoubtedly widespread in the Hymenoptera.

Pheromonal stimuli are known to regulate behavioral interactions such as food exchange, caste development, and oral grooming, to name a few, but we shall undoubtedly expose many more subtle behavioral phenomena that have pheromonal bases. It may also be anticipated that the pheromones utilized by hymenopterous queens to regulate colony homeostasis will initiate a diversity of subtle behavioral responses that are, at this juncture, only anecdotally appreciated. The ability of δ-*n*-hexadecanolactone, a pheromone produced by queens of *Vespa orientalis* Fab. (Ikan et al. 1969), to stimulate queen cell construction, demonstrates how important social responses can be demonstrated to be governed by chemical messengers. Normally, this response only occurs in the presence of the queen. Indeed, the queen substance of *V. orientalis* emphasizes the need to examine the many facets of chemical sociality as a function of caste-specific pheromones which may affect the social responses of only selected members of the colony.

Aside from the pheromones utilized by female reproductives in the milieu of the colony, caste-specific exocrine compounds have an unpredictable occurrence in hymenopterous species. The flight initiation pheromones of *Camponotus* males (Brand et al, 1973) are indeed sex limited, as are the mandibular gland products of certain species of *Lasius* males (Law et al. 1965). Although the function of the compounds produced by the latter species is unknown, it is nevertheless attractive to suggest that the presence of caste-specific compounds reflects their use in a reproductive context. Thus, males as well as alate females and queens produce alarm pheromones in ant species in the genera *Atta* (Moser et al. 1968) and *Crematogaster* (Crewe et al. 1970), and, in at least one species of colletid bee, both sexes produce the same compounds in their mandibular glands (Blum and Bohart 1972). Alarm pheromones have no known function in promoting sexual responses and the presence of these compounds in both males and females is not necessarily surprising. When caste-specific compounds are determined to be present in a species, their role in mediating the specific concourse of behavioral reactions exhibited by individuals of the species should be critically examined. Only in this way will the many facets of both the viability and intricacy of insect societies be comprehended as an integrated whole.

References

Akre, R. D. and C. W. Rettenmeyer (1968) Trail-following by guests of army ants (Hymenoptera: Formicidae: Ecitonini). J. Kansas Entomol. Soc. 41, 165–174.

Ayre, G. L. (1968) Comparative studies on the behaviour of three species of ants. I. Prey finding, capture and transport. Can. Entomol. 100, 165–172.

Ayre, G. L. and M. S. Blum (1971) Attraction and alarm of ants (*Camponotus* spp. Hymenoptera: Formicidae) by pheromones. Physiol. Zool. 44, 77–83.

Bergström, G. and J. Löfqvist (1968) Odour similarities between the slave-keeping ants *Formica sanguinea* and *Polyergus rufescens* and their slaves *Formica fusca* and *Formica rufibarbis*. J. Insect Physiol. 14, 995–1011.

Bergström, G and J. Löfqvist (1970) Chemical basis for odour communication in four species of *Lasius* ants. J. Insect Physiol. 16, 2353–2375.

Bergström, G. and J. Löfqvist (1971) *Camponotus ligniperda* Latr. – A model for the composite volatile secretions of Dufour's gland in formicine ants. *In*: Chemical Releasers in Insects, Proc. 2nd Int. *IUPAC* Congr., Tel Aviv, Israel, 1971, vol. 3; ed. A. S. Tahori (Gordon and Breach, N. Y.), pp. 195–223.

Bergström, G. and J. Löfqvist (1972) Similarities between the Dufour's gland secretions of the ants *Camponotus ligniperda* (Latr.) and *Camponotus herculeanus* (L.) (Hym.). Ent. Scand. 3, 225–238.

Bevan, C. W. L., A. J. Birch and H. Caswell (1961) An insect repellent from black cocktail ants. J. Chem. Soc. p. 488.

Blum, M. S. (1966a) The source and specificity of trail pheromones in *Termitopone, Monomorium*, and *Huberia*, and their relation to those of some other ants. Proc. Roy. Entomol. Soc. London Ser. A 41, 155–160.

Blum, M. S. (1966b) Chemical releasers of social behavior. VIII. Citral in the mandibular gland secretion of *Lestrimelitta limao*. Ann. Entomol. Soc. Am. 59, 962–964.

Blum, M. S. (1969) Alarm pheromones. Ann. Rev. Entomol. 14, 57–80.

Blum, M. S. and G. E. Bohart (1972) Neral and geranial: Identification in a colletid bee. Ann. Entomol. Soc. Am. 65, 274–275.

Blum, M. S. and C. A. Portocarrero (1964) Chemical releasers of social behavior – IV. The hindgut as the source of the odor trail pheromone in the Neotropical army ant genus *Eciton*. Ann. Entomol. Soc. Am. 57, 793–794.

Blum, M. S. and C. A. Portocarrero (1966) Chemical releasers of social behavior. X. An attine trail substance in the venom of a non-trail laying myrmicine, *Daceton armigerum* (Latreille). Psyche 73, 150–155.

Blum, M. S. and G. N. Ross (1965) Chemical releasers of social behaviour. V. Source, specificity and properties of the odour trail pheromone of *Tetramorium guineense* (F.) (Formicidae: Myrmicinae). J. Insect Physiol. 11, 857–868.

Blum, M. S. and E. O. Wilson (1964) The anatomical source of trail substances in formicine ants. Psyche 71, 28–31.

Blum, M. S., R. E. Doolittle and M. Beroza (1971) Alarm pheromones: Utilization in evaluation of olfactory theories. J. Insect Physiol. 17, 2351–2361.

Blum, M. S., J. C. Moser and A. D. Cordero (1964) Chemical releasers of social behavior. II. Source and specificity of the odor trail substances in four attine genera. (Hymenoptera: Formicidae). Psyche 71, 1–7.

Blum, M. S., F. Padovani and E. Amante (1968) Alkanones and terpenes in the mandibular glands of *Atta* species. Comp. Biochem. Physiol. 26, 291–299.

Blum, M. S., R. M. Crewe, J. H. Sudd and A. W. Garrison (1969) 2–Hexenal: isolation and function in *Crematogaster* (*Atopogyne*) sp. J. Ga. Entomol. Soc. 4, 145–148.

Blum, M. S., S. L. Warter, R. S. Monroe and J. C. Chidester (1963) Chemical releasers of social behavior. I. Methyl-*n*-amyl ketone in *Iridomyrmex pruinosus* (Roger). J. Insect Physiol. 9, 881–885.

Blum, M. S., R. M. Crewe, W. E. Kerr, L. H. Keith, A. W. Garrison and M. M. Walker (1970) Citral in stingless bees: isolation and functions in trail-laying and robbing. J. Insect Physiol. 16, 1637–1648.

Brand, J. M., R. M. Duffield, J. G. MacConnell, M. S. Blum and H. M. Fales (1973) Caste-specific compounds in male carpenter ants. Science 179, 388–389.

Brown, W. L. , Jr. (1954) Remarks on the internal phylogeny and subfamily classification of the family Formicidae. Insectes Soc. 1, 21–31.

Butenandt, A., B. Linzen and M. Lindauer (1959) Über einen Duftstoff aus der Mandibeldrüse der Blattschneiderameise *Atta sexdens rubropilosa* Forel. Arch. Anat. Microsc. Morphol. Exp. 48, 13–19.

Butler, C. G., D. J. C. Fletcher and D. Watler (1969) Nest-entrance marking with pheromones by the honeybee, *Apis mellifera* L., and by a wasp, *Vespula vulgaris* L. Anim. Behav. 17, 142–147.

Calam, D. H. (1969) Species and sex-specific compounds from the heads of male bumblebees (*Bombus* spp.). Nature (London) 221, 856–857.

Casnati, G., A. Ricca and M. Pavan (1967) Sulla secrezione difensiva delle glandole mandibolari di *Paltothyreus tarsatus* (Fabr.). Chim. Ind. (Milan) 49, 57–61.

Cavill, G. W. K. and H. Hinterberger (1962) Dolichoderine ant extractives. Proc. Int. Congr. Entomol., 11th (1960) 3, 53–59.

Chadha, M. S., T. Eisner, A. Monro and J. Meinwald (1962) Defense mechanisms of arthropods. VII. Citronellal and citral in the mandibular gland secretions of the ant *Acanthomyops claviger* (Roger). J. Insect Physiol. 8, 175–179.

Crewe, R. M. and M. S. Blum (1970a) Identification of the alarm pheromones of the ant *Myrmica brevinodis*. J. Insect Physiol. 16, 141–146.

Crewe, R. M. and M. S. Blum (1970b) Alarm pheromones in the genus *Myrmica* (Hymenoptera: Formicidae). Z. Vergl. Physiol. 70, 363–373.

Crewe, R. M. and M. S. Blum (1972) Alarm pheromones of the *Attini*: their phylogenetic significance. J. Insect Physiol. 18, 31–42.

Crewe, R. M., M. S. Blum and C. A. Collingwood (1972) Comparative analysis of alarm pheromones in the genus *Crematogaster*. Comp. Biochem. Physiol. 43B, 703–716.

Crewe, R. M., J. M. Brand, D. J. C. Fletcher and S. H. Eggers (1970) The mandibular gland chemistry of some South African species of *Crematogaster*. J. Ga. Entomol. Soc. 5, 42–47.

Cruz, C. Da Costa (1960) Contribuição ao estudo da evolução das abelhas. Author's edition. 75 pp. Rio Claro, Brazil.

Fales, H. M., M. S. Blum, R. M. Crewe and J. M. Brand (1972) Alarm pheromones in the mandibular glands of *Manica*. J. Insect Physiol. 18, 1077–1088.

Fletcher, D. J. C. (1971) The glandular source and social functions of trail pheromones in two species of ants (*Leptogenys*). J. Entomol. (A) 46, 27–37.

Fletcher, D. J. C. and J. M. Brand (1968) Source of the trail pheromone and method of trail laying in the ant *Crematogaster peringueyi*. J. Insect Physiol. 14, 783–788.

Gehlbach, F. R., J. F. Watkins and J. C. Kroll (1971) Pheromone trail-following studies of typhlopid, leptotyphlopid, and colubrid snakes. Behavior 40, 282–294.

Ghent, R. L. (1961) Adaptive refinements in the chemical defensive mechanisms of certain Formicinae. Ph.D. Thesis (Cornell Univ., Ithaca, N. Y.) 88 pp.

Hangartner, W. (1969) Trail laying in the subterranean ant, *Acanthomyops interjectus*. J. Insect Physiol. 15, 1–4.

Hölldobler, B. (1971a) Homing in the harvester ant *Pogonomyrmex badius*. Science 171, 1149–1151.

Hölldobler, B. (1971b) Recruitment behavior in *Camponotus socius* (Hym. Formicidae). Z. Vergl. Physiol. 75, 123–142.

Hölldobler, B. and U. Maschwitz (1965) Der Hochzeitsschwarm der Rossameise *Camponotus herculeanus* (Hym. Formicidae). Z. Vergl. Physiol. 50, 551–568.

Hölldobler, B. and E. O. Wilson (1970) Recruitment trails in the harvester ant *Pogonomyrmex badius*. Psyche 77, 385–399.

Ikan, R., R. Gottlieb, E. D. Bergmann and J. Ishay (1969) The pheromone of the queen of the Oriental hornet, *Vespa orientalis*. J. Insect Physiol. 15, 1709–1712.

Ishay, J. (1972) Thermoregulatory pheromones in wasps. Experientia 28, 1185–1187.

Kerr, W. E., A. Ferreira and N. S. De Mattos (1963) Communication among stingless bees – Additional data (Hymenoptera: Apidae). J. N. Y. Entomol. Soc. 71, 80–90.

Kullenburg, B. (1953) Some observations on scents among bees and wasps (Hymenoptera) Entomol. Tidskr., Stockholm. 74, 1–7.

Kullenburg , B., G. Bergström and S. Stallberg-Stenhagen (1970) Volatile components of the cephalic marking secretion of male bumblebees. Acta Chem. Scand. 24, 1481–1483.

Law, J. H., E. O. Wilson and J. A. McCloskey (1965) Biochemical polymorphism in ants. Science 149, 544–545.

Leuthold, R. H. (1968) A tibial gland scent-trail and trail-laying behavior in the ant *Crematogaster ashmeadi* Mayr. Psyche 75, 233–248.

Lin, N. (1972) Territorial behavior among males of the social wasp *Polistes exclamans* Viereck. Proc. Entomol. Soc. Wash. 74, 148–155.

Lindauer, M. and W. E. Kerr (1958) Die gegenseitige Verständigung bei den stachellosen Bienen. Z. Vergl. Physiol. 41, 405–434.

McGurk, D. J., J. Frost, E. J. Eisenbraun, K. Vick, W. A. Drew and J. Young (1966) Volatile compounds in ants: identification of 4-methyl-3-heptanone from *Pogonomyrmex* ants. J. Insect Physiol. 12, 1435–1441.

Maschwitz, U. (1964) Gefahrenalarmstoffe und Gefahrenalarmierung bei sozialen Hymenoptera. Z. Vergl. Physiol. 47, 596–655.

Moser, J. C. (1964) Inquiline roach responds to trail-marking substance of leaf-cutting ants. Science 143, 1048–1049.

Moser, J. C. and M. S. Blum (1963) Trail-marking substance of the Texas leaf-cutting ant: source and potency. Science 140, 1228.

Moser, J. C. and R. M. Silverstein (1967) Volatility of trail marking substance of the town ant. Nature (London) 215, 206–207.

Moser, J. C., R. G. Brownlee and R. M. Silverstein (1968) The alarm pheromones of *Atta texana*. J. Insect Physiol. 14, 529–535.

Pasteels, J. M., R. M. Crewe and M. S. Blum (1970) Etude histologique et examen au microscope électronique à balayage de la glande sécrétant la phéromone de piste chez deux *Crematogaster* nord-americains (Formicidae, Myrmicinae). C. R. Acad. Sci. 271D, 835–838.

Pavan, M. (1955) Studi sui Formicidae. I. Contributo alla conoscenza degli organi gastrali nei Dolichoderinae. Natura (Milano) 46, 135–145.

Plsek, R. W., J. C. Kroll and J. F. Watkins II (1969) Observations of carabid beetles, *Helluomorphoides texanus*, in columns of army ants and laboratory experiments on their behavior. J. Kansas Entomol. Soc. 42, 452–456.

Regnier, F. E. and E. O. Wilson (1968) The alarm-defense system of the ant *Acanthomyops claviger*. J. Insect Physiol. 14, 955–970.

Regnier, F. E. and E. O. Wilson (1971) Chemical communication and 'propaganda' in slavemaker ants. Science 172, 267–269.

Rettenmeyer, C. W. (1961) Arthopods associated with Neotropical army ants with a review of the behavior of these ants (Arthropoda: Formicidae: Dorylinae). Ph.D. Thesis (Univ. Kansas, Lawrence) 605 pp.

Rettenmeyer, C. W. (1962) The behavior of millipeds found with Neotropical army ants. J. Kansas Entomol. Soc. 35, 377–384.

Sonnet, P., E. and J. C. Moser (1972) Synthetic analogs of the trail pheromone of the leaf-cutting ant, *Atta texana* (Buckley). Agr. Food Chem. 20, 1191–1194.

Torgerson, R. L. and R. D. Akre (1970) The persistence of army ant chemical trails and their significance in the Ecitonine-Ecitophile association (Formicidae: Ecitonini). Melanderia 5, 1–28.

Trave, R. and M. Pavan (1956) Veleni degli insetti. Principi estratti dalla formica *Tapinoma nigerrimum* Nyl. Chim. Ind., Milan 38, 1015–1019.

Tumlinson, J. H., J. C. Moser, R. M. Silverstein, R. G. Brownlee and J. M. Ruth (1972) A volatile trail pheromone of the leaf-cutting ant, *Atta texana*. J. Insect Physiol. 18, 809–814.

Tumlinson, J. H., R. M. Silverstein, J. C. Moser, R. G. Brownlee and J. M. Ruth (1971) Identification of the trail pheromone of a leaf-cutting ant, *Atta texana*. Nature (London) 234, 348–349.

Watkins, J. F. (1964) Laboratory experiments on the trail-following of army ants of the genus *Neivamyrmex* (Formicidae: Dorylinae). J. Kansas Entomol. Soc. 37, 22–28.

Watkins, J. F., T. W. Cole and R. S. Baldridge (1967) Laboratory studies on interspecies trail following and trail preference of army ants (Dorylinae). J. Kansas Entomol. Soc. 40, 146–151.

Weber, N. A. (1958) Evolution in fungus-growing ants. Proc. Int. Congr. Entomol. 10th (1956) 2, 459–473.

Wilson, E. O. (1958) A chemical releaser of alarm and digging behavior in the ant *Pogonomyrmex badius*. Psyche 65, 41–51.

Wilson, E. O. (1962) Chemical communication among workers of the fire ant *Solenopsis saevissima* (Fr. Smith). I. The organization of mass foraging. Anim. Behav. 10, 134–147.

Wilson, E. O. (1963) The social biology of ants. Ann. Rev. Entomol. 8, 345–368.

Wilson, E. O. and W. H. Bossert (1963) Chemical communication among animals. Recent Prog. Horm. Res. 19, 673–716.

Wilson, E. O. and M. Pavan (1959) Source and specificity of chemical releasers of social behavior in the dolichoderine ants. Psyche 66, 70–76.

CHAPTER 13

Pheromones in the termite societies

B. P. MOORE

13.1. Introduction

All known termites (Isoptera) live in colonies that exhibit a well marked division of labor associated with the presence of several distinctive castes. They therefore form a unique group of insects although in terms of morphology they rank amongst the more primitive orders, with an incomplete metamorphosis. Their nearest relatives are certainly the cockroaches (Blattodea) and comparative morphological, physiological and ethological studies of examples from each order leave us in little doubt that termites represent a specialized social offshoot of an early blattoid stock. Pheromones have evidently played a crucial role in their evolution and the resulting behavioral convergence between termites and social Hymenoptera is so striking that it perhaps tends to de-emphasize the fundamental differences separating these two very distinct groups of insects.

Termite societies are always bisexual, although one sex may be dominant (or even exclusive) in a few of the sterile castes (sect. 13.2.2). Moreover, in lower termites at least, stationary immature forms (pseudergates) habitually play an active and important role in the running of the colony. This is in marked contrast with the adult-female dominated hierarchies of the Hymenoptera. Such added complications in the termite societies have certainly hindered progress in the elucidation of the complex and varied modes of caste differentiation and control that are known to exist there and our knowledge of the chemical agents likely to be involved can only be described as rudimentary. No primer pheromone has yet been fully characterized from any termite species, although the existence of a substantial number may be inferred from the results of rearing and behavioral studies with manipulated laboratory colonies.

Releaser pheromones in termites are somewhat better known, but even here the picture is still very incomplete. Therefore, what follows in the present chapter will, of necessity, be largely conjectural or speculative in nature, but it is to be hoped that it will at least provide an outline of the probable role of pheromones in termite biology and at the same time indicate some of the more important and promising lines for future research.

13.2. *Caste differentiation and control*

13.2.1. *Patterns of caste development*

The mode of differentiation and the ultimate caste distribution pattern vary rather widely in termites but two basic systems may be described. In the first, which is characteristic of the lower termites (families Mastotermitidae (Watson 1971), Kalotermitidae, Rhinotermitidae and Hodotermitidae (Miller 1969)), no truly terminal worker caste exists, but its functions are performed by a group of stationary juveniles termed pseudergates (= false workers). In balanced colonies, such pseudergates are very numerous and continue to molt at intervals and grow, but without any significant change of form. Nevertheless, they retain a competence to metamorphose (via one or more further molts) into alates (future reproductives), replacement (secondary) reproductives or soldiers in response to any caste imbalance that may occur in the colony. This competence is apparently limited to a certain critical period within each molting cycle. In this critical period the pseudergate is primed, as it were, to react to any change in extrinsic factors within the colony (such as nutritional level, numerical depletion, etc.) and its further development will then be

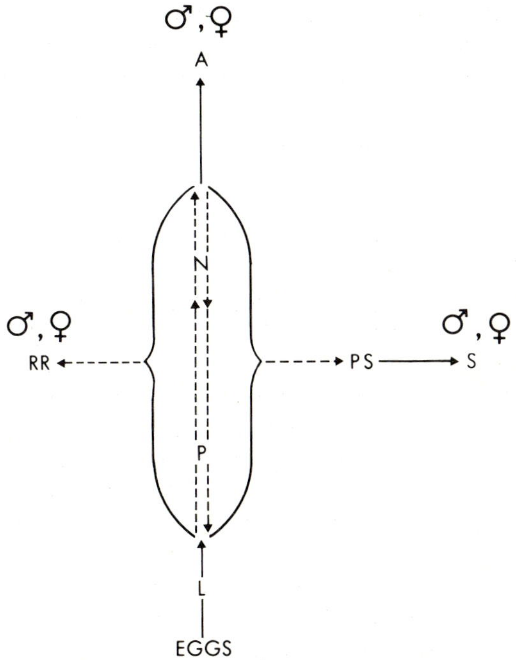

Fig. 13.1. Generalized scheme for caste development in lower termites. Full arrows indicate obligatory paths; broken arrows signify alternatives. A, alates; L, larval stadia; N, nymphal stadia; P, pseudergates; RR, replacement reproductives; PS, presoldiers; S, soldiers.

determined to meet the particular need. A generalized scheme for the lower termites is given in fig. 13.1.

The caste system is less plastic in higher termites of the large family Termitidae and a truly terminal worker form invariably occurs (Noirot 1969). Such workers apparently cease to molt when fully mature. Soldiers are produced from larvae or early-stage workers (often from only one sex) and the nymph-alate line is already differentiated at the very early second stadium. Replacement reproductives are usually derived from nymphs, or sometimes unflown alates, within the nest but in certain rare cases, workers in the early stages can give rise to morphologically distinct 'ergatoid' reproductives. However, some termitids (e.g., *Cubitermes fungifaber* (Sjöstedt) (Noirot 1969)) appear to have lost all ability to produce secondary reproductives and the life-span of the colony is then essentially that of the royal pair. A generalized scheme for higher termites is given in fig. 13.2.

Many variations of these basic schemes are possible and most are observable either in natural colonies or in those cultured under conditions of artificial stress. For example, there may be wide differences in the proportions of the various castes present between species or between colonies of a given species, according to size and age structure, or within a single colony according to the season. There may be marked polymorphism within a caste, especially the soldiers, with major and minor forms occurring together in fixed or varying proportions and fulfilling different

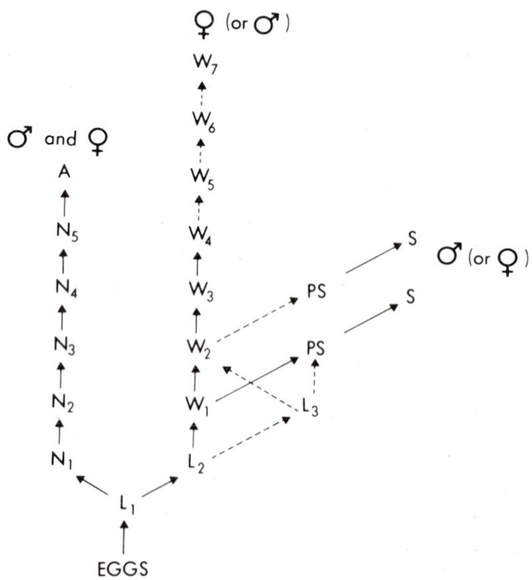

Fig. 13.2. Generalized scheme for caste development in higher termites. Full arrows indicate usual paths of development; broken arrows signify uncommon variants. A, alates; L, larval stadia; N, nymphal stadia; PS, presoldiers; S, soldiers; W, workers.

functions. The role of secondary reproductives shows remarkable shifts of emphasis, often between species of closely related groups. These secondaries may occur in large numbers and function as supplements to the primary royal pair. More often they are known only as individual replacements for lost primaries and in some species, as mentioned above, they may never be produced at all.

Although a purely genetic mechanism was at one time canvassed as the basis for caste differentiation, its inadequacies soon became apparent and by the turn of the century most workers had come to accept the alternative view that newly hatched termites were genetically equivalent, except in terms of sex, and had the potential to develop into any caste. Differentiation was ascribed to the intervention of variable extrinsic factors, such as nutrition, environmental conditions and, perhaps, influential secretions. Pickens (1932) was the first to propose an inhibition theory, in which he suggested that a functional queen might produce a substance that regulated the development of all nymphs within the colony, although he did not extend his idea to the soldier caste. Pickens' early concept of chemical mediation received considerable support from the experimental work of Castle (1934), who was able to show that isolated nymphs of *Zootermopsis angusticollis* (Hagen) gave rise to a much higher proportion of secondary reproductives than was possible on the basis of chance occurrence of genetically determined forms. Moreover, this development was delayed or inhibited by the administration of extracts of functional primaries with the food. Castle was also able to show that the presence of a soldier in incipient colonies inhibited the production of further members of its caste. Later researches by Light (1942–44) on the same species and especially by Lüscher on *Kalotermes flavicollis* (F.) (for a summary, see Lüscher 1961), established beyond reasonable doubt the validity of the inhibition theory and did much to elucidate the complex pathways of caste differentiation in lower termites.

Unfortunately, the difficulties associated with the culture of higher termites have greatly hindered progress in this group. However, in spite of the complications resulting from the existence of a true worker caste (Noirot 1969), anatomical and biological studies indicate that the basic facts of caste differentiation are analogous.

13.2.2. Pheromones as mediators in caste control

Social regulation may be seen as a balance between two independent mechanisms, namely the production and the elimination of members of a given caste. The precise outcome of this balance will be governed not only by intrinsic attributes of the species but also by extrinsic variables, such as size, age and nutritional level of the colony, together with climatic and seasonal factors. This will account for the great plasticity of termite societies in nature. Pheromones may be implicated in both of these opposing mechanisms, as is most clearly indicated by Lüscher's extended work on *K. flavicollis*.

By closely observing marked individuals, Lüscher (1952a, b) was soon able to show that pseudergates of this species are able to follow any one of several lines of further development or, in the absence of any appropriate stimulus, to undergo stationary molts for extended periods. Secondary reproductives were produced only in colonies deprived of their existing reproductives. Competence to respond to this stimulus was highest in recently molted pseudergates and it declined exponentially thereafter (Lüscher 1956a) until the onset of the succeeding molt. A primer pheromone, derived from the functional reproductives, is clearly implicated in inhibiting such development. This follows from the fact that competent colonies temporarily deprived of such reproductives for as little as 24 hours still produced their quota of replacements 6–10 days later. However, in the renewed presence of the functional reproductives, these replacements were soon recognized as being superfluous and were eaten by the pseudergates. The two mechanisms were neatly separated (Lüscher, 1952a) by dividing termite colonies with wire screens. A group isolated from reproductives in this way duly produced replacements, but these were soon eliminated if established reproductives could be detected through the screen by antennal contact. In the presence of a wider screen, which still permitted the passage of odors but prevented antennal contact, the new reproductives survived as they would in an isolated colony. Apparently antennal contact is necessary for recognition of the royal pair but whether the mechanism is purely tactile or involves non-volatile 'surface pheromones' is still unclear. However, after studying closely the elimination of reproductives in experimental colonies, Ruppli (1969) was led to favor the latter explanation.

Further insight into the source and nature of the inhibitory primer pheromone came from experiments (Lüscher 1955) in which a queen was fixed in a solid screen between two colonies so that the head was in contact with one and the abdomen with the other. Provided a male was present, development of secondaries was inhibited only in the compartment containing the abdomen. Systematic examination of the effects of varnishing various parts of the queen's abdomen disclosed the anus as the source of the inhibitory pheromone.

According to Lüscher (1964), a single queen, without her partner, will inhibit the production of female replacements to some extent, but a single king shows no corresponding effect. Two functional males significantly inhibit the production of male replacements, but complete inhibition of all sexual development requires the presence together of both king and queen. Isolated kings, in orphaned colonies, appear to evolve a factor that stimulates the production of female replacements but no corresponding activity could be demonstrated in isolated queens.

The activity of the inhibitory pheromones is evidently of very short duration, since it decays to below the threshold in colonies orphaned for 24 hours or more. In balanced colonies, there must exist a continuous metabolic turnover of these pheromones and their dissemination from the royal chamber must be extremely efficient. In large colonies at least, the time scale involved would not permit all members to have access to the primary pair and it follows that the royal attendants must be responsible for distribution of pheromones received there. In order to test this probability, Lüscher (1956b) fixed pseudergates in screens between two colonies, in such a way that the heads were in contact with the colony possessing a royal pair and the abdomens reached an orphaned group. Inhibition was quite significant in the latter group but male pseudergates seemed to pass on only the female primer pheromone and vice versa. These pseudergates evidently absorbed the pheromone appropriate to their own sex during the course of their metabolism, which was thereby regulated accordingly.

These complex interactions between the sexes provide termites with an extremely flexible means of reproductive control, but their full elucidation, and particularly the isolation of the pheromones involved, are matters of great difficulty. Lüscher's scheme for *Kalotermes*, which is incorporated in fig. 13.3, has not yet received support from isolation studies but in earlier work with *Zootermopsis angusticollis*, Light (1944) had more success in directly demonstrating the existence of an inhibitory pheromone in functional reproductives. Standard groups of larvae were reared on filter-paper impregnated with water or methanol extracts of parts of female secondary reproductives, which are more readily available in this species. The development of further secondaries was noted after three weeks. Almost complete inhibition was observed with extracts of head plus thorax but not with other parts. More recently, Lebrun (1972) has succeeded in blocking metamorphosis in nymphs of *Kalotermes flavicollis* by implantation of mandibular glands from functional reproductives of the species. The combined researches of these authors tend to confirm that reproductives of these lower termites produce inhibitory pheromones (probably in the mandibular glands) that, when passed through the anus, serve to regulate the production of others of their kind. Such a regulation is most likely achieved by interference with the recipients' endocrine systems, thereby blocking what would otherwise be an automatic avenue of development. The recent detection of 9-oxodec-*trans*-2-enoic acid in the heads of queen *Odontotermes assmuthi* Holmgren (Sannasi and George 1972) strongly suggests that the termite queen substance may be identical with that of the honey bee, but the nature of the termite king substance is entirely unknown.

Regulation of soldier production is also likely to be mediated by pheromones but the evidence for the existence of an inhibitory pheromone in this caste is far from adequate. Castle (1934) first observed that incipient colonies of *Zootermopsis augusticollis* produce one soldier from the earliest brood, but no further members of this caste during the first year. However, if the first soldier is removed, another is often quickly reared and the process may be repeated several times. On the other hand, artificial implantation of a soldier effectively inhibited the process. Similar results were obtained by Light and Weesner (1955) with *Reticulitermes hesperus* Banks, although their findings were less clear-cut. *Mastotermes darwiniensis* (Froggatt) (Watson, J. A. L., unpublished), *Hodotermes mossambicus* (Hagen) (Hewitt et al 1969) and other lower termites appear to follow the same

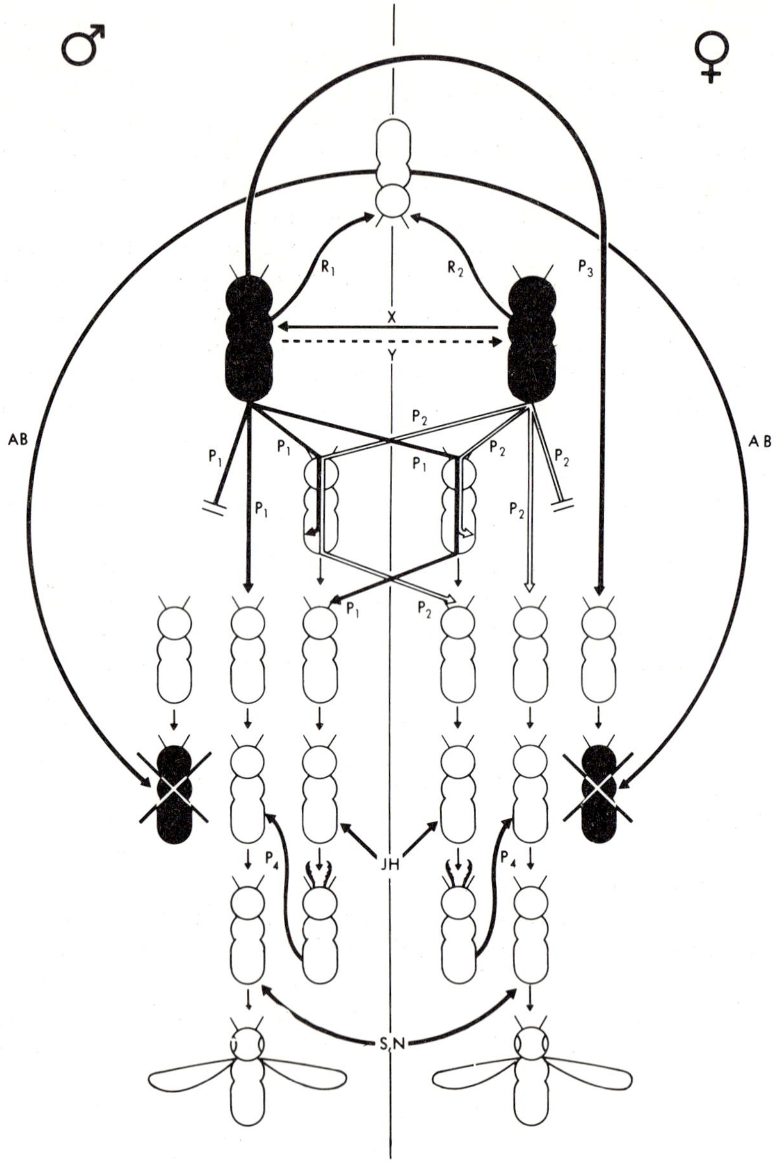

Fig. 13.3. Tentative representation of the major control mechanisms of caste differentiation in lower termites. Reproductives are shown in black, sterile castes and alates in white. The short, thin arrows represent single or multiple molts. Males are on the left of the diagram, females on the right. P_{1-4} primer pheromones; R_{1-2} releaser pheromones; AB, aggressive behavior; X, Y, stimuli of unknown nature; JH, high juvenile hormone titre; S, N, seasonal and nutritional factors. (Adapted from Lüscher, 1961).

pattern. Supplementary pre-soldiers may occasionally appear, but they are never allowed to develop further. The situation in higher termites has been examined by Gay and Moore (in: Moore 1969) working with *Nasutitermes exitiosus* (Hill), where the natural proportion of soldiers in mature mounds is about 15%. Artificial colonies that had been deprived of all soldiers reared significant numbers of this caste in a space of eight weeks, but attempts to inhibit such activity by administration of soldier extracts with the food gave rather variable results.

The production of soldiers is evidently associated with high titres of juvenile hormone (JH) in the colony, since such development may readily be induced in competent pseudergates of *Kalotermes* by implantation of corpora allata from functional reproductives in which these glands are large and active (Lüscher and Springhetti 1960). Similar treatment of nymphs, with corpora allata derived from cockroaches, gives rise to fertile intercastes (Lebrun 1970). JH activity has been shown to be widespread in various higher termites and their fungus gardens (Sannasi et al. 1972) and feeding experiments with JH analogues has led to development of very large numbers of superfluous soldiers in *Reticulitermes lucifugus* (Rossi) (Hrdý and Křeček 1972).

The balance in soldier numbers struck in nature shows great interspecific variation but is relatively constant within a species and in colonies of comparable size and age. Such balances may be envisaged as the outcome of a specifically varying (and perhaps intermittent) JH-impelled drive towards soldier production, opposed by a density-dependent titre of soldier-inhibitory pheromone and modulated by some soldier-recognition factor that promotes elimination by workers or pseudergates of superfluous members of the caste. Cases where soldiers are limited to one sex, which are rather common in higher termites (Noirot 1969), may be explained in terms of sexual differences in threshold response to JH titre. In many such cases, soldiers of the opposite sex may occasionally be produced under conditions of exceptional stress.

The production of nymphs and their development into alates are not well understood, but such factors as colony size, vigor, nutritional levels and seasonal triggers are clearly involved. In lower termites there appears to be no true elimination of nymphs, but when necessary, these can undergo regressive molts leading back to the pseudergate condition – a process that could conceivably be triggered by increasing titres of a nymph-specific pheromone. Determination for the nymph-alate line of development occurs very early in higher termites, certainly not later than the first larval stage and possibly as early as oogenesis of the queen (Noirot 1969). The controlling mechanism here is not understood and it may well vary between species with differing flight patterns. Thus in some species the onset of nymph development occurs soon after loss of the current alate population by swarming, whereas in others there is a delay of several months. In *Cephalotermes rectangularis* (Sjöstedt), which frequently produces two flights of alates in one year, young nymphs may appear before the swarming of the earlier generation has occurred (Noirot, 1969).

Alate-derived pheromones need scarcely be invoked in such cases, since seasonal and environmental factors are evidently so important, but the production of alate swarms may be seen as the culmination in natural ontogenesis of the extensive metabolic reserves accruing to the efficient termite society. The fact that some metabolism has been shunted, as it were, into the complex and nicely balanced secondary circuitry of the sterile caste system is evidently more than offset by the evolutionary advantages of the social way of life.

13.3. Pheromones in colony foundation and integration

Colony foundation in termites, well reviewed by Nutting (1969), is normally the result of union between a pair of alates after the swarming flight, but alternative mechanisms are known in a few species involving fragmentation ('budding') of existing colonies followed by independent production of secondary reproductives. (Harris 1958). The latter occurs mostly in species with diffuse colonies where outlying sections may lose pheromonal contact with the main body and then behave as orphaned groups. However, a very special type of fragmentation, described as 'sociotomy' by Grassé and Noirot (1951), involves a deliberate migration by the royal pair, plus a retinue of workers and soldiers, after the manner of swarming in honey bees. Such a migration must certainly depend upon aggregation pheromones for its cohesion, but the trigger mechanism responsible for this unusual behavior is not known.

After the short swarming flight, alates descend to earth to seek their mates. Females of many species apparently emit a short-range sex attractant. They adopt a 'calling' attitude with the tip of the abdomen raised and sometimes moving from side to side. Males quarter the ground at random, but on encountering a calling female are immediately attracted to her. The pair then begin to parade in tandem, with the male so closely following the female as to appear coupled to her. Temporary loss of contact causes the male to make searching movements, whilst the female resumes the calling posture. The male is apparently not following a scent-trail, but is responding directly to a short-range, air-borne attractant. Nothing is yet known of the nature of this pheromone. Buchli (1960), who investigated closely the behavior in *Reticulitermes lucifugus*, suggested that the attractant might be produced by the female's accessory genitalic glands. Other observers have stressed the importance of visual cues in tandem formation.

Eventually, the pair enter the ground, or timber as the case may be, and construct a royal cell ('copularium') where mating first takes place. Short-range pheromones with attractant and perhaps aphrodisiacal, properties presumably play an important role in maintaining the pair-bond during this crucial phase as, indeed, throughout the life span. These cohesive factors become particularly important when, with increasing size of the colony, the queen becomes immobilized through physogastry. She is then entirely dependent upon her attractive properties for retaining the attentions of the still mobile king. These properties are particularly apparent to the observer in freshly broken nests, when the reluctance of the king to leave his helpless mate is very obvious.

In the incipient colony, the first brood is nourished exclusively by the royal pair, but workers or their equivalent soon take over all such duties and the activities of the king and queen become entirely restricted to reproduction on an increasing scale. The colony slowly grows in size and numbers until, at maturity, it is capable of producing all castes characteristic of the species – a capability it may retain for many tens of years before decline and, ultimately, death set in.

Apart from their crucial role in maintaining caste balance (which has already been discussed), pheromones are also implicated in many of the day-to-day activities of the colony. Short-range pheromones are probably important mediators in mutual recognition, grooming and especially trophallaxis, the exchange of nutrients and essential secretions that are the very fabric of social insect life. These latter are spread throughout the colony with amazing speed and efficiency, as can readily be demonstrated by the use of radioactive tracer techniques (McMahan 1969).

Selective cannibalism can be important to termites in times of nutritional hardship and it is the usual mechanism for disposal of the injured and supernumerary members of any caste. The process generally appears to commence in overintensive grooming resulting in leakage of haemolymph. A pheromone in the latter presumably then triggers the full train of events. Many termites also consume their dead but others, such as *Amitermes laurensis* Mjöberg, construct special cemeteries within their mounds. Although such necrophoric behavior has not been thoroughly investigated, pheromones resulting from the decay of fats (oleic and ricinoleic acids) may be implicated much as they are in ants (Wilson et al. 1958).

The existence of distinctive colony-odors, even within a given species, is easily demonstrated by mixing individuals from two sources, when a fight to death will normally ensue. Such odors are obviously important in the maintenance of colony cohesion, independence and in the recognition of intruders. They have not been closely investigated but are believed to be complex blends of volatile metabolites, together with food and environmental components. Although not entirely constant in composition, these odors change only slowly so that all members of a colony remain accommodated. However, when a colony is divided the odors of the two sections slowly drift apart and after a period of three months are sufficiently distinct to cause antagonism upon reunion (Stuart, 1969). Colonies may nevertheless be successfully combined if they are cooled to complete immobility beforehand (Dropkin 1946). Under these circumstances, the two odors presumably become blended before the termites can react to them.

13.4. Defense and alarm

Termites are subject to attack by a wide variety of predators ranging from other arthropods to mammals and they have evolved an intriguing repertoire of defensive tactics to counter these diverse threats. Their small size inevitably limits their effectiveness in combat with the larger predators, against which passive measures are generally adopted. The building of impervious or inaccessible galleries and the very resilience of the colony in recouping heavy numerical losses are examples. Defense against the smaller arthropods (particularly ants) is largely the function of the soldier caste, which has evolved for this specific purpose. In most termites the soldiers show exaggerated development of the mandibles and many of the larger kinds are able to incapacitate intruders by inflicting savage bites. Smaller soldiers achieve much the same result by permanent attachment via their pincer-like mandibles. In many species, a sticky secretion is also produced (from buccal or cephalic glands) and is applied to the adversary when the soldier strikes.

A chemical mode of defense is relied upon entirely in the Nasutitermitinae (family Termitidae). The mandibles in these highly specialized soldiers are atrophied and useless but the cephalic gland is enormous and occupies most of the head capsule. In combat the defensive secretion is forcibly discharged as a sticky thread, from a gun-like nozzle on the forehead. In this way intruders are soon immobilized. The chemistry of the secretion is quite complex, containing both volatile and resinous terpenes (Moore 1968).

Alarm signals form a very important and integral part of defense in social insects. They serve to alert the entire colony to the presence of danger and offer an effective and rapid means of summoning reinforcements to the site of an attack. Pheromones are often implicated in these signals and have been particularly well studied in ants (ch. 12). The active compounds involved are usually rather volatile and have high thresholds and high diffusion rates, properties ensuring the rapid transmission of signals that will soon decay in the absence of reinforcement (Bossert and Wilson 1963). This is an essential requirement if prolonged periods of tension are to be avoided. However, some alerting pheromones in primitive ants seem to function in trace amounts (Robertson 1971).

When disturbed many termites exhibit curious oscillatory movements that soon catalyze greatly increased activity throughout the colony (Howse 1965). In lower termites such movements are often associated with the laying of a scent-trail, the means of recruitment in these species (Stuart 1963). The mechanism is clearly one of alarm. In some higher termites, particularly those with active and pugnacious soldiers, the oscillatory movements are accompanied by emission of an alarm pheromone from the cephalic gland. Such a mechanism has been detected in the Australian harvester termites *Drepanotermes rubriceps* (Froggatt) and *D. perniger* (Froggatt) (Moore 1968, and unpublished) and the pheromone involved is (+)-limonene (fig. 13.4a). Artificial presentation of this substance to the soldiers triggers the onset of a short-lived snapping and biting frenzy. Similarly, the alarm pheromone of *Amitermes herbertensis* Mjöberg has been identified as terpinolene (fig. 13.4b).

Comparable alarm reaction cannot be demonstrated in species of *Nasutitermes*, since nasute soldiers are much less excitable. However, Ernst (1959) has shown that these soldiers are stimulated to fire their shots when presented with glass rods loaded with their defensive secretion. In *N. exitiosus* and other Australian species, α-pinene (fig. 13.4c) is the major volatile component of this secretion (Moore 1968) and presentation of this material causes a similar response. It is probably best regarded as an alerting pheromone.

The association of alarm or alerting activity with components of a defensive secretion seems entirely logical, since the two functions are closely connected, but the emphasis placed upon one role or the other varies widely between different species of Termitidae. Thus nasute soldiers, with their massive glands and copious secretion, are concerned primarily with defense, and alerting is a subsidiary role. Some Amitermitinae (such as *Amitermes vitiosus* Hill) also produce relatively large amounts of a sticky and highly odorous secretion (based upon terpenes) that appears to cover both functions, whereas the *Drepanotermes* species emit only comparatively small amounts of the volatile alarm pheromone. Species of several other termitid genera do not produce any such materials in detectable quantities (Moore

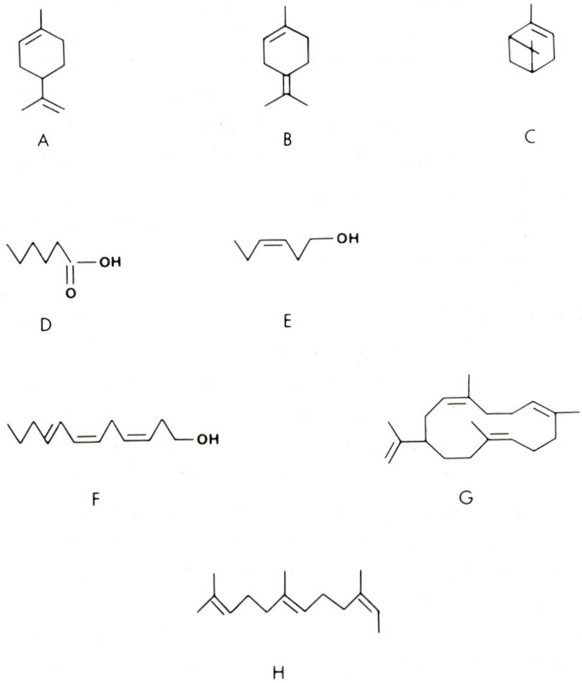

Fig. 13.4. Some identified termite pheromones and attractants. A, limonene; B, terpinolene; C, α-pinene; D, *n*-hexanoic acid; E, *n-cis*-hex-3-en-1-ol; F, *n-cis*-3, *cis*-6, *trans*-8-dodecatrien-1-ol; G, nasutene (neocembrene-A); H, 10-*cis*-2,6,10-trimethyldodeca-2,6,10-triene.

1968) and these presumably rely upon purely mechanical methods of alarm communication.

13.5. Foraging and feeding

So far as is known, all termites possess a sternal gland that is the source of a pheromone used in laying scent-trails. This gland is found at the base of the fifth abdominal sternite in most species. In some primitive termites, such as *Zootermopsis* (Hodotermitidae) which live entirely within the food-timber, trail-laying is facultative and is used solely as a means of recruitment for defense purposes (Stuart 1963). Such termites normally travel with the abdomen raised, but when alarmed they drag the area of the sternal gland across the substrate, to lay a short-lived scent-trail. Other individuals are then induced to follow the trail towards the source of disturbance. The substance largely responsible for this activity in the secretion of *Z. nevadensis* (Hagen) has been identified as *n*-hexanoic (caproic) acid (fig. 13.4d) (Hummel and Karlson 1968). Farnesol and other substances not present in the termites also show pronounced trail-laying activity towards this species.

The primitive *Mastotermes darwiniensis* and especially many of the more advanced termites seek their food at some distance from the nest. These species have adapted the trail-laying mechanism as an aid to foraging. The highly evolved Nasutitermitinae have a very diffuse sternal gland. Its secretion spreads spontaneously over the body, along with the cuticular waxes and is applied to the substrate at every contact. Thus these species appear to be obligatory trail-layers and the trail they lay is very persistent. The constant jostling of large numbers of the termites, backwards and forwards along their main foraging arteries, is quite sufficient to mark out and maintain an effective and long-lasting directional guide.

The receptors that mediate trail-following are probably located on the antennae since termites deprived of these organs do not respond to the pheromone. Close observation of termites on artificial trails shows that they do not follow its path directly but rather pursue a zigzag course crossing it repeatedly. They are evidently responding to relative changes in feedback signal as each antenna in turn sweeps across the concentration gradient. Termites with only one antenna can still follow scent-trails but their performance in perceiving sharp changes in direction is inferior. If presented with artificially overloaded trails, termites may follow an offset path where the pheromone concentration is more favorable or if saturation of their receptors occurs, they may not react at all. Thus, in testing pure substances for trail-laying activity, it is always necessary to examine a range of several ten-fold dilutions.

Termites are known to be attracted to a wide variety of food odors, particularly those associated with lignin-breakdown products and others in fungus-infected wood (Becker 1964). In many cases, extracts of such materials show pronounced activity in the trail-laying test. The leaf alcohol, *cis*-hex-3-en-l-ol (fig. 13.4e) shows such activity (Verron and Barbier 1962) and the substance has been detected in *Kalotermes flavicollis*, although it has not been positively identified as the scent-trail pheromone of the species. On the other hand, the complex, unsaturated alcohol, n-*cis*-3, *cis*-6, *trans*-8-dodecatrien-1-ol (fig. 13.4f), that occurs in large quantities in wood infected with the fungus *Lenzites trabea* Pers. (Matsumura et al. 1968, 1969) definitely appears to be the substance used for trail-laying by the several species of *Reticulitermes* that feed on this material.

The scent-trail pheromone of several Australian species of the widespread genus *Nasutitermes* was first isolated from *N. exitiosus* (Moore 1966). Later named nasutene (or more systematically, neocembrene-A), this compound had the constitution of a diterpene hydrocarbon, $C_{20}H_{32}$, but the complete determination of its structure proved a difficult chemical problem that has only recently been resolved (Birch et al. 1972). The pheromone has a curious 14-membered ring structure (fig. 13.4g) and is surprisingly stable for a compound of its class. The same substance has been detected in several other species of *Nasutitermes*, towards which it also shows trail-laying activity, and in *Coptotermes lacteus* (Froggatt), which registers no such response. Although it has not yet been positively identified as a constituent of the food-timber, extracts from the fresh termite-susceptible timber of *Eucalyptus regnans* certainly show trail-laying activity towards *Nasutitermes* species. Moreover, an apparently identical compound has been isolated in relatively large quantities from the Indian incense cedar, *Commiphora mukul* (Hooker *ex* Stocks) (family Burseraceae) by Sukh Dev and his associates (Patil et al. 1973). The latter isolate, named cembrene-A by its discoverers, is indistinguishable, physiochemically, from nasutene and it shows identical behavior in the trail-laying test. On the other hand, the attractant for *Nasutitermes exitiosus* first detected in oil from the western Australian sandalwood (*Santalum* (= Eucarya) *spicatum* R. Br.) (Moore 1966) and recently identified as a sesquiterpene hydrocarbon, $C_{15}H_{26}$ (fig. 13.4h), related to farnesene (Birch et al. 1970), has only about one-thousandth of this activity. It appears to be no more than a moderately effective molecular mimic.

Species-specificity in termite scent-trails based upon the same basic pheromone is apparently achieved through the presence of secondary components of greater volatility. Thus, in laboratory tests of interspecific activity, trails laid from extracts of one species of *Nasutitermes* were initially repellent to another, but they became increasingly more acceptable after periods of airing (Moore unpublished). By contrast, trails prepared from purified nasutene showed no such period of induction. Now that the pheromone has been identified and is readily available from the Indian plant source, it would be of interest to determine whether it forms the basis of trail-laying in any of the numerous exotic species of Nasutitermitinae. Meanwhile, it is at least clear that this substance plays a key role in the biology of both terrestrial and arboreal species, in the Australian fauna.

The present limited data do not afford a complete perspective of the evident interplay between food odors and those of special secretions in termite foraging behavior, but it would appear reasonable to assume that in at least some and perhaps many species a constituent of the favored food material has been adopted as the primary component of the scent-trail pheromone. Concentrated through the agency of the termites' special sternal gland, garnished with appropriately volatile and specific secondary components and applied continuously to the foraging trails, these salient plant constituents evidently provide an effective (and logical) extension of the short-range odor-cues through which all termites ultimately detect their food.

References

Becker, G. (1964) Termite-anlockende Wirkung einiger bei Basidomyceten-Angriff in Holz enstehender Verbindungen. Holzforsch. 18, 168–172.

Birch, A. J., K. B. Chamberlain, B. P. Moore and V. H. Powell (1970) Termite attractants in *Santalum spicatum.* Aust. J. Chem. 23, 2337–2341.

Birch, A. J., W. V. Brown, J. E. T. Corrie and B. P. Moore (1972) Neocembrene-A, a termite trail pheromone. J. Chem. Soc. Perkin Trans. I, 1972, 2653–2658.

Bossert, W. H. and E. O. Wilson (1963) The analysis of olfactory communication among animals. J. Theor. Biol. 5, 443–469.

Buchli, H. (1960) Les tropismes lors de la pariade des imagos de *Reticulitermes lucifugus* R. Vie et Milieu 11, 308–315.

Castle, G. B. (1934) An experimental examination of caste differentiation in *Zootermopsis angusticollis.* In: Termites and Termite Control, 2nd ed.: C. A. Kofoid (Univ. of California Press, Berkeley) pp. 292–310.

Dropkin, V. H. (1946) The use of mixed colonies of termites in the study of host-symbiont relations. J. Parasitol. 32, 247–251.

Ernst, E. (1959) Beobachten beim Spritzakt der Nasutitermes-Soldaten. Rev. Suisse Zool. 66, 289–295.

Grassé, P.-P. and Ch. Noirot (1951) La sociotomie: migration et fragmentation de la termitière chez les *Anoplotermes* et les *Trinervitermes.* Behaviour 3, 146–166.

Harris, W. V. (1958) Colony formation in the Isoptera. Proc. Int. Cong. Entomol., 10th M., 1956 2, 435–439.

Hewitt, P. H., J. J. C. Nel and S. Conradie (1969) Preliminary studies on the control of caste formation in the harvester termite *Hodotermes mossambicus* (Hagen). Insectes Soc. 16, 159–172.

Howse, P. E. (1965) On the significance of certain oscillatory movements in termites. Insectes Soc. 12, 335–346.

Hrdý, I. and J. Křeček (1972) Development of superfluous soldiers induced by juvenile hormone analogues in the termite *Reticulitermes lucifugus santonensis.* Insectes Soc. 19, 105–109.

Hummel, H. and P. Karlson (1968) Hexansäure als Bestandteil des Spurpheromons der Termite *Zootermopsis nevadensis* Hagen. Hoppe-Seyler's Z. Physiol. Chem. 349, 725–727.

Lebrun, D. (1970) Intercastes experimentaux de *Calotermes flavicollis* Fabr. Insectes Soc. 17, 159–172.

Lebrun, D. (1972) Effets de l'implantation de glandes mandibulaires sur la différenciation imaginale de *Calotermes flavicollis* Fabr. C. R. H. Acad. Sci. Ser. D, 274, 2077–2079.

Light, S. F. (1942–43) The determination of the castes of social insects. Quart. Rev. Biol. 17, 312–326; 18, 46–63.

Light, S. F. (1944) Experimental studies on ectohormonal control of the development of supplementary reproductives in the termite *Zootermopsis* (formerly *Termopsis*). Univ. Calif. (Berkeley) Publ. Zool. 43, 413–454.
Light, S. F. and F. M. Weesner (1955) The production and replacement of soldiers in incipient colonies of *Reticulitermes hesperus* Banks. Insectes Soc. 2, 347–354.
Lüscher, M. (1952a) Die Produktion und Elimination von Ersatzgeschlechtstieren bei der Termite *Kalotermes flavicollis* Fabr. Z. Verg. Physiol. 34, 123–141.
Lüscher, M. (1952b) Untersuchungen über das individuelle Wachstum bei der Termite *Kalotermes flavicollis* Fabr. (Ein Beitrag zum Kastenbildungsproblem). Biol. Zentralbl. 71, 529–543.
Lüscher, M. (1955) Zur Frage der Übertragung sozialer Wirkstoffe bei Termiten. Naturwissenschaften 42, 186.
Lüscher, M. (1956a) Entstehung von Ersatzgeschlechtstiere bei der Termite *Kalotermes Flavicollis.* Insectes Soc. 3, 119–127.
Lüscher, M. (1956b) Hemmende und fordernde Faktoren bei der Entstehung der Ersatzgeschlechtstiere bei der Termite *Kalotermes flavicollis* Fabr. Rev. Suisse Zool. 63, 261–267.
Lüscher, M. (1961) Social control of polymorphism in termites. In: Insect Polymorphism Symposium no. 1, Royal Entomological Society of London; ed.: J. S. Kennedy pp. 57–67.
Lüscher, M. (1964) Die spezifische Wirkung männlicher und weiblicher Ersatzgeschlechtstiere auf die Entstehung von Ersatzgeschlechtstieren bei der Termite *Kalotermes flavicollis* (Fabr.). Insectes Soc. 11, 79–90.
Lüscher, M. and A. Springhetti (1960) Untersuchungen über die Bedeutung der Corpora allata für die Differenzierung der Kasten bei der Termite *Kalotermes flavicollis* F. J. Insect. Physiol. 5, 190–212.
McMahan, E. A. (1969) Feeding relationships and radioisotope techniques. In: Biology of Termites 1; eds.: K. Krishner and F. M. Weesner (Academic Press, New York) pp. 387–406.
Matsumura, F., H. C. Coppel and A. Tai (1968) Isolation and identification of termite trail-following pheromone. Nature (London). 219, 963–964.
Matsumura, F., A. Tai and H. C. Coppell (1969) Termite trail-following substance, isolation and purification from *Reticulitermes virginicus* and fungus-infected wood. J. Econ. Entomol. 62, 599–603.
Miller, E. M. (1969) Caste differentiation in the lower termites. In: Biology of Termites, 1; eds.: K. Krishner and F. M. Weesner (Academic Press, New York) pp. 283–310.
Moore, B. P. (1966) Isolation of the scent-trail pheromone of an Australian termite. Nature (London) 211, 746–747.
Moore, B. P. (1968) Studies on the chemical composition and function of the cephalic gland secretion in Australian termites. J. Insect Physiol. 14, 33–39.
Moore, B. P. (1969) Biochemical studies in termites. In: Biology of Termites, 1; eds.: K. Krishner and F. M. Weesner (Academic Press, New York) pp. 407–432.
Noirot, Ch. (1969) Formation of castes in the higher termites. In: Biology of Termites, 1; eds.: K. Krishner and F. M. Weesner (Academic Press, New York) pp. 311–350.
Nutting, W. L. (1969) Flight and colony foundation. In: Biology of Termites 1; eds.: K. Krishner and F. M. Weesner (Academic Press, New York) pp. 233–282.
Patil, V. D., U. R. Nayak and Sukh Dev (1973) Chemistry of ayurvedic crude drugs-II, guggulu (resin from *Commiphora mukul*)-2: diterpenoid constituents. Tetrahedron (in press).
Pickens, A. L. (1932) Observations on the genus *Reticulitermes* Holmgren. Pan-Pac. Entomol. 8, 178–180.
Robertson, P. L. (1971) Pheromones involved in aggressive behaviour in the ant *Myrmecia gulosa* J. Insect Physiol. 17, 691–715.

Ruppli, E. (1969) Die Elimination überzähliger Ersatzgeschlechtstiere bei der Termite *Kalotermes flavicollis* (Fabr.). Insectes Soc. 16, 235–248.

Sannasi, A. and C. J. George (1972) Termite queen substance: 9-oxodec-*trans*-2-enoic acid. Nature (London) 237, 457.

Sannasi, A., P. K. Sen-Sarma, C. J. George and S. Basalingappa (1972) Juvenile hormone activity from various sources of termite castes and their fungus gardens. Insectes Soc. 19, 81–85.

Stuart, A. M. (1963) Studies on the communication of alarm in the termite *Zootermopsis nevadensis* (Hagen). Physiol. Zool. 36, 85–96.

Stuart, A. M. (1969) Social behavior and communication. In: Biology of Termites, 1; eds.: K. Krishner and F. M. Weesner (Academic Press, New York) pp. 193–232.

Verron, H. and M. Barbier (1962) L'héxène-3-o1-1, substance des termites *Calotermes flavicollis et Microcerotermes edentatus.* C. R. Acad. Sci., 254, 4089–4091.

Watson, J. A. L. (1971) The development of 'workers' and reproductives in *Mastotermes darwiniensis* Froggatt (Isoptera). Insectes Soc. 18, 173–176.

Wilson, E. O., N. I. Durlach and L. M. Roth (1958) Chemical releasers of necrophoric behavior in ants. Psyche 65, 108–114.

Section II

Vertebrate pheromone systems

CHAPTER 14

Pheromones in fish and amphibia

Wolfgang PFEIFFER

14.1. Introduction

In contrast to insects and mammals, little is known about the pheromones of non-mammalian vertebrates. A complete summary of the literature on pheromones will not be attempted; rather, certain aspects will be considered in some detail, particularly the fishes. This reflects the main interest of the present author and also emphasizes the fact that fish pheromones are much more studied than those of other non-mammalian vertebrates. Although little is known on pheromones in amphibia and reptiles, the fright reaction of some anuran tadpoles is recognized and will be discussed in some detail and compared with that of fishes. Concerning the reptiles, there are some observations on snakes. The massing of the prairie rattlesnake in Colorado described by Klauber (1936) may be based on the chemical senses. Species identification by olfaction in the snakes *Storeria* and *Thamnophis* has been described by Noble (1937). More recently Gehlbach et al. (1971) have demonstrated that olfactory marks may help blind snakes (*Leptotyphlops*, *Sonora*, *Tantilla*, and *Virginia*) find food, housing, conspecifics and mates. Olfaction in birds has been reviewed by Wenzel (1971) but their pheromones are completely unstudied. A very few species of birds, such as the kiwi and some vultures, seem to have a well developed olfactory sense, but recent birds rely on visual and auditory cues rather than the olfactory system. Chemoreception in fish has been reviewed by Hasler (1957), Teichmann (1962), Kleerekoper (1969), Hara (1971), Pfeiffer (1971) and by Bardach and Atema (1971). Migration and orientation, in which the chemical senses may play an important role, were reviewed by Harden Jones (1968) and Hasler (1971) and the analysis of behavior was treated by Baerends (1971). These studies should be consulted for information on chemoreception and behavior in fish.

14.2. Pheromones in fish: schooling and reproduction

Pheromones in fish may play a role in attraction and recognition of the other sex, the offspring or the parents; they may maintain a fish school during the night, or guide anadromous fish migrating upstream toward the odor of their landlocked conspecifics on the spawning site. The examples are numerous but the origin and the chemistry of the presumed pheromones are unknown; indeed, their existence is often doubtful since in all these cases the fish may simply respond to the odor of conspecifics as they do to other odors such as food, plants and predators. It was shown by Wrede (1932) and Göz (1941) that a species-specific odor emanates from the individuals of a fish school and that this odor can be recognized by them. The European minnow, *Phoxinus phoxinus* (L.), in a free-choice situation, showed a preference for an aquarium-compartment in which the odor of conspecifics lingered. In an experimental arrangement *Phoxinus* could be conditioned to discriminate the odor of various species of fish, and between different individuals of its own species. Yellow bullheads, *Ictalurus natalis* (Le Sueur), also recognized individuals of their own species chemically (Todd et al. 1967). Chemical discrimination between conspecifics and other species was found by Kühme (1964a, b) in very young free-swimming jewel cichlids, *Hemichromis bimaculatus* (Gill). An isolated fish swims to the water from its own species rather than to the water from the five-spotted cichlid, *H. fasciatus* (Peters). Blinded minnows (*Phoxinus*) and rudd, *Scardinius erythrophthalmus* (L.), stay in the vicinity of other individuals of the same species provided their olfactory organ is intact (Keenleyside 1955). At night a school of the roach, *Rutilus rutilus* (L.), does not completely disintegrate and it is assumed that olfactory cues maintain contact between individuals (Hemmings 1966). Chinook salmon, *Oncorhynchus tshawytscha* (Walbaum), showed olfactory bulbar responses to the water which had previously evoked only a slight response if individuals of the same species were placed in it. Keeping coho salmon, *O. kisutch* (Walbaum), under the same condition did not make the water as stimulating (Oshima et al. 1969). Orientation of anadromous char, *Salvelinus alpinus* (L.), toward their breeding sites may also be influenced by the odor of their conspecifics (Nordeng 1971).

The females of the blenny, *Blennius pavo* Risso, are said to be attracted by secretions from their males (Eggert 1931). Ripe females of the Mexican blind cave-fish (*Anoptichthys*) stimulate their males by an odorous secretion from the anal region (Wilkens 1972). Female guppy, *Poecilia reticulata* Peters, assume an inclined position of 30 to 70° with the horizontal, usually head upward, in response to a substance released by the males (Jaski 1939). Sex discrimination by olfaction seems likely in the brown bullhead, *Ictalurus nebulosus* (Le Sueur), according to Breder (1935). The same may be true for the blind goby, *Typhlogobius californiensis* Steindachner (MacGinitie 1939). Courtship occurs within 10 seconds when a male goby, *Bathygobius soporator* (Cuvier and Valenciennes), is kept in isolation and water is introduced from a second tank with a gravid female. The active substance is located in the ovarium fluid and exuded through the urogenital papillae. Anosmatic males fail to respond to the specific substance and show fighting behavior. The substance not only elicits courtship but inhibits fighting (Tavolga

1956), effective in both at extreme dilutions, and may eventually be classified as a pheromone. According to Losey (1969), males of the genus *Hypsoblennius* Gill were attracted by a pheromone from other males of this genus. Chemoreception plays a role in parental care, as was shown for cichlids *Hemichromis bimaculatus* by Kühme (1963) and *Cichlasoma nigrofasciatum* (Günther) by Myrberg (1966). *Hemichromis* showed typical parental behavior toward water containing their own larvae. The fanning behavior lasted 3 weeks. When the advanced young were replaced by fresh larvae, the female fish responded again with fanning behavior.

In most cases, chemical perception of other fish is by olfaction. However, taste may also play a role. The very motile filamentous pelvic fins of gouramis (*Colisa*, *Trichogaster*) have a gustatory function (Scharrer et al. 1947). Catfish may recognize one another by taste (Todd et al. 1967). Carp taste nerves increase their response frequencies when stimulated with fish slime and water in which fish had resided (Konishi and Zotterman 1963). Myrberg (1966) claimed that adult mouthbreeding cichlids recognize their young by taste.

14.3. Pheromones in fish: fright reaction

The only fish pheromone known with certainty is the alarm substance. It was tentatively classified as a pheromone by Karlson and Lüscher (1959a, b) and by Karlson (1960), and has since been proven a pheromone according to their definition.

14.3.1. The fright reaction

Discovering the fright reaction: Von Frisch (1938) accidentally discovered the fright reaction (Schreckreaktion) from two casual observations while experimenting with the European minnow, *Phoxinus phoxinus* (L.). The first was associated with the introduction of a surgically operated minnow into a school of normal individuals. Von Frisch had marked one fish by severing the nervus sympathicus near the tail, thus producing a darkening of the skin caudal to the incision. When the fish was introduced into the normal school, some of the individuals retreated rapidly and the school was obviously frightened. The second observation was made when Von Frisch released a struggling fish which had become jammed under the rim of a metal feeding tube. As it swam away, the rest of the school became alarmed and fled. Such behavior was curious enough to call for further investigation. The account given here is based on the original studies of Von Frisch (1938, 1941a, b) and his students Schutz (1956) and Pfeiffer (1960a,b, 1962a,c,d, 1963a,c, 1966a, 1967a,b, 1969a, 1970; Pfeiffer et al. 1971; Pfeiffer and Lemke 1973; Reutter and Pfeiffer 1973). Additional information was provided by Verheijen (1956, 1959a,b, 1962, 1963), Thines and Vandenbussche (1966), Gandolfi (1968), Gandolfi et al. 1968a,b), and Verheijen and Reuter (1969). Some aspects of the fright reaction and alarm substance in fish were reviewed earlier by Von Frisch (1961) and Pfeiffer (1962b, 1963b, 1966c).

Description of the fright reaction: Von Frisch (1938, 1941a,b) confirmed repeatedly his casual observations both in field and laboratory experiments. In the field, a small feeding table with a tube through which chopped earthworm could be dropped onto the table was placed near the shore of a lake. The minnows soon learned of this source of food. A school of fish was first enticed to the feeding tray and five minutes later test substances were introduced through the tube. An active test substance induced a fright reaction in 30–60 sec. Fish which had assembled at the feeding tray seemed terrified and fled a short distance in confusion; they then crowded together and retreated. Confidence returned after variable intervals of many minutes, hours or days. In the laboratory, an aquarium was furnished with a hiding place, a food tube, a wire for the introduction of food into the tube, and usually ten minnows. When first placed in such an environment, minnows are timid and flee into the hiding place. They must be conditioned to the experimental aquarium until they no longer flee when a person approaches the tank but remain near the food tube. The conditioning time varies from three days to three weeks. The behavioral changes during conditioning and the subsequent fright reaction during the experiments are quantified and the tests made objective by recording the number of minnows in the feeding area at intervals of 15 seconds for five minute periods after each feeding or the introduction of test materials. In the aquarium the fright reaction is similar to that observed in field experiments. An excellent documentation of the fright reaction in the minnow and the experimental procedure has been recorded on film by Von Frisch (1955). The intensity of the fright reaction varies. Von Frisch (1941b) distinguished seven different situations. These are arbitrary stages and many intermediate phases may be observed ranging from the most intense reaction where all fish are suddenly frightened to a scarcely visible intimidation. These categories permit useful quantitative evaluations and have been used by Von Frisch and his students Schutz and Pfeiffer in their many experiments: 1) Most intense reaction with sudden fright and rapid swimming into the hiding place, but immediately coming out and rapidly swimming around the tank, avoiding the feeding place for a long time. 2) Intense reaction as above, but fish do not leave the hiding place. Sometimes, after several minutes, some fish return to the feeding place and timidly snatch bits of food before quickly retreating. 3) Clearly frightened; the school retreats toward or more often into the hiding place but quietens down within 5–10 minutes and then approaches the feeding area more or less confidently. Sometimes fish may remain longer in the hiding place, but without showing extremely timid movements while there. 4) Only slightly frightened with somewhat confused and excited swimming; often dense crowding together and retreating to the bottom but soon quietening down if nothing further happens; occasionally retreating to the hiding place. 5) Intimidated; less confident and more cautious at the feeding tube; less frequent crowding together and retreating to the bottom; no retreat toward the hiding place. 6) Slightly uneasy with some crowding together in the area of the feeding tube, but the reaction soon disappears and the fish never leave the feeding area. 7) No reaction whatever.

This description of the fright reaction in *Phoxinus phoxinus* (L.) applies equally well to many other species of schooling Cypriniformes. Some species, however, behave in quite a different manner when alarmed. The tench, *Tinca tinca* (L.), and the crucian carp, *Carassius carassius* (L.), swim excitedly with their heads against the bottom and with their bodies at an angle of about 60° to the floor of the aquarium. In their natural habitat, this behavior disturbs the mud and debris on the bottom so that they are concealed in the turbid water. Other species, the gudgeon, *Gobio gobio* (L.), the loach, *Noemacheilus barbatulus* (L.), and the sucker, *Catostomus catostomus* (Forster), become motionless and show no movement for several minutes. They are cryptically colored and thus by 'freezing' may avoid their enemies (Schutz 1956; Pfeiffer 1963a). This type of reaction is better developed in the adults than in the young. The hornhead chub, *Hybopsis biguttata* Kirtland sinks to the bottom and starts spitting gas for a considerable time as a reaction to the alarm substance (Verheijen 1963). A few species of fish, particularly the genus *Esomus* ('flying barbs') flee to the surface when they are alarmed; they crowd together there and swim hastily, frequently jumping out of the water (Schutz 1956). Hatchetfish (Gasteropelecidae), normally swimming close to the water surface, flee toward the depth where they form a dense school when frightened by the alarm substance. When chased they may jump out of the water (Pfeiffer 1963c).

Searching for the causal agent: Von Frisch (1941b) first investigated the sense of hearing as a possible receptor in the fright reaction. Minnows were captured from a lake with a hand net, placed in a tank, then returned to the lake where they were observed to associate freely with the fishes in the lake. No fright reaction was evident. Other tests were made with narcotized minnows. Small incisions were made in the skin of narcotized and operated fish. The narcotized and operated fish were suspended in a test school. The school was obviously frightened, thus showing that it was the injury itself which frightened the uninjured minnows. The possibility of a visually induced fright reaction was eliminated by chopping bits of minnows into small pieces and introducing these as food. The schools of fish first snapped at the food but within 30 seconds showed a strong fright reaction, indicating chemical induction of the reaction. A possible involvement of the optical sense was further eliminated by preparing filtered extracts of minnows and showing that these were extremely potent in the initiation of a fright reaction. The effective chemical substance was named *Schreckstoff* ('alarm substance') and the reaction *Schreckreaktion* ('fright reaction'). In further experiments Von Frisch showed that only injured skin produced consistent and strong reactions. Minnows killed without injury of the skin produced no fright reaction. Extracts or pieces of stomach, gut, liver, spleen and muscles were ineffective. The age of the minnow and its habitat had no effect on the fright reaction. Skin from different areas of the body was compared and no differences between the dorsal skin (containing much melanin and yellow pigment) and the ventral skin (rich in guanin and red pigment) could be established. Minnows were permitted to struggle in moist filter paper or were rubbed with filter paper after narcotizing with urethane. The strong fright reaction shown to extracts of the filter paper thus prepared indicated that the epithelium was rich in alarm substance.

14.3.2. Alarm substance

Origin: The epidermal cells responsible for the alarm substance have been localized. From a histological comparison of the species which produce an alarm substance and other species which do not, the presence of certain 'club cells' could be associated with this substance (Pfeiffer 1960b). Histologically, teleost fish skin shows two types of epidermal secretory cells: the mucus cells (*Becherzellen*) and the club cells (*Kolbenzellen*). The former open onto the surface of the skin and pour out their mucus as from a beaker; the latter vary in distribution and appearance in different kinds of fishes. In *Phoxinus* club cells are not connected to the surface. Injury to the skin releases the contents of these cells and only in this way does the alarm substance reach the surface. Pfeiffer (1960b) has suggested the name *Schreckstoffzellen* ('alarm substance cells'). The alarm substance cells of the Ostariophysi (fig. 14.1) differ from the club cells of most other Teleostei both in morphology and function. Similar cells have been found only in the Gonorhynchiformes and in the Galaxiidae (Pfeiffer 1967b, 1969a), despite intensive search in many other orders and families. The club cells of the Gonorhynchiformes are alarm substance cells like those of the Ostariophysi. The Galaxiidae have not yet been tested and it is still unknown whether or not they have the fright reaction. Alarm substance cells are present in most species of the Ostariophysi; they are absent in the Gymnotoidei, Loricariidae, Aspredinidae, several Characoidei (*Chilodus*) (Pfeiffer 1963c, 1970). In some ostariophysean species (*Hemiodus*, several Siluriformes) the club cells differ in structure (fig. 14.2). Whether all club cells in the Siluriformes function as alarm substance cells cannot be decided until more families are tested. The uniform distribution of the club cells confirms Von Frisch's (1941b) observation that the skin in all regions contains the same amount of alarm substance. Further evidence that the club cells produce alarm substance was found in comparisons of skin samples containing different numbers of club cells. The Asian glass catfish (*Kryptopterus bicirrhis* Cuvier and Valenciennes) showed no fright reaction to barbel extracts (lacking club cells) but a strong reaction to extracts of the body skin (containing club cells). Finally, the alarm substance cells were found histologically in all species which contain the alarm substance according to the behavior experiment. Contrast species without the alarm substance also lack the alarm substance cells (Pfeiffer 1960b, 1963c, 1967b). Recently, the alarm substance cells from *Phoxinus* were investigated by means of more advanced techniques. The histochemical studies of alarm substance cells by Pfeiffer et al. (1971) are in complete agreement with the ultrastructural findings (fig. 14.3). Perinuclear ribosomes, mitochondria, and a Golgi complex are demonstrated. A tubular network radiates from the Golgi complex. Histochemically, glycogen granules are occasionally seen near the nucleus. Consistently, a strong RNA reaction can be shown as well as succinic-dehydrogenase activity, lactic-dehydrogenase activity, and in some cells glucose-6-phosphate-dehydrogenase activity. Leucyl-aminopeptidase activity exists in the

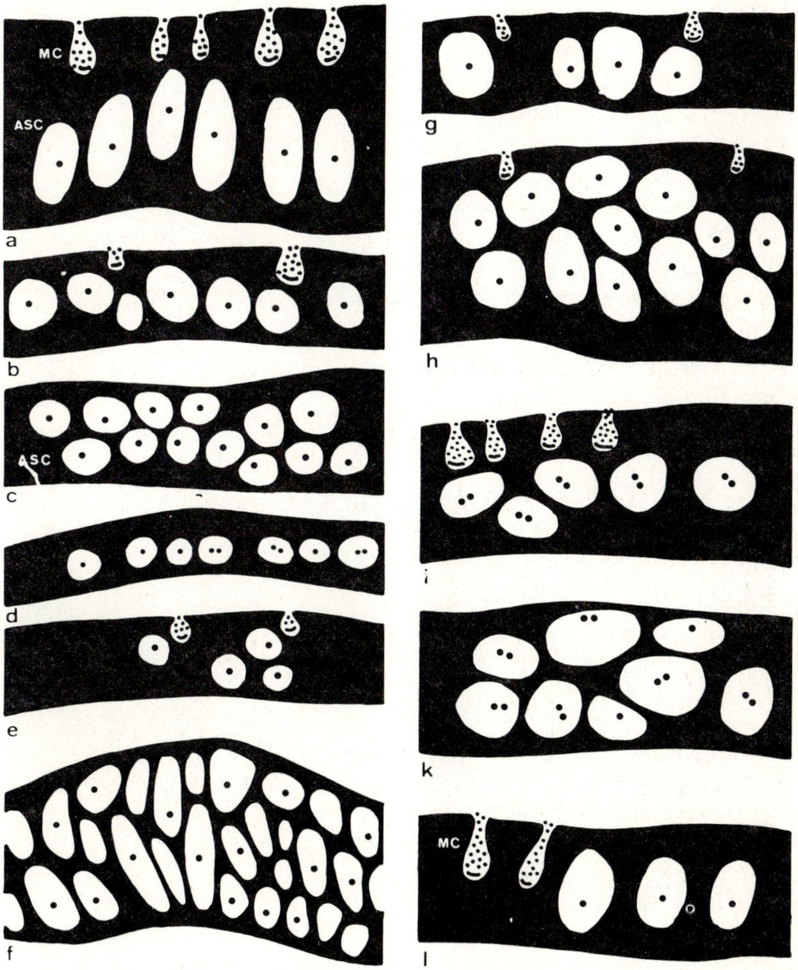

Fig. 14.1. Number and position of alarm substance cells in the epidermis of: a) *Phoxinus*; b) *Catostomus*; c) *Tribolodon*; d) *Moenkhausia*; e) *Hyphessobrycon*; f) *Homalopterus*; g) *Gyrinocheilus*; h) *Kryptopterus*; i) *Ictalurus*; k) *Etropiella*; l) *Phractolaemus*. ASC, Alarm substance cell; MC, Mucus cell. Original, after data from Pfeiffer (1960b, 1963a,c, 1967b).

cytoplasm; its maximum occurring in the vicinity of the nucleus. Proteins and diastase-resistant polysaccharides are not found in cytoplasm adjacent to the nucleus. The results indicate a secretory activity of the alarm substance cells. Finally, Pfeiffer and Lemke (1973) isolated the alarm substance from *Phoxinus* and showed that it was fluorescent when dissolved in water. This result stimulated Reutter and Pfeiffer (1973) to look for a direct demonstration of alarm substance in the alarm substance cells by fluorescent microscopy. Alarm substance cells were found to be autofluorescent after freezing (at −160 °C) and drying (at −35 °C) of

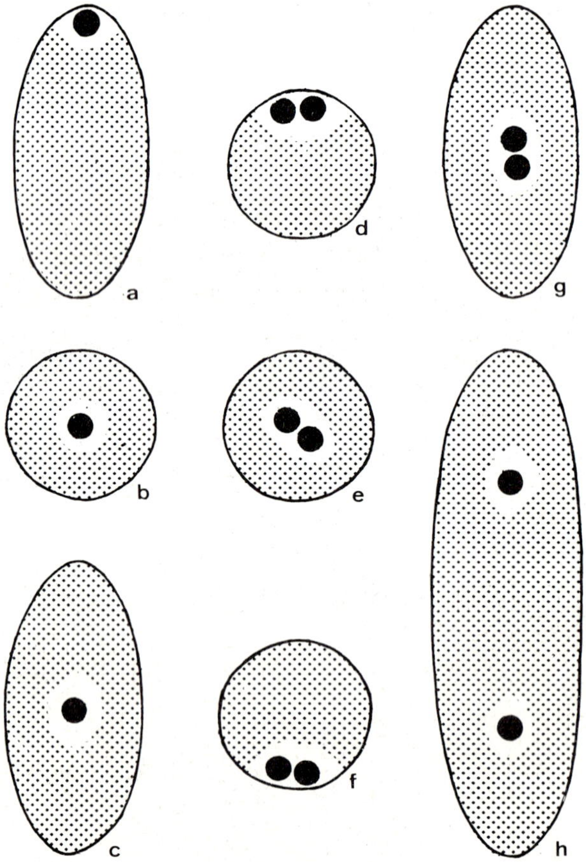

Fig. 14.2. Position and number of the nuclei in the alarm substance cells of a) *Hemiodus*; b,c) *Phoxinus*, most other Cypriniformes, all Gonorhynchiformes, some Siluridae and Trichomycteridae; d,e,f) some Amphiliidae, Ariidae, Bagridae, and Schilbeidae; e,g) most Siluriformes, and some Cypriniformes; g,h) some Bagridae, Mochokidae, and Schilbeidae. Original, after data from Pfeiffer (1960b, 1963a,c, 1967b, 1970).

the skin. The autofluorescence of the alarm substance is maximally excited at 360–380 nm; the maximum of emission lies about 515 nm. The fluorescence of an alarm substance cell was compared with the autofluorescence of the isolated alarm substance by using a microspectrophotofluorometer. The maxima of emission are separated only about 10 nm from one another, and the curves of relative fluorescence intensity are almost identical. These results confirmed Pfeiffer's (1960b) concept that the alarm substance cells of the Cypriniformes produce the alarm substance.

Potency: Von Frisch (1941b) developed a standard procedure for the preparation of the skin extracts and this procedure has been followed in many later experiments. A 0.2-g sample of fresh skin (equivalent to the skin of a seven cm

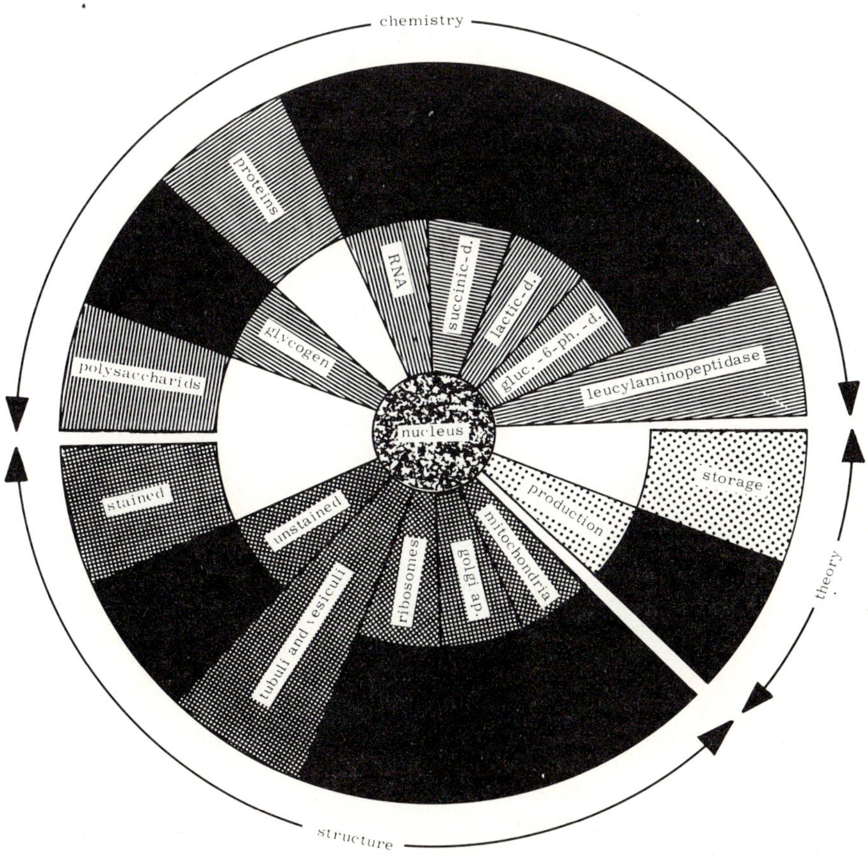

Fig. 14.3. Morphological and histochemical properties of an alarm substance cell from *Phoxinus*. The halo around the nucleus differs markedly from the rest of the cytoplasm. Original, after data from Pfeiffer et al. (1971).

Phoxinus) is cut with scissors 150 times and diluted with 200 ml water. It is shaken at five-min intervals for 30 min and filtered. Appropriate dilutions may then be made from this standard extract. In any test, 100 ml of liquid are poured through the feeding tube during about 45 sec. In earlier experiments, Von Frisch (1941b) found that the standard extract could be diluted considerably without losing its effectiveness. Schutz (1956) and Pfeiffer (1960b) found that *Phoxinus* and *Tribolodon* still respond at a dilution of 1:50,000. Sucker (*Catostomus*) reacted to a dilution of 1:100; the characid *Aphyocharax rubropinnis* Pappenheim responded very well to a dilution of 1:2000, and the hybrids of *Anoptichthys* and *Astyanax* did so at a dilution of 1:1000. Schutz (1956) related the intensity of the fright reaction to the surface area of fish skin. He found that the extract from 1/100 mm^2 of skin (0.002 mg skin) of a three-cm *Phoxinus* was sufficient to repel a school from the feeding place in a 14-liter aquarium. The isolation of the alarm substance (Pfeiffer and Lemke 1973) permitted a determination of the threshold of alarm substance eliciting the fright reaction. The isolated alarm substance produced a fright reaction at a dilution of 0.05 μg/ml, when five ml of the fluid were poured into a 20-liter aquarium with *Danio malabaricus* (Jerdon) (unpublished data of the author). However, the substance used was not pure and would, moreover, be diluted immediately when poured into the aquarium. Thus, the actual threshold will be much lower and the concentration reaching the fish considerably less.

Chemistry: Hüttel (1941) suggested that the alarm substance of the minnow was a purine- or a pterin-like substance. However, purines and pterins were supposed to be highly concentrated in the xanthophores (Ziegler-Günder 1956) which are most numerous in the dorsal skin, and it has been established that ventral skin is as effective as dorsal skin in eliciting the fright reaction (Von Frisch 1941b). Recently Tucker and Suzuki (1972), in an effort to characterize the alarm substance, have studied the olfactory stimulating effect of skin extracts from white catfish, *Ictalurus catus* (L.). Electric potentials from the olfactory lamella were recorded. Crude extracts of skin and seven fractions from gel chromatography with Sephadex G-25 were tested. However, the enhancement of biological activity was quite modest. Salmon skin extracts were almost equally effective on catfish, although the alarm substance is absent in Salmonidae. In an effort to isolate and identify the alarm substance of *Phoxinus* Pfeiffer and Lemke (1973) tested skin extracts on the behavior of several hundred schools of the giant danio, *Danio malabaricus* (Jerdon), in 100 aquaria under identical conditions. Later, the alarm substance of both species were shown to be identical. Lyophilized skin could be stored for at least six months without loss of activity. No reduction of the activity was observed after the solvent solution was drawn off in the evaporator at 30 °C when compared with the concentration by freeze drying. After separation over Diaflo membranes in ultrafiltration cells the total activity was in the solution that ran through the last membrane (UM 05). Four spots fluoresced blue at 360 nm under the quartz lamp. After preparative separation, the main spot and one of the accessory spots elicited a fright reaction. A comparison with isoxanthopterin showed that isoxanthopterin also elicited the fright reaction. The results of Pfeiffer and Lemke (1973) indicate that the alarm substance of the Cypriniformes is probably a pterin. Comparative investigations with a characid, *Alestes longipinnis* (Günther), were in complete agreement with the results on the cyprinids *Phoxinus* and *Danio*. Chemical work on the alarm substance is presently being performed by Professor Viscontini at the University of Zürich while the behavioral experiments continue in our laboratory.

Olfactory detection: The alarm substance is detected only by the sense of smell; the sense of taste is not involved. Von Frisch (1941b) removed the nervus olfactorius and bulbus olfactorius in 10 schools of *Phoxinus* and kept the minnows in isolation until they recovered. The removal of the olfactory bulb prevented regeneration of the olfactory organ. Operated fish did not respond to the alarm substance. The reaction was not reduced in four schools of sham-operated controls in which the roof of the skull had been opened, folded back, then closed again without injuring the olfactory nerve and olfactory bulb.

14.3.3. Visual transmission of the fright reaction

When *Phoxinus* which showed the fright reaction were moved to another aquarium and placed with fish which were not affected by alarm substance, the behavior of the latter group varied with the number of minnows introduced. If relatively few fish were introduced, the resident minnows were not disturbed, but rather seemed to produce a quieting effect on their alarmed associates. If the introduced minnows were equal or greater in number, the resident fish became intimidated. This experiment indicated that the movements associated with the fright reaction could initiate a reaction in fish which did not have direct contact with the alarm substance. Another type of experiment was performed with blinded minnows. Blind fish cannot school. When exposed to alarm substance they swim to the bottom of the aquarium and often show fright movements. However, each fish reacts as an individual, and there is no group response. In another experiment three minnows with the olfactory organ destroyed were associated in an aquarium with three unoperated fish and tested with minnow skin extract. The unoperated fish promptly showed the expected fright reaction and, within a few minutes, the operated minnows were also alarmed and the entire school showed the effects of the reaction for several days (Von Frisch 1941b). The visual transmission of the fright reaction was further demonstrated by the following experiments. Two aquaria were placed side by side and the interiors arranged as mirror images of each other. The same number of *Phoxinus* was placed in each aquarium. In one of the aquaria, the minnows were exposed to alarm substance and the reactions were observed in both tanks. When no hiding place was provided and a strong reaction was induced, so that the alarmed minnows swam hastily to and fro, then the fish in the neighboring aquarium displayed the characteristic fright reaction. Many observations of Schutz (1956) and

Verheijen (1956) confirmed that the alarm substance frightens the first individuals having contact with it, while the other members of the school respond to the behavior of these fish. In nature, this behavior would have obvious survival value.

14.3.4. Ontogeny and variations in the fright reaction

Ontogeny: Since the fright reaction is so similar in fish of different geographic origin and habitats, Von Frisch (1941b) assumed it to be innate. Schutz (1956) and Pfeiffer (1963b, 1966a) established this in various species. The European minnow *Phoxinus phoxinus* (L.), the bitterling *Rhodeus sericeus* Bloch, the dace *Leuciscus leuciscus* (L.), the redside shiner *Richardsonius balteatus* (Richardson), the zebra fish *Brachydanio rerio* (Hamilton-Buchanan), and hybrids of the characids *Astyanax bimaculatus* (L.) and *Anoptichthys antrobius* Alvarez were hatched in the laboratory and tested for the presence of the alarm substance and for their ability to respond to it at various times during development. Recently hatched fish showed no fright reaction. It appeared in *Brachydanio* at 28 days, in *Richardsonius* at 42 days, in the characid hybrids at 46 days, in *Phoxinus* at 51 days, and in *Leuciscus* at 59 days after hatching. In *Rhodeus* it was first observed 40 days after the young left the mussel where they developed. By contrast, schooling behavior appeared much earlier than the fright reaction. Young *Brachydanio* schooled at 20 days, *Phoxinus* at 25 days, *Leuciscus* at 28 days, and *Rhodeus* when they left the mussel. It was also shown that the alarm substance was present in the skins of these small fish one to two weeks prior to their first reaction.

Variations in the fright reaction: Because of the variability in the reaction, valid conclusions can only be based on large numbers of experiments. Von Frisch (1941b) found it necessary to perform 438 tests with schools of *Phoxinus* to establish the nature of the fright reaction. Pfeiffer (1966b), studying the genetics of the fright reaction, tested individually 308 hybrids of *Astyanax* and *Anoptichthys.* Pfeiffer and Lemke (1973), isolating the alarm substance, performed more than 400 experiments with *Danio.* Under seemingly identical conditions Von Frisch (1941b) sometimes obtained positive results at high dilutions while on other occasions schools might not respond to the undiluted extract. In these experiments it became apparent that several factors may contribute to this variability while others have no obvious effect. Comparisons of skin extracts show that fish tested at different seasons, fish from different waters, males and females and different individuals from healthy schools all have approximately the same content of alarm substance in their skin. Temperature has also been ruled out as a source of variability in the results. Thus it seems evident that much of the variability in the reactions depends on 'the readiness' of the school to respond. It has frequently been observed that fish from the same catch, after the same treatment with the same alarm substance at the same dilution, may react totally differently. These individual differences in the schools are difficult to explain, but several contributing factors have been noted. It is evident that the readiness to respond generally decreases with repeated testing. Therefore, comparisons must be based on first reactions. The period of residence and the actual size of the tank also modify the results. As might be expected because of the dilution factor, the reactions are more marked in smaller tanks. Familiarity with the experimental tank is particularly important (Von Frisch 1941b). Minnows are easily alarmed by a great variety of stimuli when first placed in an aquarium. Later they become tame and fail to show any reaction to the usual disturbances in the laboratory. Von Frisch (1941b) has observed that the schools of *Phoxinus* which require a longer period for habituation show the strongest response to alarm substance. Since schools which become habituated more slowly have been in the tanks longer, there are two possibilities: differences in the schools of fish (more 'timid' fish perhaps always reacting more strongly) or actual length of time spent in the aquarium (greater familiarity with the surroundings resulting in increased stimulus susceptibility). The general health and condition of the fish might be expected to modify the response. Individuals which are obvious sick show little or no reaction to the alarm substance. Von Frisch (1941b) showed that starvation had a marked effect on the content of alarm substance in minnow skin. Thines and Vandenbussche (1966) studied the effects of the alarm substance on the cohesion of four schools of the harlequin fish *Rasbora heteromorpha* Duncker in light and darkness at different times in the 24 hour cycle. The fright reaction was more marked during daytime. It was suggested that a diurnal fluctuation exists in the responsiveness of the fish to the alarm substance. The effect was greater during the day, even when the tests were carried out under dark conditions. The data indicate a lowering of responsiveness to the alarm substance during nighttime independently of light conditions. Gandolfi et al. (1968b) assumed the existence of both sensitive and indifferent individuals of the same species. This suggestion seems to be based on a misinterpretation of Schutz (1956) and Verheijen (1956) who both found that it is unnecessary for every individual to have contact with the alarm substance; the visual stimulus caused by alarmed fish will induce a typical response in the other members of the school. However, this does not mean that visually alarmed fish will not be frightened by the alarm substance if they have contact with it, or that these fish cannot smell the alarm substance. Accordingly, Gandolfi et al. (1968b) did not discover individuals of *Brachydanio rerio* which were indifferent to the alarm substance.

14.3.5. The fright reaction in different species

Von Frisch (1938, 1941b) extended his investigations of the fright reaction to several other species of fish. He demonstrated it readily in *Leuciscus cephalus* (L.), *Rhodeus sericeus* Bloch, *Scardinius erythrophthalmus* (L.), and *Danio malabaricus* (Jerdon), but in repeated experiments failed to find it with the perch (*Perca fluviatilis* L.). Von Frisch noted that all species which showed positive results were schooling cyprinids; he therefore suggested that the fright reaction was either characteristic of certain groups of fishes (for example, the Cyprinidae) or of schooling behavior. Von Frisch's survey has been extended to include numerous species of fishes from many families and different social habits (Schutz 1956; Pfeiffer 1960b, 1963c, 1967b). Schutz found the fright reaction in 19 species of Cyprinidae, one species of Cobitidae, and three species of Characidae. Pfeiffer found the fright reaction in several families of the Siluriformes (1960a,b, 1962c, 1963c), and in several families of the Characoidei (Anostomidae, Citharinidae, Gasteropelecidae), in most families of the Cyprinoidei, i.e., the Catostomidae, Gyrinocheilidae, Homalopteridae (1962a,d, 1963a,c) and finally (1967a,b) in the Gonorhynchiformes (Kneriidae, Phractolaemidae). These experiments clearly demonstrated that the fright reaction is not confined to schooling fishes. Schutz obtained negative results with Salmonidae; Verheijen (1959a) and Pfeiffer (1960b) found no fright reaction in schooling Clupeidae. An extended series of tests involving numerous species of marine fishes added further proof that the reaction occurs only within groups having certain taxonomic affinities. Pfeiffer (1960a,b) in some 250 experiments examined 66 species of marine fishes representing 32 different families. None of the marine species examined had a fright reaction. On the basis of these tests, the presence of the fright reaction in any marine species was naturally questioned. The Japanese cyprinid *Tribolodon hakonensis taszanowskii* (Steindachner) is one of the few representatives of the Cypriniformes that lives in marine and brackish habitats, entering fresh water only at the time of reproduction. In a series of experiments it was demonstrated that this cyprinid shows the fright reaction in sea water as well as in fresh water, and that the reaction is of the same order as that of *Phoxinus*. Table 14.1 summarizes the number of species, families, and orders studied. Most species were listed by Pfeiffer (1960b, 1963c, 1967b, 1968a, 1970). The fright reaction exists only in the Ostariophysi and the Gonorhynchiformes (fig. 14.4); moreover, it is associated with these groups of fishes and not with any particular habitat or type of social behavior (Pfeiffer 1967b). The Ostariophysi are distinguished by a row of small bones known as the Weberian apparatus, which connects the inner ear with the swim bladder and adds considerably to the auditory sensivity and range. They contain 5000 species, mostly fresh-water fishes. The Gonorhynchiformes only contain seven genera with some African and two Indopacific species. Pfeiffer (1963c), in some 350 experiments involving 75 species of Ostariophysi found some species that lack the fright reaction. Two groups could be distinguished: a) fishes that do have alarm substance, but in which the fright reaction is absent (*Anoptichthys*, Serrasalminae, Mylinae); b) fishes that lack both the alarm substance and the fright reaction to alarm substance from other species (*Chilodus*, Nannostominae, Gymnotoidei, Loricariidae, Aspredinidae). As the fright reaction occurs in the Cypriniformes plus the Siluriformes, it is concluded that the ostariophysean species without the fright reaction have lost it during phylogeny. Ostariophysean species that lack the fright reaction differ markedly from the cyprinid way of life: blind

TABLE 14.1

Number of species, families, and orders of fishes that have been studied with respect to their fright reaction and/or alarm substance cells. Teleostei in ( )

	Number of		
	Orders	Families	Species
a) Studied with respect to both the fright reaction and the alarm substance cells	19 (16)	69 (66)	183 (180)
b) Studied only with respect to the fright reaction	0 (0)	0 (0)	25 (25)
c) Studied only with respect to the alarm substance cells	8 (2)	56 (49)	138 (127)
d) Sum of those studied with respect to the fright reaction (a + b)	19 (16)	69 (66)	208 (205)
e) Sum of those studied with respect to the alarm substance cells (a + c)	27 (18)	125 (115)	321 (307)
f) Existing Teleostei	~30	~420	~20,000
g) Percentage of Teleostei studied with respect to the fright reaction plus the alarm substance cells	~50%	~15%	~1%

cave-fish, piranha, headstander, pencilfish, armored catfish, and electric knife fish.

The fright reaction of fishes has been repeatedly misinterpreted. The statement of Hasler (1957) that the fright reaction was first discovered by Noble (1939) is wrong, since Noble himself cites Von Frisch (1938) and writes: 'in *Tilapia macrocephala*, the same reaction occurs, but only in juvenile fish'. Certainly Noble's *Tilapia* responded to other stimuli, but not to any alarm substance since this is absent in the Cichlidae. Many hundreds of tests with percomorph fishes were negative (Von Frisch 1941b; Schutz 1956; Pfeiffer 1960b). Noble's conclusion was criticized by Pfeiffer (1963b). Later Skinner et al. (1962) reported an alarm reaction in the top smelt *Atherinops affinis* (Ayres). Pfeiffer (1963b) criticized their conclusions and Rosenblatt and Losey (1967) reexamining *A. affinis* did not observe the reported alarm reaction; these workers interpret the reaction reported by Skinner et al. (1962) as an experimental artifact. In the other Atherinidae studied, the fright reaction is also absent (Schutz 1956; Pfeiffer 1960b). Contradictory results exist with the Cyprinodontiformes (Heintz, 1954; Schutz, 1956; Pfeiffer, 1960b). Until these experiments with Cyprinodontiformes are repeated, it cannot be definitely stated whether they have a reaction analogous to the fright reaction of the Ostariophysi or not. Analogous fright reactions to the body odor from conspe-

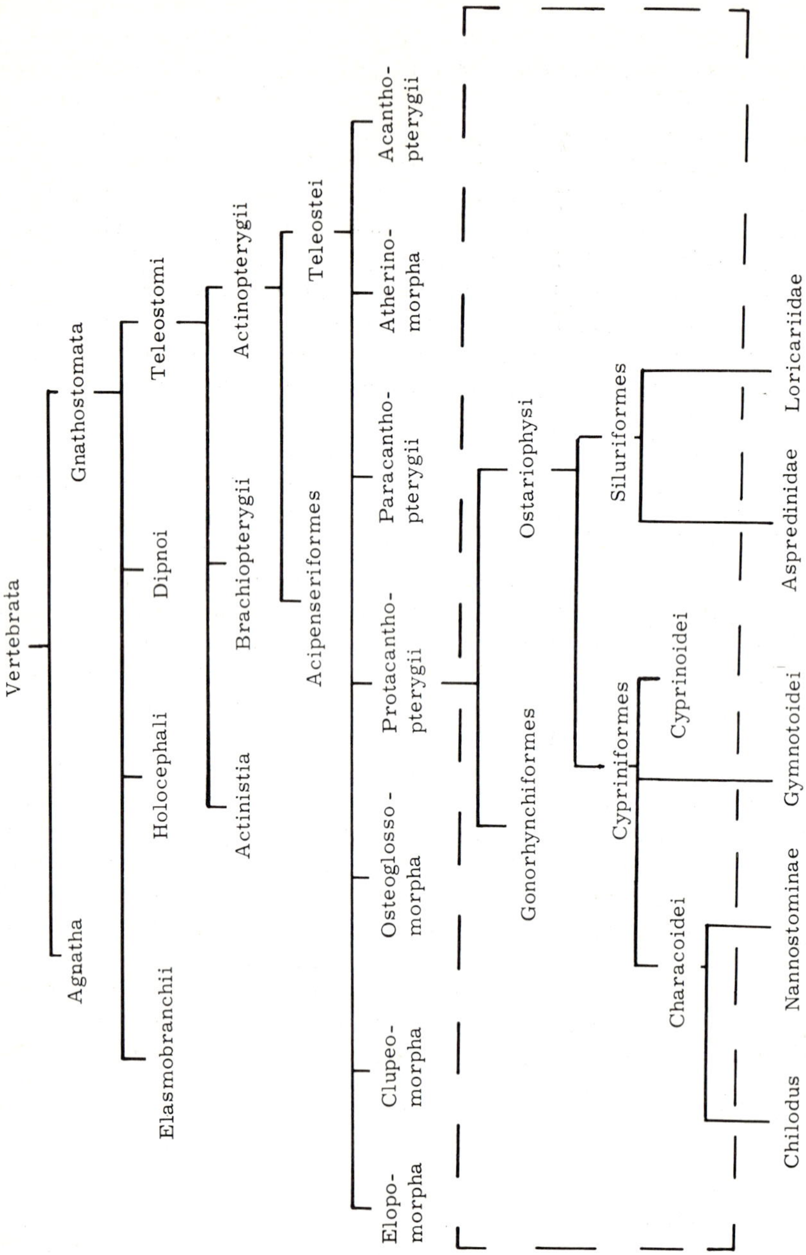

Fig. 14.4. Distribution of the fright reaction in fishes; it is confined to the groups framed and is primarily absent in the upper groups but secondarily absent in the lower ones. Original, after data from Pfeiffer (1960b, 1962b, 1963b,c, 1967b).

cifics occur in tadpoles and in snails (Snyder 1967). Parallel evolutions in other groups of fishes cannot be excluded without prior performance of critical experiments. Hara (1971), reviewing Reed (1969), mentions the reaction of various minnows to the odor of pike and other predaceous fishes in connection with the fright reaction. That the odor of pike may influence the behavior of minnows was described by Von Frisch (1941b) and Göz (1941). However, this is a reponse to the repellant odor of an enemy and completely different from the fright reaction. In accordance with the definition proposed by Von Frisch, we call only substances which communicate the presence of danger 'alarm substance', provided that they are produced by members of the same species. This does not exclude that the substance of a closely related species may also be effective. Pike odor does not produce any fright reaction in conspecifics or closely related fishes since there is no alarm substance in the pike.

Interspecific tests: Von Frisch (1941b), studying Cyprinidae, first noted an interspecific reaction to the alarm substance and many subsequent tests have confirmed his finding. Within the Ostariophysi and the Gonorhynchiformes there is evidently a strong similarity in the alarm substance (Pfeiffer 1967b). However, there may be differences in the substance. According to Schutz (1956) the most marked response is obtained with the alarm substance from the same species. Many tests have shown that interspecific reactions are especially strong in taxonomically close species. According to present evidence, the alarm substance is universally effective within the Cypriniformes *sensu* Greenwood et al. (1966) provided that: 1) the skin-extract of the species possesses alarm substance; and 2) the species tested possesses the ability to respond to the alarm substance. Comparisons of the alarm substance of *Phoxinus* and *Danio* (Cyprinidae) with *Alestes longipinnis* (Günther) (Characidae) indicated that the alarm substance of all three species was identical (Pfeiffer and Lemke 1973). Further, the results with *Kneria* and *Phractolaemus* on the one hand and *Gymnocorymbus* and *Puntius* on the other indicate that the alarm substance from Gonorhynchiformes is effective in the Ostariophysi and vice versa (table 14.2) (Pfeiffer 1967b). There are various reasons for investigating interspecific reactions: 1) whether interspecific reactions occur (Von Frisch 1941b), and how strong they are (Schutz 1956); 2) whether species which do not react to their own skin extract possess the alarm substance or lack the ability to respond; 3) whether the ability to respond to the alarm substance is inherited (Pfeiffer 1963c, 1966a).

14.3.6. Genetics of the fright reaction

The characid *Astyanax bimaculatus* (L.) has a well developed fright reaction. However, the ability to respond to the alarm substance seems to be absent in the cave-fishes *Anoptichthys* (Schutz 1956; Pfeiffer 1963c). The blind cave-fishes can be crossed with the eyed river fish. Since the F_1 hybrids are completely fertile,

TABLE 14.2

Summary of the tests performed between families. Skin extract of the one family produced a fright reaction in members of the other family (to which the arrow is pointing). Data (1b, 4a, b) from Schutz (1956) and (the others) from Pfeiffer (1963c, 1967b).

1) Within the Cyprinoidei:			
a)	Cyprinidae	⇄	Catostomidae
b)	Cyprinidae	→	Cobitidae
2) Within the Characoidei:			
a)	Characinae	→	Tetragonopterinae
b)	Glandulocaudinae	→	Tetragonopterinae
c)	Pyrrhulinae	→	Tetragonopterinae
d)	Serrasalminae	→	Tetragonopterinae
e)	Mylinae	→	Tetragonopterinae
f)	Anostomidae	→	Characidae
g)	Gasteropelecidae	→	Characidae
3) Between Cyprinoidei and Characoidei:			
a)	Cyprinidae	⇄	Characidae
4) Between Cypriniformes and Siluriformes:			
a)	Cyprinidae	→	Ictaluridae
b)	Cyprinidae	←	Callichthyidae
5) Within the Gonorhynchiformes:			
a)	Kneriidae	⇄	Phractolaemidae
6) Between Ostariophysi and Gonorhynchiformes:			
a)	Characidae	⇄	Kneriidae
b)	Cyprinidae	⇄	Kneriidae

both the cave-fishes and the river fish may be considered as ecological races or highly differentiated populations of *Astyanax bimaculatus*. More than 300 fish, hybrids between *Astyanax* and *Anoptichthys antrobius* Alvarez, were tested individually with the alarm substance to study the inheritance of the response to this substance (Pfeiffer 1966a). All 43 F_1 hybrids tested responded to the alarm substance. From 210 F_2 hybrids only 197 showed the fright reaction. There was no correlation with the size of the eye or with the degree of pigmentation. From 55 R hybrids (i.e., the backcross from F_1 x *Anoptichthys*) only 47 responded to the alarm substance. It is presumed that fish which did not respond to the alarm substance lack the ability to respond. The result with the F_1 hybrids indicates that the river fish is homozygous for the reaction, and that the cave-fish is homozygous for the absence of the ability to react. Approximately one-sixteenth of the fish in the F_2 did not react, which indicates that there are two dominant factors which are segregating independently from each other. The dominant alleles are responsible for the reaction, and the recessive alleles are responsible for the lack of reaction. A single dominant allele seems to be required for the reaction. The result with the R hybrids fits this hypothesis. The number of non-responding fish was relatively greater than in the F_2 generation. It would be interesting to know whether fish which fail to respond do not smell the substance or are not capable of reacting. To me the second assumption seems more plausible. As a result of recessive mutation one link in the chain from the perception of the alarm substance to the reaction is lost in the non-responding blind cave-fishes.

14.3.7. Contribution of the fright reaction to taxonomy

Greenwood et al. (1966) revised the taxonomy of the Teleostei on the basis of the osteology of recent species (fig. 14.5a). The following were the major changes: 1) the order of Isospondyli is divided since it is considered a polyphyletic assemblage; 2) the Gonorhynchiformes are considered a separate order; 3) the Gonorhynchiformes are considered as derived from salmonoids; 4) the Ostariophysi are

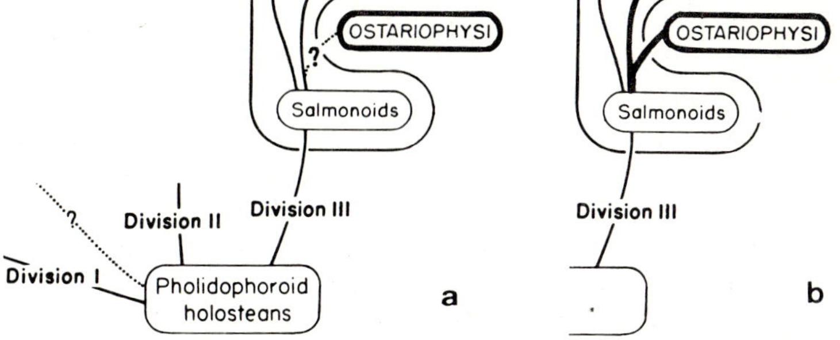

Fig. 14.5. Concepts of the relationship of the Ostariophysi with the other fishes. Uncertain relationships are shown by broken line and question mark. a) From Greenwood et al. (1966); b) modification according to the results with the fright reaction by Pfeiffer (1967b).

considered as possibly derived from salmonoids with a question mark in Greenwood's figure. Thus it is clearly indicated that the Ostariophysi have common ancestors with the Gonorhynchiformes. Characteristics common to both Gonorhynchiformes and Ostariophysi were detected with the fright reaction, the alarm substance and the alarm substance cells (Pfeiffer 1967c). The alarm substance cells (visible histologically) and the alarm substance (demonstrated in behavioral experiment) are closely connected with each other, since the alarm substance is derived from the alarm substance cells. In contrast, the presence of the alarm substance in the skin and the ability to respond to it are independent of each other (Pfeiffer 1960b, 1963c). Their coincidence is of functional significance: the fright reaction will appear only if both components are present. Alone, each component lacks biological significance. The fright reaction may be considered one complex feature. The alarm substance of the Gonorhynchiformes and Ostariophysi is similar or identical; otherwise it would not be effective reciprocally in both orders. Consequently, the ability to respond to the alarm substance must be similar or identical in both orders. The fright reaction demonstrates that the Ostariophysi and Gonorhynchiformes form a natural group and derive from common ancestors. The questionable systematic position of the Ostariophysi in the classification of Greenwood et al. (1966) is now beyond question according to findings with the fright reaction (fig. 14.5b). Since the Ostariophysi and Gonorhynchiformes are derived from salmonoid like fishes the fright reaction might have evolved within the salmonoids. Actually, club cells which are very similar in shape to the alarm substance cells of the Gonorhynchiformes and Ostariophysi were found in the epidermis of *Galaxias attenuatus* (Jenyns) (Galaxiidae, Salmoniformes) by Pfeiffer (1969a). However, whether they are alarm substance cells, must await experiments on the fright reaction with the Galaxiidae.

14.3.8. Biological significance of the fright reaction

Von Frisch (1941b) postulated that such a widespread reaction must have profound biological significance, and an understanding of its meaning was a primary objective of many of his experiments. The group of fishes which show this reaction are mostly social; they lack defensive structures and are generally non-predaceous. Von Frisch assumed that the damage to a minnow's skin by the sharp teeth of a pike would be sufficient to elicit the fright reaction and thus to protect other members of the school. This aspect of the problem was investigated. The water in an aquarium, where a pike (*Esox lucius* L.) lived, was tested for the presence of alarm substance before and after the pike had eaten a minnow (*Phoxinus*). These studies showed clearly that the capture of a minnow by a pike created damage sufficient to initiate a fright reaction. Recently Verheijen and Reuter (1969) confirmed that enough alarm substance was given off when a pike swallowed a minnow. The odor of the pike, by itself, did not provoke a fright reaction in schools of minnows that had not had previous experiences with the predaceous activities of pike. However, Göz (1941) showed that minnows quickly learn the odor of pike and that pike odor alone will produce a marked reaction in fish which have experience with pike odor in combination with the alarm substance. Göz used blinded minnows which showed no initial response to pike odor. After some of the blinded members had been attacked by a pike, the remainder showed alarm reactions to pike odor in absence of alarm substance. Recently Reed (1969) reports predator odor capable of eliciting an alarm response in local prey species in the American pike and various Perciformes. Von Frisch (1941b) has shown that a school of minnows reacts more intensely to the alarm substance if the water also contains the odor of the pike. Immature individuals of the predaceous northern squawfish, *Ptychocheilus oregonense* (Richardson), showed a marked fright reaction after eating a smaller conspecific, and it was proven that alarm substance was released (passively, of course!) (Pfeiffer 1962d). It is evident, however, that a pike with its sharp teeth injures its prey more than a toothless cyprinid does.

In field experiments, Von Frisch (1941b) noted repeatedly that minnows which became alarmed in the region of the feeding tube would subsequently feed much less readily there than in nearby areas. The fright reaction changes the behavior of the fish fundamentally; they not only swim away, but their vigilance and readiness to flee are increased and they are particularly wary of the area where they were frightened. Twice Von Frisch observed the fright reaction under natural conditions: once when a perch captured a member of a school of minnows, and again when a bittern caught and dropped a member of a school of bleaks. Another aspect of the value of the reaction is seen in ontogenetic relationships. Very young minnows possess the alarm substance in their skins but fail to respond until they are about 4–6 weeks old. An older fish, after eating or injuring a very small individual, will be alarmed, swim away and avoid the schools of small fish. Consequently, the small juveniles may be protected from the cannibalistic attacks of the adults (Schutz 1956). Verheijen (1962), admitting that it is difficult to provide direct evidence pro or contra this supposed function of the alarm substance, was cautious about accepting the theory that alarm substance prevents intra-specific predation. Verheijen (1959b) assumed that if the alarm substance was absent, as for example in the Clupeidae, the fish would not be protected from cannibalism. This is an incorrect assumption since schools of fish may be alarmed by visual, auditory and other cues as well as by olfactory ones. The fright reaction elicited by the alarm substance is only one type of alarm reaction found among fishes. Under certain conditions *Phoxinus* are cannibalistic (Von Frisch 1941b). A number of Cyprinidae are well known to be predaceous when adult. In the American northern squawfish (*Ptychocheilus*) intraspecific predation is common under certain circumstances, although young individuals of this species have a well developed fright reaction (Pfeiffer 1963a). Gandolfi et al. (1968a) suggest that, at high dilutions of the alarm substance, only a minority of the individuals of a school react to it while the rest of the shoal depends on visual signals. However, there is no evidence that this assumption is justified. Further, Gandolfi et al. (1968a) believe that the individuals which respond to the alarm substance itself would be at a disadvantage, attracting the attention of the predator. Actually, this assumption is based upon experiments with models under artificial conditions. An alarmed fish will swim to and fro wriggling its tail as Gandolfi's model did only in the aquarium; in nature an alarmed fish will flee, i.e., swim hastily and immediately be followed by its conspecifics. There is no reason to assume that the more sensitive individuals would be at a disadvantage. On the contrary, the opposite is very probably; the more sensitive individual may be at an advantage.

Thus, in several ways the evolution of the fright reaction in the Ostariophysi and Gonorhynchiformes is an important insurance against predation. The alarm substance does not protect the individual but serves for the protection of its school. It is of greatest value in social life. The strong schooling tendencies, especially in juveniles, become more understandable with the demonstration of this reaction. Obviously all species of the Ostariophysi without the fright reaction differ markedly from a cyprinid-like fish. Blind cave-fish, predaceous piranha, armored catfish and electric knife fishes are end stages of different lines of evolution. It seems important to me that the fright reaction was found in all cyprinid-like species studies. The biological significance of the fright reaction for the great majority of the Ostariophysi seems to be demonstrated by the fact that an ostariophysean species cannot afford to lose the fright reaction without compensating for it by another ability or a different way of life. The fright reaction has probably contributed markedly to the biological success of the Ostariophysi–the group which constitutes the majority of fresh-water fishes and consists in some 5000 to 6000 known species. The present distribution of the fright reaction suggests an evolution of the reaction prior to the divergence of the Gonorhynchiformes and Ostariophysi. This would indicate an evolution of the alarm substance and the fright reaction as early as the Cretaceous or Jurassic.

14.4. *Pheromones in amphibia: fright reaction*

Eibl-Eibesfeldt (1949) and Hrbacek (1950) described a fright reaction in the tadpoles of *Bufo bufo* (L.) and the tadpole reaction was more completely investigated by Kulzer (1954) and Pfeiffer (1966b). It is a similar reaction to that of the Ostariophysi and Gonorhynchiformes, produced by a pheromone released from injured animals.

14.4.1. *The fright reaction*

The fright reaction of the tadpoles of the common toad *Bufo bufo* was studied by Kulzer (1954) both in the field and in the laboratory. In 23 field experiments a crushed tadpole was brought near a tadpole school and a strong fright reaction resulted. The animals closest to the extract became disturbed and swam into deeper water, while the neighboring animals turned or tried to avoid the place occupied by the crushed tadpole. The oriented, parallel-swimming, schooling pattern was disturbed. The method in the tadpole experiments was analogous to that applied in the minnow experiments. After skin-extract had been poured into the tank, some animals immediately left the feeding area; all animals left within a few minutes. The tadpoles swam toward the bottom or to the corner of the tank opposite the feeding place. The effect of the extract diminished after two minutes and the tadpoles then began to return slowly to the feeding area. The reactions were consistent. The alarm substance is perceived by the olfactory organ only. When the olfactory nerve was transected the tadpoles no longer responded. More recently Pfeiffer (1966b) studied the fright reaction of anuran tadpoles in more than 100 experiments with as many different experimental groups belonging to the Bufonidae, Pipidae, Discoglossidae, Hylidae, and Ranidae. It was observed in tadpoles of *Bufo bufo* and of the natterjack toad, *Bufo calamita* Laurenti. However, a fright reaction was not found in any anurans that did not belong to the Bufonidae: i.e., *Xenopus leavis* Wagler, *Alytes obstetricans* (Laurenti), *Bombina variegata* (L.), *Hyla arborea* (L.), *Rana temporaria* L., *Rana esculenta* L., and *Rana pipiens* Schreber. Eibl-Eibesfeldt (1962) reports a fright reaction for the tadpoles of *Discoglossus pictus* Otth. However, since the reaction is absent in all relatives of *Discoglossus* studied (i.e., *Alytes*, *Bombina*, *Xenopus*) its existence in *Discoglossus* is questioned. It is suspected that the fright reaction commonly occurs in the genus *Bufo* or in the family Bufonidae and that it is confined to this systematic group. The alarm substance from *Bufo bufo* was effective with *Bufo calamita* while tadpoles of *Bufo bufo* responded to the alarm substance from *Bufo calamita*. Anurans not belonging to the Bufonidae did not respond to the alarm substance from bufonid tadpoles while the bufonid tadpoles did not respond to the skin extracts from nonbufonids (Pfeiffer 1966b). Thus the nonbufonids lack both the alarm substance and the ability to respond.

14.4.2. Alarm substance

Skins from all anuran species tested were compared histologically (Pfeiffer 1966b). It was found that the bufonid tadpoles have large cells in their epidermis that are absent in the skin of the nonbufonids. Because of the size and uncertain function of these cells, the name 'Riesenzellen' (giant cells) was proposed. The giant cells extend to the surface of the epidermis but have no external opening; they are probably glandular. They are distributed uniformly over the body surface. There are at least two arguments against the multicellular glands as the source of the alarm substance: a) they open to the surface of the epidermis, whereas the alarm substance is secreted only when the skin is damaged; b) they develop during metamorphosis and are absent in young tadpoles, but young tadpoles have the alarm substance as soon as they are free swimming. Nevertheless, it is possible that the giant-cells of *Bufo* may produce alarm substance since: 1) giant-cells are restricted to the systematic group that has the alarm substance; 2) they do not open on the epidermal surface; and 3) they are present in very young tadpoles. We know little about the chemistry of the alarm substance of tadpoles. It seemed possible that the alarm substance might be identical with poisonous secretions of the toad. However, extracts of parotic gland were tested and found to be less effective than skin extracts. Kulzer (1954) tested a series of substances, some of which were not effective while others produced some response. The effectiveness of bufotoxin and gama-bufotoxin ('gama' is Japanese and means 'toad') could not be distinguished from that of skin extracts. Two mg of each of the substances were diluted in two ml of water. This solution retained its effectiveness after repeated dilution; 0.05 ml diluted in 500 ml water was still effective. Paper chromatograms of skin extracts showed similar distributions for both the alarm substance and the bufotoxin or gama-bufotoxin. In addition, absorption spectra of both substances were similar, but these results did not prove that both substances were identical.

14.4.3. Factors influencing the fright reaction

In contrast to the fish, tadpoles did not respond to fright movements of their associates. Kulzer (1954) placed two aquaria side by side and poured alarm substance in one tank. Only the tadpoles exposed to the alarm substance fled. In contrast to very young fish, newly hatched tadpoles immediately reacted to the extract of their companions which were the same age. Before metamorphosis, the intensity of the reaction became maximal. The tadpoles during metamorphosis responded to the alarm substance as long as they came to the feeding place in the aquarium. Also, the skin of small toads contained an effective alarm substance. It was demonstrated that neither food nor the duration of captivity has any influence on the responsiveness of tadpoles. In contrast to fish, the reaction of the tadpoles is more vigorous in warm water. Further, fish often become unresponsive to the alarm substance after a few tests, while this is not the case with tadpoles. Normal responsiveness to alarm substance is present within a day after a test. The effect of the minnow (*Phoxinus*) alarm substance on tadpole schools (*Bufo*) and the effect of the tadpole alarm substance on minnow schools was studied by Kulzer (1954) and Schutz (1956) with negative reactions in both cases. Thus, the fright reaction of *Bufo* tadpoles is convergent with that of the Ostariophysi and Gonorhynchiformes. From existing evidence, we may assume that the fright reaction of anuran tadpoles is an important insurance against predation. The schooling tendency of the bufonid tadpoles becomes more understandable with this reaction. The alarm substance protects the shoal; it is logically of greatest value in species exhibiting social life.

References

Baerends, G. P. (1971) The ethological analysis of fish behavior. In: Fish Physiology. vol. 6; eds.: W. S. Hoar and D. J. Randall (Academic Press, New York and London) pp. 279–370.

Bardach, J. E. and J. Atema (1971) The sense of taste in fishes. *In*: Handbook of Sensory Physiology. vol. 4, part (2); eds.: H. Autrum, R. Jung, W. R. Loewenstein, D. M. Mackay and H. L. Teuber (Springer-Verlag, Berlin, Heidelberg, New York) pp. 293–336.

Breder, C. M. (1935) The reproductive habits of the common catfish, *Ameiurus nebulosus* (Le Sueur), with a discussion of their significance in ontogeny and phylogeny. Zoologica 19, 143–185.

Eggert, B. (1931) Die Geschlechtsorgane der Gobiiformes und Blenniiformes. Z. wiss. Zool. 139, 249–558.

Eibl-Eibesfeldt, I. (1949) Über das Vorkommen von Schreckstoffen bei Erdkrötenquappen. Experientia 5, 236.

Eibl-Eibesfeldt, I. (1962) Die Verhaltensentwicklung des Krallenfrosches (*Xenopus laevis*) und des Scheibenzünglers (*Discoglossus pictus*) unter besonderer Berücksichtigung der Beutefanghandlungen. Z. Tierpsychol. 19, 385–393.

Frisch, K. Von (1938) Zur Psychologie des Fisch-Schwarmes. Naturwissenschaften 26, 601–606.

Frisch, K. Von (1941a) Die Bedeutung des Geruchsinnes im Leben der Fische. Naturwissenschaften 29, 321–333.

Frisch, K. Von (1941b) Über einen Schreckstoff der Fischhaut und seine biologische Bedeutung. Z. Vergl. Physiol. 29, 46–145.

Frisch, K. Von (1955) Schreckstoffwirkung bei der Elritze. Film von 1939 (Institut für den Wissenschaftlichen Film, Göttingen).

Frisch, K. Von (1961) Gerüche als Lock- und Schreckstoffe. *In*: Ausgewählte Vorträge 1911-1969; ed.: K. Von Frisch, (BLV München, Basel, Wien, 1970) pp. 203–214.

Gandolfi, G. (1968) Reazione di paura nel cyprinide *Brachydanio rerio*: variazioni della reattività indotte sperimentalmente. Arch. Zool. Ital. 53, 245–259.

Gandolfi, G., D. Mainardi and A. C. Rossi (1968a) La reazione di paura e lo svantaggio individuale dei pesci allarmisti (esperimenti con modelli). Rend. Inst. Lomb. Sci. Lett. B 102, 8–14.

Gandolfi, G., D. Mainardi and A. C. Rossi (1968b) The fright reaction of zebra fish. Atti Soc. Ital. Sci. Natur. 57, 74–88.

Gehlbach, F. R., J. F. Watkins and J. C. Kroll (1971) Pheromone trail-following studies of typhlopid, leptotyphlopid, and colubrid snakes. Behaviour 40, 282–294.

Göz, H. (1941) Über den Art- und Individualgeruch bei Fischen. Z. Vergl. Physiol. 29, 1–45.

Greenwood, P. H., D. E. Rosen, S. H. Weitzman and G. S. Myers (1966) Phyletic studies of teleostean fishes, with a provisional classification of living forms. Bull. Am. Mus. Nat. Hist. 131, 339–455.

Hara, T. J. (1971) Chemoreception. *In*: Fish Physiology. vol. 5; eds.: W. S. Hoar and D. J. Randall (Academic Press, New York and London) pp. 79–120.

Harden Jones, F. R. (1968) Fish Migration (Edward Arnold Ltd. London).

Hasler, A. D. (1957) Olfactory and gustatory senses of fishes. *In*: The Physiology of Fishes; vol. 2; ed.: M. E. Brown (Academic Press, New York) pp. 187–209.

Hasler, A. D., (1971) Orientation and fish migration. In: Fish Physiology. vol. 6; eds.: W. S. Hoar and D. J. Randall (Academic Press, New York and London) pp. 429–510.

Hemmings, C. C. (1966) Olfaction and vision in fish schooling. J. Exptl. Biol. 45, 449–464.

Hrbacek, J. (1950) On the flight reaction of tadpoles of the common toad caused by chemical substances. Experientia 6, 100–102.

Hüttel, R. (1941) Die chemische Untersuchung des Schreckstoffes aus Elritzenhaut. Naturwissenschaften 29, 333–334.

Jaski, C. J. (1939) Ein Oestruszyklus bei *Lebistes reticulatus* (Peters). Proc. Ned. Akad. Wetensch. 42, 201–207.

Karlson, P. (1960) Pheromones. Ergebn. Biol. 22, 212–225.

Karlson, P. and M. Lüscher (1959a) 'Pheromone', ein Nomenklaturvorschlag für eine Wirkstoffklasse. Naturwissenschaften 46, 63–64.

Karlson, P. and M. Lüscher (1959b) 'Pheromones': a new term for a class of biologically active substances. Nature (London) 183, 55–56.

Keenleyside, M. H. A. (1955) Some aspects of the schooling behaviour of fish. Behaviour 8, 183–248.

Klauber, L. M. (1936) A statistical study of rattlesnakes. Occas. Pap. S. Diego Soc., 1–24.

Kleerekoper, H. (1969) Olfaction in Fishes (Indiana University Press, Bloomington, London).

Konishi, J. and Y. Zotterman (1963) Taste function in fish. *In*: Olfaction and Taste. Proc. First Int. Symp. Wenner-Gren Center, Stockholm, Sept. 1962; ed.: Y. Zotterman (Pergamon Press, New York) pp. 215–233.

Kühme, W. (1963) Chemisch ausgelöste Brutpflege und Schwarmreaktionen bei *Hemichromis bimaculatus* (Peters). Z. Tierpsychol. 20, 688–704.

Kühme, W. (1964a) Eine chemisch ausgelöste Brutpflegereaktion bei Cichliden (Pisces). Naturwissenschaften 51, 20–21.

Kühme, W. (1964b) Eine chemisch ausgelöste Schwarmreaktion bei jungen Cichliden (Pisces). Naturwissenschaften 51, 120–121.

Kulzer, E. (1954) Untersuchungen über die Schreckreaktion bei Erdkrötenkaulquappen (*Bufo bufo* L.) Z. Vergl. Physiol. 36, 443–463.

Losey, G. S. (1969) Sexual pheromone in some fishes of the genus *Hypsoblennius* Gill. Science 163, 181–183.

MacGinite, G. E. (1939) The natural history of the blind goby, *Typhlogobius californiensis* Steindachner. Amer. Midl. Natur. 21, 489–505.

Myrberg, A. A. (1966) Parental recognition of young in cichlid fishes. Anim. Behav. 14, 565–571.

Noble, G. K. (1937) The sense organs involved in the courtship of *Storeria*, *Thamnophis* and other snakes. Bull. Am. Mus. Nat. Hist. 73, 673–725.

Noble, G. K. (1939) The experimental animal from the naturalist's point of view. Am. Natur. 73, 113–126.

Nordeng, H. (1971) Is the local orientation of anadromous fishes determined by pheromones? Nature (London) 233, 411–413.

Oshima, K., W. E. Hahn and A. Gorbman (1969) Olfactory discrimination of natural waters of salmon. J. Fish. Res. Can. 26, 2111–2121.

Pfeiffer, W. (1960a) Über die Verbreitung der Schreckreaktion bei Fischen. Naturwissenschaften 47, 23; also in: Bull. St. Biol. Arcach. 12.

Pfeiffer, W. (1960b) Über die Schreckreaktion bei Fischen und die Herkunft des Schreckstoffes. Z. Vergl. Physiol. 43, 578–614; also in: Bull. St. Biol. Arcach. 13.

Pfeiffer, W. (1962a) Die Verbreitung der Schreckreaktion bei nord-amerikanischen Fischen. Naturwissenschaften 49, 141.

Pfeiffer, W. (1962b) The fright reaction of Fish. Biol. Rev. Cambridge Phil. Soc. 37, 495–511; also in: Bull. St. Biol. Arcach. 15; shortened also in: C. L. Kutcher ed., Readings in Comparative Studies of Animal Behavior, 1971 (Xerox College Publishing, Waltham, Massachusetts - Toronto).

Pfeiffer, W. (1962c) Uber die Verbreitung der Schreckreaktion bei Salmlern (Characidae) und Welsen (Siluroidea). Naturwissenschaften 49, 614.

Pfeiffer, W. (1962d) The fright reaction in American fish. Am. Zool. 2, 437.
Pfeiffer, W. (1963a) The fright reaction in North American fish. Can. J. Zool. 41, 69–77.
Pfeiffer, W. (1963b) Alarm substances. Experientia 19, 113–123.
Pfeiffer, W. (1963c) Vergleichende Untersuchungen über die Schreck-reaktion und den Schreckstoff der Ostariophysen. Z. Vergl. Physiol. 47, 111–147.
Pfeiffer, W. (1966a) Über die Vererbung der Schreckreaktion bei *Astyanax* (Characidae, Pisces). Z. Vererbungslehre 98, 97–105.
Pfeiffer, W. (1966b) Die Verbreitung der Schreckreaktion bei Kaulquappen und die Herkunft des Schreckstoffes. Z. Vergl. Physiol. 52, 79–98.
Pfeiffer, W. (1966c) Die Schreckreaktion der Fische und Kaulquappen. Naturwissenschaften 53, 565–570.
Pfeiffer, W. (1967a) Schreckreaktion und Schreckstoffzellen bei Kneriidae und Phractolaemidae (Isospondyli, Pisces). Naturwissenschaften 54, 177.
Pfeiffer, W. (1967b) Schreckreaktion und Schreckstoffzellen bei Ostariophysi und Gonorhynchiformes. Z. Vergl. Physiol. 56, 380–396.
Pfeiffer, W. (1968a) Die Fahrenholzschen Organe der Dipnoi und Brachiopterygii. Z. Zellforsch. 90, 127–147.
Pfeiffer, W. (1968b) Über die Epidermis von *Latimeria chalumnae* J. L. B. Smith 1939 (Crossopterygii, Pisces). Z. Morphol. Tiere. 63, 419–427.
Pfeiffer, W. (1968c) Das Geruchsorgan der Polypteridae (Pisces, Brachiopterygii). Z. Morphol. Tiere 63, 75–110.
Pfeiffer, W. (1969a) Kolbenzellen in der Epidermis der Galaxiidae, *Galaxias attenuatus* (Salmoniformes). Experientia 25, 432.
Pfeiffer, W. (1969b) Der Geruchssinn der Polypteridae (Pisces, Brachiopterygii). Z. Vergl. Physiol. 63, 151–164.
Pfeiffer, W. (1969c) Das Geruchsorgan der rezenten Actinistia und Dipnoi (Pisces). Z. Morphol. Tiere 64, 309–337.
Pfeiffer, W. (1970) Über die Schreckstoffzellen der Siluriformes (Ostariophysi, Pisces). Anat. Anz. 126, 113–119.
Pfeiffer, W. (1971) Bau, Leistung und biologische Bedeutung des Geruchsorgans der Knochenfische . Naturwissenschaftliche Rundschau 24, 417–423.
Pfeiffer, W. and J. Lemke (1973) Untersuchungen zur Isolierung und Identifizierung des Schreckstoffes aus der Haut der Elritze, *Phoxinus phoxinus* (L.) (Cyprinidae, Ostariophysi, Pisces). J. Comp. Physiol. 82, 407–410.
Pfeiffer, W., D. Sasse and M. Arnold (1971) Die Schreckstoffzellen von *Phoxinus phoxinus* und *Morulius chrysophakedion* (Cyprinidae, Ostariophysi, Pisces). Histochemische und elektronenmikroskopische Untersuchungen. Z. Zellforsch. 118, 203–213.
Reed, J. R. (1969) Alarm substances and fright reaction in some fishes from the southeastern United States. Trans. Am. Fish. Soc. 98, 664–668.
Reutter, K. and W. Pfeiffer (1973) Fluoreszenzmikroskopischer Nachweis des Schreckstoffes in den Schreckstoffzellen der Elritze, *Phoxinus phoxinus* (L.) (Cyprinidae, Ostariophysi, Pisces). J. Comp. Physiol. 82, 411–418.
Rosenblatt, R. H. and G. S. Losey (1967) Alarm reaction of the top smelt, *Atherinops affinis*: re-examination. Science 158, 671–672.
Scharrer., E., S. W. Smith and S. L. Palay (1947) Chemical sense and taste in the fishes, *Prionotus* and *Trichogaster*. J. Comp. Neurol. 86, 183–198.
Schutz, F. (1956) Vergleichende Untersuchungen über die Schreckreaktion bei Fischen und deren Verbreitung. Z. Vergl. Physiol. 38, 84–135.
Skinner, W. A., R. D. Mathews and R. M. Parkhurst (1962) Alarm reaction of the top smelt, *Atherinops affinis* (Ayres). Science 138, 681–682.

Snyder, N. F. R. (1967) An alarm reaction of aquatic gastropods to intraspecific extract. Cornell University, Agricultural Experiment Station, New York State College of Agriculture, Ithaca, New York, Memoir 403.

Tavolga, W. N. (1956) Visual, chemical and sound stimuli as cues in the sex discriminatory behavior of the gobiid fish, *Bathygobius soporator*. Zoologica 41, 49–64.

Teichmann, H. (1962) Die Chemorezeption der Fische. Ergeb. Biol. 25, 177–205.

Thines, G. and E. Vandenbussche (1966) The effects of alarm substance on the schooling behaviour of *Rasbora heteromorpha* Duncker in day and night conditions. Anim. Behav. 14, 296–302.

Todd, J. H., J. Atema and J. E. Bardach (1967) Chemical communication in social behavior of a fish, the yellow bullhead (*Ictalurus natalis*). Science 158, 672–673.

Tucker. D. and N. Suzuki (1972) Olfactory responses to Schreckstoff of catfish. *In*: Olfaction and Taste 4. Proc. 4th Int. Symp. held in Starnberg, Germany, August 2-4, 1971; ed.: D. Schneider (Wissenschaftl. Verlagsges. mbH, Stuttgart) pp. 121–127.

Verheijen, F. J. (1956) Transmission of a flight reaction amongst a school of fish and the underlying sensory mechanisms. Experientia 12, 202–204.

Verheijen, F. J. (1959a) Absence of alarm substance in some clupeids. Publ. Sta. Zool. Napoli, 31, 146–152.

Verheijen, F. J. (1959b) Aquarium studies: A new outlook in Sardine research. World scientific meeting on the biology of Sardines and related species. Rome, 14–21 September 1959. Experience Paper No. 10.

Verheijen, F. J. (1962) Alarm substance and intra-specific predation in Cyprinids. Naturwissenschaften 49, 356.

Verheijen, F. J. (1963) Alarm substance in some North American cyprinid fishes. Copeia 1963, 174–176.

Verheijen, F. J. and J. H. Reuter (1969) The effect of alarm substance on predation among cyprinids. Anim. Behav. 17, 551–554.

Wenzel, B. M. (1971) Olfaction in birds. *In*: Handbook of Sensory Physiology. vol. 4, part (1); eds.: H. Autrum, R. Jung, W. R. Loewenstein, D. M. Mackay and H. L. Teuber (Springer-Verlag, Berlin, Heidelberg, New York) pp. 432–448.

Wilkens, H. (1972) Über Präadaptationen für das Höhlenleben, untersucht am Laichverhalten ober- und unterirdischer Populationen des *Astyanax mexicanus* (Pisces). Zool. Anz. 188, 1–11.

Wrede, W. L. (1932) Versuche über den Artduft der Elritzen. Z. Vergl. Physiol. 17, 510–519.

Ziegler-Günder, I. (1956) Untersuchungen über die Purin- und Pterin-pigmente in der Haut und in den Augen der Weissfische. Z. Vergl. Physiol. 39, 163–189.

CHAPTER 15

The role of odor in the social biology of small mammals

D. Michael STODDART

15.1. Introduction

The existence of olfactory communication in many, or more probably most, mammal species cannot now be doubted (Mykytowycz 1970, 1972; Ralls, 1971; inter alia), but little experimentation with, and analysis of, odors has yet taken place. Until it does, the levels of dependence of naturally occurring rodent and other small mammal species upon olfactory communication cannot accurately be assessed. If odors are used for social purposes one might expect that the range of messages to be exchanged would be as large as the range of visual signals observed in social groups of large mammals. This is a point of fundamental importance that appears implicit in many recent writings on scent communication in mammals. The object of this chapter is to review the existing evidence supporting this assumption and to illuminate the areas deserving the attention of ethologists and ecologists wherein further supporting evidence should be sought.

Before considering the components of social organization it would be expedient for us to generalize on the way of life of most small mammals. By far the greatest proportion live either beneath the surface of the ground, or actually on the surface itself. Those living well above the surface, or in habitats where visual or acoustic social communication is possible, most frequently possess visual or acoustic adornment (e.g. Balph and Balph 1966; Ewer 1968). For the large majority of small mammals the denseness of the habitat precludes the use of visual or acoustic communication for many components in the repertoire of the social behavior. No doubt visual and acoustic signals are used in close range behavior patterns such as are seen in courtship and mating, but they would be likely to be less efficient for 'tele-advertizements' relating to dominance status, sexual condition, territory or range ownership. This argument is not to say that visual and acoustic signalling is more highly advanced in an evolutionary sense than olfactory signalling, but rather more to say that natural selection has favored the spread of species with well developed scent producing organs in habitats which tend to preclude the use of visual and acoustic signals.

Rodents and other small mammals are indeed richly endowed with odor producing organs of a specific nature (i.e. excluding any intrinsic olfactory 'benefit' derived from normally produced sweat, urine or feces, with or without any microbial decomposition (Shelley 1956)), but it would be unwise at the present state of our understanding of olfactory communication to suggest that small mammals possess more scent organs, or organs of greater complexity, than do large mammals. The principal sources of odors in small mammals are glands and gland complexes lodged in the skin.

It is not the place of this chapter to delve into the literature concerning gland sites and structure. Full details may be found in Dieterlen (1959), Eibl-Eibesfeldt (1953), Flowerdew (1971), Lehmann (1962, 1966, 1967, 1969a, b), Martan (1962), Niethammer (1969), Pearson (1946), Quay (1965 and 1968), Schultze-Westrum (1965), Stoddart (1972a, b), Vrtiš (1930, 1932), Wallin (1967), and others. Suffice it to say that glands are found at a wide variety of sites on the body in both rodent and insectivore species. Six zones seem to be particularly widely used, namely: the flank (and hip) in *Sorex*, many microtines including *Microtus*, *Pitymys*, *Arvicola*, *Alticola* and *Lagurus*, *Cricetus* and *Mesocricetus*; the sternal region – *Meriones*, *Rattus* spp.; the tail – *Perognathus*, *Dicrostonyx* and *Apodemus*; the head – *Petaurus*, possibly *Lemmus* and several others; the rump – *Lemmus* and *Cavia*; and mid-dorsal region – *Dipodomys*. Glands opening into the urinary or alimentary tract are also a source of odor in small mammals. The anal gland produces copious secretion in mustelids (Goethe 1964), ground squirrels (Sleggs 1926), marmots (Kratochvil 1964) and dormice (Koenig 1960). This gland may also be used more than is at present thought in those species which defecate at sites of social significance (e.g. *Microtus agrestis* L., *Arvicola terrestris* (L.), *Lemmus lemmus* (L.)). The preputial gland is recognized as a source of odor in rodents (Bronson and Caroom 1971) although whether the odor is expelled in the urine or not is still a matter of some debate. If it is expelled, the gland producing the taint may assume an enhanced social significance in those species urinating at specific sites. Although the structure of scent organs found in small mammals will not be reviewed here, a brief comment may be useful. Most of the glands and gland complexes opening onto the surface of the skin are modified sebaceous glands. Usually they are holocrine in production, the dead cell being expelled with the secretion (Lipkow 1954; Quay 1954; Stoddart 1972b; Vrtiš 1930) but frequently apocrine glands are also found in conjunction with the sebaceous glands (Pearson 1946). A point of fundamental importance to note is that usually the odor producing glands occur in discrete patches, or associations in the skin. Mykytowycz (1970) suggests that communication may not be the only role fulfilled by the scent organs and states that sebum may be required for nourishment and protection of the hair. If this were so, then a type of behavior analogous with preening in birds would be observed. That no such behavior has been recorded in those species with specialized areas can be taken as an indication that these areas are not used as reserves of hair conditioning fluid (but see Eisenberg 1963). Their discretion has necessitated the development of particular and specific behavior patterns (Frank 1957; Schultze-Westrum 1965; Thiessen et al. 1968) derived from existing patterns of behavior (Eibl-Eibesfeldt 1958).

Cutaneous glands appear to be largely under the control of sex hormones (Martan 1962; Mitchell 1965; Stoddart 1972a) but this may not be so in every species (Pearson 1946). Castration, followed by hormone implant or injection therapy causes the glands to continue functioning normally, as far as is known. Lack of this therapy causes atrophy and involution of the glands.

15.2. Chemical studies

Regrettably, rather little emphasis has been placed by ethologists and ecologists on the chemical composition of olfactory signals. This is one of the largest and most persistent gaps in our knowledge. We can not say with certainty that the same, or similar, groups of compounds occur in the olfactory secretions from even closely related species. All the known chemical analytical techniques have been employed to investigate the chemical composition of odors. Gas–liquid chromatography is favored by many workers since organic mixtures are readily separated, and this method allows the odor as produced by the animal to be examined. A wide variety of substances have been found, few, however, from small mammals. Working on the anal gland secretion of the red fox, Albone and Fox (1971) identified twelve volatile substances, including a base and a series of carboxylic acids (C_2 to C_6). Müller and Lamperle (1964) indicated twelve compounds in the orbital gland secretion of male red deer and seven compounds in the anal gland secretion of male alsatian dogs. Brownlee et al. (1969) isolated the main component of the tarsal gland secretion of *Odocoileus hemionus* (Rafinesque) and identified it to be *cis*-4-hydroxydodec-6-enoic acid lactone. Recently, Goodrich and Mykytowycz (1972) examined the compounds produced by various skin glands in the rabbit (*Oryctolagus cuniculus* L.). This is a particularly useful study since it combines the results of gas chromatography, thin layer chromatography and electrophoresis on agar and polyacrylamide gels. Anal and chin glands, sebum from the inguinal pouches, and whole inguinal gland homogenates were examined. The chin glands produce primarily proteins and carbohydrates and the concentration of them is far higher in males than it is in females. The inguinal gland is composed primarily of lipids, with much monoglyceride, diglyceride and triglyceride material present. Goodrich and Mykytowycz point out that sex differences and individual differences also occur, although they give no specific information of the latter.

As yet, few workers have examined the chemical composition of odors produced by rodents. Lederer (1950) pointed out that *castoreum* from the beaver (*Castor fiber* L.) contained no less than 45 different substances. Stevens and Erickson (1942) identified the main components of the musk from the musk-rat (*Ondatra zibethicus* (L.) as cyclopentadecanol and cycloheptadecanol and their corresponding ketones. While these studies may prove a useful basis of knowledge, it is a matter of considerable regret that no sound work has been conducted on the odors less attractive to the perfume industry, for it is in rats, mice and related species that most of the observations have been made of social behavior involving odors. Work is currently in progress on the composition of the odors produced by the flank organs of the water vole (*Arvicola terrestris*) and it would appear that not only are the odors of extreme complexity, but that the most complex odors are found in samples from male specimens (Stoddart, unpublished).

15.3. Behavioral, physiological and developmental studies

The literature on small mammals contains many records of specific patterns of behavior associated with the laying of scent gland secretions. Before describing the main patterns, it would be useful for us to reflect on the social roles of male and female mammals. Whatever else he may do, the principal role of the male is to compete amongst his fellows for a mate, since theoretically just one individual male of any species is probably capable of producing sufficient sperm to fertilize all the females of his species. In this way his role is the chief controlling factor in population regulation (Wynne-Edwards 1962). The social role of the female is not primarily to compete, but to live a more self-centered life than her mate and to rear young. Within the animal kingdom there are a myriad examples of the male being 'adorned' in some way such that intraspecific competition can reach its zenith of intensity prior to mating. The occurrence of visual adornments is quite acceptable to us – manes, tusks, horns and the like – but the occurrence of olfactory adornments is less so. It is to be hoped that increasing familiarity with this idea will bring about a change. The fact that odor producing organs are found in females of some species as well as males suggests that odor is not produced exclusively for male–male interaction. One must not exclude attractant odors used to establish or maintain the pair bond. The studies of Schultze-Westrum (1965), Goodrich and Mykytowycz (1972), Stoddart (unpublished) and others have demonstrated unequivocally that a greater repertoire and intensity of odors are produced by male animals. As far as is known, there is no species in which the female produces a greater quantity or a more complex odor than the male.

Several distinct and purposeful scent setting behaviors are known, all derived from primitive movement patterns. Since scent production appears to be seasonal (Quay 1953; Stoddart 1972a), these behaviors may not be observed at all times of the year and may only be exhibited at times when scent glands are active. The most important motor patterns with the ability to be canalized into marking behavior are those associated with stretching (i.e. an extension of the body and limbs followed by a flexion); ventral rubbing and side rubbings (left and right); those associated with the perineal drag (movement pattern occurring when a small mammal leaves its nest); and those associated with body grooming. It does not follow that social olfaction occurs only in those species with associated patterns of behavior, for many species appear to set scent passively from special organs.

The behavior of various Heteromyid rodents has been well described by Eisenberg (1963). Of these some have well defined discrete organs (*Perognathus*-Quay 1965) while others (*Microdipodops* and *Dipodomys*) have no discrete patch but an overall copious sebaceous secretion. The place where an animal has sand-bathed (side and ventrum rubbing) is often attractive to another animal. After examination, and sniffing, the spot is usually overmarked. It cannot be doubted that such loci act as information centers.

Although shrews (*Blarina*, *Sorex*, and *Suncus*) possess well defined lateral organs and a ventral organ (Dryden and Conaway 1967; Pearson 1946), there does not appear to be any special behavior associated with the setting of the scent. The lateral organs are positioned on the flanks immediately behind the ribs and are supposed by Pearson to mark passively the walls of the burrows as the animal passes along. A flank organ occurs in both sexes of the microtine *Arvicola terrestris* (Vrtiš 1930), but in this species a specialized form of scent setting behavior has been reported. The vole employs a modification of the normal grooming behavior to stroke the flank organ with a hind foot. The foot is then stamped onto the ground in a marking drumming behavior (Frank 1957). *A. terrestris* is an interesting species in that the spatial organization of populations remains very constant for long periods of time. The degree of constance implies that there is a well defined communication for spacing behavior (Stoddart 1970). Further, the secretory output from the flank organs varies during the year reaching a peak at the time the first born of the year are weaned (Stoddart 1972a; Vrtiš 1930). Flank organs are observable from four days of age (Vrtiš 1930), and young voles are able to obtain, and successfully retain, an individual range from 21 days old – shortly after the age at which weaning occurs. Stoddart (1971) has shown that the young born in the first litter of the year are much more likely to survive until the following breeding season than young born in later litters. Considering that secretory output is maximal at the time the first litter becomes independent, it is tempting to suggest that the weanlings are in command of a complex olfactory repertoire from a very early age and are able to seize the available individual range sites so effectively that later aspirants are prevented from settling. Studies are in progress to verify these suggestions.

From his careful developmental study of the scent glands of the short-tailed shrew (*Blarina brevicauda* Say) Pearson (1946) states that both lateral organs and the ventral organ are visible at an age of 5 days. In adult males the lateral organs are usually thicker (and more productive?) than the ventral, while the reverse is usually true for females. The lateral organs of pregnant females are greatly reduced and are sometimes only visible histologically. They are slightly better developed during lactation and when the shrew is in estrus. During winter, and in an estrus, the organs are well developed with little size difference between males and females. Pearson concludes that the organs are used in some social context, but was unable to investigate marking behavior or when the scent was set.

The relationship between scent organ productivity and the breeding season has now been demonstrated sufficiently frequently for there to be little doubt as to its validity. In all species of *Dipodomys*, except *elephantinus* Grinnel, *margaritae* Merriam and *mitchelli* Mearns, the mid-dorsal organ is maximally productive during the breeding season and comparatively quiescent during the non-breeding time. In each of the species studied in depth (Quay 1953: *merriami* Mearns, *agilis* Gambel, *heermanni* Le Conte, *deserti* Stephens and *ordi* Woodhouse) a higher proportion of males than females was found to be secreting at all times of the year and the size (area) of the organ in females only rarely surpassed that of males.

Sebaceous gland organs occur in the flanks of several species of cricetid and microtid rodents (*Cricetus cricetus* L., *Mesocricetus auratus* Waterhouse, *Microtus xanthognatus* Leach, *M. chrotorrhinus* Miller, *Neofiber alleni* True, *Chilotus* and *Lagurus*). Eibl-Eibesfeldt (1953) reports that both sexes of *Cricetus cricetus* possess flank organs, the secretions of which are rubbed on the inner walls of the burrows and on the burrow entrances. The bases of grass tussocks and flat stones are also marked and the secretion may be so plentiful on the latter as to be quite visible. The position of the organs in this species appears to be well suited for its role in passive marking. Lipkow (1954) regards the position of the flank organ in *Mesocricetus auratus* as an adaptation to the hamster's partially subterranean way of life. Regrettably, little is known about any specialized behaviors associated with the flank organs in *Microtus*, *Neofiber*, *Chilotus* and *Lagurus*, but it is thought that these rodents transfer secretion in a passive manner.

Little can be said about integumentary scent glands in the murids, or the behavioral context in which they are used. Mice of the genus *Apodemus* have a well formed sebaceous gland complex in the skin of the ventral aspect of the proximal third of the tail (Niethammer 1969; Flowerdew 1971; Stoddart, 1972b), and mice of the genus *Perognathus* have a similar organ in a similar position (Quay 1965). No specific behavior has been observed to be associated with odor spreading, but possibly odor is deposited during the perineal drag following defecation and urination. Preliminary work on the caudal organ of *Apodemus* spp. (Stoddart unpublished) shows that much greater chemical complexity exists in a homogenate of the proximal third of the tail of adult male *A. flavicollis* than in the central or distal thirds (fig. 15.1). Mice of the genus *Mus* have no discrete scent organs. However, behaviorally active substances are known to be present in the urine and in secretions from the preputial gland (Bronson and Caroom 1971) and these play an important role in reproductive and other activities. Neither *Rattus rattus* L. nor *R. norvegicus* (Berkenhout) bear discrete odor producing sites, but, as in mice, a variety of glandular systems are capable of tainting urine (Krames et al. 1969). Eleven species of *Rattus* from the south Pacific have been shown to possess a

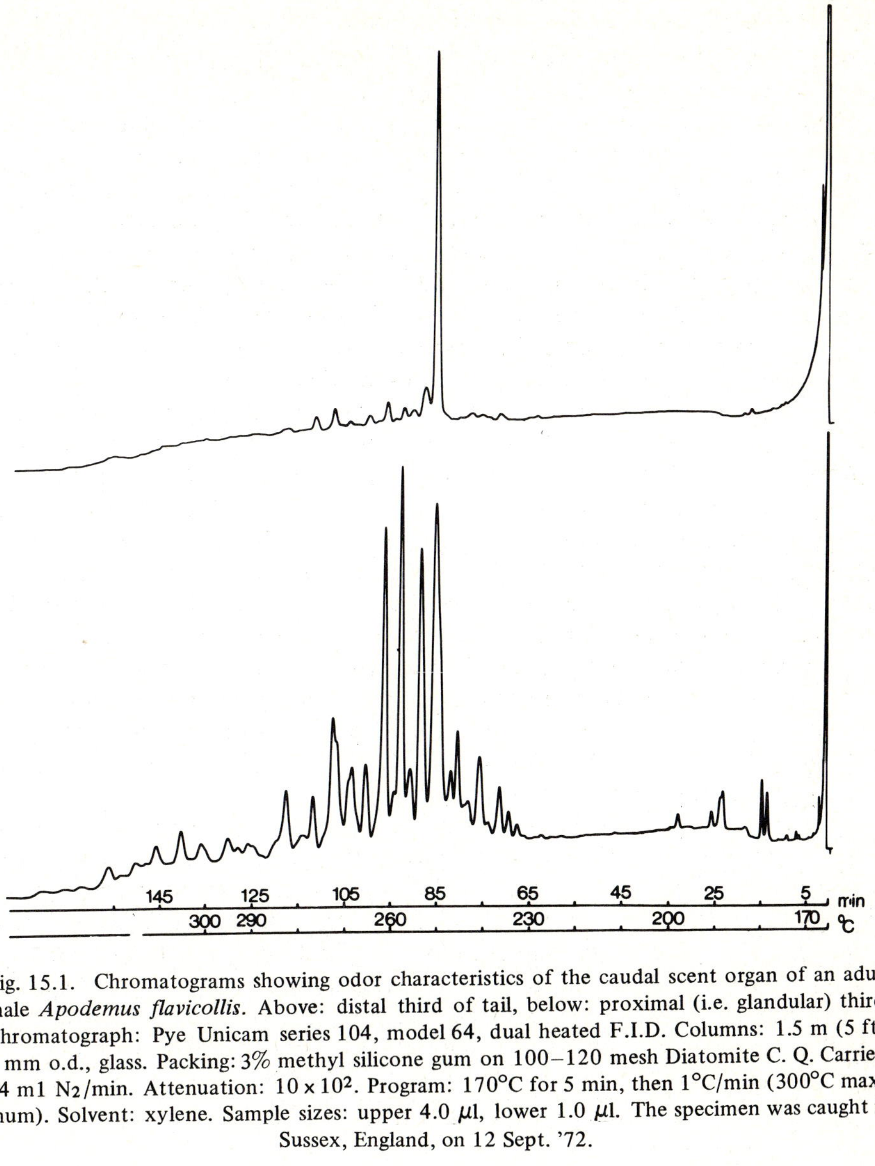

Fig. 15.1. Chromatograms showing odor characteristics of the caudal scent organ of an adult male *Apodemus flavicollis*. Above: distal third of tail, below: proximal (i.e. glandular) third. Chromatograph: Pye Unicam series 104, model 64, dual heated F.I.D. Columns: 1.5 m (5 ft), 6 mm o.d., glass. Packing: 3% methyl silicone gum on 100–120 mesh Diatomite C. Q. Carrier: 54 ml N_2/min. Attenuation: 10×10^2. Program: 170°C for 5 min, then 1°C/min (300°C maximum). Solvent: xylene. Sample sizes: upper 4.0 μl, lower 1.0 μl. The specimen was caught in Sussex, England, on 12 Sept. '72.

ventral gland complex (*R. exulans* Peale, Quay and Tomich 1963; *R. annandalei* Bonhote, *muelleri* Jentink, *sabanus* Thomas, *rajah* Thomas, *surifer* Kloss, *cremoriventer* Miller, *canus* Miller, *edwardsi* Thomas, *bowersi* Andersen, *r. jalorensis* Bonhote, Rudd 1966). This is an elongated narrow strip, up to 5 x 67 mm in *R. bowersi*, extending from the preputials to the base of the sternum. It appears to be present in both sexes, but by far the greatest development occurs in adult males. In *R. exulaus* it develops rapidly at the onset of sexual maturity. Observations on how the secretion is transferred to the gound have not yet been reported, but it is likely that a modified stretching behavior is utilized, perhaps analogous with the ventral rub of many Heteromyids.

Mid-ventral glandular organs occur in both sexes of *Cricetus* (Vrtiš 1932), *Cricetulus*, *Mesocricetus*, *Phodopus* and *Sigmodon* (Vorontsov and Gurtovoi 1959), in *Neotoma* (Howell 1926), in *Peromyscus* (Richmond and Roglund 1952) and in *Meriones* (Thiessen et al. 1958). Only in the last mentioned species have detailed observations been made on the way in which the organ is used. During transference the animal uses a ventral rub, with first the throat and then the belly sliding over the object receiving the scent. Both sexes possess a mid-ventral glandular organ, but males display scent spreading behavior at least twice as frequently as females.

From the above it is clear that male small mammals have better developed scent organs than females and use them more frequently, though it is not always certain for what purpose. The implications of this are overwhelming when the sociological role of the male is recalled. As further evidence of complexity of male odor compared with female odor, fig. 15.2 shows the preliminary characterization of caudal organ odors of *Apodemus flavicollis* Melchior (Stoddart, unpublished). Several peaks peculiar to the male are present and their identification and isolation are the subject of continuing studies.

Mention was made above of the dual role played by the scent producing apparatus of some small mammals. There seems little doubt that cutaneous glands play an active role in mate attraction. If this is not known from direct observation it is at least inferred from the fact that many such glands decrease in size during the period of sexual quiescence (Quay, 1953; Mitchell 1965, 1967; Stoddart, 1972a). The fact that they operate for other purposes which, if not sexual, must be social, is shown by the fact that many, if not *all* species have scent organs active throughout the whole year. Little is known from field studies about the effects of old age on the scent organs, but in the laboratory post reproductive *Arvicola* lose their scent organs altogether. In *Mesocricetus* a great reduction of secretory activity occurs (Lipkow; 1954 Vrtiš 1930). Ecological studies on small mammals seldom reveal senility, but when it does occur the effect of the scent organs is presumably similar to that of removal of the site of sex hormone production. This results in a drying up and cessation of function of the glandular tissue (Martan 1962; Mitchell 1965; Stoddart 1972a; Thiessen 1968).

Although scent organs may play a large part in the bringing together of two indivi-

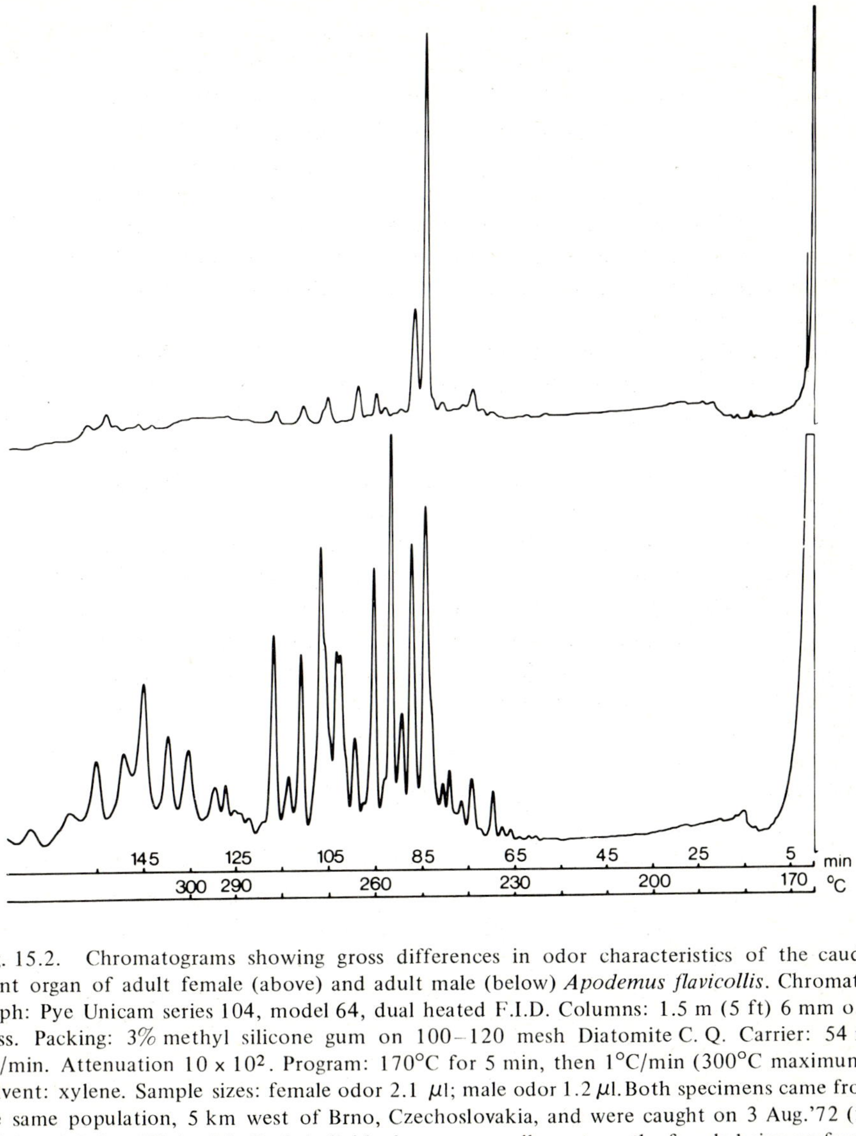

Fig. 15.2. Chromatograms showing gross differences in odor characteristics of the caudal scent organ of adult female (above) and adult male (below) *Apodemus flavicollis*. Chromatograph: Pye Unicam series 104, model 64, dual heated F.I.D. Columns: 1.5 m (5 ft) 6 mm o.d. glass. Packing: 3% methyl silicone gum on 100–120 mesh Diatomite C. Q. Carrier: 54 ml N_2/min. Attenuation 10 x 10^2. Program: 170°C for 5 min, then 1°C/min (300°C maximum). Solvent: xylene. Sample sizes: female odor 2.1 μl; male odor 1.2 μl. Both specimens came from the same population, 5 km west of Brno, Czechoslovakia, and were caught on 3 Aug.'72 (female) and 5 Aug.'72 (male). Both individuals were sexually mature, the female being perforate and the male having scrotal testes averaging 14.5 mm in length.

duals to mate, there is no evidence that lack of the scent organs prevents successful breeding. There have been few studies conducted to investigate this, but one, using *Meriones unguiculatus* Milne-Edwards, has shown conclusively that presence of the mid-ventral scent organ is not essential to normal successful breeding (Mitchell 1967). This is not to say that scent is unimportant in mating. Indeed anosmic male hamsters show no copulatory behavior towards receptive females (Lisk et al. 1972) and anosmic rats show impaired sexual behavior (Larsson 1971). However, the most obvious odor producing organs are not primarily for use in the intimate behavior surrounding mating.

There can be little doubt that olfaction offers the main pathway of social communication within populations of small mammals. Two factors above all others point to this. Firstly, glandular development is more enhanced in the male than in the female and his odor may contain more compounds than that of the female. Secondly, there is a high degree of specialized scent setting behaviour shown by many species of small mammals. If the odor was required *only* in the context of intimate behaviour there would be no need for a broadcasting behaviour. However, in several mainly subterranean species, a passive form of odor spreading has been adopted. These two factors leave us with little doubt that it is important for information about one individual in the population to be made known to the others, or at least some, and that this information has considerable social value. Before discussing odor as a factor in the social biology of populations, it should be re-emphasized that more studies are needed now on populations under natural conditions, in order to indicate which olfactory messages are employed at times of greatest dynamic change in the population. Such indications would constitute a major breakthrough in small mammal population biology.

15.4 The social effects of odor

Let us return to our basic assumption, that if odors are to be used for social integration in small mammals that are unable to use visual and acoustic signals, we might expect that the total range of messages to be transmitted is as wide as it is in those species able to use visual and acoustic signals. Surprisingly little attention has been paid to the social organization of populations of small mammals under natural conditions, but this is probably due to the difficulties of such study. As a corollary, even less attention has been paid to the communication necessary to maintain the organization. Wherever observations have been made on social organization of natural populations (e.g. Sadleir, 1965), it is clear that a strong supporting network of communication exists.

All aspects of life within a society require communication between individuals. These aspects can conveniently be discussed under four headings: Reproduction; Aggression and social dominance; Individual range and territory maintenance; Family and clan cohesion. In reviewing what is known about these we shall have to dwell to a considerable extent on the results of laboratory investigations. These have been, for the most part, very thorough, but have not been confirmed by field observations. In terms of real social communication their interpretation must be treated with considerable caution.

15.4.1. Reproduction

Little is to be said here about the effects and influences of odors on reproductive patterns, since this is the substance of a later chapter (Bronson, Ch. 18). As Bronson (1971) points out, most of the work has been carried out on rodents, primarily the house mouse, with little attention spared elsewhere. In most of these studies the site of origin, let alone the composition of the odor is not known, although its association with urine is not in doubt. It may prove that odors involved in strange male implantation block and related phenomena (Bruce 1960; Clulow and Clarke 1968; Bronson 1971) emanate from a variety of sites. The need for further experimentation in this field is great.

15.4.2. Aggression and social dominance

There have been enough investigations conducted into aggressive interactions in mice for it to be accepted that a factor, or some factors ('Angstgeruch' Müller-Velten 1966; Mackintosh and Grant 1966; Ropartz 1968) inducing fear or attack in others can be produced in mice. Such a substance or substances appears to be taken up by the surroundings of mice and remains active for seven to eight hours. Müller-Velten accedes that the source of 'Angstgeruch' may also be the skin glands, or the feces, but it has been positively identified as occurring in the urine. Individuals of one sex react to the urine from others of that sex and in addition females react to the urine of males. Males react to the urine of females not by flight, but by investigative behavior. This suggests that urine may be the site of several sorts of messages. Even mice owning territory within laboratory colonies show a high degree of peace towards intruding females which is not shown to males (Mackintosh 1970). Dixon and Mackintosh (1971) were able to show that urine from an adult female significantly reduces the amount of aggression when one male or a two male partnership is daubed with urine. The authors consider that the substance acts directly to inhibit aggression, since there is a concomitant increase in sexual and non-social behavior.

It is possible that urination in mice replaces the specialized scent setting behaviors in other species, since it appears to be under a certain degree of social control. Reynolds (1971) estimated the amount of urination occurring in encounters between cage owning mice and visitors of both sexes to home cages by measuring the area of urine, as revealed by the blot on the absorbent paper lining of the floor of the cage. Urination was greatest in adult male/adult female encounters. It was thought unlikely that this was a fear response since no fighting occurred in these interactions. Urination was scanty in female/female encounters, but was more abundant in cage owning males than in their male visitors. It seems logical to argue that in mixed sex encounters the continued proximity of a partner has an obvious biological advantage, and that the ample supply of urine excreted produces the communicatory wherewithall for this advantage to be exploited. Urination might then exert an influence in social structure and ecological stability of the population, involving the now well known effects of male odor on female reproductive cycles. Here we can detect one of many paradoxes resulting from a wide interpretation of closely controlled laboratory experiments. Bruce (1960) pointed out over a decade ago that presence of a strange male, or even his urine in the cage of a newly fertilized female, caused termination of the pregnancy by resorption. It is hard to see the adaptive significance of this phenomenon which acts to reduce population density and increase strain and possible malaise to the individual female. Reynolds' (1971) work suggests that there is a strong biological advantage to be gained by contrived proximity of a partner of the opposite sex, yet, if the Bruce effect is to occur, this advantage must (or possibly, depending on stage of pregnancy) include the sacrifice of a litter. The ecological and evolutionary issues here are complex and there is insufficient space to discuss them more fully. As has been said before, the social implications of these laboratory studies cannot fully be gauged until populations living in natural, or near natural, conditions have been studied.

The level of social dominance achieved by individual mammals in populations has been much studied by workers on large mammals. Few studies have been conducted into olfactory transmission of status information in small mammals. Krames et al. (1969) demonstrated the occurrence of a status signal produced by laboratory rats. Rats of known hierarchical status, measured by the amount of time spent guarding the only food pot in a cage housing four individuals, were presented with cardboard cylinders that had previously held either a dominant or a submissive male for one hour. Their response was assessed by the length of time they spent investigating the cylinder. Dominant rats paid little heed to the odor of other dominants and great heed to the odor of submissives. Submissive rats divided their time more equally spending only a little longer at the source of 'submissive' odor than at the source of 'dominant' odor. No attempt was made to identify the precise location of the origin of the odor nor, regrettably, what the active ingredient for dominance is in the total odorous output of the rat.

Thiessen et al. (1968) report that dominant gerbils 'ventral rub' their environment more frequently than subordinates. Ralls (1971) quotes the unpublished work of Johnston on golden hamsters in which dominant males apply their scent organs to the arena many times more often than do subordinates. She quotes similar results of work with rabbits, sugar gliders, marmosets, Maxwell's duikers and pangolins. The need to express dominance is thus as strong in small mammals as it is in large and there can be no other explanation of these results.

15.4.3. *Individual range and territory maintenance*

The question of territorial and individual range marking and related issues is also the subject of a separate communication in this volume (Mykytowycz ch. 17) and will not be dealt with here. The main questions for further research must involve a critical analysis of exactly what messages are conveyed by the odor used in marking and the identification of the active ingredients responsible for each message.

15.4.4. *Family and clan cohesion*

Cohesion of the social group, whether it be family or clan, appears to depend upon olfactory communication. Indeed the mother rat has been shown to recognize the odor of her young and selectively choose her own from a large group (Beach and Jaynes 1956). The existence of a 'maternal pheromone' has been identified in lactating mice and rats (Cowley and Wise 1970; Leon and Moltz 1971, respectively). This substance emitted from the female has an attractant effect on pre-weanling juveniles. Given the choice between an air stream tainted by a lactating rat and untainted air, a strong selection is made for the tainted air. Rat pups moved as readily towards any lactating female as towards their mother, thus demonstrating that the cue is not litter specific. In an extension of this work, Leon and Moltz (1972) showed that the substance is first emitted on about the 14th day of lactation at which time the pups are starting to leave the nest. By testing whether young of various ages from one to 41 days choose to go towards their own mother or a nulliparous female, it appears that by 14 days the young begin to approach their own mother preferentially. The preference is lost by 41 days. By testing young of 16 days with lactating females at different stages of lactation, it appears that they start emitting the substance at about the time the young are able to perceive it and cease to produce it at the time the young are no longer able to perceive it. Since it is known that a sharp decline in retrieving behavior by the mother occurs at about 14 days, it is thought that the pheromonal bond serves to attract the young to the mother for the remaining two weeks of lactation. The site of production of the maternal pheromone is not known, but the mammary glands cannot be overlooked as a possible site. (It is interesting to note in passing that components in human and pig milk occur in the same proportions throughout lactation, but in the echidna, platypus and kangaroo the ratio of high palmitic acid/C_{18} unsaturated acids in early milk changes to a low one in late milk. In these species at least, the mammary gland is constantly able to change the composition of its secretory output (Griffiths et al. 1972).) Cowley and Wise (1970) showed that the activity of 6-day old baby mice is reduced if they are kept in the presence of soiled sawdust or urine from a lactating female, whereas activity increases if they are kept in the presence of stock sawdust. The adaptive significance of this phenomenon is clearly to maintain cohesion in the nest during the preweaning period.

The concept of the small social group or clan smell has now been well investigated in at least two rodent and one small marsupial species. Barnett (1963) describes how one member of a tightly knit wild rat clan, under laboratory conditions, is set about by his former allies if he is removed from their proximity and kept in an empty cage for some time. Death usually follows such attacks. If the expatriate is allowed to keep some of his original bedding material during his exile, the harassment does not occur on re-introduction. Similarly, strangers can be accepted by the clan if they have first been daubed with urine, feces and bedding of clan members. Thus the active ingredient indicating clan membership cannot be genetically determined. Possibly it has something to do with the quality of the food eaten by the group (c.f. human garlic eaters), or with the constant social sniffing within the group. There are many important questions raised by Barnett's observations that prospective field workers would be well advised to consider. Godfrey (1958) examined olfactory relationships within the taxonomically complex group of *Clethrionomys.* He investigated wild populations which, he concluded, were in a great state of taxonomic flux since he could recognize different and distinct behavior patterns in different races. When presented with females of their own and other races, male *Clethrionomys* showed a strong mating selection for their own race. The results of his 'Y' maze experiments confirmed that the males were making their choices on the basis of the odor they received from the female. Godfrey's observations, including those on viability of hybrids from inter race matings, provoke many questions on the benefit of deme formation and subspeciation. This need not concern us here. What does concern us is the clearly indicated presence of a racial or subspecific smell emanating from the body of females and perceived by males. Godfrey himself suggests that geographic differences in scent 'may have arisen as a result of selection for the pleiotropic effect of gene substitutions that control differences in scent'. What these gene substitutions are is still a matter of conjecture. Kalkowski (1967) working with laboratory colonies of white mice demonstrates that the degree of discrimination among the community is very great, with individuals knowing their position in a social hierarchy of many members. He seems not to have known the work of Godfrey (1958), for he concludes that discrimination of a particular nest smell or scent of some determined community seems unnecessary, except perhaps for orientation on returns back to the community from excursions abroad.

In his work on the flying phalanger (*Petaurus breviceps* Thomas) Schultze-Westrum (1965) states that young animals recognize others as belonging to a particular group before they are able to recognize them as individuals. It is not known which of the three possible sites of origin is concerned, head, sternum and anal region, but Schultze–Westrum was able to show that a distinctively different odor was produced by the different glands. Odors of foreign groups of flying phalangers are partly, but not wholly responsible for the release of aggressive behavior and if they are missing such behavior cannot be released by visual or acoustic signals. Thus olfactory communication underlies the organization of the group and tends to reduce fraternization between communities. How far this trend can be taken under natural conditions is not known and although in the long term it may inhibit refreshment of gene pools it is likely in the short term to aid individual survival. Natural selection will favor any mechanism that prevents overoccupation and concomitant overexploitation of resources. Olfactory communication appears to play an important part in this mechanism.

Working on individual recognition in mice Bowers and Alexander (1967) used the familiar 'Y' maze apparatus to show that mice were able to discriminate between the sexes by odor cues alone and between two species, *Mus musculus* L. and *Peromyscus maniculatus* (Wagner). They argue that individual discrimination could have arisen as a by product of interspecific discrimination which would need to have been acute to allow more than one species to live in the same ecological community. It is a pity that Bowers and Alexander did not use two species more closely related (e.g. *P. maniculatus* and *P. leucopus* Rafinesque) within which there is a greater amount of genetic similarity. What is shown for the purposes of our argument is that recognition through olfactory cues is possible at the individual level.

15.5. Conclusion

There can be little doubt, under controlled conditions at least, that small mammals depend for the integration of their populations upon olfactory communication. It would indeed be interesting to know if this dependence was greater in totally subterranean forms which often lack eyes, than in the surface dwelling forms. Moles and mole rats (e.g. *Spalax*, *Bathyergus*, *Talpa*) appear not to have attracted this sort of attention as yet (but see Lehmann 1969b). However, we must recognize that the artificial conditions produced in the laboratory may be sufficient to show effects which would not normally be expressed under natural conditions. It is unlikely, however, that captive conditions would establish a communication pathway or central nervous network that was not present in natural conditions. It is more likely that captive conditions draw out responses not normally present in the wild, as they often represent extremes of normally encountered ecological conditions.

There is need for more investigation into such laboratory observed or even induced phenomena, but in order to understand the social functioning of a species in nature there is an even greater need for studies to be carried out on naturally occurring social groups. The difficulties of such studies are great, but not insuperable, and the time is ripe for an integrated approach to the concepts of social biology. A thorough understanding of the ecology of the species is essential to this integration. This is the link between the environment and its resources, and the social processes operating to regulate natality, mortality, immigration, emigration, dispersal, dispersion, survival, etc., etc.. The communicatory bridges achieving population stability in rodent pest species offer an exciting challenge to workers interested in pest control and as far as small mammal pests are concerned the need for new approaches has never been greater.

Acknowledgment

I am grateful to Miss M. J. Wood for having read and commented on a draft of this contribution.

References

Albone, E. S. and M. W. Fox (1971) Anal gland secretion of the red fox. Nature (London) 233, 569–570.

Balph, D. M. and D. F. Balph (1966) Sound communication of Uinta ground squirrels. J. Mammal. 47, 440–450.

Barnett, S. A. (1963) A Study in Behaviour (Methuen & Co., London) 288 pp.

Beach, F. A. and J. Jaynes (1956) Studies on maternal retrieving in rats. III. Sensory cues involved in the lactating female's response to her young. Behaviour. 10, 104–125.

Bowers,J. M. and B. K. Alexander (1967) Mice: Individual recognition by olfactory cues. Science 158, 1208–1210.

Bronson, F. H. (1971) Rodent pheromones. Biol. of Reprod. 4, 344–357.

Bronson, F. H. and D. Caroom (1971) Preputial gland of the male mouse; attractant function. J. Reprod. Fert. 25, 279–282.

Brownlee, R. G., R. M. Silverstein, D. Müller–Schwarze and A. G. Singer (1969) Isolation, identification and function of the chief component of the male tarsal scent in black-tailed deer. Nature (London) 221, 284–285.

Bruce, H. M. (1960) A block to pregnancy in the mouse caused by proximity of strange males. J. Reprod. Fert. 1, 96–103.

Clulow, F. V. and J. R. Clarke (1968) Pregnancy-block in *Microtus agrestis* an induced ovulator. Nature (London) 219, 511.

Cowley, J. J. and D. R. Wise (1970) Pheromones, growth and behaviour. In:Chemical Influences on Behaviour. CIBA Foundation Study Group No. 35; eds.: R. Porter and J. Birch, (Churchill, London) pp. 144–170.

Dieterlen, F. (1959) Das Verhalten des syrischen Goldhamsters (*Mesocricetus auratus* Waterhouse). Z. Tierpsychol. 16, 337–338.

Dixon, A. K. and J. H. Mackintosh (1971) Effects of female urine upon the social behaviour of adult male mice. Anim. Behav. 19, 138–140.

Dryden, G. L. and C. H. Conaway (1967) The origin and hormonal control of scent production in *Suncus murinus*. J. Mammal. 48, 420–428.

Eibl-Eibesfeldt, I. (1953) Zur Ethologie des Hamsters (*Cricetus cricetus* L.). Z. Tierpsychol. 10, 204–254.

Eibl-Eibesfeldt, I. (1958) Das Verhalten der Nagetiere. Handb. Zool. 8 (10:12), 1–88.

Eisenberg, J. F. (1963) A comparative study of sandbathing behaviour in heteromyid rodents. Behaviour 22, 16–23.

Ewer, R. F. (1968) Ethology of Mammals (Logos, London) 418 pp.

Flowerdew, J. R. (1971) The subcaudal glandular area of *Apodemus sylvaticus*. J. Zool. (London) 165, 525–527.

Frank, F. (1957) Das Duftmarkieren der Grossen Wühlmaus *Arvicola terrestris* (L.). Z. Säugetierk. 21, 172–175.

Godfrey, J. (1958) The origin of sexual isolation between bank voles. Proc. Roy. Phys. Soc. Edinburgh, 27, 47–55.

Goethe, F. (1964) Das Verhalten der Musteliden. Handb. Zool. 8(10:37), 1–80.

Goodrich, B. S. and R. Mykytowycz (1972) Individual and sex differences in the chemical composition of pheromone-like substances from the skin glands of the rabbit, *Oryctolagus cuniculus*. J. Mammal. 53, 540–548.

Griffiths, M. the late D. L. McIntosh and R. M. C. Leckie (1972) The mammary glands of the red kangaroo with observations on the fatty acid components of the milk triglycerides. J. Zool. (London) 166, 265–275.

Howell, A. B. (1926) Anatomy of the wood rat. Mon.Am. Soc. Mammal., No. 1 (Williams and Wilkins, Baltimore).

Kalkowski, W. (1967) Olfactory bases of social orientation in the white mouse. Folia Biol. 15, 69–87.

Koenig, L. (1960) Das Aktionssystem des Siebenschläfers (*Glis glis* L.). Z. Tierpsychol. 17, 427–505.

Krames, L., W. J. Carr and B. Bergmann (1969) A pheromone associated with social dominance among male rats. Psychon. Sci. 16, 11–12.

Kratochvil, J. (1964) Das mänliche Genitalsystem des europäischen Bergmurmeltieres *Marmota marmota latirostris* Krat. 1961. Z. Säugetierk. 29, 290–304.

Larsson, K. (1971) Impaired mating performances in male rats after anosmia induced peripherally or centrally. Brain, Behav. Evol. 4, 463–471.

Lederer, E. (1950) Odeur et parfums des animaux. Fortschr. Chem. Org. Naturst. 6, 87–153.

Lehmann, E. von (1962) Uber die Seitendrüsen der mitteleuropäischen Rötelmaus (*Clethrionomys glareolus* Schreber). Z. Morph. Oekol. Tiere 51. 335–344.

Lehmann, E. von (1966) Über die Seitendrüsen der mitteleuropäischen Wühlmäuse der Gattung *Microtus* Schrank. Z. Morphol. Oekol. Tiere 56, 436–443.

Lehmann, E. von (1967) Die Seitendrüsen der Feldmaus (*Microtus arvalis*). Z. Morphol. Oekol. Tiere 59, 436–438.

Lehmann, E. von (1969a) Über die Hautdrüsen der Schneemaus (*Chionomys nivalis nivalis* Martins 1842). Bonn. Zool. Beitr. 4, 373–377.

Lehmann, E. von (1969b) Die Rückendrüse des Europäischen Maulwurfs (*Talpa europaea*). Z. Säugetierk. 34, 358–361.

Leon, M. and H. Moltz (1971) Maternal pheromone: Discrimination by preweanling albino rats. Physiol. Behav. 7, 265–267.

Leon, M. and H. Moltz (1972) The development of the pheromonal bond in the albino rat. Physiol. Behav. 8, 683–686.

Lipkow, J. (1954) Über das Seitenorgan des Goldhamsters (*Mesocricetus auratus auratus* Waterh.). Z. Morphol. Oekol. Tiere. 42, 333–372.

Lisk, R. D., J. Zeiss and L. A. Ciaccio (1972) The influence of olfaction on sexual behavior in the male golden hamster (*Mesocricetus auratus*). J. Exptl. Zool. 181, 69–78.

Mackintosh, J. H. (1970) Territory formation by laboratory mice. Anim. Behav. 18, 177–183.

Mackintosh, J. H. and E. C. Grant (1966) The effect of olfactory stimuli on the agonistic behaviour of laboratory mice. Z. Tierpsychol. 23, 584–587.

Martan, J. (1962) Effect of the castration and androgen replacement on the supracaudal gland of the male guinea pig. J. Morphol. 110, 285–297.

Mitchell, O. G. (1965) Effect of castration and transplantation on ventral gland of the gerbil. Proc. Soc. Exptl. Biol. Med. 119, 953–955.

Mitchell, O. G. (1967) The supposed role of the gerbil ventral gland in reproduction. J. Mammal. 48, 142.

Müller, D. and E. Lamperle (1964) Objectivierung und Analyse olfaktorischer Signale der

Säugetiere mit Hilfe der Gaschromatographie. Naturwissenschaften 51, 346–347.

Müller-Velten, H. (1966) Über den Angstgeruch bei der Hausmaus (*Mus musculus*L.). Z. Vergl. Physiol. 52, 401–429.

Mykytowycz, R. (1970) The role of skin glands in mammalian communication. In: Advances in Chemoreception, vol. I, Communication by chemical signals; eds.: J. W. Johnston, D. G. Moulton and A. Turk, (Appleton-Century-Crofts, N.Y.). pp. 327–360.

Mykytowycz, R. (1972) The behavioural role of the mammalian skin glands. Naturwissenschaften 59, 133–139.

Niethammer, J. (1969) Eine artspezifische Schwanzdrüse der männlichen Gelbhalsmaus (*Apodemus flavicollis* Melchior, 1834). Bonn. zool. Beitr. 1. 30–37.

Pearson, O. P. (1946) Scent glands of the short-tailed shrew. Anat. Rec. 94, 615–625.

Quay, W. B. (1953) Seasonal and sexual differences in the dorsal skin gland of the kangaroo rat, *Dipodomys*. J. Mammal. 34, 1–14.

Quay, W. B. (1954) The dorsal holocrine skin gland of the kangaroo rat. Anat. Rec. 119, 161–176.

Quay. W. B. (1965) Variation and taxonomic significance in the sebaceous caudal glands of pocket mice (Rodentia: Heteromyidae). Southwest. Nat. 10, 282–287.

Quay, W. B. (1968) The specialised posterolateral sebaceous glandular regions in microtine rodents. J. Mammal. 49, 427–445.

Quay, W. B. and P. Q. Tomich (1963) A specialized mid-ventral sebaceous glandular area in *Rattus exulans*. J. Mammal. 44, 537–542.

Ralls, K. (1971) Mammalian scent marking. Science 171, 443–449.

Reynolds, E. (1971) Urination as a social response in mice. Nature (London) 234, 481–483.

Richmond, N. D. and H. R. Roglund (1952) A mid-ventral gland in *Peromyscus maniculatus*. J. Mammal. 33, 103–104.

Ropartz, P. (1968) The relation between olfactory stimulation and aggressive behaviour in mice. Anim. Behav. 16, 97–100.

Rudd, R. L. (1966) The midventral gland in Malaysian murid rodents. J. Mammal. 47, 331–332.

Sadleir. R. M. F. S. (1965) The relationship between agonistic behaviour and population changes in the deermouse *Peromyscus maniculatis* (Wagner). J. Anim. Ecol. 34, 331–352.

Schultze–Westrum, T. (1965) Innerartliche Verständigung durch Düfte beim Gleibeutler *Petaurus breviceps papuanus* Thomas (Marsupialia, Phalangeridae). Z. Vergl. Physiol. 50, 151–220.

Shelley, W. B. (1956) The role of apocrine sweat in the production of axillary odor. J. Soc. Cosmet. Chem. 7, 171–175.

Sleggs, G. (1926) The adult anatomy and histology of the anal glands of the Richardson ground–squirrel, *Citellus richardsonii* Sabine. Anat. Rec. 32, 1–43.

Stevens, P. S. and J. L. E. Erickson (1942) American Musk I. The chemical composition of the musk of the Louisiana muskrat. J. Am. Chem. Soc. 64, 144–147.

Stoddart, D. M. (1970) Individual range, dispersion and dispersal in a population of water voles (*Arvicola terrestris*(L.)). J. Anim. Ecol. 39, 403–425.

Stoddart, D. M. (1971) Breeding and survival in a population of water voles. J. Anim. Ecol. 40, 487–494.

Stoddart, D. M. (1972a) The lateral scent organs of *Arvicola terrestris* (Rodentia: Microtinae). J. Zool. (London) 166, 49–54.

Stoddart, D. M. (1972b) An examination of the caudal organ of *Apodemus agrarius*, *A. flavicollis*, *A. microps*, and *A. sylvaticus*, from Moravia (ČSSR). Zool. listy 21, 39–42.

Thiessen, D. D. (1968) The roots of territorial marking in the Mongolian gerbil: A problem of the species-common topography. Behav. Res. Meth. Instr. 1, 70–76.

Thiessen, D. D., H. C. Friend and G. Lindzey (1968) Androgen control of territorial marking in the Mongolian gerbil. Science 160, 432–434.

Vorontsov, N. N. and N. N. Gurtovoi (1969) Structure of the mid-abdominal gland of the true hamster (Cricetini, Cricetinae, Rodentia, Mammalia). Dokl. Biol. Sci. (Sects. Akad. Nauk, SSSR) 125. 385–388.

Vrtiš, V.. (1930) Glandular organ on the flanks of the water rat, their development and changes during breeding season. Biol. Spisy vys. Šk. zvěrolék Brno 4.

Vrtiš, V. (1932) The cutaneous umbilical glandular organ of the Hamster *Cricetus cricetus* (L.). Biol. Spisy vys Šk. zvěrolék Brno 13.

Wallin, L. (1967) The dorsal skin gland of the Norwegian lemming. Z. Morphol. Oekel. Tiere 59, 83–90.

Wynne-Edwards, V. C. (1962) Animal Dispersion in Relation to Social Behaviour. (Oliver and Boyd, Edinburgh.) 653 pp.

CHAPTER 16

Olfactory recognition of species, groups, individuals and physiological states among mammals

Dietland MÜLLER-SCHWARZE

16.1. Introduction

Odors produced by a mammal may affect the behavior of other individuals of the same or related species, or of predators and prey in a variety of ways. Here we are concerned only with intraspecific responses. An odor may identify (to its conspecifics) the species, group or family membership, individuality, and long- and short-term physiological state of a given individual. The same odor may also simultaneously prescribe a certain course of action. The answer to the question 'Who is there? ' can carry with it instructions on 'what to do'.

Two types of experimental approach must be distinguished in demonstrating the ability to discriminate odors. One type uses the spontaneous response to, or choice of, an experimentally presented odor, without a direct behavioral consequence (reward or punishment) being part of the design of the experiment. The odor stimulus, however, may have its own reinforcing properties. Under these circumstances it is usually assumed that the response will change very little with repeated stimulation, so long as intervals between exposures are long enough to avoid habituation, or to maintain the response at a certain level after initial habituation. The second type of experiment employs conditioning techniques, whereby an animal is rewarded and/or punished for its responses. Here, a change or 'improvement' in the ability to discriminate is expected with repeated stimulation, the subject being driven by the experimenter to the limits of its ability to discriminate under the given conditions. The discriminatory acuity may vary with differing experimental conditions. Thus, the exclusion of other senses in controlled laboratory tests will often produce a higher acuity of the olfactory sense, in much the same way as blind and deaf-mute persons can 'cultivate' their chemical and tactile senses. Mammalian populations in the wild respond to odor stimuli with and without recognizable reinforcement although the reinforcing properties of the stimulus situation are still obscure in most cases. This treatment discusses selected examples of odor discriminations which were achieved in both types of experimental approaches.

16.2. Olfactory recognition of species and subspecies

Perhaps the most basic discrimination task for an animal is to identify members of its own species, using individual or combined signals in all sensory modalities. Only examples of proven species discrimination by odors will be discussed here, since in virtually all cases where the responses to odors of related *versus* own species have been investigated, clear discrimination has been demonstrated.

One of the first succesful inquiries into recognition of the odor of conspecifics was that by Heitzenroeder (1913) even though it lacked certain controls. He presented airstreams carrying the odors of three drops of the urine of a bitch, of a chicken bone, of vanillin, of musk, of eight other chemicals and several species of flowers to a male dog (8-year old Spitz). He then measured the frequency and amplitude of respiratory movements by means of a rubber belt around the dog's chest and a kymographion. The dog increased his frequency of respiration from 4/15 sec to 76/15 sec within 12 sec in response to the odor of bitch urine. Urine of a male dog and the odor of a chicken bone released a weaker response. Musk and vanillin released a response, while flower odors did not. This early experiment showed a strong 'spontaneous' response to an odor produced by a conspecific of the opposite sex, in the absence of the donor.

Most subsequent controlled laboratory experiments have been carried out with rodents. Godfrey (1958) studied the role of odors in the sexual isolation of bank voles (*Clethrionomys*). He confronted males with odors of females of different subspecies in a Y-shaped choice apparatus. Typically a male preferred the odor of a female of its own subspecies to that of another subspecies. Rauschert (1963) repeated these experiments with three species, six subspecies, and four hybrid forms of *Clethrionomys*. Males recognized and preferred the odor of a female of their own species. On the level of the subspecies, however, the results varied. In one instance the males preferred females of their own subspecies, but in three other subspecies no such preferences were observed. Moore (1965) investigated sexual isolation by odors in two species of white-footed mice (*Peromyscus*). The experimental animals were *P. maniculatus rufinus** from New Mexico and *P. polionotus leucocephalus* from an island in Florida. A test animal could choose between two chambers, in each of which an odor donor of one of the two species had been confined for eight hours and then removed. The crossings into each chamber were recorded automatically during eight hours of darkness. Males of *P. maniculatus* preferred to stay in the chamber with the odor of a female of its own species for the initial period of the experiment. The same pattern held for females responding to male odors. In *P. polionotus*, however, odor of conspecifics was not preferred at a statistically significant level. Females of *Peromyscus maniculatus bairdi* in estrus prefer the odor of males of their own species to that of males of *P. leucopus novebora-*

* Many authors' names are seldom used in the literature. They are therefore omitted in this chapter rather than add to the confusion or add new mistakes.

censis. Non-estrous females do not show a preference (Doty 1972). House mice *Mus musculus* of the strain C57B1 distinguished the odor of their own species from that of *Peromyscus maniculatus* (Bowers and Alexander 1967). Gerbils (*Meriones unguiculatus*) discriminated between the odor of their own species and that of *Rattus norvegicus*, *Mus musculus*, *Mesocricetus auratus*, or *Dicrostonyx groenlandicus* (Dagg and Windsor 1971).

Among ungulates, two subspecies of *Odocoileus hemionus*, the Rocky Mountain mule deer (*O. h. hemionus*) and the black-tailed deer (*O. h. columbianus*), respond more to tarsal scent of their own subspecies than to that of the other (Müller-Schwarze unpublished). In these, as in previous experiments, the mule deer were less mobile and active than the black-tailed deer. Thus, in response to the preferred tarsal scent of its own subspecies, the mule deer were less active than the black-tailed in response to their own tarsal scent. This is a point which has not been taken into account in other odor discrimination studies, where equal manifestations of responsiveness have been assumed in the various species or subspecies used.

16.3. Olfactory recognition of sex

There are numerous examples of recognition of sex odors among mammals. Often only the males possess specialized skin glands and consequently a peculiar odor (as, for instance, the subauricular and dorsal glands in the male pronghorn), while the odor indicating estruş is confined to the females. In the golden hamster, experimental transfer of vaginal secretions of intact females onto castrated males or ovariectomized females causes males to treat the experimental animals like intact females, with intensified mounting attempts (Johnston 1972). Wild house mice (*Mus musculus*) can be readily captured in traps containing the odor of the opposite sex (Rowe 1970). In encounters between two laboratory mice, a maximum of urination occurs if the two individuals are of opposite sex. The male will then contribute most of the urine discharged by the pair. It is assumed that this behavior serves in attraction and recognition of the sexes (Reynolds 1971).

16.4. Olfactory recognition of physiological stages

LeMagnen (1952) showed that male white laboratory rats prefer the odor of receptive females over that of non-receptive females. The olfactory discrimination of estrous from non-estrous females has been known for dogs for a long time and has also been demonstrated experimentally in sheep (Kelly 1937; Lindsey 1956; Banks et al. 1963) and cattle (Donovan 1967). In Long-Evans rats, sexually satiated polygamous males prefer the odor of a novel female over one with which they have copulated; monogamous males do not show that preference (Carr et al. 1970a). Polygamous females, however, did not discriminate between the odor of the original male and that of a novel one. Adult, experienced, male Long-Evans rats preferred the odor of receptive females to that of non-receptive ones. Experienced and naive receptive females preferred the odor of intact males to that of castrates (Carr et al. 1965). Immature males also preferred the odor of normal males over that of castrated ones. In females, sexually inexperienced receptive individuals preferred the odor of non-receptive females over that of receptive ones (Carr et al. 1970c).

The chemical basis for the typical odor of estrous females has been investigated in the rhesus monkey. Six fatty acids present on the vulva serve as sex attractants for males. These acids are: acetic, propionic, *iso*-butyric, *n*-butyric, *iso*-valeric and iso-caproic acids (Michael et al. 1971; see Epple ch. 19). Synthetic mixtures of these fatty acids increased the number of mounting attempts by male rhesus monkeys (Curtis et al. 1971; Michael et al. 1971).

Laboratory rats and mice can distuinguish stressed conspecifics by odor. Rats have been trained to discriminate the odor of stressed rats from non-stressed ones (Valenta and Rigby 1968). Stressed mice produce an odor which is avoided by other mice. Females are more sensitive to this 'fright substance' than males (Müller-Velten 1966). Male mice prefer the odor of non-shocked males and females over that of shocked members of both sexes. Male mice also prefer the odor of victors over that of defeated mice, except when the odor donor had defeated the test animal (Carr et al. 1970b). In Mongolian gerbils (*Meriones unguiculatus*), defeated animals avoid the odor of the victor (Nyby et al. 1970).

16.5. *Group odors*

Mammals that touch each other frequently and/or use communal nest sites, dens, etc. invariably exchange individual odors and thus produce a group odor. In addition to accidental transfers of odoriferous material, stereotyped behavior patterns may ensure the spread of glandular secretions and urine. Such behavior-based marking of conspecifics has been termed 'allomarking', but a word of pure composition is to be preferred. In analogy to the word 'trophallaxis' for exchange of food in insect colonies, the term 'osmallaxis', meaning exchange of odor, is suggested here. Osmallaxis is a broad term and could be subdivided into 'stereotyped osmallaxis' (social marking) and 'accidental osmallaxis' (general odor transfer).

Sugar glider (*Petaurus breviceps papuanus*) males rub their frontal glands against the sternal glands of females in their group, thus producing a clan-specific odor (Schultze-Westrum 1965). African dwarf mongooses (*Helogale undulata rufula*) mark one another with their anal glands. This behavior seems to be important for the maintenance of social bonds (Rasa 1973).

Rats (*Rattus norvegicus* and *R. rattus*) 'crawl under' and 'walk over' members of their colony (Barnett 1963). During these contacts the individual on top often deposites a drop of urine on the other rat. This occurs particularly in heterosexual encounters, and most of the marking is performed by the male (Oldham and Müller-Schwarze, in preparation). These three forms of social marking are examples of 'stereotyped osmallaxis'. Sheppard and Yoshida (1971) investigated the recognition of young sibling Richardson's ground squirrels (*Spermophilus richardsoni*). In paired encounters, siblings exhibited less agonistic behavior and more sniffing and 'cohesive' behavior than did non-siblings. From this, a 'group odor' is inferred. Rabbits (*Oryctolagus cuniculus*) maintain group odors in their territories because several members of a colony, especially males, defecate on communal piles of fecal pellets. These 'marking pellets' differ from dispersed pellets by carrying the scent of the anal glands (Mykytowycz 1968). Female rabbits will tolerate their own young, harass those of other females in the same colony and kill kittens of another colony. Olfactory cues are determinative in this behavior (Mykytowycz and Dudzinski 1972).

In vicuñas (*Vicugna vicugna*) family groups, which are territorial, maintain dung piles to which all members contribute. Thus the dung piles carry a group odor which is assumed to aid the resident group's orientation in space. Also, the dung piles may separate neighbors at territory borders, although other, non-neighboring groups will enter a territory in the absence of the resident group (Franklin 1973).

Geist (1971) assumes that in Dall's sheep (*Ovis dalli*) a group odor results from the young males' rubbing against the antorbital glands of old rams. Another form of stereotyped osmallaxis in ungulates is the pressing together of the maxillary glands in Maxwell's duikers (*Cephalophus maxwelli*). In this species, social marking between males is the prelude to a fight (Ralls 1969).

16.6. Recognition of individual odors

Groups of adults: In a group of adult black-tailed deer, hostile encounters particularly between strangers, may start with a sniffing of the tarsal organs of another individual (Müller-Schwarze 1971). Here, as in many other cases, the various sensory modalities will contribute to individual recognition; thus, an individual may be recognized by its group-mates with the aid of a combination of smell, posture, gait, etc. Laboratory experiments have demonstrated that two individuals can be discriminated by odor even if the donors and the responding animal have never met. Laboratory mice (*Mus musculus*, strain C57B1) were able to discriminate between the odors of two males of their own strain with which they had not previously been associated (Bowers and Alexander 1967). Receptive female laboratory rats can discriminate the odors of different males (Krames 1970). Two male white mice living together can be made more aggressive toward one another by rubbing the ano-genital region of a strange male on one or both of the males. Conversely, a strange male will be attacked less if he is treated with the odor of one of the two resident males (Mackintosh and Grant 1966). Mongolian gerbils discriminate among the odors of different males (Dagg and Windsor 1971). African dwarf mongooses (*Helogale undulata rufula*) mark objects with their cheek glands and immediately afterwards with their anal glands. The anal gland secretions, but not the cheek gland secretions of different individuals can be distinguished by conspecifics (Rasa 1973). In rabbits, one animal will take longer to identify another if the inguinal glands of the latter have been extirpated (Mykytowycz 1972).

Territorial individuals: Pronghorn males (*Antilocapra americana*) mark their territories with their subauricular glands and maintain dung sites, where pawing, urinating and defecation take place. Captive pronghorn have distuinguished among subauricular scent marks of different males, including their own (Müller-Schwarze and Müller-Schwarze 1972). They can also clearly distinguish their own dung from that of other males with whom they are familiar (Müller-Schwarze et al. 1973).

Mother–young relations: In a number of mammalian species, mothers recognize their own young by the olfactory sense. This is true for laboratory rats (Beach and Jaynes 1956; Meyer 1964), mouflon (*Ovis aries musimon*) (Tschanz 1962), sheep (Smith 1965), black-tailed deer (*Odocoileus heminous columbianus*) (Müller-Schwarze, unpublished), and rabbits (Mykytowycz 1972). Goats recognize their own young by olfaction and taste (Klopfer and Gamble 1966).

In rats, the retrieving response was used to demonstrate discrimination between own and alien young. Own young are retrieved sooner than strange ones (Beach and Jaynes 1956). Olfaction is important in this discrimination. Rats will kill their own young, if they are sealed in polyethylene bags or masked with artificial odors (Meyer 1964). Mouflon and black-tailed deer recognize their young by sniffing the anal and tail region. In both species the bleating of the young activates the mother, but does not serve in individual recognition. When mouflon lambs wore small plastic pants over their anal area, their mothers did not recognize them. On the other hand, application of tail scent of her own lamb to a strange one would convince a mouflon mother to accept it as her own (Tschanz 1962). In domestic sheep, a ewe will smell the hind quarters or flanks of a lamb before accepting it. Lindsay and Fletcher (1968) found that ewes recognized their lambs by visual cues, but expected smell to be important in allowing a lamb to suckle. In rabbits a mother will recognize her young after smelling them at the rear and head areas. She will attack her own young if they have been smeared with secretion from inguinal glands of a strange female. Anal gland secretion does not release this effect (Mykytowycz and Dudzinski 1972). The reverse has also been demonstrated. Shapiro and Salas (1970) showed that rat pups recognize the odor of their mother. When exposed to the maternal odor, the locomotor activity of the pups is inhibited. Similarly, cat kittens, when displaced before the age of eye opening, use olfactory stimuli emanating from their nest for finding their way back home. They crawl toward their nest if displaced but cease locomotion when placed in the nest area (Rosenblatt et al. 1969).

16.7. *The establishment of social odor preferences*

The establishment of social odor preferences or 'olfactory imprinting' has been investigated experimentally in only a few cases. In altricial mammals, early olfactory stimulation has profound effects on later social behavior. Marr and Gardner (1965) rubbed pups of laboratory rats daily with cologne odor or methyl salicylate from birth to four weeks of age. The cologne-treated rats later preferred cologne-smelling rats. The rats treated with methyl salicylate did not show any preferences. Female mice (*Mus musculus*) are imprinted by their fathers (Mainardi 1963). Mainardi et al. (1965) sprayed mice parents with perfume. This treatment, or absence of the father in early infancy led to lack of sex discrimination in the adult. Quadagno and Banks (1970) confirmed that female mice learn species recognition in the nest, but males do not. Among mice reared with their mother and three siblings of the same sex, males at weaning age preferred the odor of males while females spent more time at odor of females of another strain. When adult, the males preferred female odor, while estrous females preferred odor of males of another strain. Anestrous females showed no preference (Landauer and Banks 1972). Fox and Himwich (1965) treated the mammae of lactating bitches with aniseed oil and found that the pups then made positive response to aniseed oil from birth to five days of age.

Precocial mammals: Carter and Marr (1970) raised guinea pigs (*Cavia porcellus*) with differently scented mothers and litter-mates. Later these animals preferred the scent with which they had been raised. The scents used were natural guinea pig odor, ethyl benzoate, and acetophenone. When exposed for 15 or 20 days after birth, the animals showed a clear preference at 16 or 23 days of age respectively. When exposed for only six days, the responses decreased, but during days 1–6 the animals were more sensitive to the treatment than later. Exposure for only three days was less effective than six days; but during days 1–3 they were more sensitive than during days 4–6. However, when tested at 60 days of age, all groups preferred the natural odor of guinea pigs. This experiment clearly demonstrates three points; 1) sensitivity to olfactory stimuli in a social context changes during the first weeks of life in guinea pigs; 2) early effects are reversible; 3) the tendency is strong to revert to preferring the natural odor of their own species.

In domestic goats, the first five minutes of olfactory and gustatory contact between the mother and her newborn kid suffice to establish a specific bond–the mother will reject young other than her own. If the mother had been rendered anosmic during parturition, she would accept any young. Thus, manifestation of general maternal behavior and discrimination of own and alien young are two separate processes (Klopfer and Gamble 1966).

Olfactory imprinting has also been demonstrated in black-tailed deer. A small fawn raised for the first 15 days after birth with a surrogate mother scented with pronghorn ischiadic scent learned to prefer this odor over deer scents. He also preferred a live pronghorn female over live mule and black-tailed deer (Müller Schwarze and Müller-Schwarze 1971). When three more fawns were raised in isolation with scented surrogate mothers, a male showed some preferences for social odors experienced in early life, while the females did not (Müller-Schwarze et al. in preparation).

Although it is difficult to prove, it has been postulated repeatedly that even in man, early exposure to body odors may have an imprinting effect. Wenzel (1954) suggested that the clinical psychologist may benefit from patients' reports on olfactory hallucinations evoking early childhood memories. Bieber (1959) assumes that a child is capable of identifying the sources of sex odors and that olfactory experiences are important for the organization of heterosexual behavior, which occurs between two and five years of age. Similarly Kalogerakis (1963) suggests that the sense of smell may play a role on the development of the Oedipus complex and in the establishment of sexual identity. He describes the case of a boy who was attracted to heterosexual odors but repelled by ipsisexual odors between the ages of three and five and a half years.

16.8. Conclusion

The ability of mammals to communicate by odors has attracted increasing interest among researchers during the last decade. Although there is currently considerable flux in this field and only a few species are being studied, a few generalizations can be made:

1) Though olfactory stimuli are important in nearly all aspects of the social life of most terrestrial mammals, they are only one part of multi-sensory complex stimuli directing behavior. An olfactory stimulus may trigger only one step in a chain of behavioral events, or simultaneous stimuli from several modalities may be necessary to release a single behavior pattern. Therefore, in experiments with social odors, often only partial responses are obtained. If, for instance, the vaginal secretion of a female golden hamster is applied to a white clay model of a hamster, males investigate the object but do not show sexual behavior. Other stimuli are necessary: when the same vaginal secretion is applied to an anesthetized male hamster, it is mistaken as a female and arouses sexual behavior in other males (Devor and Murphy 1972).

2) Some biologically significant odors are learned in early life, as shown by experiments with artificial scenting of mothers, dummies or nests. Once acquired, this knowledge has to be maintained by frequent 'refreshing' of the specific experience. In the absence of maintaining stimuli social odors can be re-learned. It is particularly easy to revert to the natural odor(s) of the own species.

3) Olfactory recognition of species, groups, individuals, etc. is typically achieved only over short distances (a few centimeters) or by direct contact.

4) The distinguishing of one's own scents from those of others serves vital functions, not only in orientation and territorialism, but in many different con-

texts. When encountering odors of other individuals, an animal will adjust its behavior in preparation for encounters to come. If only its own odor is present, it will be more 'at ease' and more likely to rest or feed and thus will conserve energy.

5) The responses to some social odors depend on the physiological state of a mammal. We expect little change in sensivity to alarm pheromones; but responses to sex odors vary with the reproductive state. In *Peromyscus* (Doty 1972) and laboratory mice (Landauer and Banks 1972) anestrous females show less odor preferences than estrous ones.

References

Banks, E. M., R. Bishop and H. W. Norton (1963) The effect of temporary anosmia on courtship in the ram (*Ovis aries*). Proc. XVI Int. Congr. Zool. 2, 25.

Barnett, S. A. (1963) A Study in Behaviour (Methuen, London) 288 pp.

Beach, F. A. and J. Jaynes (1956) Studies of maternal retrieving in rats. I. Recognition of young. J. Mammal. 37, 177–180.

Bieber, I. (1959) Olfaction in sexual development and adult sexual organization. Am. J. Psychotherap. 13, 851–859.

Bowers, J. M. and B. K. Alexander (1967) Mice: Individual recognition by olfactory cues. Science 158, 1208–1210.

Carr, W. J., L. S. Loeb and M. L. Dissinger (1965) Responses of rats to sex odors. J. Comp. Physiol. Psychol. 58, 370–377.

Carr, W. J., L. Krames and D. J. Constanzo (1970a) Previous sexual experience and olfactory preference for novel versus original sex partners in rats. J. Comp. Physiol. Psychol. 71, 216–222.

Carr, W. J., R. D. Martorano and L. Krames (1970b) Responses of mice to odors associated with stress. J. Comp. Physiol. Psychol. 71, 223–228.

Carr. W. J., N. R. Wylie and L. S. Loeb (1970c) Responses of adult and immature rats to sex odors. J. Comp. Physiol. Psychol. 72, 51–59.

Carter, C. S. and J. N. Marr (1970) Olfactory imprinting and age variables in the guinea pig, *Cavia porcellus*. Anim. Behav. 18, 238–244.

Curtis, R. F., J. A. Ballantine, E. B. Keverne, R. W. Bonsall and R. P. Michael (1971) Identification of primate sexual pheromones and the properties of synthetic attractants. Nature (London) 232, 396–398.

Dagg, A. I. and D. E. Windsor (1971) Olfactory discrimination limits in gerbils. Can. J. Zool. 49, 283–285.

Devore, M. and M. R. Murphy (1972) Social agnosia produced by peripheral olfactory blockage in hamsters. Am. Zool. 12, 653.

Donovan, C. A. (1967) Some clinical observations on sexual attraction and deterrence in dogs and cattle. Vet. Med. Small. An. Clinician 62, 1047–1048.

Doty, R. L. (1972) Odor preferences of female *Peromyscus maniculatus bairdi* for male mouse odors of *P. m. bairdi* and *P. leucopus noveboracensis* as a function of estrous state. J. Comp. Physiol. Psychol. 81, 191–197.

Fox, M. W. and W. A. Himwich (1965) Olfactory imprinting: a measure of early learning in the neonate dog. Fed. Proc. Am. Soc. Exptl. Biol. 24, 522.

Franklin, W. L. (1973) Vicuna behavioral ecology. In: The Behaviour of Ungulates and its Relation to Management; eds.: V. Geist and F. Walther (in press).

Geist, V. (1971) Mountain sheep. A Study in Behavior and Evolution. (Univ. Chicago Press, Chicago and London) 142 pp.

Godfrey, J. (1958) The origin of sexual isolation between bank voles. Proc. Roy. Phys. Soc. Edinburgh 27, 47–55.

Heitzenroeder, C. (1913) Über das Verhalten des Hundes gegen einige Riechstoffe. Z. Biol. (Munich) 62, 491–507.

Johnston, R. E. (1972) Sex pheromones of the golden hamster, Am. Zool. 12, 662.

Kalogerakis, M. G. (1963) The role of olfaction in sexual development. Psychosom. Med. 25, 420–432.

Kelley, R. B. (1937) Studies in fertility of sheep. Bull. Counc. Sci. Ind. Res. (Melbourne) 112, 1–67.

Klopfer, P. H. and J. Gamble (1966) Maternal 'imprinting' in goats: the role of chemical senses. Z. Tierpsychol. 23, 588–592.

Krames, L. (1970) Responses of female rats to the individual body odors of male rats. Psychonomic Sci. 20, 274–275.

Landauer, M. R. and E. M. Banks (1972) The influence of early olfactory experience on social preference in mice (*Mus musculus*). Am. Zool. 12, 652.

Lemagnen, J. (1952) Les phénomènes olfacto-sexuels chez le rat blanc. Arch. Sci. Physiol. 6, 295–331.

Lindsay, D. R. (1965) The importance of olfactory stimuli in the mating behavior of the ram. Anim. Behav. 13, 75–78

Lindsay, D. R. and I. C. Fletcher (1968) Sensory involvement in the recognition of lambs by their dams. Anim. Behav. 16, 415–417.

Macintosh, J. H. and E. C. Grant (1966) The effect of olfactory stimuli on the agonistic behaviour of laboratory mice. Z. Tierpsychol. 23, 584–587.

Mainardi, D. (1963) Un esperimento nella parte attiva svolta dalla femina nella selezione sessuale in *Mus musculus*. Arch. Sci. Biol. 47, 227–237.

Mainardi, D., M. Marsan and A. Pasquali (1965) Causation of sexual preferences of the house mouse. The behaviour of mice reared by parents whose odour was artificially altered. Atti Soc. Ital. Sci. Nat. 104, 325–338.

Marr, J. N. and L. E. Gardner, Jr. (1965) Early olfactory experience and later social behavior in the rat. Preference, sexual responsiveness and care of young. J. Genet. Psychol. 107, 167–174.

Meyer, J. S. (1964) Stimulus control of mouse-killing rats. J. Comp. Physiol. Psychol. 58, 112–117.

Michael, R. P., E. B. Keverne and R. W. Bonsall (1971) Pheromones; Isolation of male sex attractants from a female primate. Science 172, 964–966.

Moore, R. E. (1965) Olfactory discrimination as an isolation mechanism between *Peromyscus maniculatus* and *Perymuscus pelionotus*. Am. Midl. Nat. 73, 85–100.

Müller-Schwarze, D. (1971) Pheromones in black-tailed deer (*Odocoileus hemionus columbianus*). Anim. Behav. 19, 141–152.

Müller–Schwarze, D. and C. Müller-Schwarze (1971) Olfactory imprinting in a precocial mammal. Nature (London) 229, 55–56.

Müller-Schwarze, D. and C. Müller-Schwarze (1972) Social scents in hand-reared pronghorn (*Antilocapra americana*). Zool. Afr. 7, 257–271.

Müller-Schwarze, D., C. Müller-Schwarze and W. L. Franklin (1973) Factors influencing scent marking in the pronghorn (*Antilocapra americana*). Verh. Deut. Zool. Ges. (Mainz) 1972 (in press).

Müller-Velten, H. (1966) Über den Angstgeruch bei der Hausmaus (*Mus musculus*). Z. Vergl. gl. Physiol. 52, 401–429.

Mykytowycz, R. (1968) Territorial marking by rabbits. Sci. Am. 218, 116–126.
Mykytowycz, R. (1972) The behavioural role of the mammalian skin glands. Naturwissenschaften 59, 133–139.
Mykytowycz, R. and M. L. Dudzinski (1972) Aggressive and protective behaviour of adult rabbits *Oryctolagus cuniculus* (L.) towards juveniles. Behaviour 43, 97–120.
Nyby, J., D. D. Thiessen and P. Wallace (1970) Social inhibition of territorial marking in the Mongolian gerbil (*Meriones unguiculatus*) Psychon. Sci. Sect. Anim. Physiol. Psychol. 21, 310–312.
Oldham, J. and D. Müller-Schwarze, Urine marking in rats (in preparation).
Quadagno, D. M. and E. M. Banks (1970) The effect of reciprocal cross fostering on the behaviour of two species of rodents, *Mus musculus* and *Baiomys taylori ater*. Anim. Behav. 18, 379–390.
Ralls, K. (1969) Scent marking in Maxwell's duiker, *Cephalophus maxwelli*. Am. Zool. 9, 1071.
Rasa, O. A. E. (1973) Marking behaviour and its social significance in the African dwarf mongoose, *Helogale undulata rufula*. Z. Tierpsychol. 32, 293–318.
Rauschert, K. (1963) Sexuelle Affinitat zwischen Arten und Unterarten von Rotelmausen (*Clethrionomys*). Biol. Zentralbl. 82, 653–664.
Reynolds, E. (1971) Urination as a social response in mice. Nature (London), 234, 481–483.
Rosenblatt, T. S., G. Turkewitz and T. C. Schneirla (1969) Development of home orientation in newly born kittens. Trans. N. Y. Acad. Sci. II, 31, 231–250.
Rowe, F. P. (1970) The response of wild house mice (*Mus musculus*) to live-traps marked by their own and by a foreign mouse odour. J. Zool.. (London) 162, 517–520.
Schapiro, S. and M. Salas (1970) Behavioral response of infant rats to maternal odor. Physiol. Behav. 5, 815–818.
Schultze-Westrum, T. (1965) Innerartliche Verständigung durch Düfte beim Gleitbeutler *Petaurus breviceps papuanus* Thomas (Marsupialia, Phalangeridae). Z. Vergl. Physiol. 50, 151–220.
Sheppard, D. H. and S. M. Yoshida (1971) Social behavior in captive Richardson's ground squirrels. J. Mammal. 52, 793–799.
Smith, F. V. (1965) Instinct and learning in the attachment of lamb and ewe. Anim. Behav. 13, 84–86.
Tschanz, B. (1962) Über die Beziehungen zwischen Muttertier und Jungen beim Mufflon. Experientia 18, 187–190.
Valenta, J. E. and M. K. Rigby (1968) Discrimination of the odor of stressed rats. Science 161, 599–601.
Wenzel, B. M. (1954) Problems of odor research from the viewpoint of a psychologist. Ann. N. Y. Acad. Sci. 58, 58–61.

CHAPTER 17

Odor in the spacing behavior of mammals

R. MYKYTOWYCZ

17.1. Introduction

The complex and often controversial question of the use of space by animals and man has been repeatedly dealt with in the past and recently attention was again focused on this subject during the International Symposium on 'Behavior and Environment' held at the 1968 meeting of the American Association for the Advancement of Science in Dallas, Texas. The Proceedings of this meeting, during which a variety of views was expressed, provide a particularly good source of information (Esser 1971). In order to aid documentation of the involvement of scent in the use of space by vertebrates some brief general introductory remarks are made here to their spacing behavior.

The characteristic relationship of many species to the space which they occupy has been noticed by many of those interested in the life of animals. The writings of Aristotle and Pliny already contain references to space ownership by birds. However, at the time when our knowledge of the behavior of animals was limited, too much emphasis was placed on the phenomenon of 'territoriality' and the concept of defense and aggression associated with it. Because of the endless varieties of 'territoriality' in different species no one has yet formulated a single, clear and generally valid definition of this phenomenon and the emphasis placed on the importance of aggression and the complete exclusion of conspecifics from an occupied area has diverted attention away from numerous other forms of socially motivated behavior in relation to space.

Hediger more than anyone else has contributed toward the formation of our current ideas concerning the relationship of animals to the space which they occupy by emphasizing that the animals form an inseparable unit with their space. It was he who introduced the view that animals, like man, reserve separate sections of their home ranges for different purposes. Thus there are places which are used for specific purposes like sleeping, resting, sheltering, eating, food storage, drinking, defecation, urination, basking, rubbing, and wallowing, and still others where young ones are deposited and kept during infancy. Further, it was Hediger who firmly expressed the idea that animals use visual, acoustic and olfactory methods to mark the possession of space (Hediger 1944, 1949, 1950, 1955, 1956). The role of odor in the behavior of animals generally, and in territoriality particularly, has been reviewed recently (Gleason and Reynierse 1969; Ewer 1968; Mykytowycz 1970, 1972; Ralls 1971).

Scent deposited in the space becomes a substitute for the animal itself and continues to be an effective message in the absence of the signalling animal. In the behavior of primitive man odor is not only used in many cases for object marking, but also for placing of a spell or taboo – as defense measures against rivals and demons. Medicinemen in the bazaars of Morocco sell tarry preparations in short lengths of sheep intestine which the Berbers apply to the four corners of their huts or houses to ward off evil spirits (Hediger 1955). Among the desert Arabs the sense of smell still plays an important role. While other cultural groups–for instance the southern Europeans–fear the 'evil-eye', the Bedouins fear nothing so much as the 'evil smell' (Musil quoted by Brill 1932).

Although the social space of animals is usually viewed as an area defined by visual or olfactory signals which affect the movements of individuals, there is evidence available that the overall physiology of animals is influenced by the 'atomosphere' of the owned space so that their moods are affected and they become predisposed to particular behavioral activities (Mykytowycz 1973). Strange space may have the opposite effect on the animals' behavior. The aim of this chapter is to emphasize that apart from territory in the strict sense of its meaning animals possess a whole range of space requirements superimposed upon one another which complicate and confuse the overall picture of space utilization. In all spatial requirements odor marking is characteristically used and plays an important role in defining the different types of areas.

The different space requirements of mammals are matched by their ability to mark differentially the separate types of living space. There is an indication that the size and secretory activity of odor producing organs change in relation to sex, reproductive state, age, social status and behavioral status generally. Thus the production of odor is strengthened by the urge of the individual to distribute it. There are also changes in the chemistry of secretions functioning for marking purposes related to the same factors. Variations occur not only in the ability of animals to produce but also to perceive odors which undoubtedly affect their behavior towards different types of social space. At different stages in the reproductive cycle individuals have different space requirements and it has been reported for some species, including man, that changes in the olfactory system and the ability to detect certain odors are correlated with the reproductive cycles (Mykytowycz 1970). Age, social status and other factors also affect the relationship of the individual to different types of social space. For instance, at the height of the breeding season of the wild European rabbit, *Oryctolagus cuniculus* (L.), when territoriality is strictly observed by adults, some juveniles display a tendency to disperse and disregarding territorial boundaries move into new group territories. Of course aggression is not entirely absent in these movements, but it is to the benefit of the species that some young individuals become integrated into new social groups.

In the insect world pheromones attain a highly specific role. Whole populations respond uniformly and unconditionally to odor messages which are usually highly specific. Considering the sharply defined requirements of insects and their short life span, it is essential that messages related to vitally important factors should be promptly acted upon.

In the life of mammals the importance of odor signals is not of the same magnitude. Usually there is no need for all individuals in a given population to participate equally strongly in all activities, particularly not in reproduction. It is not in the interests of the species that all mature individuals should breed unrestrictedly. As mentioned above, at a given time within a given population there will be a range of individuals which will react differently to the same signal. These differences may be induced by genetic make-up, social status, physiological state, previous experience – learning, and amongst other things by a varying degree of olfactory acuity. There will rarely be a uniform reaction towards any signals, including olfactory ones. Space marking with odors in mammals is a mechanism functioning to assure a certain order within the population for the smooth operation of social relationships. It is, however, only one of many factors and not solely responsible for the survival of an individual and population. In the event of the failure of odor marking, it is possible that other systems may take its place to preserve the important patterns of social behavior of the species.

Despite recognition of the importance of the olfactory marking of social space by mammals and the frequent references to it, surprisingly few detailed studies have been carried out on the marking behavior of any species. Some of the more detailed work, unfortunately, has been done with laboratory animals whose natural spatial requirements and social structures are completely unknown. The Mongolian gerbil, *Meriones unguiculatus* Milne-Edwards, is an example. Its marking behavior, involving the ventral gland, has been intensively studied by Thiessen and associates who paid particular attention to the effect of gonadal hormones on the intensity of secretion and its application (Thiessen et al. 1971). There is a need for more controlled studies of the role of odor in the space marking of free-living mammals. However, due to the inherent difficulties associated with studying natural populations over long periods the task will not always be simple.

17.2. Spacing behavior of the wild rabbit, Oryctolagus cuniculus

In Australia prolonged studies of the wild rabbit, *Oryctolagus cuniculus*, living in natural and experimental conditions have provided an opportunity to determine the pattern of social organization of the species and its relationship to the occupied space. The brief picture of the rabbit's territorial behavior given below is based on information reported in a series of earlier published papers (Myers and Poole 1959; Mykytowycz 1958, 1968; Myers et al. 1971). The whole system of the rabbits' social behavior is the result of the domination of one individual by another. Social relationships are constantly reinforced by aggressive displays or by avoidance. Hence, it is legitimate to refer to territoriality in its strict sense of meaning in connection with most of the forms of utilization of space by rabbits.

The wild rabbit is a gregarious species which forms social entities – colonies – occupying their own warren systems and grazing grounds. Colonies consist of separate groups each of which confines its activities to a group territory. Groups are made up of a few males and females among which a social hierarchy develops separately for each sex. The dominance hierarchy typical for the rabbit is indeed largely an organized spacing behavior. Each member of the group confines its activity to a particular space. These spaces of individuals overlap and those of the dominant males are the most extensive, tending to coincide with the group's territory. Dominant females, because of frequent breeding, are the most sedentary and their territories are the smallest. Females give birth to their kittens in breeding chambers dug as extensions to the existing warren system. However, among members of the same group, competition for breeding space within the commonly used section of the warren, is present and consequently, under the pressure of dominant females, some individuals are forced to deposit their litters in hastily dug 'breeding stops' at a distance from the warren. There are unattached individuals, mostly males, which do not acquire permanent membership of one group, but which, although they live outside the colony's territory, do not sever contact with it and regularly visit it. Some changes in the space occupied by groups may occur as the kittens mature, but more extensive and clearly defined re-arrangements take place at the onset of the breeding season. The size of the area around a rabbit which it can keep free of others and the extent to which an individual can penetrate into the personal space of another one is a reliable indicator of the social position of an individual within a group. The operation of the 'individual distance' phenomenon (Hediger 1955) is very clearly demonstrated by the aggressive approaches of dominants and the avoidance by subordinate animals. These are the most characteristic and most commonly seen forms of behavior during the observation of any colony of rabbits.

As in other species, notably domestic cats (Leyhausen 1971), the same space may be used by different rabbits at different times, so that direct social interaction may never occur between two individuals.

The space occupied by a mammal changes because the overall motivational state varies with circadian, seasonal and other rhythms and also through interference from non-rhythmic factors (Leyhausen 1971; McBride 1971). Thus during feeding activities relatively wider distances between rabbits are preserved and each animal confines its activities to its own territory. However, during alarm or resting actual bodily contact may be tolerated.

In rabbit populations the size and quality of space interacts with behavior – particularly their breeding behavior. The effect of space on sociality and health of rabbits has also been specifically studied experimentally. Harmful physiological changes have been demonstrated where living space was restricted; aggressive behavior increased and reproductive capacity decreased; and there were adverse changes in the condition of embryos, nestlings and young animals (Myers 1966; Myers et al. 1971). In conjunction with observations on the spacing behavior of rabbits studies have been made on the role of olfaction. The results of these studies, published in detail in a series of earlier papers to which references are made in the body of this chapter, form the basis of this text. In addition, relevant information for other species is mentioned.

17.3. Sources of odor used by mammals in marking space

The odors used by animals to demarcate their own space may come from various sources – urine, feces, saliva and most importantly from special odor-producing skin glands, the secretions from which may increase the communicative power of feces and saliva (Hediger 1949; Mykytowycz 1970, 1972).

In the rabbit, there are two externally secreting skin glands which seem to function for territorial purposes: the submandibular and the anal glands. Together with the inguinal gland, which also functions in the rabbit for behavioral purposes, these glands have been the subject of a series of ethological, histological, and chemical investigations (Mykytowycz 1965, 1966a, b; Goodrich and Mykytowycz 1972). The secretion from the submandibular gland is applied precisely to various objects when a rabbit touches its chin to them. The scent from the anal gland coats the hard fecal pellets as they pass through the end portion of the rectum; the characteristic 'rabbity' smell of feces comes from the secretion of this gland. Feces in the rabbit, as in many other species of vertebrates, are used for communicative purpose. Dung-hills – special sites in the rabbits' home range on which feces are regularly deposited – are important objects in the territorial behavior of the species (Mykytowycz and Gambale 1969).

There is a close correlation between the degree of development and the secretory activity of the odor-producing skin glands, and the social position of individuals, particularly their involvement in marking and defense of the social space. Thus male rabbits generally, and dominant ones in particular, possess the largest glands. The dominant females, however, which are also strongly territorial, may have glands just as large as non-dominant males (Mykytowycz and Dudzinski 1966).

The chemical composition of the skin glands of rabbits has been analysed using gas-chromatography, thin-layer chromatography, and electrophoresis. Differences occur in the composition of secretions from the separate types of glands and there may be variations related to sex and individual within the same type of gland. The secretion from the chin glands contains protein components as well as carbohydrate. The anal gland secretion contains protein as well as lipid – both free and protein-bound. The free lipid, with a 'rabbity' odor, accounts for approximately one percent of the total secretion. It is composed mostly of hydrocarbon together with an as yet unidentified component which has a mobility on thin-layer chromatography similar to aliphatic esters (Goodrich and Mykytowycz 1972).

17.4. Specific odor of the space occupied by a given species

In earlier discussions of social spacing attention has usually been paid to the repelling force of markings. However, it is not always in the interest of individual animals or of the species as a whole that conspecifics should be kept apart. Each species possesses a specific social distance, i.e. the maximum distance between individuals of any group. On this basis Hediger (1955) differentiates between 'contact animals' and 'distance animals'. The 'contact animals' are mainly gregarious species. Gregariousness of the wild rabbit has been dealt with elsewhere (Mykytowycz and Fullagar 1973) and it has been emphasized that basically there is no tendency to disperse even in the presence of ample space. Rabbits will try to associate themselves with an existing warren and consequently create conditions which support social frictions. This behavior adversely affects a proportion of the population, usually the subordinate animals. Conditions in any warren, while detrimental to some individuals, are beneficial to the species by acting as a density regulating mechanism. Imprinting to the odor of its own species is undoubtedly a factor attracting an individual to an area occupied by conspecifics.

Odor associated with the space occupied by animals can be perceived even by man. It is not difficult to detect rat or mouse infested premises from the characteristic odors or to tell a horse stable from a dairy shed. These odors are derived from the spontaneously deposited metabolic products as well as from deliberate space marking activities. Different patterns of spatial distribution of sympatric genetically related species, capable of breeding under laboratory conditions, assist speciation. Young rabbits still at nestling stage, when given the choice between artificial nests with and without rabbit odor, display a preference for the nests which had the scent of their own species (Gambale and Dudzinski, unpublished).

17.5 Specific odor of a social unit

There is ample evidence that when animals enter the area of a strange population they can detect it because of its characteristic odor.

Many people claim that they can distinguish the smell of different colonies of mice or rats. The characteristic odors are both intrinsic and extrinsic in origin. The intrinsic odor may be affected by food. Thus rats inhabiting a pig-sty smell differently from those living in a cold store, which carry the scent of trimethylamine or from a fish curing room, which smell of buccoline (Steinbrecher 1962).

The behavior of a rabbit entering the home range of a strange colony suggests that it is reacting to olfactory cues. It adopts a characteristic body posture, moves cautiously, exploring olfactorily the surroundings. It suspends eating and marking, displays a submissive posture to all permanent residents of the ground and is ready to withdraw at the slightest aggressive provocation. In the course of an experimental study of the aggressive behavior of adult female rabbits towards immature individuals, it has been demonstrated that kittens born within a strange colony were more severely attacked than kittens born to members of the same group. When the adult females were blindfolded it became clear that olfactory identification was involved (Mykytowycz and Dudzinsky 1972). Considering the high level of aggression of adult females to the kittens born to members of strange groups, it is important for the young rabbits early in their lives to recognize the characteristic odor of their own groups so that they can confine their movements to the area in which they remain protected from attacks by strange does and individuals of their own age (Mykytowycz and Ward 1971; Mykytowycz and Dudzinski 1972). Formation of group odors has been discussed elsewhere (Mykytowycz 1973) and it has been suggested that in the rabbit as in other species, e.g. sugar glider, *Petaurus breviceps papuanus* Thomas (Schultze-Westrum 1969), all members of a group add towards the characteristic odor, but that the dominant males are the most important contributors as they are the best equipped to produce scent and are most actively engaged in its distribution.

17.6. *Marking of breeding space*

There are various reasons why young individuals may be kept isolated from other members of their social group by being confined to special sites. Thus they may need better protection from predators and adverse climatic conditions or may have to be kept closer to sources of food and water or protected from deliberate or accidental injury by conspecifics.

During the course of amatory behavior prior to mating in the Indian rhinoceros, *Rhinoceros unicornis* L., the bulls and estrous females become engaged in wild chases which continue for days around the group's territory. Prior to this period, cows with young calves abandon the common territories and in small groups consisting of up to eight to ten mothers with their progeny, move into smaller calving grounds at a distance of approximately half a mile. There they remain safe until the end of the mating period when they rejoin the rest of the group (Ullrich 1967).

Rabbit litters are deposited in specially dug breeding chambers which, prior to parturition are lined with grass which is usually dry, and fur which the doe plucks from her belly, chest and flanks. Presumably this fur carries the scent of the mother, particularly the inguinal scent, with which the kittens become familiar very early in their lives. The mother also deposits a few fecal pellets in the nest. Experiments have shown that kittens learn to recognize the anal odor of the mother and at an early age display more attraction towards it than to any other natural rabbit odor (Mykytowycz and Ward 1971). A rabbit mother suckles her nestlings very briefly once per day for the first three weeks. Outside the feeding time the entrance to the breeding chamber is blocked by the female with a soil plug which is packed down with the forefeet and nose. On the soil plug the female deposits a few fecal pellets and a small quantity of urine.

In the course of prolonged studies of rabbit populations during which regular inspections of warrens were carried out, it was found that usually burrows containing young kittens were not entered by other members of the group. Interference by conspecifics may take place, however, when population pressures rise and territoriality crumbles. In situations when social stress increases, under both experimental and natural conditions, young kittens are frequently killed by other females. Although marking is obviously an effective method of protection it does not offer complete security to the kittens and the physical presence of the mothers may be very important in certain situations. Indeed it has been seen repeatedly that mothers excluded other rabbits from the vicinity of the nest and feeding grounds of their young progeny (Mykytowycz 1959).

Olfactory communication between nestling albino rats and their mothers has been reported. The lactating females start to emit a pheromone at about 14 days post-partum and cease to produce it at about 27 days, which coincides with the loss of responsiveness of the young ones towards it. The existence of the maternal pheromone seems to assure the reunion of the progeny with their mothers at the time when they are still dependent and yet display mobility (Leon and Moltz 1972). The pheromone seems to be contained in the feces (Leon, personal communication).

17.7. Scent marking of paths

The path is significant in the spacing behavior of animals not only because it connects points of importance and interest in the home range but more so because, irrespective of its dimensions, it is part of the animal's life. All changes in the animal's distance relationships develop along paths (Fischer 1971). A system of paths running across the home range of an animal imposes a standard pattern of movement. Space, time, and the behavior of animals interact closely and this dependence of one factor on another can clearly be seen in the movements of animals along their paths (Hediger 1967; Walther 1967). Man the hunter realized this a long time ago and took advantage of it.

When animals move regularly from one point to another, especially in numbers, they leave traces, or tracks, which have definite spatial delineations that can be recognized visually. For example, hippo paths become furrows 60 cm wide with a typical crest in the center; bison 30 cm and mice 3 cm wide (Walther 1967). On the other hand paths may be recognized olfactorily. Wildebeest in Masailand leave a characteristic odor on the ground from interdigital glands which allow not only conspecifics, but also man to track their movements (Talbot and Talbot 1963).

The marking of paths can, however, be much more complex and the house mouse provides a good example. Along its paths the mouse establishes urinating 'posts', originating on a fecal pellet, and with the accumulation of dust and debris cemented by urine these 'posts' reach considerable dimensions. Their distribution pattern suggests some symmetry; in one instance the distances between 'posts' were measured and found to be approximately 5 cm (Welch 1953). Rats establish similar 'posts' along their paths. Individuals of both sexes rub their urogenital regions on the 'posts' leaving clearly recognizable traces of mucus in addition to urine. This results in the mixing of secretions, desquamated skin, hairs and sebum from glands located at the base of the tail. This mixture of protein, mucin and fatty acids, undergoes oxidation and bacterial decomposition.

It has been suggested that bacterial strains which can as a rule be found in normal rat's urine may play an important role in shaping the odor of individual animals (Reiffe 1956). The tracks established by rats and mice within their home ranges facilitate not only their own orientation and movements but also those of newcomers. The wolf also displays a similar habit of marking with urine. Scent stations are established on or around stumps, sticks and logs. On a wide open expanse such as a frozen lake any conspicuous object may become a scent post. Sometimes several wolves of a pack will wait in line to urinate at the same place. They may repeat this each time they pass by and as a result a large amount of frozen urine accumulates on such a station over a winter. The scent posts may provide information on the number and size of social units (Mech 1970) and it is obvious from the behavior of wolves that scent posts have some meaning to animals outside the pack that makes them.

Not only the species mentioned above but many others also use urine to mark the space which they occupy (Hediger 1944; Wickler 1966).

The role of the path is particularly well understood in the life of the Indian rhinoceros. Their paths connect biologically important places within the home-range such as feeding, wallowing, bathing and sleeping sites. Some sections are used by all members of the group, shorter sections leading to feeding and sleeping places are private possessions and are protected. Rhino paths are 40–50 cm wide and often run through tunnels in the elephant grass. At the points where the tunnels start at the edge of clear grass-areas, fecal marking is practiced by all members of the group on the sides of the path. Even when in flight an individual will stop to contribute towards the dung-hills. Gradually the deposition may grow up to 70 cm in height. It has been suggested that for rhinos, which seemingly have very poor sight, the dung-hills indicate the entrances to tunnels and permit them to find the shortest way. They are formed only in the situations where there is a transition from tall grass to open land. After a fire in which the tall cover is destroyed this form of behavior is not practised. Similar marking is retained by rhinos in zoological gardens where openings occur in their enclosures (Ullrich 1967).

Paths are obvious in the rabbit's home-range. The most convincing demonstration of the complete confidence with which a rabbit uses its own paths is the fact that when released in its home range after being captured a rabbit will aim for a path and follow it to shelter. This it does apparently blindly, since the placing of an obstacle in the path will not be noticed and the animal will collide with it. This has been utilized when catching rabbits in experimental enclosures. Rabbits fleeing towards their burrows readily ran into long handled nets placed across the paths.

17.8. Special places for the exchange of information with conspecifics

Wynne-Edwards (1962), while discussing the problem of homeostasis, i.e. self regulation of natural populations of animals, introduced the concept of 'epideictic displays'. He suggested that these are necessary to allow animals to regulate their numbers and that the special sites on which animals deposit their scent are part of these displays. Most frequently these special sites for scent deposition are dung-hills. Many species of animals form dung-hills (Altmann 1969; Mykytowycz and Gambale 1969) which may not only be small discrete points, but in some species cover a considerable area, as for instance in the case of the hyena, *Crocuta crocuta* Kaup, up to a quarter of an acre (1012 m^2). The number of these special sites also varies from species to species depending on their need to communicate. Some like vicuna and alpacas maintain only one or two within their range, while for hippos 84 dung-hills were counted on a 350 m stretch of river bank.

As these special places are centres of communication it is necessary that as many animals as possible, even non-members of the group, come to gather the information deposited on them. The fact that they are connected by paths which are often commonly used, assures regular access to them. To avoid a meeting between opponents on these special sites a different time schedule may be employed. This happens with domestic cats and dogs.

It has been suggested that olfactory marking may function in some ways like railway signals. A fresh mark denotes 'section closed'; less fresh, 'proceed with caution'; old 'go ahead' (Leyhausen 1971). Naturally many other messages can be read simultaneously from the information sites.

The behavior of wild rabbits on their dung-hills has been studied both experimentally and in natural populations (Mykytowycz and Gambale 1969; Mykytowycz and Hesterman 1970). It has been found that the dung-hills are visited by all the males, but only by a few of the females occupying the area. When at the dung-hills, the rabbits examine them olfactorily and deposit their own scent in the form of fecal pellets coated with secretion from the anal gland. Sometimes they also deposit secretion from the chin gland. It has been demonstrated that the fecal pellets produced for marking possess a stronger 'rabbity' odor than those produced at other times (Hesterman and Mykytowycz 1968). Rabbit dung-hills are not distributed randomly, but are concentrated at points which are most exposed to contact or invasion from neighbors. Some observations on the distribution of fecal pellets have been carried out also in holding pens. Four pens 3 x 4 meters in size were built of wire mesh, allowing visual and olfactory communication between adjacent pens. On the floors three separate zones were marked. Counting the fecal pellets deposited in these zones indicated that the removal of feces from the pens increased the deposition of fecal pellets, and that deposition was most intense in the zones bordering onto other pens.

Not only fecal deposition sites, but as mentioned above in the case of wolves, cats and dogs, urination 'posts' also serve as permanent communication centers.

In the brown bear, *Ursus arctos* L., the use of another system of communication – 'rubbing place' – has been described. Members of this species select special places, usually trees for their rubbing activities and scents emanating from these sites play a role in social organization. There are main and subsidiary rubbing places in the bears' home ranges (Tschanz et al. 1968). The European bison also has demarcation trees, to which it applies its scent marks (Hediger 1955).

Species which do not hold a fixed area to which the traditional definition of territory could be applied also use communication point systems to regulate their spacing. A study of the interactions of groups of cheetah, *Acinonyx jubatus* Schreber, revealed that both sexes marked with their urine selected objects which stood out from the immediate environment. In open areas large trees, shrubs and stones were selected, and in heavily vegetated regions plants which contrasted with the homogeneous prevailing background. Anatomically, cheetah, in common with other cats, are highly specialized for marking with urine. They closely examine and react to markings left by other conspecifics. A 'time plan' system similar to that of domestic cats operates through marking points to prevent meetings between opponents occupying the same area (Eaton 1970).

As emphasized earlier it is not always in the interest of the species to prevent meetings between conspecifics. For the smooth functioning of a community there is a need for individuals to come together. Cats, seemingly solitary species, also have their social gatherings. At night they leave their territories and gather at certain places, sitting around looking at one another but not engaging in any other social activities. After 1–2 hours they disperse (Leyhausen 1971). A daily 'general assembly' of the strictly territorial rabbits has also been reported. For a short time each day all members of a group would gather around the main warren disregarding their normal individual territorial ranges (Mykytowycz 1958).

17.9. Personal space

Hediger (1955) also introduced another concept of the spacing of animals – the individual distance, i.e. the minimum distance within which animals of the same species may approach one another. This is not a fixed physically measurable area but a space surrounding an individual. This concept is probably more evident in the behavior of man than in any other species. There is often a tendency to emphasize the significance of odor in man's sexual behavior (Comfort 1971a, b, ch. 20 this volume). However, this is not the only situation in which smell plays an important role in our social relationships, particularly not in 'class' societies. It has been suggested that human odor is actually responsible for separating human beings (Brill 1932). We are aware of this in our everyday life and actually adjust our individual distances according to our needs. We use both our signalling and perceiving olfactory capacities to a different extent depending upon our personal and cultural habits. The use of perfume by women and in Western societies shaving lotion by men is not necessarily an expression of the desire to become more sexually attractive but rather the wish to be readily accepted by others or to make one's own presence more apparent.

Individual distance as any other social space varies with the needs or requirements of an individual at a given time. As the production of odor from the skin glands is under the control of sex hormones, individual distances of aggressive animals or those in a reproductive state will be increased automatically with a repelling or attracting effect depending on their physiological state. Thus for instance the individual distance of an estrous female rabbit will be narrower, i.e. she will be more approachable, more attractive in relation to males, and wider, i.e. she will be less approachable, more repelling, in relation to females.

Apart from the spontaneous variation of the individual distances of animals released by seasonal or long-lasting physiological changes, there are numerous examples of deliberate efforts by animals to change them in different behavioral situations. The aggressive display of the wild rabbit offers a good example. The dissemination of an individual's own odor in various forms precedes and accompanies the fighting of two male rabbits. Individuals seem to make a deliberate attempt to surround themselves with their own odor. Thus prior to actual physical contact, which in many cases never takes place, the two opponents become engaged in scratching the surface of, and chinning, the ground. They also chin intensively on any other objects and often defecate. Simultaneously they erect their tails prominently exposing the inguinal glands and partly extruding the anus. Analysis of film records of rabbits in aggressive interactions shows clearly that individuals prominently displaying the white undersurface of the tail invariably emerged as the victors. The subordinate, less aggressive rabbits, much as inhibited dogs, press their tails down tightly, presumably suppressing the dissemination of their odors. Thus it seems that there is a deliberate attempt by animals of many species to surround themselves with their own odor and by this means to widen their safety zone.

A good example of the manipulation of social distance by the use of odor comes from a report on the behavior of the hippopotamus. According to Verheyen (1954, quoted by Frädrich 1967), two hippos, confronting one another aggressively, become engaged in the production of their own odor. They defecate and expel gases through their mouths. The one which produces the larger amount of feces emerges as the victor.

Urine also plays a very important role in the manipulation of social distance. It is used by rabbits of both sexes in the course of aggression as well as in mating behavior. Enurination in the rabbit was originally reported by Southern (1948), and enurination of does by bucks is an integral part of the precopulatory behavior of the species (Myers and Poole 1961). In this way not only the males but also their sexual partners carry the olfactory signal demonstrating their sphere of influence. Chinning and enurination of young individuals, which is a very common form of behavior of males, produce the same effect and thereby strengthens the social claims of the individual identified with a given scent. Self enurination, so frequently reported amongst animals, particularly ungulates (Hediger 1944), is another example of the re-inforcement of individual distances. Males of many species during the breeding season urinate on their chest, abdomen, and legs with the result that their characteristic odor can be detected at a distance even by man. Some species of primates rub urine onto various parts of their body after urinating on their hands.

Enurination as a component of aggression and sexual behavior has been reported in many animals and Eibl-Eibesfeldt (1958) suggested that this is a 'symbolic takeover' of the sexual partner and should be regarded as an extension of the male's territorial marking. Kirchshofer (1960), who studied enurination in the mara, *Dolichotis patagonum* Desmarest, rejected this idea in view of the occurrence of enurination in species which do not use urine for territorial marking. The operation of individual distance in the mara is, however, obvious from her reference to aggressive competition for access to feeding places and to the existence of a social hierarchic order. Hence it is conceivable that even in this species communication about the presence and the intentions of an individual are necessary. If the distinction between territory and personal space is kept in mind the two views expressed above by the different workers are not contradictory.

17.10. *Confidence-giving effect of the odor of an individual's own space*

The confidence-giving effect of an individual's own territory is not an entirely new idea. In the past the thought has often been expressed that the individual's territory, familiar space, isolates it from harmful social frictions and effects its total behavior. Recently the importance of home environment on the reproductive behavior of rabbits has been discussed at length and special emphasis has been placed on the role of odor in shaping it (Mykytowycz 1973). It has been stressed that the behavior of rabbits and many other species is such that they permeate the environment in which they live with their own odor both passively and deliberately. This applies just as much to man although in his case many of the odors used are not necessarily his own natural ones.

Within the space in which its own or familiar odors prevail an animal acquires a physiological state which allows it to complete various biologically important functions and notably to participate in various stages or reproduction. The confidence giving effect of an animal's own and familiar odor has been demonstrated experimentally with rabbits. Rabbits were introduced in pairs into a neutral space and simultaneously the fecal pellets, or chin gland secretion, of one of them were also placed in the area. In a new neutral environment, but in the presence of its own or familiar odor, one individual dominates another. It moves confidently, attacks first and usually emerges as the winner. When the circumstances are reversed the outcome of the confrontation is also reversed with the original loser becoming dominant (Mykytowycz 1973). It should be emphasized that the presense of urine did not have an equally strong effect and the inguinal gland secretion had no effect at all on such confrontations. This indicates once more the behavioral specialization of different odors in the same individual.

17.11. Summary

Observations mainly on the behavior of the wild rabbit, *Oryctolagus cuniculus*, are used to show that animals possess different spatial requirements which assure the smooth functioning of social relationships. These include group and individual home ranges and territories; feeding, watering and food storage areas; resting, wallowing and sleeping sites; paths and special centers for the exchange of information – urinating posts and dung-hills; spaces reserved for young individuals and individual zones. Olfactory signals are used to delineate the various types of space and are derived from feces, urine and specialized odor-producing skin glands.

Changes in the ability to produce and perceive odors match the animals' spatial requirements. Although the repelling role of spacing is usually emphasized, its attractive functions are just as important. While it is assumed that odor of occupied space is mainly for communication with conspecifics there is evidence that it is of importance primarily to the owner of the space itself.

The distinction between the role played by pheromones in the lives of insects and mammals is emphasized. The uniform reaction of insects to pheromones is rarely seen in mammals, because at a given time a mammalian population consists of behaviorally heterogenous individuals which will never react in the same way to a particular signal. Olfactory marking by mammals of the occupied space preserves the typical pattern of social relationships and is part of the mechanism for self-limitation of the population.

Acknowledgments

Helpful criticism of the manuscript by Messrs. B. V. Fennesy and E. R. Hesterman (Division of Wildlife Research CSIRO) and Dr. B. S. Goodrich (Division of Animal Health, CSIRO) is appreciated.

References

Altmann, D. (1969) Harnen und Koten bei Säugetieren. (Ziemsen, Wittenberg Lutherstadt.) 104 pp.

Brill, A. A. (1932) The sense of smell in the neuroses and psychoses. Psychoanalytic Qu. 1, 7–42.

Comfort, A. (1971a) Communication may be odorous. New. Sci. 49, 412–414.

Comfort, A. (1971b) Likelihood of human pheromones. Nature (London) 230, 432–433.

Eaton, R. L. (1970) Group interactions, spacing and territoriality in cheetahs. Z. Tierpsychol. 27, 481–491.

Eibl-Eibesfeldt, I. (1958) Das Verhalten der Nagetiere. Handb. Zool. 8 (10:13), 1–88.

Esser, A. H. (1971) Behavior and Environment. The Use of Space by Animals and Men. (Plenum Press, New York–London) 411 pp.

Ewer, R. F. (1968) Ethology of Mammals. (Logos Press, London) 418 pp.

Fischer, F. (1971) Ten phases of the animal path: behavior in familiar situations. In: Behavior and Environment; ed.: A. H. Esser (Plenum Press, New York-London) pp. 9–21.

Frädrich, H. (1967) Das Verhalten der Schweine (Suidae, Tayassuidae) und Flusspferde (Hippopotamidae). Handb. Zool. 8 (10:26), 1–44.

Gleason, K. K. and J. H. Reynierse (1969) The behavioral significance of pheromones in vertebrates. Psychol. Bull. 71, 58–73.

Goodrich, B. S. and R. Mykytowycz (1972) Individual and sex differences in the chemical composition of pheromone-like substances from the skin glands of the rabbit *Oryctolagus cuniculus* (L.). J. Mammal. 53, 540–548.

Hediger, H. (1944) Die Bedeutung von Miktion und Defäkation bei Wildtieren. Schwiz A. Psychol. 3, 170–182.

Hediger., H. (1949) Säugetier-Territorien und ihre Markierung. Bijdr. Dierk. 28, 172–184.

Hediger, H. (1950) Wild Animals in Captivity (Butterworth, London) 207 pp.

Hediger, H. (1955) Studies of the Psychology and Behavior of Captive Animals in Zoos and Circuses (Butterworth's Scientific Publications, London) 166 pp.

Hediger, H. (1956) Instinkt und Territorium. In: L'instinct dans le Comportement des Animaux et de l'Homme. (Masson, Paris) pp. 521–543.

Hediger, H. (1967) Strassen der Tiere. (Vieweg, Braunschweig) 313 pp.

Hesterman, E. R. and R. Mykytowycz (1968) Some observations on the odour of anal gland secretions from the rabbit, *Oryctolagus cuniculus* (L.). CSIRO Wildl. Res. 13, 71–81.

Kirchshofer, R. (1960) Über das 'Harnspritzen' der Grossen Mara (*Dolichotis patagonum*). Z. Säugetierk. 25, 112–127.

Leon, M. and H. Moltz (1972) The development of the pheromonal bond in the albino rat. Physiol. Behav. 8, 683–686.

Leyhausen, P. (1971) Dominance and territoriality as complemented in mammalian social structure. In: Behavior and Environment; ed.: A. H. Esser (Plenum Press, New York-London) pp. 22–33.

McBride, G. (1971) Theories of animal spacing: the role of flight, fight and social distance. In: Behavior and Environment; ed.: A. H. Esser (Plenum Press, New-York-London) pp. 53–68.

Mech, L. D. (1970) The Wolf: The Ecology and Behavior of an Endangered Species. (Natural History Press, New York) 384 pp.

Myers, K. (1966) The effects of density on sociality and health in mammals. Proc. Ecol. Soc. Aust. 1, 40–64.

Myers, K. and W. E. Poole (1959) A study of the biology of the wild rabbit, *Oryctolagus cuniculus* (L.), in confined populations. I. The effects of density on home range and the formation of breeding groups. CSIRO Wildl. Res. 4, 14–26.

Myers, K. and W. E. Poole (1961) A study of the biology of the wild rabbit, *Oryctolagus cuniculus* (L.), in confined populations. II. The effects of season and population increase on behaviour. CSIRO Wildl. Res. 6, 1–41.

Myers, K., C. S. Hale, R. Mykytowycz and R. L. Hughes (1971) The effects of varying density and space on sociality and health in animals. In: Behavior and Evironment; ed.: A. H. Esser (Plenum Press, New York-London) pp. 148–187.

Mykytowycz, R. (1958) Social behaviour of an experimental colony of wild rabbits, *Oryctolagus cuniculus* (L.). I. Establishment of the colony. CSIRO Wildl. Res. 3, 7–25.

Mykytowycz, R. (1959) Social behaviour of an experimental colony of wild rabbits, *Oryctolagus cuniculus* (L.). II. First breeding season. CSIRO Wildl. Res. 4, 1–13.

Mykytowycz, R. (1965) Further observations on the territorial function and histology of the submandibular cutaneous (chin) glands in the rabbit, *Oryctolagus cuniculus* (L.). Anim. Behav. 13, 400–412.

Mykytowycz, R. (1966a) Observations on odoriferous and other glands in the Australian wild rabbit, *Oryctolagus cuniculus* (L.) and the hare, *Lepus europaeus* P. I. The anal gland. CSIRO Wildl. Res. 11, 11–29.

Mykytowycz, R. (1966b) Observations on odoriferous and other glands in the Australian wild rabbit, *Oryctolagus cuniculus* (L.) and the hare, *Lepus europaeus* P. II. The inguinal glands. CSIRO Wildl. Res. 11, 49–64.

Mykytowycz, R. (1968) Territorial marking by rabbits. Sci. Am. 218, 116–126.

Mykytowycz, R. (1970) The role of skin glands in mammalian communication. In: Advances in Chemoreception. vol. I. Communication by Chemical Signals; eds.: J. W. Johnston, D. G. Moulton and A. Turk (Appleton-Century-Crofts, New York) pp. 327–360.

Mykytowycz, R. (1972) The behavioural role of the mammalian skin glands. Naturwissenschaften 59, 133–139.

Mykytowycz, R. (1973) Reproduction of mammals in relation to environmental odours. J. Reprod. Fert., Suppl. 19, 431–444.

Mykytowycz, R. and M. L. Dudzinsky (1966) A study of the weight of odoriferous and other glands in relation to social status and degree of sexual activity in the wild rabbit, *Oryctolagus* (L.). CSIRO Wildl. Res. 11, 31–47.

Mykytowycz, R. and M. L. Dudzinsky (1972) Aggressive and protective behaviour of adult rabbits, *Oryctolagus cuniculus* (L.) towards juveniles. Behaviour 43, 97–120.

Mykytowycz, R. and P. J. Fullagar (1973) Effect of social environment on reproduction in the rabbit, *Oryctolagus cuniculus* (L.). J. Reprod. Fert., Suppl. 19, 501–520.

Mykytowycz, R. and S. Gambale (1969) The distribution of dung-hills and the behaviour of free-living rabbits, *Oryctolagus cuniculus* (L.) on them. Forma Functio 1, 333–349.

Mykytowycz, R. and E. R. Hesterman (1970) The behaviour of captive wild rabbits, *Oryctolagus cuniculus* (L.) in response to strange dung-hills. Forma Functio 2, 1–12.

Mykytowycz, R. and M. M. Ward (1971) Some reactions of nestlings of the wild rabbit, *Oryctolagus cuniculus* (L.) when exposed to natural rabbit odors. Forma Functio 4, 137–148.

Ralls, K. (1971) Mammalian Scent Marking. Science 171, 443–449.

Reiff, M. (1956) Untersuchungen über natürliche und synthetische Geruchstoffe die bei Ratten und Mäusen eine stimulierende Wirkung auslösen. Acta Trop. 13, 289–318.

Schultze-Westrum, T. G. (1969) Social communication by chemical signals in flying phalangers (*Petaurus breviceps papuanus*). In: Olfaction and Taste. Proceedings of the third Intern. Symp; ed. : C. Pfaffman (Rockefeller Univ. Press, New York) pp. 268–277.

Southern, H. N. (1948) Sexual and aggressive behaviour in the wild rabbit. Behaviour 1, 173–195.

Steinbrecher, N. (1962) Die Duftwahl von Wander-und Hausratten. Z. Angew. Zool. 49, 301–349.

Talbot, L. M. and M. H. Talbot (1963) The wildebeest in western Masailand, East Africa. Wild. Monogr. No. 12.

Thiessen, D. D., K. Owen and G. Lindzey (1971) Mechanisms of territorial marking in the male and female Mongolian gerbil (*Meriones unguiculatus*). J. Comp. Physiol. Psychol. 77, 38–47.

Tschanz, B., M. Myer-Holzapfel and S. Bachmann (1968) Das Informationssystem bei Braunbären. Z. Tierpsychol. 25, 47–72.

Ullrich, W. (1967) Nashornstrassen in Assam. In: ed.: H. Hediger, Die Strassen der Tiere (Vieweg, Braunschweig) pp. 56–67.

Verheyen, R. (1954) Monographie étologique de l'hippopotame. Inst. Parc Nat. Congo, Explor. Parc Nat. Albert.

Walther, F. (1967) Tierstrassen in Afrika. In: Die Strassen der Tiere; ed. H. Hediger (Vieweg, Braunschweig) pp. 19–45.

Welch, J. F. (1953) Formation of urinating 'posts' by house mice (*Mus*) held under restricted conditions. J. Mammal. 34, 502–503.

Wickler, W. (1966) Ursprung und biologische Deutung des Genitalpräsentierens männlicher Primaten. Z. Tierpsychol. 23, 422–437.

Wynne-Edwards, V. C. (1962) Animal Dispersion in Relation to Social Behavior (Oliver and Boyd, Edinburgh) 653 pp.

CHAPTER 18

Pheromonal influences on reproductive activities in rodents

F. H. BRONSON

18.1. Introduction

As a generality, our knowledge about mammalian pheromones is neither as richly diverse nor as ecologically detailed as that provided by entomologists. Scientists and non-scientists alike have long been aware of the importance of chemical communication in mammals but a reasonably broad research thrust into this area dates only from the early 1960's. This effort has involved reproductive physiologists, ethologists, and psychologists; it has not included ecologists, chemists or neurophysiologists to nearly as great an extent. As a consequence, our detailed knowledge in this field can quickly be summarized as largely laboratory animal-oriented, most often set within the framework of laboratory rather than field ecology, and with an emphasis on behavior and reproductive physiology at the expense of neural mediation and pheromone chemistry.

Regardless of such limitations, real progress has been made and many solid generalities have emerged. For one, mammals apparently do communicate via specific volatile compounds and in a manner satisfying the classic definition of a pheromone (Kalmus 1964; Regnier 1970). For another, when addressing the subject of pheromones in mammals, we are apparently talking primarily, and possibly exclusively, about odors and olfactory reception. There are several possible sensory routes available for chemical perception in mammals, e.g., through receptors in the olfactory epithelium, via the vomeronasal organ, by way of unspecialized nerve endings in the nasal cavity leading to the trigeminal nerve, and, of course, taste. No real evidence associating pheromonal function with gustatory processes has yet been forthcoming. The possible importance of the trigeminal and the vomeronasal routes has been inadequately examined. A role for the latter, however, is strongly suggested in some species showing a 'Flehmen' response, that is a contraction of the lips, most often elicited when in close sexual association, and which could function to transport materials to the vomeronasal organ (see Eisenberg and Kleiman 1973). Functional participation by the trigeminal innervated area of the nasal epithelium has been suggested by human studies using standard odor tests (Henkin and Hoye

1966). The importance of volatile, air-borne compounds and participation by the olfactory epithelium and bulbs, on the other hand, is more than suggestive; it is unequivocal.

By way of a third generality, a dichotomy of mammalian pheromonal function, modelled after entomological constructs, has proven quite useful: i.e. a) signalling pheromones that result in a more or less immediate change in motor activity on the part of the recipient animal; and b) priming pheromones that trigger neuroendocrine and endocrine activity. A response to a signalling pheromone (e.g., a sex attractant), if it does occur, will be behavioral and is most apt to occur shortly after reception of the information. An example of a mammalian primer is a factor in male urine, the smell of which passively induces neural and hormonal changes in females which culminate in ovulation and sexual behavior 48–72 hours later. All mammalian priming functions so far documented are associated in some way with the process of reproduction. Signalling pheromones apparently have diverse functions, but again most are associated with behaviors modulated by the reproductive hormones. Probably at this time we are wise to assume relatively few complex functions for signalling pheromones; primarily those of identification of species (race and/or colony?), individual, age, sex, sexual state, and fear. Unfortunately no mammalian primers and only a few signalling pheromones have been isolated and identified. Reasonable identification of signals has been accomplished for a tarsal gland pheromone in the black-tailed deer (Müller-Schwarze 1971) and for a vaginal sex attractant in the rhesus monkey (Michael et al. 1971). A third pheromone, an attractant found in the boar's preputial, has been inclusively documented (e.g., Dutt et al. 1958; Sink 1967; Katkov and Gower 1968). Pheromonal sources have been localized in a variety of other species, however, and include urine and a variety of glands such as specialized and non-specialized sebaceous glands in the skin, eye and buccal cavity glands and sex accessory glands such as the preputial. Feces are often cited as a pheromone source but critical work is too often lacking. While good field work is severely limited, some of the natural functions postulated for such presumed pheromones seem quite reasonable and, in terms of pheromone chemistry, there is every reason to assume an ability to isolate and synthesize many of these important factors.

As still another generality, an important and uniquely interesting feature of many pheromonal systems in mammals is their modifiability. One would suspect, a priori, that most comparisons between mammalian and insect pheromonal systems, for example, would approximate the relationship between the capacities of their two distinctly different types of nervous systems. While it is no longer in vogue to refer to all of the insects' behavioral repertoire as 'stereotyped', 'stimulus-bound', or other such terminology inferring inflexibility and complete programming by genetics, the mammalian nervous system nevertheless is decidedly more flexible and its behavior definitely more experience-determined. Responses to pheromones among mammals are likewise decidedly variable and often experience-oriented.

There are, for example, situations known for both signalling and priming pheromones where the response must be conditioned in association with the pheromone. There are other instances where olfactory experiences encountered early in the mammal's life function to determine adult response to odors; both of these situations being quite typical of much non-pheromonally stimulated mammalian behavior. As an additional and more specific example of the modifiability of mammalian systems, a female sex attractant may elicit an immediate response that varies considerably in strength, a response that may be positive or negative, or no response at all depending upon a variety of experiences and, hence, competing drives in the recipient male; e.g., his dominance status, the nearby presence of other males, sexual satiation, etc. Because of the strong interaction with experience in at least some mammalian phenomena, the term *signalling* rather than *releasing* seems a more reasonable modifier for that category of pheromones yielding an immediate effect on behavior (Bronson 1968). The former term, while admittedly somewhat redundant, implies only the passage of information without demanding a response.

Two additional problems leading to still further complexity in mammals should be mentioned at this time. Both stem from the fact that many mammals rely heavily on a combination of senses in their continual assessment of their surroundings. Thus olfactory cues are usually not used exclusively as determinants of a particular behavioral response and, in addition, an exceedingly large variety of olfactory cues used by mammals do not fit the restricted concept of specific allomones or pheromones. As an example of the first of these problems, rats are known to make strong use of olfactory cues during their pre-copulatory sexual behavior, yet loss of their sense of smell usually results in no absence of this behavior, only a stronger dependence on visual and tactile cues. As another example, boar odor functions to arouse an estrous sow and result in her adoption of a mating posture; 90% will do so given the sound and smell of a boar and the pressure of a handler's hand, all three factors acting in a more or less additive fashion to reach that figure with sound being of less importance than pressure or smell (Signoret and Du Buisson 1961). Again, the paramount rule in mammals would seem to be the simultaneous use of many sensory systems to accomplish a particular behavioral task. As an example of the second problem mentioned above, mice can be trained to discriminate between two other mice of the same sex, age, and highly inbred strain (Bowers and Alexander 1967). It is difficult to visualize the use of anything other than the broadest possible spectrum of individual odors in this phenomenon and, hence, unreasonable either to apply the strict concept of a pheromone or attempt its isolation in such a situation.

Because of the problems discussed above, the term pheromone has probably been over-used by investigators working with mammals. Invocation of the concept of a pheromone would seem useful only where natural functions are obvious and where it seems reasonable to predict isolation, identification, and synthesis of a discrete compound or, at the most, a restricted mixture of odors. Even then such specific volatile signals are often used only in conjunction with other sensory activity; the ultimate behavioral or physiological response being determined only after integration of all possible sensory information.

As a summary of all that has been said so far concerning generalities and problems, then: a) mammals make heavy use of olfactory cues, most often in conjunction with other sensory modalities; b) some of these cues satisfy a restricted concept of pheromonal communication and, furthermore, can be functionally dichotomized with relative ease into priming or signalling categories; and finally c) social experience adds an important dimension of variability to these behavioral systems. The purpose of the rest of this chapter is to discuss in a more detailed fashion the role of pheromones in mammalian, particularly rodent, reproductive physiology and behavior. As a final comment before undertaking this discussion, one could say that, while the field of mammalian pheromones is decidedly under-researched, it is just as decidedly over-reviewed. An interested reader can turn to any of a large number of recent reviews to find up-to-date bibliographies concerning almost all facets of this broad subject: Bronson (1968, 1971); Bruce (1966, 1967, 1970); Cheal and Sprott (1971); Eisenberg and Kleiman (1973); Gleason and Reynierse (1969); Mykytowycz (1970); Ralls (1971); Schultz and Tapp (1973); Whitten (1966); and Whitten and Bronson (1970). Because of these extensive efforts, no attempt will be made in the present chapter to cite other than the latest or most relevant references.

18.2. Pheromones and reproduction in mice

When one considers the known pheromonal systems in mammals, undoubtedly the best documented and the most detailed is that encompassing the behavioral and physiological activities involved in reproduction in laboratory mice. More is known about priming pheromonal action in this species than in any other and, in addition, while field work involving mice is limited, considerable laboratory experimentation relevant to olfactory signals has been accomplished. It is my intention in this chapter to use a detailed discussion of the interrelated phenomena pertaining to mouse reproduction as a model system for generalizing to other pheromonal systems and functions in other species of mammals. Before discussing the impact of pheromones on this particular set of events, however, we must first consider reproductive activities in the mouse in their entirety. Behaviorally we shall consider sexual behavior, maternal care, and aggression; the latter acting as a mechanism for population dispersal during the reproductive season. Physiologically we shall be interested in puberty and the regulation of the infertile cycle as well as early pregnancy and maternal phenomena. A general text on reproduction (e.g.. Van Tienhoven 1968) can be consulted for details but, briefly, house mice may show profound seasonal variation in their reproductive efforts in the field but breed throughout the year in the constant environment of the laboratory. Basic regulatory mechanisms rely on the neural ramifications of external cues such as photoperiodic changes or priming pheromones. Of particular interest are mechanisms at the level of the hypothalamus, whose activity regulates the secretion of the gonadotropins, follicle-stimulating hormone (FSH) and luteinizing hormone (LH), from the anterior pituitary. With regard to non-pregnant, female mice, the secretion of gonadotropins is cyclic over a period of days (the estrous cycle); i.e., every few days the female ovulates and, for a period of hours at this time, will accept a male. There is strong circadian involvement since ovulation and mating almost always occur in the dark phase of the animal's day. FSH and LH act in concert to promote ovum maturation, ovulation, and the production of the ovarian steroids, the estrogens and progesterone. In the male, secretion of the gonadotropins is relatively constant and the actions of FSH and LH are to maintain spermatogenesis and promote synthesis of testosterone and other androgenic steroids by the testes.

Fig. 18.1 attempts to illustrate the entire complexity of behavioral and physiological events relevant to reproduction in both sexes of mice. The physical and/or social environment is perceived through sense receptors. Information thus collected is processed in the brain and certain cues or combinations of cues act via the

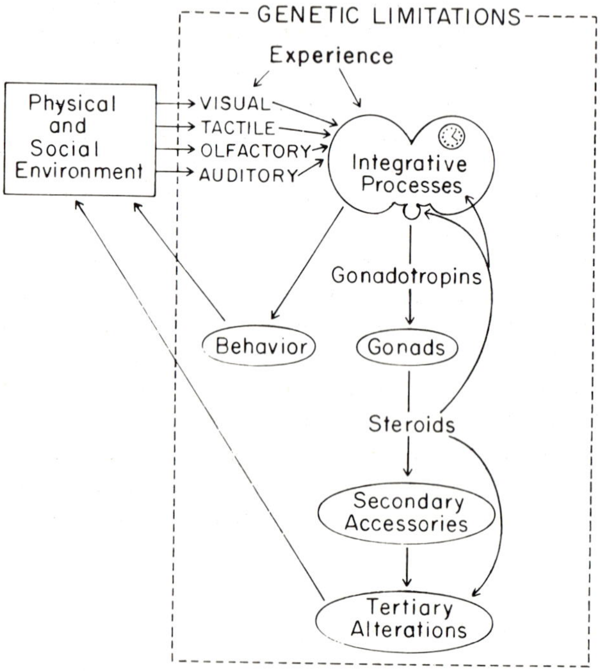

Fig. 18.1. Summarizing scheme of the complexity of behavioral and physiological events related to reproduction in both sexes of mice.

hypothalamus to ensure activity along the anterior pituitary gonadal axis. Steroid synthesis thus induced in the gonads ensures maintenance of the secondary accessory organs whose functions are necessary for reproduction but steroids are also active at a tertiary level; e.g., serving as the basis for sex differences in musculature, size, and pheromone production. Important actions of steroids occur when they feed back to brain receptors regulating gonadotropin secretion and, in addition, modulating reproductive-related behaviors such as sexual and aggressive behavior. To complete this description, both the overt behavior of the subject and some tertiary effects such as pheromone production then become external cues for other members of the same species, thus modifying the recipient's behavior and/or physiology. Finally, the past experience of the subject animal may modify the stimulus-response systems inherent in this complexity, and all of the above is set within genetic limits that have been determined by past selective processes.

What one sees in fig. 18.1, then, is a perceptual system of environmental cues resulting in hormone production which, in turn, ensures successful reproduction by a) guiding activity of the reproductive organs; and b) ensuring the potential for displaying the appropriate behavior at the correct time, given the appropriate external trigger. Thus hormones not only ensure that a female will ovulate at a particular time in her cycle but also condition her to be receptive to a male should one be available shortly before or after ovulation. Hormones also ensure that a male is more or less constantly ready, both behaviorally and physiologically, to inseminate a female and, in addition, support his aggressiveness toward other males. Importantly, all sensory modalities probably play a role sometime during this complex series of events; pheromones being only one such type of cue. Judicious laboratory experimentation, however, has allowed the separation of the various types of input into this system; hence, we can discuss the role of pheromones separately. Briefly, androgen-dependent, primer pheromones in male urine are known to accelerate the onset of puberty in females, to accelerate and regularize their estrous cycles, and to block pregnancy, all presumably by influencing the release of the female's gonadotropic hormones. A suspected female-originating primer is thought to suppress or prolong the estrous cycle in other females, presumably by partial inhibition of gonadotropin release. In addition, olfactory signals are known to be heavily used in sexual behavior, aggressive behavior, and maternal care. Finally, olfactory experiences occurring early in the life of the mouse are known to play an imprinting-like role, thus in part determining social (sexual and aggressive) choice when adult.

18.3. Mouse primer pheromones

Reproductive physiologists have been largely concerned with a series of priming effects discovered since 1955. The overall impact of olfaction on mouse reproduction is perhaps best demonstrated by the complete cessation of reproductive activity occurring in some, but not all, strains following olfactory bulbectomy (c.f. Whitten 1956a; Bruce and Parrott 1960; Gandelman et al. 1972; Rowe and Edwards 1972). Ideally this type of surgery should be useful for interrupting pheromonal transmission thereby verifying the nature of the cue in question. Unfortunately in many strains the operation itself has so many central effects that reproduction and, hence, its associated behaviors, is no longer physiologically possible, apparently because of effects on gonadotropin synthesis and/or release.

One of the best documented aspects of primer pheromone function in mammals is certainly in the control of the estrous cycle of the laboratory mouse (Whitten 1956b; 1959). While typically thought of as possessing 4 to 5-day periodicity, estrous cycles ranging up to 11–12 days may be easily produced and should be considered perfectly normal depending upon the presence or absence of male odors and the genetic strain under consideration (Bronson 1968). Two distinct phenomena interact to produce this variation; a) the suppression of estrous cycling by a poorly understood odor that is apparently produced among groups of females; and b) the acceleration or induction of cycling by a priming factor in male urine. Cycles of relatively short duration, then, are obtained in adults of some but not all strains of mice by isolation or, in most strains, by exposure to male odor regardless of whether the females are housed alone or in groups. It is interesting that all classic references on mouse reproduction have recorded the cycle length for this species as 4–5 days or, at the most six days for some strains. The mouse estrous cycle was first investigated in an era when mice were routinely kept in large numbers per cage and in large rooms containing a decided mixture of sexes and strains. Given our present knowledge about the profound effects of male urinary priming pheromone, and the reasonably low thresholds for response to this factor, it is obvious that the development of the 4–5 day dogma was the result of considerable data collection in poorly ventilated animal rooms where females were always subjected to male odors. The use of more modern animal rooms, typically smaller in size and with one-way air flow, coupled with better separation of the sexes, were important factors leading to the elucidation of the ability of primers to regulate this cycle.

With specific regard to the phenomena of estrus-suppression by grouping of females in the absence of male odor, this presumed pheromonal action may result in either a prolongation of the quiescent phase of the estrous cycle (Whitten 1959) or spontaneous pseudopregnancy (Lee and Boot 1956). Thus depending upon the strain under investigation, the density of the population of grouped females, and/or probably some other unknown factors, grouped females tend to cycle slowly and erratically and may even become pseudopregnant. Even two females housed together tend to suppress each other's cycles to some degree (Champlin 1971). The evidence for a pheromonal basis for such cycle-lengthening rests on reports that suppression is alleviated by olfactory bulbectomy and is independent of vision, audition, and physical contact (Whitten 1959; Biancifiori and Caschera 1963). In addition, Champlin (op. cit.) has succesfully slowed the cycle of the isolated females by housing them on bedding previously soiled by other females. These observations seem most easily explained by postulating a female primer; each female having the ability to accommodate to her own pheromone but not to those produced by other females. Thus, as is presumed for the pregnancy blocking effect which will be discussed later, some aspect of individuality must be associated with the primer. Whether this is a coupling of individual odors with a core primer pheromone or not remains to be seen.

The presence of a pheromone has been better established as the stimulus associated with a male that can override the suppressive effects of all-female grouping and, therefore, synchronize the estrous cycles and, hence, ovulation among a group of females (Whitten 1956b). The odor of male urine of the appropriate species induces estrous synchrony in both mice and deermice (Bronson and Marsden 1964; Marsden and Bronson 1964). The mouse pheromone is apparently of small enough molecular size to be transported at least eight feet on a 0.25-mph air current (Whitten et al. 1968). As little as 0.1 ml of male urine per day for two days (applied to the bedding) will effectively accelerate cycling among groups of wild house mouse females; 0.01 ml is effective in deermice (Bronson 1971). Additionally, it has been shown that just the presence of males in the same animal room is sufficiently stimulating to influence cycle duration in wild house mouse females (Chipman and Fox 1966). Bladder urine has proven as effective in inducing estrus as externally voided urine, thus apparently ruling out participation by a variety of sex accessory glands. The pheromone is either an androgen metabolite or the product of androgen-maintained tissue since castration removes it from urine and testosterone replacement returns it to castrates of either sex (Bronson and Whitten 1968). Saline homogenates of mouse testes are ineffective in inducing estrus (Bronson unpublished observations). An active fraction of urine has been obtained from a Sephadex column, but isolation and identification have not yet been accomplished (Whitten personal communication). Finally it should be noted that species specificity has been established for the urinary priming pheromone within the limited framework of deermice, several inbred house mouse strains, and human male urine (Bronson and Whitten 1968).

We are thus apparently confronted with a small molecule in male urine that is androgen dependent, species-specific and, at least as tested in deermice or wild house mice in the laboratory, may act at remarkably low concentrations to initiate an estrous cycle via olfactory reception. The mechanism of action of this molecule is assumed to be by way of the hypothalamus and to cause the release of gonadotropins by the anterior pituitary. A variety of studies using intact, ovariectomized, prepubertal females, however, have so far failed to delineate the precise hormonal responses to this male odor (e.g. Bronson and Stetson 1973).

An interesting action of what could be presumed to be the same pheromone in male urine is to induce precocial puberty in young female mice. There is apparently a period of time prior to puberty in young females when the entire reproductive system is almost mature but has not yet been triggered to function. Exposure to a male or his odor during this time induces puberty, complete with ovulation and mating (Vandenbergh 1969). Unlike the ease with which the male primer acts on grouped adult females, however, grouping of prepubertal females provides a strong resistance to the male's odor (Vandenbergh et al. 1972). The response of prepubertal females to male odor, assessed in terms of uterine weight, provides an efficient, sensitive bioassay for male priming pheromone (Bronson and Stetson 1973).

The estrus-inducing compound discussed above, coupled with individual identification, provides adequate pheromonal basis to conceptualize a block to implantation resulting from exposure to a strange male; a phenomenon first described in laboratory mice by Bruce (1959). Removal of the stud from an inseminated female's home cage and replacement with another male results in both a failure to implant and a return to the infertile cycle. This effect is absent in anosmic females and may be duplicated by exposing the inseminated female to pooled urine, providing the urine is collected from a normally or experimentally androgenized mouse (Bruce 1965; Dominic 1965). Such a response to a male would seem to be similar to the estrus-induction phenomenon previously described, given: a) accommodation on the part of the female to the pheromones of the original stud but not to those of the stranger, and b) the hormonal responses to male odor possibly being somewhat different in inseminated females than they are during the infertile cycle. The former supposition would seem to be of prime importance since re-exposure to the original stud male does not result in a blocked pregnancy. Additionally, the efficiency of blockage is enhanced if stud and strange males are of different genetic strains (Parkes and Bruce 1961). Thus the key concept would appear to be discrimination on the part of the female between the odors of the two males; a discrimination allowing her to cease responding to the stud after his original induction of her estrous cycle but to react to the new male by hormonal changes leading to a return to estrus at the expense of implantation. Such a process implies a role for experience and signalling pheromonal differences (individual identification of males) as well as sensory, central integrative, and steroidal influences on the part of the female, none of which are well understood. Lott and Hopwood (1972) have challenged the idea that accommodation to the stud is an aspect of the blocking mechanism. They provide data suggesting that, indeed, the action of the stud mouse is to *sensitize* the female to further male exposure.

Regardless of this conflict, the obvious physiological effect of strange male exposure is to prevent functionalization of the corpus luteum, i.e., that component of the ovary primarily responsible for producing quantities of progesterone which, in turn, allow uterine development to a point where implantation can occur. Formation of the corpus luteum is at least in part due to increased secretion of a hormone, prolactin, from the anterior pituitary in the mouse. Protection from the block may be obtained by injecting prolactin concurrently with male exposure (Bruce and Parkes 1960; Dominic 1966) suggesting that the primary effect of the male is to enhance the normal tonic inhibition of prolactin release. On the other hand, Hoppe and Whitten (1972) induced similar blocks to pregnancy by injecting pregnant mare's serum, an FSH-like hormone, and Chapman et al. (1972) reported a decrease in pituitary LH (and, hence, presumably a release of LH) preceding any effect on pituitary prolactin content in inseminated females as a consequence of strange male exposure. To further confuse the picture, adrenalectomy protects against the block in one stock of laboratory mice (Snyder and Taggert 1967) and greatly increased levels of circulating corticosterone have been reported in inseminated deermice during the initial stages of strange male exposure (Bronson et al. 1969). In the latter case, however, adrenalectomy offered no protection against an implantation failure and even pharmacological doses of the pituitary principal controlling the adrenal cortex, ACTH, did not decrease the probability of implantation.

In summarizing the priming effects in house mice, one could say that there is certainly adequate evidence on hand to indicate that volatile compounds acting via olfactory reception can have profound effects on several pituitary hormones. Considerable work remains to be done. The few genetic studies accomplished so far have indicated that the inheritance of these phenomena may be reasonably simple (Chapman and Whitten 1968; Eleftheriou et al. 1972) thus possibly providing good tools for answering relevant problems. Regardless of approach, however, the prime problems would seem to remain: a) careful elucidation of the physiological action of primers in the brain and on the pituitary, b) isolation and identification of the primers; and c) conceptualizing the individualistic aspects of these primers which are seen in the all-female suppressing effect and in the pregnancy-block discrimination.

18.4. Mouse signalling pheromones

To understand the importance of olfactory signals in intra-population communication among mice, one must emphasize that these are nocturnal animals with individuals in the population often being widely spaced both geographically and temporally. Under such circumstances, signalling pheromones would certainly be suspected of playing an important communicative role and many studies have now documented this obvious relationship. With regard to reproduction, numerous studies have shown the importance of olfaction in sexual, aggressive, and maternal behaviors. The presence of sex attractants, however, is incompletely documented in mice. A female-originating pheromone acting as an attractant for males has, surprisingly, received only cursory attention despite the fact that such a signal is a known suspected component of the urine of so many mammals. The opposite attraction is better documented. Female mice become more active when in the presence of odor drawn from a cage of males (Ropartz 1968a), and, additionally, Scott and Pfaff (1970) have shown that females prefer urine collected from intact males to that obtained from castrates. The male's preputial gland lipids have been implicated in this phenomenon (Bronson and Caroom 1971), with one report of such pheromonal activity in the free-fatty acid fraction (Gaunt 1968).

Experience is a strong modifier of the response to preputial attractant; sexual experience being a necessary prerequisite for almost any degree of responsiveness under laboratory conditions (Bronson and Caroom 1971). The female's responsiveness is somewhat enhanced by estrogen and is blocked by progesterone; pregnant females are not attracted to the male's preputial odor (Caroom and Bronson 1972). Considerable chemistry has been done on the normal male gland (Sansone and Hamilton 1969; Spener et al. 1969), and it is probable that this will be the first mouse pheromone to be isolated and identified. A word of caution is necessary, however, concerning the concepts of attraction and arousal as determined in the laboratory. What is actually known, with respect to the preputial gland, is that saline homogenates or lipid extracts of these glands are preferred by sexually-experienced females in a two- or four-choice test situation and, additionally, that such preparations will more or less instantly awaken females from a sound sleep. It is not known, for example, whether the preputial lipids are attractive to both sexes nor is it known how other species react to them. Interestingly enough, there is a suggestion that the attraction for male urine may actually be stronger among diestrus females than for those in estrus (Scott and Pfaff 1970).

Several authors have documented the loss of aggressiveness in male mice following olfactory bulbectomy (Ropartz 1968b; Rowe and Edwards 1971). A re-examination of this phenomenon, however, using topical application of zinc sulfate rather than surgery showed no depression in fighting, possibly indicating more central effects of bulbectomy rather than simple interruption of cue transmission in this type of experiment (Edwards et al. 1972; see also Bandler and Chi 1972). Both 'aggression-inducing' and 'aggression-inhibiting' pheromones have been postulated in mice. The basis for assuming the presence of an inhibitor is the fact that males whose fur has been rubbed in female urine are not attacked as frequently as expected (Mugford and Nowell 1970; Dixon and Macintosh 1971). The general repellent action of the odor of one male upon another has been known for some time (Chanel and Vernet-Mary 1963) and several workers have shown that the odor of strange male urine will elicit attack among normally compatible groups of males. Techniques of demonstrating this latter phenomenon have included the use of soiled bedding (Archer 1968) and rubbing urine from a strange male onto the fur of one member of a usually or expected compatible pair of males (Macintosh and Grant 1966; Mugford and Nowell 1970). Strange male urine is decidedly more effective in eliciting attack if obtained from an intact rather than from a castrate male (Mugford and Nowell 1970). Androgenized females elicit considerable aggression from normal males and, on the basis of experimental evidence, it has been suggested that these females were producing two androgen-dependent pheromones, one in the urine and the other from the preputial gland, both stimulating attack by normal males (Mugford and Nowell 1971). Somewhat confusing, but indicative of the importance of the preputial gland, is the report that preputialectomized males fight more frequently than expected when housed with intact males (McKinney and Christian 1970). In addition, the preputial gland apparently grows during the process of attaining social dominance and is decreased in size (and presumably altered in function) among subordinate males (Bronson 1973). There can be little doubt, then, that mice make ready use of urinary signals, and possibly a specific androgen-dependent lipid(s) from the preputial gland, in their assessment of a potentially aggressive encounter. Mice do apparently display a territorial organization of their inter-male social behavior under some conditions (Mackintosh 1970) but the possibility of scent-marking to reinforce this organization has not been investigated in any depth.

Maternal relationships provide an example of another social situation in mice where pheromones are apparently heavily used. It must be emphasized, in addition, that pheromonal communication is active both from parent to young and vice versa. The strong dependence upon chemical cues on the mother's part is shown by experiments in which olfactory bulbectomy is followed by an absolute absence of maternal care and, in fact, the anosmic mother often eats her young (Gandelman et al. 1972). Female rats react the same way but, unlike mice, cannibalism can be prevented by experiential factors; i.e., either the hormonal experience of pregnancy or pre-exposure (sensitization) to young rats will prevent the anosmic mother from eating her young (Schlein et al. 1972; see also Herrenkohl and Rosenberg 1972). The mother is likewise providing chemical information to the young mice. Of particular importance here is an imprinting-like action of the parental (and possibly the siblings') odors. Thus Mainardi (1963) found that the normal adult sexual preferences of one subspecies of *Mus* for males of the same subspecies was eliminated if no adult males were present during the pre-weaning period. Furthermore Mainardi et al. (1965) showed that perfuming the mother altered the later expected pattern of mating preferences by the females in her litter but not the males. Thus odors encountered early in life play a strong role in determining the correct species choice when adult.

In summary, it can be stated that the potent influences of pheromones on mouse reproductive activities, both specifically and in toto, have been sufficiently well documented to provide probably the best model pheromonal system available among the mammals. Mice make strong use of priming pheromones to regulate the secretion of their reproductive hormones. These actions have dramatic overt effects such as inducing precocial puberty, blocking pregnancy, and regulating the frequency of ovulation. Signalling pheromones are heavily utilized in the evocation of many specific hormone-modulated and reproductively-related social behaviors such as those occurring in sexual, aggressive, and maternal behavior. In terms of absolute dependence of these behaviors on olfactory cues, however, it is highly probable that, like most mammalian systems, experience plays a strong role in both priming and signalling phenomena and, in addition, multiple sensory input is usually the rule.

As suggested earlier, mouse signalling pheromones are most obviously serving identification functions: identification of individual, species, age, sex, sexual state, and presence of fear. Following an argument which restricts the use of the term pheromone to situations where chemical isolation seems reasonable, we are possibly searching for only a few specific signals: a) a female-originating message that both attracts males, blocks their attack, and denotes age and sexual state by concentration; b) a male signal that provokes attack, attracts females, and also denotes age and/or sexual state by concentration; and c) a fear substance (discussed later). Individual identification is undoubtedly dependent upon a melange of odors; species-identification remains an entirely open question. It is also conceivable that mouse primers and signals might on occasion be the same compound; the dichotomy used here being functionally rather than chemically-based.

18.5. Other mouse pheromonal systems

Signalling pheromones are thought to play a role in some behaviors not so obviously related to reproductive activities in mice. The best documented phenomenon in this category would seem to be the use of a fear substance. The presence of a postulated urinary pheromone functioning to communicate fear or danger is based upon evidence that mice stressed by blowing air upon them, or by electroshock, excrete urine whose smell causes avoidance by other mice or which otherwise interferes with conditioning experiments (Müller-Velten 1966; Sprott 1969; Carr et al. 1970; see also Carr et al. 1971). Mice do learn to cease avoiding such odors after a period of time thus confirming the typical lack of stereotypy of mammalian responses to signalling pheromones. Importantly the phenomenon is species specific as tested within a three-species framework (Müller-Velten 1966). Rats are also known to discriminate between the urine of shocked and unshocked rats (Valenta and Rigby 1968; Morrison and Ludvigson 1970). It thus seems reasonable to suspect a relatively specific signalling pheromone in the urine of stressed animals which would function to communicate danger to other members of the same species in a natural population.

Another area where odors apparently operate is to influence the general locomotor activity of individuals, although the following observations could probably be as easily discussed within the context of population organization of aggressive activity. Specifically, a correlated behavioral result of exposure to strange male odor is a general increase in motor activity. Importantly, no increase in activity is found if a group's own odor is passed back onto themselves in a control experiment (Ropartz 1967a). Ropartz has implicated two odor sources in the activity change: a urinary factor traceable to the coagulating glands and a secretion by the plantar glands in the soles of the feet (Ropartz 1967a). The former is apparently produced only among males found in groups while the latter is thought of as a type of individual identification. Of particular interest within this context is a possible primer effect; strange male odor causes an increase in adrenal weight and a decrease in adrenal ascorbic acid among isolated male mice (Archer 1969; Ropartz 1966). Ether extracts of coagulating glands cause an increase in adrenal weight (Ropartz 1967a), but odors from cages of females also increase adrenal weight in males (Ropartz 1967b). The full story on these interesting observations is, of course, yet to come, but the need to precisely measure changes in activity and aggression as well as to investigate the possible adrenal-activating primer at the same time in the same experimental program is obvious.

18.6. Priming pheromones in other mammals

The question of uniqueness of priming pheromonal usage among mammals is of obvious importance since it is on this basis that such pheromones will be accorded greater or lesser importance in the overall picture of mammalian biology. The reproductive priming phenomena that have been discussed have been documented in only one of the 19 possible orders of mammals, the rodents. Physiologic information leading one to suspect their functional presence may be found for three additional orders, but the nature of this evidence is tenuous. Direct relationships between olfactory stimulation or ablation and reproductive function have been documented for cats, pigs, and rabbits (David et al. 1952; Signoret and Mauleon 1962; Franck 1966). Estrous cycles of two species, sheep and goats, are known to be synchronized by the presence of a male but the role of olfaction in this regard is not known (Schinckel 1954; Shelton 1960; Hulet 1966; Morgan et al. 1972). The CNS arousing effect of male urine in pigs is again worthy of note (Signoret and Du Buisson 1961).

Probably the most convincing argument that priming pheromones are more widespread than now documented, at least among rodents, rests on the fact that all of the priming phenomena known to exist in mouse reproduction also occur and seem to function identically in the prairie deermouse (*Peromyscus*) (Bronson and Eleftheriou 1963; Bronson and Marsden 1964; Bronson and Dezell 1968). *Mus* and *Peromyscus* belong to different families of rodents and, while one evolved in Asia (*Mus*), the evolution of the other has apparently been limited to North America. Thus, the similarity between priming functions in these two species could simply be an interesting case of convergent evolution, but considering the few species which have actually been investigated, it is more probable that they are indeed representative of a large number of species and that future work with a wider spectrum of mammals should thus prove rewarding. Important in this respect is the necessity for looking beyond our normal laboratory or domestic stocks of animals since these are end products of long, and often unintentional, selection for reproductive efficiency and, hence, probable selection against pheromonal effects. The loss of pregnancy blocking capacity in many inbred strains of mice is a case in point (Marsden and Bronson 1965). Indirect evidence of priming effects does exist for many other rodents. Two species of voles (*Microtus*, sp.) show a post-insemination pregnancy block when exposed to strange males but the role of olfaction has not been explored (Clulow and Clark 1964; Clulow and Langford 1971). The induction of estrous cycling and, hence, ovulation in response to a male has also been shown in a vole (*M. ochrogaster*) and, here, the evidence for a primer pheromone is better since the male can be replaced with his soiled bedding (Richmond and Conaway 1969). Estrous cycling is profoundly influenced in both the pocket mouse (*Peronathus*, Ostwald et al. 1972) and the cuis (*Galea*) by the male's presence although, in the latter case, physical contact seems necessary (Weir 1971). Finally, even the highly domesticated, common laboratory rat can be suspected of primer pheromonal phenomena. Female rats do not suppress their cycles when grouped but many studies by Cooper and co-workers (e.g., Cooper et al. 1972) have shown that the presence of an intact but not a castrate male will regularize estrous cycles made aberrant by under-feeding. In addition, a variety of studies have shown that neither anosmia nor blinding exert strong effects on pituitary gonadotropin content by themselves but in combination these procedures can drastically alter hormonal secretion in rats (e.g. Donofrio and Reiter 1972; see also Orbach and Kling 1966). Apparently then the rat has the capacity to use male- but not female-originating primers but long domestication has ensured that their reproduction is not dramatically dependent upon them. Studies in wild rats would be particularly interesting in this regard.

18.7. *Signalling pheromones in other mammals*

A wealth of observational information on a host of mammalian species attests to the fact that olfactory signals are heavily utilized by many mammals for intra-population communication. A review of this literature reveals a hodgepodge of species examined, some under carefully controlled laboratory conditions, some in the field, and some in semi-natural environments. It is indeed unfortunate that many of the best-controlled studies take place in the limited confines of the laboratory and involve only the common laboratory animals, while far too many field studies provide only the minimum of documentation and/or experimental manipulation. While correlative-type observations made under field conditions are thus legion, too many provide little more than suggestions concerning the importance of olfactory cues. Notable studies done under field or semi-natural conditions include those on the rabbit in Australia (Mykytowycz 1965), a marsupial, the sugar glider (Schultze-Westrum 1969), and the black-tailed deer (Müller-Schwarze 1969; 1971). Worthy of note regarding laboratory approaches is a large series of studies on scent marking by the Mongolian gerbil (e.g., Thiessen et al. 1970).

As of now the simple framework of limited functions and numbers of signals which was established earlier for the mouse is probably not a bad guide for examining signalling pheromones in mammals as a whole; that is, identification of species, race, individual, age, sex, sexual state, and fear with single compounds able to accomplish more than one of these functions depending upon concentration and, in addition, variation in response being dependent upon experience and sex of the recipient. Given a broader spectrum of species and possibilities, however, it is expected that some inadequacies will be apparent in this scheme. Much attention, for example, has been given to scent marking, an unknown phenomenon in mice (reviewed by Ralls 1971; Eisenberg and Kleiman 1973). Scent marking could be included in the mouse system either under the aggressive or sexual categories, probably most often under the former since its function in most mammals seems to be associated either with dominance or territory.

Within the above framework, then, individual recognition has been experimentally demonstrated using conditioning techniques in rats as well as mice (Husted and McKenna 1966; Krames 1970). Gerbils can discriminate between the urinary odors of two other gerbils of the same sex even when the test urines are diluted 1000-fold (Dagg and Windsor 1971). Species preferences based on olfactory cues have been documented for a variery of rodents, e.g., voles (Godfrey 1958) and deermice (Doty 1972). Examples of olfactory attraction to a receptive female are reported for dogs (Beach and Gilmore 1949), deer (Golley 1957), deermice (Doty 1972), and rats (Lemagnen 1952). Sexual attraction is a two-way process; for example, estrous ewes will succesfully seek out a ram without the use of visual cues (Lindsay 1966). A series of papers by Carr and his associates (Carr and Caul 1962; Carr et al. 1965; 1966) has examined the relative roles of gonadal state and past sexual experience as modifiers of identification-attraction responses in rats. Ability of rats of either sex to detect odors of sexually active members of the opposite sex is independent of their own gonadal state. Attraction to that odor, on the other hand, requires that females be either sexually experienced or under the influence of estrogen while positive responses by males require both androgen and sexual experience. Lydell and Doty (1972), also working with rats, confirmed the role of sexual experience in male-attraction phenomena and, in addition, showed that aged (24 hr +) urine from females was not as preferred as fresh urine (see also Stern 1970). Orsulak and Gawienowski (1972) have shown a strong attraction on the part of sexually-experienced females for homogenates of male rat preputials and, in addition, documented the increased activity of the females when in the presence of preputial odor.

Other than scent marking, the experimental testing of the role of odors in intra-specific fighting has largely been limited to mice. The importance of odors in the early imprinting of species-recognition, however, has been documented in rats (Marr and Lilliston 1969) and guinea pigs (Cartier and Marr 1970), both studies using a procedure of applying artificial odors to mothers and/or siblings. Cross-fostering studies involving two species of rodents have also successfully confirmed the presence of early maternal imprinting (Quadagno and Banks 1970; Stark and Hazlett 1972). It should be noted here that Leon and Moltz (1972) have suggested the presence of a specific 'maternal pheromone' produced in rats between 14 and 27 days post-partum and acting to attract the young. Thus species-imprinting could also involve a highly specific pheromone. Finally, olfactory recognition at the species level has been documented surprisingly few times (e.g., Doty 1972) despite the fact that this form of communication obviously provides one of the best possible modalities for sexual and other types of isolation. 'Colony' (Barnett 1963) or racial isolation provides another untrammelled area of research in mammals.

References

Archer, J. E. (1968) The effect of strange male odor on aggressive behavior in male mice. J. Mammal. 49, 572–575.

Archer, J. E. (1969) Adrenocortical responses to olfactory stimuli in male mice. J. Mammal. 50, 836–841.

Bandler, R. J. and C. C. Chi (1972) Effects of olfactory bulb removal on aggression: a reevaluation. Physiol. Behav. 8, 207–211.

Barnett, S. A. (1963) The Rat, a Study in Behavior (Aldine, Chicago) 288 pp.

Beach, F. A. and R. Gilmore (1949) Response of male dogs to urine from females in heat. J. Mammal. 30, 391–392.

Biancifiori, C. and F. Caschera (1963) The effect of olfactory lobectomy and induced pseudopregnancy on the incidence of methylcholanthrene-induced mammary and ovarian tumors in C3Hb mice. Brit. J. Cancer 17, 116–118.

Bowers, J. M. and B. K. Alexander (1967) Mice: Individual recognition by olfactory cues. Science 158, 1208–1210.

Bronson, F. H. (1968) Pheromonal influences on mammalian reproduction. In: Reproduction and Sexual Behavior; ed.: M. Diamond (Indiana Univ. Press, Bloomington) pp. 341–361.

Bronson, F. H. (1971) Rodent pheromones. Biol. Reprod. 4, 344–357.

Bronson, F. H. (1973) Establishment of social rank among grouped male mice: Relative effects on circulating FSH, LH, and corticosterone. Physiol. Behav. 10, 947–951.

Bronson, F. H. and D. Caroom (1971) Preputial gland of the male mouse: attractant function. J. Reprod. Fert. 25, 279–282.

Bronson, F. H. and H. E. Dezell (1968) Studies on the estrus-inducing (pheromonal) action of male deermouse urine. Gen. Comp. Endocrinol. 10, 334–343.

Bronson, F. H. and B. E. Eleftheriou (1963) Influence of strange males on implantation in the deermouse. Gen. Comp. Endocrinol. 3, 515–518.

Bronson, F. H., B. E. Eleftheriou and H. E. Dezell (1969) Strange male pregnancy block in deermice; prolactin and adrenocortical hormones. Biol. Reprod. 1, 302–306.

Bronson, F. H. and H. M. Marsden (1964) Male-induced synchrony of estrus in deermice. Gen. Comp. Endocrinol. 4, 634–637.

Bronson, F. H. and M. H. Stetson (1973) Gonadotropin release in prepubertal female mice following male-exposure: A comparison with the adult cycle. Biol. Reprod. (in press)

Bronson, F. H. and W. K. Whitten (1968) Oestrus-accelerating pheromone of mice: assay , androgen-dependency, and presence in bladder urine. J. Reprod. Fert. 15, 131–134.

Bruce, H. M. (1959) An exteroreceptive block to pregnancy in the mouse. Nature (London) 184, 105.

Bruce, H. M. (1965) The effect of castration on the reproductive pheromones of male mice. J. Reprod. Fert. 2, 138–142.

Bruce, H. M. (1966) Smell as an exteroreceptive factor. J. Anim. Sci. 25, 83–89.

Bruce, H. M. (1967) Effects of olfactory stimuli on reproduction in mammals. Ciba Found. Study Group 26, 29–42.

Bruce, H. M. (1970) Pheromones. Brit. Med. Bull. 26, 10–13.

Bruce, H. M. and A. S. Parkes (1960) Hormonal factors in exteroreceptive block to pregnancy in mice. J. Endocrinol. 20, 29–30.

Bruce, H. M. and D. M. V. Parrot (1960) Role of olfactory sense in pregnancy block by strange males. Science 131, 1526.

Caroom, D. and F. H. Bronson (1971) Responsiveness of female mice to preputial attractant: Effects of sexual experience and ovarian hormones. Physiol. Behav. 7, 659–662.

Carr, W. J. and W. F. Caul (1962) The effect of castration in rats upon discrimination of sex odors. Anim. Behav. 10, 20–27.

Carr, W. J., L. S. Loeb and M. L. Dissinger (1965) Responses of rats to sex odors. J. Comp. Physiol. Psychol. 59, 370–377.

Carr, W. J., L. S. Loeb and N. R. Wylie (1966) Responses to feminine odors in normal and castrated male rats. J. Comp. Physiol. Psychol. 62, 336–338.

Carr, W. J., R. D. Martorano and L. Krames (1970) Responses of mice to odors associated with stress. J. Comp. Physiol. Psychol. 71, 223–228.

Carr, W. J., P. Roth and M. Amore (1971) Responses of male mice to odors from stressed vs. nonstressed males and females. Psychon. Sci., Sect. Anim. Physiol. Psychol. 25, 275–276.

Carter, C. S. and J. N. Marr (1970) Olfactory imprinting and age variables in the guinea pig, *Cavia porcellus*. Anim. Behav. 18, 238–244.

Champlin, A. K. (1971) Suppression of oestrus in grouped mice: the effects of various densities and the possible nature of the stimulus. J. Reprod. Fert. 27, 233–241.

Chanel, J. and E. Vernet-Maury (1963) Détermination par un test olfactif des inter-attractions chez la souris. J. Physiol. (Paris) 55, 121–122.

Chapman, V. M. and W. K. Whitten (1969) The occurrence and inheritance of pregnancy block in laboratory mice. Genetics 61, 49 (abstract).

Chapman, V. M., C. Desjardins and W. K. Whitten (1970) Pregnancy block in mice: Changes in pituitary LH and LTH and plasma progestin levels. J. Reprod. Fert. 21, 333–337.

Cheal, M. L. and R. L. Sprott (1971) Social olfaction: a review of the role of olfaction in a variety of animal behaviors. Psychol. Rep. 29, 195–243.

Chipman, R. K. and K. A. Fox (1966) Oestrus synchronization and pregnancy blocking in wild house mice (*Mus musculus*). J. Reprod. Fert. 12, 233–236.

Clulow, F. V.. and J. R. Clarke (1964) Pregnancy-block in *Microtus agrestis*, an induced ovulator. Nature (London) 219, 511.

Clulow, F. V. and P. E. Langford (1971) Pregnancy-block in the meadow vole *Microtus pennsylvanicus*. J. Reprod. Fert. 24, 275–277.

Cooper, K. J., K. Purvis and N. B. Haynes (1972) Further observations on the ability of the male to influence the oestrous cycle of the underfed rat. J. Reprod. Fert. 28, 473–475.

Dagg, A. T. and D. E. Windsor (1971) Olfactory discrimination limits in gerbils. Can. Zool. 49, 283–285.

David, R., G. Thiery, M. Bonvallet and P. Dell (1952) Effets de la stimulation des bulbes olfactifs sur le cycle sexuel de la chatte. C. R. Soc. Biol. 146, 670–672.

Dixon, A. K. and J. H. Mackintosh (1971) Effects of female urine upon the social behaviour of adult male mice. Anim. Behav. 19, 138–140.

Dominic, C. J. (1965) The origin of the pheromones causing pregnancy block in mice. J. Reprod. Fert. 10, 469–472.

Dominic, C. J. (1966) Observations on the reproductive pheromones of mice. II. Neuroendocrine mechanisms involved in the olfactory block to pregnancy. J. Reprod. Fert. 11, 415–421.

Donofrio, R. J. and R. J. Reiter (1972) Depressed pituitary prolactin levels in blinded anosmic female rats: role of the pineal. J. Reprod. Fert. 31, 159–162.

Doty, R. L. (1972) Odor preferences of female *Peromyscus maniculatus bairdii* for male odors of *P.m. bairdii* and *P. leucopus noveboracensis* as a function of estrous state. J. Comp. Physiol. Psychol. 81, 191–197.

Dutt, R. J., E. C. Simpson, J. C. Christian and C. E. Barnhart (1959) Identification of preputial glands as the site of production of sexual odor in the boar. J. Anim. Sci. 18, 1557–1558 (abstract).

Edwards, D. A., M. L. Thompson and K. G Burge (1972) Olfactory bulb removal vs peripherally induced anosmia: differential effects on the aggressive behavior of male mice. Behav. Biol. 7, 823–828.

Eleftheriou, B. E., D. W. Bailey and M. X. Zarrow (1972) A gene controlling male pheromonal facilitation of PMS-induced ovulation in mice. J. Reprod. Fert. 31, 155–158.

Eisenberg, J. F. and D. G. Kleiman (1973) Olfactory communication in mammals. Ann. Rev. Ecol. and Syst. 3 (in press).

Franck, H. (1966) Effets de l'ablation des bulbes olfactifs chez la lapine impubère. Repercussions sur le physiologie génitale chez la lapine adulte. C. R. Soc. Biol. 160, 863–865.

Gandelman, R., M. X. Zarrow and V. H. Denenberg (1972) Reproductive and maternal performance in the mouse following removal of the olfactory bulbs. J. Reprod. Fert. 28, 453–456.

Gaunt, S. L. (1968) Studies on the preputial gland as a source of a reproductive pheromone in the laboratory mouse (*Mus musculus*). Thesis (University of Vermont).

Gleason, K. K. and J. H. Reynierse (1969) The behavioral significance of pheromones in vertebrates. Psychol. Bull. 71, 58–73.

Godfrey, J. (1958) The origin of sexual isolation between bank voles. Proc. Roy. Phys. Soc. Edinburgh 27, 47–55.

Golley, F. B. (1957) Gestation period, breeding and fawning of the Columbian black-tailed deer. J. Mammal. 38, 116–120.

Henkin, R. I. and R. C. Hoye (1966) Hyposmia secondary to excision of the olfactory epithelium: the definition of primary and accessory areas of olfaction. Life Sci. 5, 331–341.

Herrenkohl, L. R. and P. A. Rosenberg (1972) Exteroceptive stimulation of maternal behavior in the naive rat. Physiol. Behav. 8, 595–598.

Hoppe, P. C. and W. K. Whitten (1972) Pregnancy-block: initiation by administered gonadotropin. Biol. Reprod. 7, 254–259.

Hulet, C. V. (1966) Behavioral, social and psychological factors affecting mating time and breeding efficiency in sheep. J. Anim. Sci. 25, Suppl. 5–20.

Husted, J. R. and F. S. McKenna (1966) The use of rats as discriminative stimuli. J. Exptl. Anal. Behav. 9, 677–679.

Kalmus, H. (1964) Some potentialities and constraints of chemical telecommunication. Paper presented at the 2nd Intern. Congr. Endocrinol., London.

Katkov, T. and P. B. Gower (1968) The biosynthesis of 5α-androst-16-en-3-one from progesterone by boar testes homogenates. Acta Biochim. Biophys. 164, 134–136.

Krames, L. (1970) Responses of female rats to the individual body odors of male rats. Psychon. Sci. Sect. Anim. Physiol. Psychol. 20, 274–275.

Lee, S. van der and L. M. Boot (1956) Spontaneous pseudopregnancy in mice. II. Acta Physiol. Pharmacol. Neer. 5, 213–214.

Lemagnen, J. (1952) Les phénomènes olfactosexuels chez le rat blanc. Arch. Sci. Physiol. 6, 295–332.

Leon, M. and H. Moltz (1972) The development of the pheromonal bond in the albino rat. Physiol. Behav. 8, 683–686.

Lindsay, D. R. (1966) Mating behaviour of ewes and its effect on mating efficiency. Anim. Behav. 14, 419–424.

Lott, D. F. and J. H. Hopwood (1972) Olfactory-pregnancy-block in mice (*Mus musculus*): an unusual response acquisition paradigm. Anim. Behav. 20, 263–267.

Lydell, K. and R. L. Doty (1972) Male rat odor preferences for female urine as a function of sexual experience, urine age, and urine source. Horm. Behav. 3, 205–212.

Mackintosh, J. H. (1970) Territory formation by laboratory mice. Anim. Behav. 18, 177–183.

Macintosh, J. H. and E. C. Grant (1966) The effect of olfactory stimuli on the aggressive behavior of laboratory mice. Z. Tierpsychol. 23, 584–587.

Mainardi, D. (1963) Eliminazione della barriera etologica all'isolamento reproduttino tra *Mus musculus domesticus* e *M. m. bactrianus* mediante axione sull'apprendimento infantile. Rend. Ist., Lomb. Sci. Lett. B97, 291–299.

Mainardi, D., M. Marsan and A. Pasquali (1965) Causation of sexual preferences of the house mouse. The behavior of mice reared by parents whose odor was artificially altered. Atti. Soc. Ital. Sci. Nat. 104, 325–338.

Marr, J. N. and L. G. Lilliston (1969) Social attachment in rats by odor and age. Behaviour 33, 277–282.

Marsden, H. M. and F. H. Bronson (1964) Estrous synchrony in mice: alteration by exposure to male urine. Science 144, 3625.

Marsden, H. M. and F. H. Bronson (1965) Strange male block to pregnancy: its absence in inbred mouse strains. Nature (London) 207, 878.

McKinney, T. D. and J. J. Christian (1970) Effect of preputialectomy on fighting behavior in mice. Proc. Soc. Exptl. Biol. Med. 134, 291–293.

Michael, R. P., E. B. Keverne and R. W. Bonsall (1971) Pheromones: isolation of male sex attractants from a female primate. Science 172, 964–966.

Morgan, P. D., G. W. Arnold and D. R. Lindsay (1972) A note on the mating behavior of ewes with various senses impaired. J. Reprod. Fert. 30, 151–152.

Morrison, R. R. and H. W. Ludvigson (1970) Discrimination by rats of conspecific odors of reward and non-reward. Science 167, 904–905.

Mugford, R. A. and N. W. Nowell (1970) Pheromones and their effect on aggression in mice. Nature (London) 226, 967–968.

Mugford, R. A. and N. W. Nowell (1971) The preputial glands as a source of aggression-promoting odors in mice. Physiol. Behav. 6, 247–249.

Müller-Schwarze, D. (1969) Complexity and relative specificity in a mammalian pheromone. Nature (London) 223, 525–526.

Müller-Schwarze, D. (1971) Pheromones in black-tailed deer (*Odocoileus hemionus columbianus*). Anim. Behav. 19, 141–152.

Müller-Velton, H. (1966) Über den Angstgeruch bei der Hausmaus (*Mus musculus* L.). Z. Vergl. Physiol. 52, 401–429.

Mykytowycz, R. (1965) Further observations on the territorial function and histology of the submandibular cutaneous (chin) glands in the rabbit, *Oryctolagus cuniculus* (L.). Anim. Behav. 13, 400–412.

Mykytowycz, R. (1970) The role of skin glands in mammalian communication. In: Advances in Chemoreception, vol. 1; eds.: J. W. Johnson, D. G. Moulton and A. Turk (Appleton-Century-Crofts, New York) pp. 327–360.

Orbach, J. and A. Kling (1966) Effect of sensory deprivation on onset of puberty, mating, fertility and gonadal weights in rats. Brain Res. 3, 141–149.

Orsulak, P. J. and A. M. Gawienowski (1972) Olfactory preferences for the rat preputial gland. Biol. Reprod. 6, 219–223.

Ostwald, R., K. Wilken, J. Simons, H. Highstone, S. Cimino and S. Shimondle (1972) Influences of photoperiod and partial contact on estrus in the desert pocket mouse, *Perognathus penicillatus*. Biol. Reprod. 7, 1–8.

Parkes, A. S. and H. M. Bruce (1961) Olfactory stimuli in mammalian reproduction. Science, 134, 1049–1054.

Quadagno, D. M. and E. M. Banks (1970) The effect of reciprocal cross fostering on the behaviour of two species of rodents, *Mus musculus* and *Baiomys taylori ater*. Anim. Behav. 18, 379–390.

Ralls, K. (1971) Mammalian scent marking. Science 171, 443–449.

Regnier, F. E. (1971) Semiochemicals–structure and function, Biol. Reprod. 4. 309–326.

Richmond, M. and C. J. Conway (1969) Induced ovulation and oestrus in *Microtus ochrogaster*. J. Reprod. Fert. 6, 357–376.

Ropartz, P. (1966) Contributions à l'étude du détermination d'un effet de groupe chez les souris. C. R. Acad. Sci. Ser. D, 262, 2070–2072.

Ropartz, P. (1967a) Role des communications olfactives dans le comportement social des souris males. Collq. Int. Cent. Nat. Rech. Sci. 173.

Ropartz, P. (1967b) La seule odeur d'un groupe de souris femelles est capable d'induire un hypertrophie surrénalienne chez des males isolés. C. R. Acad. Sci. Ser. D 264, 2811–2814.

Ropartz, P. (1968a) Mise en évidence d'une augmentation de l'activité locomotrice des groupes de souris femelles en response à l'odeur d'un groupe de males étranges. C. R. Acad. Sci. Ser. D 267, 2341–2343.

Ropartz, P. (1968b) The relation between olfactory discrimination and aggressive behavior in mice. Anim. Behav. 16, 97–180.

Rowe, F. A. and D. A. Edwards (1971) Olfactory bulb removal: influences on the aggressive behaviors of male mice. Physiol. Behav. 7, 889–892.

Rowe, F. A. and D. A. Edwards (1972) Olfactory bulb removal: influences on the mating behaviors of male mice. Physiol. Behav. 8, 37–41.

Sansone, G. and J. G. Hamilton (1969) Glyceryl ether, wax ester and triglyceride composition of the mouse preputial gland. Lipids 4, 435–440.

Schinckel, P. G. (1954) The effect of the presence of the ram on the ovarian activity of the ewe. Aust. J. Agric. Res. 5, 465–469.

Schlein, P. A., M. X. Zarrow, H. A. Cohen, V. H. Denenberg and N. P. Johnson (1972) The differential effect of anosmia on maternal behaviour in the virgin and primiparous rat. J. Reprod. Fert. 30, 139–142.

Schultz, E. F. and J. T. Tapp (1973) Olfactory control of behavior in rodents. Psychol. Bull. (in press).

Schultze-Westrum, T. G. (1969) Social communication by chemical signals in flying phalangers (*Petaurus breviceps papuanus*). In: Olfaction and Taste; ed.: C. Pfaffman (Rockefeller Univ. Press, New York), pp. 268–277.

Scott, J. W. and D. W. Pfaff (1970) Behavioral and electrophysiological responses of female mice to male urine odors. Physiol. Behav. 5, 407–411.

Shelton, M. (1960) Influence of the presence of a male goat on the initiation of oestrous cycling and ovulation of angora does. J. Anim. Sci. 19, 368–375.

Signoret, J. P. and F. Du Mesnil du Buisson (1961) Etude du comportement de la truie en oestrus (Fourth Congr. Anim. Reprod. Artif. Insem., The Hague).

Signoret, J. P. and P. Mauleon (1962) Action de l'ablation des bulbes olfactifs sur les mécanismes de la réproduction chez la truie. Ann. Biol. Anim. Biochim. Biophys. 2, 167–174.

Sink, J. D. (1967) Theoretical aspects of sex odor in swine. J. Theor. Biol. 17, 174–180.

Snyder, R. L. and N. E. Taggart (1967) Effects of adrenalectomy on male induced pregnancy block in mice. J. Reprod. Fert. 14, 451.

Spener, F., H. K. Mangold, G. Sansone and J. G. Hamilton (1969) Long-chain alkyl acetates in the preputial gland of the mouse. Act. Biochem. Biophys. 192, 516–521.

Sprott, R. L. (1969) 'Fear communication' via odor in inbred mice. Psychiatr. Res. Rep. 25, 263–268.

Stark, B. and B. A. Hazlett (1972) Effects of olfactory experience on aggression in *Mus musculus* and *Peromyscus maniculatus*. Behav. Biol. 7, 265–269.

Stern, J. J. (1970) Responses of male rats to sex odors. Physiol. Behav. 5, 519–524.

Thiessen, D. D. G. Lindzey, S. L. Blum and P. Wallace (1970) Social interactions and scent marking in the Mongolian gerbil (*Merione unguiculatus*). Anim. Behav. 19, 505–513.

Valenta, J. E. and M. K. Rigby (1968) Discrimination of the odor of stressed rats. Science 161, 599–601.

Van Tienhoven, A. (1968) Reproductive Physiology of Vertebrates (W. B. Saunders, Philadelphia) 498 pp.

Vandenbergh, J. G. (1969) Male odor accelerates female sexual maturation in mice. Endocrinology 84, 658–660.

Vandenbergh, J. G., L. C. Drickamer and D. R. Colby (1972) Social and dietary factors in the sexual maturation of female mice. J. Reprod. Fert. 28, 397–405.

Weir, B. J. (1971) The evocation of oestrus in the cuis, *Galea musteloides*. J. Reprod. Fert. 26, 405–408.

Whitten, W. K. (1956a) The effect of the removal of olfactory bulbs on the gonads of mice. J. Endocrinol. 14, 160–163.

Whitten, W. K. (1956b) Modifications of the oestrus cycle of the mouse by external stimuli associated with the male. J. Endocrinol. 13, 399–404.

Whitten, W. K. (1959) Occurrence of anoestrus in mice caged in groups. J. Endocrinol. 18, 102–107.

Whitten, W. K. (1966) Pheromones and mammalian reproduction. In: Advances in Reproductive Physiology, vol. 1; ed.: A. McLaren (Academic Press, New York) pp. 155–177.

Whitten, W. K. and F. H. Bronson (1970) Role of pheromones in mammalian reproduction. In: Advances in Chemoreception; eds.: J. W. Johnson and D. C. Moulton and A. Turk (Appleton-Century–Crofts, New York) pp. 309–325.

Whitten, W. F., F. H. Bronson and J. A. Greenstein (1968) Estrus-inducing pheromone of male mice: transport by movement of air. Science 161, 584–585.

CHAPTER 19

Primate pheromones

Gisela EPPLE

19.1. Introduction

During recent years our knowledge on the behavioral biology of primates has advanced considerably. Experimental studies on primates in the laboratory, as well as field research on many species, have provided insight into reproductive behavior, social behavior and communication. It is characteristic for the communication systems of higher primates that they are multimodular, relying on olfactory, vocal, tactile and visual signals. While visual as well as vocal and – to some degree – tactile communication has been studied quite extensively in a variety of species (c.f. Marler 1965; Altmann 1967; Lancaster 1968), little is known about the role of the chemical senses in primate communication. This lack of knowledge might – in part – reflect a human bias: as one ascends the phylogenetic scale from the prosimians to the monkeys and apes, there is a continuous reduction in the size of the bulbus olfactorius (Stephan 1966) which appears to be correlated with an increase in the importance of visual and vocal communication and a decrease in olfactory communication. In addition, visual and vocal patterns obviously are more noticeable to the human observer, who is anatomically better equipped and may be mentally more prepared to see a display or hear a call than to smell an odor. Thus, chemical communication has often been considered of minor importance, and much more attention has been paid to visual and vocal patterns. Except for the studies of Michael and his co-workers (c.f. Michael et al. 1972) on sex attractants in *Macaca mulatta* Zimmerman, little experimental evidence for the existence and biological function of pheromones in primates is available. However, a very large number of reports on the occurrence and histological structure of specialized, odor-producing skin glands and on behavioral patterns concerned with the emission, deposition and olfactory investigation of excretions suggest that pheromones not only exist in many – if not most – primate species, but that they are also of considerable importance in regulating the daily life of the individual.

On the following pages, I shall review the evidence for the existence of pheromones in infrahuman primates and discuss their possible functions. That means, this article will mainly deal with the discussion of behavioral patterns from which the occurrence and function of pheromones can be inferred. As is to be expected on the basis of our very limited knowledge, a discussion of the biological role of primate pheromones will include some speculations which might very well prove to be entirely untrue as research in this area progresses. However, they are presented here, not only in an attempt to tie our present knowledge together but also in order to stimulate more experimental studies in this field, which is not only interesting and rewarding but also of importance for a better understanding of the biology of our own species.

Bronson (1971 and ch. 18) has recently challenged the general applicability of the term pheromone to all forms of intraspecific chemical communication in mammals. He argues that chemical communication in many mammalian species seems to rely heavily on a variety of odor cues from different sources or on a highly complex mixture of several chemical substances. Thus it seems difficult, if not at all impossible, to relate certain messages, like individual recognition, to only one, or at least a limited number of chemicals present in urine, skin gland secretions or in general body odor. He therefore proposes to limit the term pheromone to those situations where one or at least a restricted mixture of compounds can be isolated. The biological activity of these compounds should then be confirmed experimentally by a synthesized product.

These arguments seem to be especially valid in the case of 'primate pheromones'. For example: On the one hand, the sexual attractant of the female rhesus monkey consists of five volatile aliphatic acids whose biological activity can be mimicked by a synthetic mixture (Curtis et al. 1971). These 'copulins' (Curtis et al. 1971) meet all the requirements of Bronson's definition and may legitimately be called pheromones. On the other hand, our own studies on chemical communication in marmoset monkeys have shown that the secretions of scent glands, which are mixed with urine during marking behavior contain messages on the species and sex of an animal, its social status, and maybe, the reproductive state of the female, as well as provide cues for individual recognition (Epple 1971, 1972, 1973a, b and unpublished data). It is unlikely that we will be able to relate every message to one or a few chemical compounds in the highly complex mixture produced during marking.

In many primate species there is good behavioral and anatomical evidence for the existence of chemical communication. However, on the basis of our present knowledge, it is not possible to determine which ones of the chemical signals are pheromones in the stricter sense of the term proposed by Bronson (1971) and which ones are produced by a mixture of odors from various sources. Therefore, whenever the term 'pheromone' is used in this review as a synonym for any kind of chemical signal involved in primate communication, it is with the understanding that this is an over-simplification which has to be revised as our knowledge on chemical communication increases.

19.2. *Evidence for the existence of chemical communication in primates*

While the existence, biological function and chemical nature of a pheromone has been clearly demonstrated only in *Macaca mulatta* (c.f.Curtis et al. 1971; Michael et al. 1972), it is inferred in a great number of primate species. Evidence for communication by chemical signals and for their function is mainly based on three groups of facts:

1) The majority of all infrahuman primates shows olfactory and gustatory (sniffing and sometimes licking) investigation of the bodies of conspecifics and of their odor marks in different social and especially in sexual situations (c.f. Michael 1969 and many others).

2) Many species possess specialized skin glands in various body regions which often produce odoriferous secretions.

3) Many species show highly stereotyped behavioral patterns, interpreted as scent marking. These are concerned with applying feces, urine, saliva, vaginal discharge and the products of skin glands to their own body, that of conspecifics or to the environment. The behavioral context in which these marking patterns are observed (e.g. sexual or aggressive encounters, territorial defense) is often the only cue to the biological role of the chemical signals.

The frequent sniffing of the bodies, the genitals and the scent marks and excretions of sexual and social partners indicates that mainly olfaction is involved in the perception of primate pheromones. In the species which possess a functioning organ of Jacobson (Stephan 1965), this might be involved also. Seitz (1969) for instance, reports that *Nycticebus coucang* Boddaert sniffs the urine of conspecifics while showing rapid oscillating protrusions of the tongue. He remarks on the similarity of this behavior to the rhythmic tongue protrusions of lizards and snakes and argues that the behavior might serve to bring taste stimuli into the mouth as well as bring stimules molecules in contact with the organ of Jacobson through the *canales incisivi*. In several species of marmoset monkeys which also have a functioning organ of Jacobson, we frequently observe olfactory investigation of urine, scent marks and the body of conspecifics accompanied by rhythmic protrusion of the tongue, whose tip touches the stimulus (Epple 1967). *Saimiri sciureus* L. males show an almost identical behavior when sniffing the urine and the genitals of females (personal observation). In marmosets the sniffing behavior is occasionally followed by a 'Flehmen' face. Facial expressions very reminiscent of 'Flehmen', which is supposedly involved in perception of mainly sexual stimuli via the organ of Jacobson (Knappe 1964), have been observed in *Lemur catta* L. (Jolly 1966) during the investigation of chemical stimuli.

The frequency with which a few species not only sniff the various chemical stimuli provided by conspecifics, but also lick them and even ingest excretions indicates that taste might play a role in their perception and/or that there are some primate pheromones which affect the receiving organism via ingestion. For instance, tasting and drinking the urine of females in all stages of the reproductive cycle has been observed in males of two species of *Ateles* by Klein (1971) both in a captive colony and in the field.

It is impossible to review in detail all existing reports on the occurrence and structure of primate scent glands and on scent marking behavior within the framework of this article. The reader is referred to the following studies which, in turn, review earlier reports: Andriamiandra and Rumpler (1968), Arao and Perkins (1969), Dobroruka (1972), Ellis and Montagna (1963), Epple and Lorenz (1967), Machida and Giacometti (1967), Martin (1968), Rumpler and Andriamiandra (1968 , 1971), Rumpler and Oddou (1970), Schifter (1968), Sisson and Fahrenbach (1967), Sorenson (1970).

Scent marking behavior in primates is quite variable. Some of the species simply spread or rub urine, feces, or scent gland secretions on items of their environment, using simple motor patterns. Others apply glandular secretions mixed with small quantities of urine or vaginal discharge. The most spectacular marking patterns, however, involve almost ceremonial mixing and application of scent from several different sources. Thus, for instance, male *Lemur catta* rub the antebrachial glands on their lower forearms against the brachial glands above the axillae, presumably mixing the secretions of both organs. Then the male pulls his tail between his forearms bringing it in intimate contact with the antebrachial organ and anointing it with the scent mixture. He stands with his tail arched over his back and quivers the tail violently in the vertical plane, shaking its odor forward (Bolwig 1960; Jolly 1966; Evans and Goy 1968). Jolly (1966) reports that males always direct this behavior at an opponent in aggressive encounters and that these 'stink-fights' between two males may last for up to an hour. Some of the more elaborate marking patterns serve not only to mix and distribute odors but also function as visual displays. This seems certainly to be true for the 'stink-fight' displays of *Lemur catta* whose very conspicuous black and white tail is widely visible.

The vast majority of scent producing skin glands and of stereotyped marking patterns has been described in prosimians and South American monkeys . Recent studies on *Macaca mulatta* and a few other Old World primates (c.f. Gartlan and Brain 1968; Poirier 1970; Rahaman and Parthasarathy 1971; Michael et al. 1972) however, suggest that pheromones may play a more important role in the life of the Old World monkeys and apes than we have realized so far.

The circumstances under which behavior patterns related to olfactory investigation and marking of conspecifics or the environment were observed, suggest that the chemical cues involved in these behaviors play a role in a variety of non-communicatory and communicatory functions. Moreover, a chemical signal is not necessarily limited to one function alone but may serve a variety of purposes in the same individual. Not all authors have interpreted the specialized skin glands and marking behavior as evidence for the existence of pheromones, Schmidt and Seitz (1967) for instance interpreted the 'urine washing' (washing of the palms of hands and feet in their own urine) of *Saimiri sciureus* as thermoregulatory behavior while Castell and Maurus (1967) believe it is essential to keep hands and feet clean and moist. Latta et al. (1967), Baldwin (1970) and Kirchshofer (1963) on the other hand, interpreted 'urine washing' as scent marking. Cowgill (1966) observed that *Perodicticus potto* Müller produces a secretion in the circumgenital area which attracts insects eaten by the potto. The brachial glands of the slender loris (*Loris tardigradus* L.) discharge an unpleasant odor when the animal is handled. This might serve to repel predators (Seitz 1969; Petter and Hladik 1970). Since functions other than intraspecific communication are not a subject of this review, the above reports will not be discussed further. This chapter, then, will present a discussion of those functions which seem to be pheromonal, using a few selected examples reported in the literature.

19.3. Communication of information concerning the physiological and emotional condition of the individual

19.3.1. Species, sex, individual identity and social status

It seems reasonable to assume that in many species, general body odor, excretions, saliva and skin gland secretions used in marking serve as carriers of information on the species, sex, age, identity, and sexual, social and emotional state of the individual which produces them. Such messages could then have important functions in several different areas of behavior.

In many non-primate mammals, chemical communication of messages of the above type has been found (Müller-Schwarze ch. 16 this volume). In primates, however, little experimental analysis of the amount and character of information concerning the physiological and emotional condition of individuals is available. Seitz (1969) and Epple (1970) showed that *Nycticebus coucang* and *Callithrix jacchus* L. recognize species-specific odors of urine and scent marked objects. Evidence for olfactory recognition of sex and identity is provided by Seitz (1969). In tests in which he measured the time a male and a female *Nycticebus coucang* spent sniffing samples of their own urine, that of a strange male conspecific and that of a strange female, he found that the male subject discriminated between his own urine, that of another male and that of a female. The female discriminated her own urine from that of a male but did not show a sniffing preference for the urine of a strange female over her own.

In our own laboratory, we have recently started to analyze the messages contained in the complex scent marks of a species of South American marmoset monkey (*Saguinus fuscicollis* Spix)(Epple 1971, 1972, 1973a,b). This species possesses large scent glands in the circumgenital, suprapubic and sternal areas (Perkins 1966). Scent marking is performed by rubbing the glandular areas against items of the environment. When the combined circumgenital and suprapubic glands are used, a few drops of urine are applied at the same time. In this type of marking, vaginal discharge is probably also mixed into the mark. At times, the labia pudendi are vigorously rubbed against a perch. This causes them to open and brings their inner surfaces in contact with the substrate. A detailed discussion of the marking patterns, the circumstances under which they are observed, and some of their functions is given by Epple (1970, 1972, 1973b). One of the major roles of scent marking seems to be the transmission of messages about the individual who produces the marks. These messages might then be used effectively in several different areas of behavior.

In an attempt to analyze the informational content of the complex scent marks which the animal applies to its environment, we tested the ability of the marmosets to discriminate between: 1) the scent marks of adult males and the scent marks of adult females; 2) the marks of two adult individuals of the same sex, both known to the subjects; 3) the scent marks of dominant males and those of submissive males, both unknown to the subjects. In all three experiments, the adult subjects were given series of preference tests during which they received two perches of white pine of identical dimensions. Each perch had been scent marked by a donor monkey immediately prior to being presented to the subject. Both perches were simultaneously introduced into the subject's home cage for a 15-minute test. The total test period was divided into intervals of five seconds each and the subjects received a score of one per interval for contacting, sniffing and scent marking either stimulus perch. The total time the subjects spent in contact with either stimulus was recorded with stopwatches. The following results were obtained:

1) The subjects preferred wooden perches scent marked by strange males over those scent marked by strange females (Epple 1971). Their preference was expressed in a higher frequency of marking with the sternal and with the circumgenital glands on the stimulus perch which carried the odor of males ($P = 0.012$). One male subject showed a significant time preference for scent marks of females ($P = 0.01$). The preferences of the subjects for the odor of strange males cannot be interpreted as preferences for the stimulus carrying the larger or smaller amount of scent. The subjects scent marked the stimulus perch carrying male odor more frequently than that carrying female odor regardless of whether the male perch was marked by one male and the female perch was marked by two females, or vica versa, or whether both perches carried the odor of one donor only (Epple 1971 and unpublished data). Identical results were obtained when the subjects were given the choice between two perches carrying equal volumes of pooled scent marks from males and pooled scent marks from females (Epple and Burlingame unpublished data). When the animals were presented with the choice between 0.4 ml urine from males and 0.4 ml urine from females applied to wooden perches by the investigator from a pool of fresh urine and presented in the way described above, they did prefer the male perch (Epple unpublished data). The preference for the intact scent marks of males as well as for pooled material recovered from male marks shows that the

marks carry information on the sex of the animal who produced them and that this information is independent of the total amount of scent present. The question, of course, remains which one of the various excretions and secretions mixed into a scent mark by the performing monkey is the carrier of this information. As our data indicate, urine alone, which is one component of intact marks, contains the information, or has picked enough of it from the skin glands to motivate the subjects to show their usual preference. It remains up to further experimentation to test the information contained in skin secretions alone.

2) In order to test the ability of marmosets to discriminate between the scent marks of two individuals of the same sex, the subjects had to be motivated to prefer the odor of one individual over that of another. Since aggression against a conspecific was observed to stimulate great interest in the scent marks of this particular animal, it was expected that the subjects would prefer the odor of an individual with whom they had recently fought over that of another familiar animal which they had not recently met. Therefore, an individual belonging to a strange group was introduced to the subjects for 10 minutes. This resulted in an aggressive encounter between the subjects and the stranger. Later, the subjects were given the choice between a wooden perch scent marked by the stimulus animal and a perch marked by another individual of the same sex, also belonging to a strange group, against whom they had not fought recently. In these tests, the subjects spent significantly more time investigating, sniffing and marking the perches carrying the scent of those males and females with whom they had recently fought than they spent with the perches carrying the marks of familiar but 'neutral' adults of the same sex as their recent opponent (male opponents: time preference $P = 0.027$; sniffing preference $P = 0.008$; marking preference $P = 0.027$. Female opponents: time preference $P = 0.012$; sniffing preference $P = 0.004$; marking preference $P = 0.004$). This shows that they could discriminate between the scent marks of two adults of the same sex (Epple, 1973a). The preference for the marks of an opponent was shown when the scent was presented on the day of the encounter between the subjects and the donor. However, it was also shown when the subjects were tested three or more days following the most recent introduction of the opponent. This not only shows that the monkeys can remember the scent of other individuals for several days, but also controls for the possibility that the subjects preferred the scent of their recent opponent because it was characteristic for a stressed animal rather than because of its individual quality (Epple 1973a). Preliminary results obtained from tests in which the subjects received a choice of 0.4 ml urine samples rather than the intact scent marks produced by the donors indicate that urine alone does not contain enough information on the individual to motivate the preference shown for intact marks (Epple, unpublished data).

3) In a third experiment, the marmosets were offered the choice between a wooden perch marked by a dominant male and a perch carrying the odor of a submissive male, both unknown to the subjects. The subjects sniffed and scent

marked the perches carrying the odor of dominant males significantly more frequently than those carrying the odor of submissive males (P = 0.005). During the first five minutes of testing, they also had a time preference for the scent of dominant males (P = 0.0025) but this preference did not persist throughout the whole test period of 15 minutes (Epple 1973a). These results indicate that scent marks of males of different social status contain some information that enabled the subjects to discriminate between them. However, this information is likely to be based on the quantity of the scent rather on its quality. Dominant males and dominant females scent mark more frequently than submissive individuals (Epple, 1970 and unpublished data). This possibly resulted in a larger amount of odorous material on the perches marked by the dominant donors, causing the subjects to prefer them. Further experiments are necessary to check out this possibility.

The studies reviewed above demonstrate that the scent marks of *Saguinus fuscicollis* are complex mixtures of several body products which carry information on the sex, the identity and the social status of the individual. Further research will doubtlessly show that these are not the only messages contained in the marks. Observational data and some pilot experiments, for instance, indicate that the marks of females in estrus also contain sexual attractants.

19.3.2. The reproductive condition of the female

The transmission of messages on the reproductive condition of the female seems to be extremely widespread among primates. This apparently is even the case in Old World monkeys and apes where we have otherwise so little evidence of chemical communication (c.f. Michael 1969).

Many males are strongly attracted to the scent marks of females in estrus and also sniff and lick the genitalia of these females (c.f. Michael and Zumpe 1972). *Galago senegalensis* E. Geoffroy, *Loris tardigradus* and *Perodicticus potto* females produce a conspicuous vaginal discharge at the time of estrus. In *Loris* and *Perodicticus* it is mixed with urine during marking and in all three species it has an extremely strong attraction for the male, very likely informing him about the condition of the female and at the same time arousing his sexual activities (Sauer and Sauer 1963; Doyle et al. 1967; Seitz 1969). Female *Lemur catta* show a peak of genital marking during and after estrus (Jolly 1966). They press the inner surfaces of the labia against the substrate and apply vaginal mucus and probably urine (Evans and Goy 1968). In marmoset monkeys, scent marking frequency increases immediately before and after copulation (Epple 1970). Female *Callimico goeldi* (Thomas) impregnate their tails with urine and the secretions of the circumgenital scent glands with increased frequency during estrus. The male apparently keeps a check on the reproductive condition of the female by regularly smelling and licking her genital scent glands and urine. Chemical cues from the female seem to initiate courtship and mating during estrus (Lorenz 1972). In another South American monkey *Saimiri sciureus*, Latta et al. (1967) report that receptive females show increased urine washing of hands and feet and that males increasingly smell female odors during this time. Spider monkey (*Ateles belzebuth* E. Geoffroy and *Ateles geoffroyi* Kuhl) males in capitivity and under natural conditions frequently sniff, lick and even drink the urine of females in all phases of the sexual cycle, including pregnancy. They also sniff their own hands after handling the clitora of females and investigate places where females sat. Since females do not show any visual signs of cycling, Klein (1971) suggests that olfactory clues are the main transmitters of information on the reproductive condition of the female.

In Old World primates, olfactory investigation of the females' genitalia is common. Rowell (1972) points out that in species whose females do not show conspicuous visual signs of cycling, olfactory investigation of the females by males is particularly common. For instance, in *Macaca speciosa arctoides* J. Geoffroy, which shows no female sexual swelling, males – prior to copulation – insert their fingers into the female's vagina, sniffing them afterwards (Michael and Zumpe 1972). Evidence of chemical communication of sexual cycling is also found in *Macaca radiata* E. Geoffroy, again a species which does not show visual signs of female receptivity (Rahaman and Parthasarathy 1971). Even in those species whose females show visual signs of cycling, pheromonal communication might be important. Michael and Keverne (1969) showed that the stimulation of intense redness of the sexual skin of ovariectomized rhesus monkeys by topical application of estradiol did not stimulate male sexual interest in these females. The application of sex pheromones to the same females, however, resulted in a dramatic increase in sexual behavior of males.

Among all inferred primate sexual attractants the only one whose behavioral function, hormonal control and chemical nature has been analyzed in detail is the sex pheromone of the rhesus monkey, *Macaca mulatta*. Michael and Keverne (1968) trained rhesus monkey males to press a lever in order to gain access to a female partner in a free-cage situation. The males frequently worked to obtain access to ovariectomized females who were rendered receptive by injections of estrogen but did not consistently work to obtain access to ovariectomized, non-treated females. When the males were rendered anosmic by plugging the nasal olfactory area with gauze impregnated with bismuth-iodoform-paraffin paste, they were no longer able to discriminate between receptive and non-receptive females. Reversal of anosmia, however, restored their ability to do so. These experiments clearly indicated that the female's attractiveness for the male is largely dependent on olfactory cues produced by her and that the male, when deprived of these cues, does not necessarily initiate sexual interactions, although the female might be receptive and invite copulations.

In an attempt to localize the source of these olfactory cues, Michael and Keverne (1969, 1970) applied vaginal washings from estrogen treated donor females to the sexual skin of untreated, unreceptive females. Although the males had shown little interest in the non-receptive females previously, the application of vaginal secretions from receptive females immediately caused them to obtain access to the females by rapid lever pressing and to show a significant and dramatic increase in sexual behavior. This occurred in spite of the fact that the ovariectomized recipient females were totally unreceptive and did not at all encourage the males. The control application of estradiol to the sexual skin of unreceptive females produced no changes in male behavior or female receptiveness. Small dosages of estrogen administered directly into the vaginae of unreceptive females also rendered them highly attractive to males, although they did not stimulate female receptivity (Michael and Saayman 1968). These experiments demonstrated that the females produce sex pheromones of vaginal origin and that the production of these pheromones is under estrogenic control.

Curtis et al. (1971) recently succeeded by means of gas chromatography and mass spectrometry in identifying the pheromonally active constituents of vaginal washings from estrogenized females as a mixture of five aliphatic acids: acetic acid, propionic acid, *iso*-butyric acid, *n*-butyric acid and *iso*-valeric acid. A synthetic mixture of these acids was made up to match the concentrations present in a pool of twenty four vaginal washings from estrogenized females. Two-ml samples of this mixture, containing about 1.5 times the acid content of one vaginal lavage, were applied to the sexual skin of unreceptive females. The synthetic samples mimicked the behavioral effects of the natural pheromone.

Michael et al. (1972) report that vaginal washings of *Papio anubis* Lesson, *Erythrocebus patas* Schreber, *Macaca nemestrina* L., *Macaca fascicularis* Raffles, *Saimiri sciureus* and *Homo* show a similar, although not identical, content of aliphatic acids as those of the rhesus monkey. Unreceptive rhesus females, treated with vaginal washings of intact anubis baboons, stimulated the sexual activity of male rhesus monkeys significantly, indicating that there is some interspecific activity of the sex attractants.

Although the previously reviewed studies show that the sex pheromones are produced in the vagina, they do not provide information on the exact source of the attractants. However, the finding that the amount of volatile acids in vaginal washings from rhesus monkeys increased after incubation at 37 °C, but was inhibited by autoclaving or the addition of penicillin before incubation, indicates that pheromonal production depends on bacterial action within the vagina. Gonadal hormones might regulate acid production in vivo by determining the availability of the substrate or the pH of the vagina (Bonsall and Michael 1971; Michael et al. 1972).

19.4. *The role of chemical signals in some other areas of behavior*

In the previous pages, we have discussed information transmitted by chemical signals on species and individual identity and on physiological and social conditions of an animal. These messages are probably produced by many more primate species than have been studied so far and are likely to play important roles in a variety of behavioral contexts. They might function in orientation within the home range, and in the correlation of intergroup and intragroup social interactions, including consort relationships, spacing, aggression, territorial defense, and parent–infant relations. The lack of space does not permit me to review the evidence for all of these possible functions. Therefore, further discussion will be limited to a few behavioral categories where the importance of chemical signals is particularly intriguing.

19.4.1. Orientation by trail marking

Bolwig (1960), Sauer and Sauer (1963) and Seitz (1969) have suggested that one of the functions of urine marking in prosimians, especially nocturnal species, is the production of odoriferous trails which help the animal to orient itself within its home range. Seitz (1969) showed that *Nycticebus coucang* is capable of using trails of its own urine to orient itself in a totally dark test room. When he introduced subjects into a totally dark room which did not contain any urine trails, the animal showed a phase of initial orientation during which they investigated their environment, continuously sniffing and urine marking. Following the phase of initial orientation, the subjects showed less olfactory investigation and urine marking, and demonstrated that they were familiar with the new environment. When the subjects were tested under identical conditions after the investigator had applied trails of the subjects' own urine to the floor of the test room, initial orientation in a new environment took place along the artificial urine trails. After surgical blinding, a female tested in a new environment increased the time she spent sniffing the new environment to 91.6% of the total test time as compared to only 21.1% when her eyesight was intact and she was tested in an illuminated test room. Although Seitz (1969) did not eliminate the possibility that his subjects used other senses (e.g. touch or hearing) during orientation in the test environment, his experiments strongly indicate that when eyesight is eliminated, olfaction can take over and urine trails help the animal to orient itself in an unfamiliar space.

The question remains, how strongly the animals rely on their own urine marks for orientation in a natural environment, where they are hardly ever totally deprived of their ability to see. Seitz's animals may well have learned to rely on their sense of olfaction and to use urine marks in orienting within a limited space which, after repeated testing, was not altogether unfamiliar to them and which was relatively simple in its three dimensional structure. Charles-Dominique (1971a) doubts that under natural conditions lorises make much use of their urine marks in orientation. *Perodicticus potto*, for instance, travels through its whole natural territory without using fixed pathways. Moreover, urine is not deposited throughout the territory but only in particular places. Although urine marks left in some places within the territory might function as reminders during orientation, Charles-Dominique (1971a) suggests that their more important function is in territorial and social behavior, a possibility which is also discussed by Seitz (1969).

19.4.2. Territorial functions

In many primates, especially in prosimians and in New World monkeys, scent marking is thought to play a role in territorial behavior. However, only a few examples of 'territorial marking' can be reviewed here. Seitz (1969) introduced *Nycticebus coucang* into a uniformly equipped test territory, bordered at two sides by *Nycticebus* living cages, at one side by a *Loris tardigradus* cage and at the fourth side by no other animals. The males marked most frequently in the area adjacent to the living cages of the same species, less frequently in the area adjacent to the *Loris* cage and little in the center of the territory and in the area not bordered by a neighbor. Females, however, limited their marking activity to the center of the test territory. Similar observations are reported for *Galago senegalensis* in the field by Sauer and Sauer (1963). Charles-Dominique (1971b) reports that wild galagos and pottos deposit urine marks particularly in zones in which the territories of the individuals overlap. Wild *Lepilemur mustelinus* J. Geoffroy males deposit urine and feces on exposed branches of their territories which seem to serve as lookout points for observing neighbors in adjacent territories (Charles-Dominique and Hladik 1971). The highly ritualized territorial disputes among *Propithecus verrauxi* Grandidier groups in their natural environment involve a frenzy of scent marking (Jolly 1966). Marking is also a regular component of the complex and ritualized territorial ceremonies of wild Titi monkeys (*Callicebus moloch* Hoffmannseg) (Mason 1966) and is regularly seen when groups of captive marmosets engage in aggressive encounters (Epple personal observation). The first report of territorial rubbing in Old World monkeys is that of Gartlan and Brain (1968) who observed marking with the chest and the cheeks in wild and captive *Cercopithecus aethiops* L.. No scent glands have been identified histologically, so far. In the langur *Presbytis johnii* Fischer territorial battles are accompanied by excessive defecation. Poirier (1970) suspects that its overpowering odor serves as a territorial scent and that fecal odor may also serve to mark the sleeping trees of wild *Cercopithecus aethiops*.

A common concept of territorial demarcation by olfactory signals is that the inhabitants of a territory apply their scents to part or all of the territorial borders which they will defend against invaders. The odor of the residents supposedly functions as a repellent and helps to prevent strange conspecifics from invading the occupied territory. The reports on primate 'territorial marking', provide little information on whether or not this is true in any single species. The observation that an animal scent marks prominent places in its environment, applies its scent preferably at the borders of its home range or shows a high frequency of marking during territorial disputes with neighbors actually tells us little about the exact function of the chemical signals. The reports reviewed above indicate that 'territorial marking' under the observed conditions was motivated by aggression against strange conspecifics. However, though intolerance of certain conspecifics probably motivated the marking performance, the biological function of the chemical signals might vary widely among the different species. Even in the same species, territorial marking might serve more than one purpose alone. The following functions of chemical signals in territorial behavior seem possible and are indicated by observational data:

a) The application of personal scent is an act of 'self-advertisement' (Jolly 1966). It expresses self-confidence and helps to reassure the marking animal in the presence of opponents. The odor also might have a reassuring effect on other members of the group, or it might stimulate their aggression against invaders, thus correlating the motivations and displays of all group members and promoting group cohesion during territorial ceremonies. It is obvious that the expression of self-confidence by scent marking does not need to be limited to territorial encounters. It might just as well function in a variety of other behaviors, e.g. during intragroup aggression or in sexual courtship.

b) Marking gives the territory the characteristics of a 'home'. It is common knowledge that – in captivity – many primate species very actively remark their home cages after these have been washed. Moreover, the lion marmoset (*Leontopithecus rosalia rosalia* L.) shows increased scent marking after heavy rainfalls in open air enclosures (Snyder 1972). This indicates that the absence of their own odor within the home range might have a stressful effect on the inhabitants who, therefore, renew the marks frequently. Mykytowycz (1972) suggests that the presence of the personal odor within their living space is essential for many mammals to behave freely and participate in breeding activities. Where the territory of social species is marked by many group members, a characteristic group odor – as in the flying phalanger (Schultze-Westrum 1965) – might result.

c) The odor produced in territorial marking serves as a short term threat signal which intimidates opponents. This function is not limited to intergroup aggression. It is likely that odors discharged during the spectacular 'stink-fights' performed by male *Lemur catta* in intragroup conflicts (Jolly 1966; Evans and Goy) serve as threat signals directed at group mates.

d) Territorial scent is a long term manifestation of the presence of the owner(s) in the territory. It alerts invaders to the presence of the owners and might help prevent invasions. However, it depends on the motivation of the invaders whether they are intimidated by the signal or not. Martin (1968) suggests that *after* having experienced defeat during territorial encounters with a resident, they might become conditioned to avoid an area where a specific scent indicates the presence of the former opponent.

e) Finally, scent applied throughout the living space of an individual may communicate detailed information on the species, age, sex and reproductive state to conspecifics occupying adjacent territories and thus not only serve to announce the occupation of a territory but also form a bridge between individuals who rarely encounter each other personally, as in the case of solitary prosimians.

Recent field studies on *Lepilemur mustelinus* (Charles-Dominique and Hladik

1971), *Microcebus murinus* (Martin 1972), *Perodicticus potto* and *Galago demidovii* Fischer (Charles-Dominique 1971b, 1972), all of which, with the exception of *Galago*, are commonly classified as solitary, have revealed that these prosimians show various forms of 'semi-social' organizations. Individuals occupy territories which more or less overlap with the ranges of their neighbors. They engage in a limited amount of friendly social interactions, especially with neighbors of the opposite sex, and more or less defend their territories against neighbors of the same sex. In such semi-social primates, the major means of communication between individuals who rarely engage in close contact encounters might be chemical. Male *Perodicticus potto* frequently patrol the areas in which their ranges overlap with those of females. The urine marks left in these zones by the males and by the females keep the animals informed of each other's presence, identity and sexual state. Males avoid encountering other males in zones of overlap. The scent marks they leave in these zones, however, permit them to communicate with each other (Charles-Dominique 1971b).

19.4.3. Intergroup aggression and social dominance

Ralls (1971) recently reviewed mammalian scent marking and discussed the role of pheromones in the aggressive behavior of some mammals. She points out that in all species whose marking behavior has been studied experimentally there is an obvious correlation between aggressiveness, social dominance and the frequency of scent marking. This seems also to be true in primates. Although very few experimental studies on the scent marking behavior of primates exist, many observers report that the animals marked frequently in situations where they were aggressive, intolerant of conspecifics and dominant to them (Bolwig 1960; Moynihan 1964; Sprankel 1961; Jolly 1966; Epple and Lorenz 1967; Evans and Goy 1968; and many others).

In an attempt to study the correlations between social dominance, aggressive behavior and scent marking, the social interactions and the marking frequencies in three groups of common marmosets (*Callithrix jacchus*) were recorded under various conditions (Epple 1970). The groups established independent rank orders among males and among females respectively. Both dominant males and dominant females showed a higher frequency per hour of scent marking than submissive group members. However, in one group which contained only one adult female but more than one adult male, the dominant male showed the highest marking frequency while in groups which contained only one adult male but several adult females, the dominant female marked most frequently.

When a male belonging to another group of the same species was introduced to the group of subjects for a 10-minute encounter, the dominant males of the three groups were the most active among all group members in threatening, attacking and fighting the strange males. When the marking frequencies of all group members were recorded for one hour immediately following the aggressive encounters with strange males, the dominant males marked significantly more frequently than during comparable periods of undisturbed daily routine, and in two groups the two α-males marked significantly more frequently than all the other group members.

When a female belonging to another group of the same species was introduced to the subjects for a 10-minute encounter, the dominant resident females threatened, attacked and fought the stimulus female very actively. During the hour immediately following the removal of the stimulus female, the dominant females in all three groups scent marked significantly more frequently than in undisturbed situations or after aggressive interactions with strange males. In two groups, the dominant females also scent marked most frequently among all group members.

The results of this study show that in the common marmoset, aggression is mainly directed at adult members of the same sex while those of the opposite sex are more or less tolerated. The presence of an animal of the same sex stimulates the scent marking frequency of dominant males and females but not that of submissive individuals, whether this animal is a member of the subject's group or a stranger. Conspecifics not belonging to the same group stimulate strong aggression in dominant animals and there is a clear-cut covariance between aggressive behavior and the frequency of marking. Under certain social conditions the scent marking activity of an individual is a direct indication of its aggressiveness against conspecifics. It is likely that either the quantity or the quality of scent marks, or both, communicate these aggressive tendencies to conspecifics. Thus a high frequency of marking might serve to establish, maintain and demonstrate social dominance within the group as well as in intergroup encounters.

It is obvious that by marking frequently, a dominant animal saturates its environment with its own odor to a greater extent than its submissive group mates do. Since marmosets recognize the odor of individual conspecifics (Epple 1971), submissive animals are confronted with the 'presence' of a dominant group mate throughout much of their living space, even when the dominant animal is not within sight or hearing. This fact, reinforced by personal encounters with the superior group mate might severely stress submissive individuals and might result in a kind of 'psychological castration'. Baldwin (1968) even suggests the possibility that in *Saimiri sciureus* primer pheromones produced by dominant males inhibit the gonadal activity of submissive males during the breeding season.

It is not known how widespread the demonstration of dominance by chemical signals is among primates. However, the few reports cited above suggest that it might be a major function of primate pheromones.

19.4.4. Synchronization of reproduction

The idea that pheromones might be involved in synchronizing the breeding activities of seasonal primates is particularly intriguing. The most fascinating pheromonal effects reported in rodent reproduction are the induction of estrus, the blocking of pregnancy, and the acceleration of female maturation by male urinary pheromones (Bronson 1971). No experimental evidence for any such action is available in primates. Several authors, however, have speculated whether or not phenomena of behavioral and physiological synchronization of reproductive activity in seasonal primates might be, in part, controlled by pheromones.

In *Lemur catta*, Jolly (1967) reports a very short breeding season during which the group shows a high degree of behavioral synchronization, correlated with a sharp increase in sexual and social interactions and in the various patterns of olfactory marking and olfactory investigation. As Jolly (1967) points out, the great variety of olfactory marking patterns of the species and a large amount of mutual sniffing of each other's bodies and scent marks may be one of the major means of communicating the rising excitement of the breeding season among members of a *Lemur catta* group. She suggests, therefore, that synchrony of reproductive activity depends, in part, on olfactory and other social communications within the group. There is no information on whether the chemical stimuli correlate the behavioral responses only or whether 'primer' pheromones might also be involved, exerting a physiological effect on the hypothalamic-pituitary-gonadal axis.

In squirrel monkeys (*Saimiri sciureus*) Latta et al. (1967) noted increased urine washing behavior in receptive females under laboratory conditions and reported that males frequently smelled the genitalia and bodies of females and the places where they had urine washed. Baldwin (1970), who studied a seasonally breeding group of *Saimiri* under seminatural conditions, reports that there is an increase in olfactory investigation of females by males during the breeding season. Males, however, are attracted to female odors whether the female is in estrus or not, although the scent of estrus females seems to have stronger attraction. He suspects that female odors might stimulate the males and bring them into the reproductively active condition. In laboratory groups, where males and females are caged together, the males are permanently exposed to female odors. This would explain why the males of many laboratory colonies are more or less sexually active all year round (Latta et al. 1967). In free ranging groups, however, adult males travel separately from the females except during the breeding season, when they are spermatogenic (Baldwin 1968). As female odors become more attractive during the breeding season, they might motivate the males to interact with the females and thus be exposed to the stimulating effect of female pheromones (Baldwin 1970).

Vandenbergh (1969) induced sexual activity in male rhesus monkeys (*Macaca mulatta*) by exposing them to ovariectomized, estrogenized females during the nonbreeding season. The monkeys were captured from a free-ranging group on an island near Puerto Rico's southwestern coast and remained exposed to their normal environmental conditions during the experiments. No sexual behavior was recorded at the same time in the free-ranging animals not involved in the experiment. Rose et al. (1971, 1972) have recently shown that plasma testosterone levels in male rhesus monkeys increase with social rank and sexual activity. Although no direct evidence is available at this point, the stimulation of male reproductive activity through sexual interactions and the presence of receptive females might, in part, result from primer pheromones produced by the females.

Acknowledgment

Part of my own studies were supported by NSF Grant GB12 660 and were carried out while I was a Biomedical Fellow of the Population Council of the Rockefeller University.

References

Altman, S. A. (1967) The structure of primate social communication. *In*: Social Communication among Primates; ed.: S. A. Altman (The University of Chicago Press, Chicago and London) pp. 325–362.

Andriamiandra, A. and Y. Rumpler (1968) Role de la testostérone sur le déterminisme des glands brachiales et antebrachiales chez le *Lemur catta*. C. R. Soc. Biol. 162, 1651–1655.

Arao, T. and E. Perkins (1969) The skin of primates. XLIII. Further observations on the Philippine tarsier (*Tarsius syrichta*). Am. J. Phys. Anthropol. 31, 93–96.

Baldwin, J. D. (1968) The social behavior of adult male squirrel monkeys (*Saimiri sciureus*) in a seminatural environment. Folia Primatol. 9, 281–314.

Baldwin, J. D. (1970) Reproductive synchronization in squirrel monkeys. (*Saimiri*). Primates 11, 317–326.

Bolwig, N. (1960) A comparative study of the behavior of various lemurs. Mém. Inst. Sci. (Madagascar) Ser. A. 14. 205–217.

Bonsall, R. W. and R. P. Michael (1971) Volatile constituents of primate vaginal secretions. J. Reprod. Fert. 27, 478.

Bronson, F. H. (1971) Rodent pheromones. Biol. Reprod. 4, 344–357.

Castell, R. and M. Maurus (1967) Das sogenannte Urinmarkieren von Totenkopfaffen (*Saimiri sciureus*) in Abhängigkeit von umweltbedingten und emotionalen Faktoren. Folia Primatol. 6. 170–176.

Charles-Dominique, P. (1971a) Eco-éthologie des prosimiens du Gabon. Biologia Gabonica 7, 121–228.

Charles-Dominique, P. (1971b) Sociologie chez les lémuriens. Recherche (Paris) 15, 780–781.

Charles-Dominique, P. (1972) Ecologie et vie social de *Galago demidovii* (Fisher 1808, Prosimii). Z. Tierpsychol. Beiheft. 9, 7–41.

Charles-Dominique, P. and C. M. Hladik (1971) Le *Lepilemur* du sud de Madagascar: écologie, alimentation et vie sociale. Terre et la Vie. 1, 3–66.

Cowgill, U. M. (1966) *Perodicticus potto* and some insects. J. Mammal. 47, 156–157.

Curtis, R: F., J. A. Ballantine, E. B. Keverne, R. W. Bonsall and R. P. Michael (1971) Identification of primate sexual pheromones and the properties of synthetic attractants. Nature (London) 232, 396–398.

Dobroruka, L. J. (1972) Social communication in the Brown capuchin. Int. Zoo Yearb. 12, 43–45.

Doyle, G. A., A. Pelletier and T. Bekker (1967) Courtship, mating and parturition in the lesser bushbaby (*Galago senegalensis moholi*) under semi-natural conditions. Folia Primatol. 7, 169–197.

Ellis, R. A. and W. Montagna (1963) The sweat glands of the Lorisidae. *In*: Evolutionary and Genetic Biology of Primates, Vol. 1; ed.: J. Buettner-Janusch (Academic Press, New York and London) pp. 197–228.

Epple, G. (1967) Vergleichende Untersuchungen über Sexual- und Sozialverhalten der Krallenaffen (*Hapalidae*). Folia Primatol. 7, 37–65.

Epple, G. (1970) Quantitative studies on scent marking in the marmoset (*Callithrix jacchus*). Folia Primatol. 13, 48–62.

Epple, G. (1971) Discrimination of the odor of males and females by the marmoset *Saguinus fuscicollis ssp.* Proc. Int. Congr. Primat., (Zürich) 3rd. (Karger, Basel, New York) 3, 166–171.

Epple, G. (1972) Social communication by olfactory signals in marmosets. Int. Zool. Yearb. 12, 36–42.

Epple, G. (1973a) The role of pheromones in the social communication of marmoset monkeys (*Gallithricidae*). J. Reprod. Fert. Suppl. 19, 445–452.

Epple, G. (1973b) The behavior of marmoset monkeys (*Gallithricidae*). *In*: Primate Behavior, Developments in Field and Laboratory Research, vol. 3; ed.: L. A. Rosenblum (Academic Press, New York and London) (in press).

Epple, G. and R. Lorenz (1967) Vorkommen, Morphologie und Funktion der Sternaldrüse bei den *Platyrrhini*. Folia Primatol. 7, 98–126.

Evans, C. S. and R. W. Goy (1968) Social behaviour and reproductive cycles in captive Ringtailed lemurs (*Lemur catta*). J. Zool. London 156, 181–197.

Gartlan, J. S. and C. K. Brain (1968) Ecology and social variability in *Cercopithecus aethiops* and *C. mitis*. *In*: Primates. Studies in Adaptation and Variability; ed.: P. Jay (Holt, Rinehart and Winston, New York) pp. 253–292.

Jolly, A. (1966) Lemur behavior. A Madagascar field study. (University Chicago Press, Chicago and London) pp. 187.

Jolly, A. (1967) Breeding synchrony in wild *Lemur catta*, In: Social Communication among Primates; ed.: S. A. Altman (The University of Chicago Press, Chicago and London) pp. 3–14.

Kirchshofer, R. (1963) Einige bemerkenswerte Verhaltenweisen bei Saimiris im Vergleich zu anderen Arten. Z. Morphol. Antropol. 53, 77–91.

Klein, L. L. (1971) Observations on copulation and seasonal reproduction of two species of spider monkeys, *Ateles belzebuth* and *A. geoffroyi*. Folia Primatol. 15, 233–248.

Knappe, H. (1964) Zur Funktion des Jacobsonschen Organs (*Organon Vomeronasale Jacobsoni*). Zool. Gart. 28, 188–194.

Lancaster, J. B. (1968) Primate communication systems and the emergence of human language. *In*: Primates. Studies in Adaptation and Variability; ed.: P. C. Jay (Holt, Rinehart and Winston, New York). pp. 439–457.

Latta, J., S. Hopf and D. Ploog (1967) Observations on mating behavior and sexual play in the squirrel monkey (*Saimiri sciureus*). Primates 8, 229–246.

Lorenz, R. (1972) Management and reproduction of the Goeldi's monkey *Gallimico goeldii* (Thomas, 1904) Callimiconidae, Primates. *In*: Saving the Lion Marmoset, Proc. WAPT Golden Lion Marmoset Conference; ed.: (Wild Animal Propagation Trust, Oglebay Park, Wheeling, West Virginia) pp. 92–109.

Machida, H. and L. Giacometti (1967) The anatomical and histochemical properties on the skin of the external genitalia of the primates. Folia Primatol. 6, 48–69.

Marler, P. (1965) Communication in monkeys and apes. *In*: Primate Behavior. Field Studies of Monkeys and Apes; ed.: I. DeVore (Holt, Rinehart and Winston, New York) pp. 544–584.

Martin, R. D. (1968) Reproduction and ontogeny in tree shrews (*Tupaia belangeri*), with reference to their general behaviour and taxonomic relationships. Z. Tierpsychol. 25, 409–495.

Martin, R. D. (1972) A preliminary field-study of the Lesser-Mouse Lemur (*Microcebus murinus* J. F. Miller 1777). Z. Tierpsychol. Beiheft. 9, 43–89.

Mason, W. A. (1966) Social organization of the South American monkey, *Gallicebus moloch*: A preliminary report. Tulane Stud. Zool. 13, 23–28.

Michael, R. P. (1969) The role of pheromones in the communication of primate behaviour. Proc. Int. Congr. Primat. (Atlanta, Ga.) 2nd, vol 1 (Karger, Basel, New York) pp. 101–107.

Michael, R. P. and E. B. Keverne (1968) Pheromones in the communication of sexual status in primates. Nature (London) 218, 746–749.

Michael, R. P. and E. B. Keverne (1969) A male sex-attractant pheromone in rhesus monkey vaginal secretions. J. Endocrinol. 46, 20–21.

Michael, R. P. and E. B. Keverne (1970) Primate sex pheromones of vaginal origin. Nature (London) 225, 84–85.

Michael, R. P. and G. S. Saayman (1968) Differential effects on behaviour of the subcutaneous and intravaginal administration of oestrogen in the rhesus monkey (*Macaca mulatta*). J. Endocrinol. 41, 231–246.

Michael, R. P. and D. Zumpe (1972) Patterns of reproductive behavior. *In*: Comparative Reproduction of Nonhuman Primates; ed.: E. S. E. Hafez (Charles C. Thomas, Pub. Springfield, Ill.) pp. 205–242.

Michael, R. P., D. Zumpe, E. B. Keverne and R. W. Bonsall (1972) Neuroendocrine factors in the control of primate behavior. Recent Progr. Horm. Res. 28, 665–706.

Moynihan, M. (1964) Some behavior patterns of platyrrhine monkeys. I. The night monkey (*Aotus trivirgatus*). Smithson. Misc. Collect. 146, 1–84.

Mykytowycz, R. (1972) The behavioural role of the mammalian skin glands. Naturwissenschaften 59, 133–139.

Perkins, E. M. (1966) The skin of primates XXXI. The skin of the black-collared tamarin (*Tamarinus nigricollis*). Am. J. Phys. Anthropol. 25, 41–70.

Petter, J. J. and C. M. Hladik (1970) Observations sur le domaine vital et la densité de population de *Loris tardigradus* dans les forêts de Ceylon. Mammalia 34, 394–409.

Poirier, F. E. (1970) The communication matrix of the nilgiri langur (*Presbytis johnii*) of South India. Folia Primatol. 13, 92–136.

Rahaman, H. (1971) The role of the olfactory signals in the mating behavior of bonnet monkeys (*Macaca radiata*). Proc. Indian Sci. Congr. 58, 550–551.

Rahaman, R. and M. D. Parthasarathy (1971) The role of olfactory signals in the mating behavior of bonnet monkeys (*Macaca radiata*). Commun. Behav. Biol. Part A Orig. Artic. 6, 97–104.

Ralls, K. (1971) Mammalian scent marking. Science 171, 443–449.

Rose, R. M., J. W. Holaday and I. S. Bernstein (1971) Plasma testosterone, dominance rank and aggressive behaviour in male rhesus monkeys. Nature (London) 231, 366–368.

Rose, R. M., T. P. Gordon and I. S. Bernstein (1972) Plasma testosterone levels in the male rhesus: Influence of sexual and social stimuli. Science 178, 643–645.

Rowell, T. E. (1972) Female reproduction cycles and social behavior in primates. *In*: Advances in the Study of Behavior, vol. 4; eds.: D. S. Lehrmann, R. A. Hinde and E. Shaw (Academic Press, New York and London) pp. 69–105.

Rumpler, Y. and A. Andriamiandra (1968) Sur l'étude des glands brachiales et antebrachiales du *Lemur catta*. C. R. Soc. Biol. 162, 1430–1434.

Rumpler, Y. and A. Andriamiandra (1971) Étude histologique des glandes de marquage de la face antérieure du cou des Lemuriens malgaches, C. R. Soc. Biol. 165, 436–442.

Rumpler, Y. and J. H. Oddou (1970) Comportement de marquage et structure histologique des glands de marquage chez *Lemur macaco*. C. R. Soc. Biol. 164, 2686–2690.

Sauer, F. and E. Sauer (1963) The African bushbaby of the *Galago senegalensis* group. J. South West Afr. Sci. Soc. (Windhoek) 16, 5–36.

Schifter, H. (1968) Zucht und Markierungsverhalten von Wollaffen im Zoologischen Garten Zürich. Zool. Gart. 36, 107–132.

Schmidt, U. and E. Seitz (1967) Waschen mit Harn zum Zweck der Thermorengulation bei Totenkopfaffen (*Saimiri sciureus* L.). Anthropol. Anz. 30, 162–165.

Schultze-Westrum, T. (1965) Innerartliche Verständigung durch Düfte beim Gleitbeutler *Petaurus breviceps papuanus* Thomas (*Marsupialia, Phalangeridae*). Z. Vergl. Physiol. 50, 151–220.

Seitz, E. (1969) Die Bedeutung geruchlicher Orientierung beim Plumplori, *Nycticebus coucang* Boddaert 1785 (Prosimii, Lorisidae). Z. Tierpsychol. 26, 73–103.

Sisson, J. K. and W. H. Fahre Bach (1967) Fine structure of steroidogenic cells of a primate cutaneous organ. Am. J. Anat. 121, 337–368.

Snyder, P. A. (1972) Behavior of *Leontopithecus rosalia* (the golden lion marmoset) and related species: A review. *In*: Saving the Lion Marmoset. Proc. WAPT Golden Lion Marmoset Conference; ed.: D. D. Bridgwater (Wild Animal Propagation Trust, Oglebay Park, Wheeling, West Virginia), pp. 23–49.

Sorenson, M. W. (1970) Behavior of tree shrews. *In*: Primate Behavior. Developments in Field and Laboratory Research, vol. 1; ed.: L. A. Rosenblum (Academic Press, New York and London) pp. 141–193.

Sprankel, H. (1961) Histologie und biologische Bedeutung eines jugosternalen Duftdrüsenfeldes bei *Tupaia glis* (Diard 1820) in Gefangenschaft. Verh. Deut. Zool. Ges. (Saarbrücken) pp. 198–206.

Stephan, H. (1965) Der Bulbus olfactorius accessorius bei Insektivoren und Primaten. Acta Anat. 62, 215–253.

Stephan, H. (1966) Grössenänderungen im olfaktorischen und limbischen System während der phylogenetischen Entwicklung der Primate. *In*: Evolution of the Forebrain; eds.: R. Hassler and H. Stephan (Georg Thieme Verlag, Stuttgart) pp. 377–388.

Vandenbergh, J. G. (1969) Endocrine coordination in monkeys: Male sexual responses to the female. Physiol. Behav. 4, 261–264.

CHAPTER 20

The likelihood of human pheromones*

Alex COMFORT

20.1. Introduction

The likelihood that there are functional human pheromones has been both asserted (Wilson 1963; Wiener 1966, 1967a, 1967b) and denied (Gleeson and Reynierse 1969), both without direct experimental evidence: the finding of clear pheromonal effects in monkeys (Michael and Saayman 1967; Michael and Keverne 1970) and the recent observation of menstrual synchronization between close friends (McClintock 1971) re-open the possibility more definitely, and make direct experiment obligatory.

The practical importance of such research lies in the possibility of primer control over human endocrine cycles and reproduction generally; if this exists, it might open a new chapter in reproductive pharmacology at a time when it is badly needed. Compared with drugs, pheromones are strikingly economical in quantity, many operating at a level of molecules rather than milligrams. Even the study of simple 'releaser' effects could clarify a field of human, and especially developmental, biology which has been so far suspected rather than elucidated. Odor fingerprinting techniques and gas chromatography (Dravnieks and Krotoszynski 1970) now make the detection and preparation of human pheromonal agents feasible if they exist.

20.2. Developmental effects

Sexual releaser effects of odor in man have been recognized throughout human experience, even in cultures which found the idea embarrassing, and the richness of human olfactosexual behavior was fully documented by Havelock Ellis (1905). All release effects in man tend to be more variable than in lower animals because of the large variety of human signal systems and the size of the override from learned or

* Adapted from an article of the same title by A. Comfort, Nature (London) (1971) 230, 432–433, 479, with extracts from 'Communication may be odorous' which first appeared in New Scientist (1971) 49, 412–415.

conditioned behavior, which is such that not even the human sex object is irrevocably fixed. The large observed individual variation in conscious olfactory awareness is almost certainly in part genetic, but psycho-analytic writers have both suggested and documented the possibility of a special role for odor in infant psychosexual development (Brill 1932; Daly and White 1930; Bieber 1959; Fitzherbert 1959; Kalogerakis 1963). According to this view, attraction to the odor of the opposite-sex parent and avoidance as a threat of the odor of the same-sex parent act as biological triggers for the Oedipal responses, an idea of much biological interest. This would represent a case intermediate between releaser and primer conditions, and possibly a programmed 'temporary organ'.

We have the observation of several workers, notably Kalogerakis (1963) and Bieber (1959) that odor plays an important part in infantile psychosexual development. At the stage in development when dominance-competition between son and father appears, the 'oedipal phase', it is accompanied by a marked awareness of the sexual odor of adults, with a distaste for that of the same-sex parent. A biological psychoanalyst could not fail to note that three regions in man are provided with odor glands and large, odor-diffusing hair tufts – the breast-axilla complex, and the anal and the genital regions, all imprinting points in human development. The odor of the areolar glands, which adults cannot perceive, could be our first impression in life. The sequence of associations is biologically interesting.

Groddeck (1925) argued that man is as macrosmatic as the dog, but represses the capacity in adult life for psychosexual reasons. Without accepting this view, it is still credible that some part of human olfactosexual response may be confined to infancy and childhood, and subsequently 'turned off', or altered in direction, either by a process of repression or, as in other mammals, by the advent of adult sex hormone status, most adult pheromone response being either androgen or estrogen-dependent. The complexity of human psychosexual development is likely to produce unique effects on adult-response not seen in other mammals. 'Even the most learned man', said Groddeck, 'has to let his nose decide for him in matters of love'. For some people this is consciously true. Unfortunately for simple analysis, we tend to 'imprint' releasers from past experience – musk, human or animal, is a 'releaser', but so, for some people, is the odor of gasoline rubber, through a conditioned association with contraceptives. Babies can be readily conditioned to like the smell of codliver oil (Welch and Hayes 1957).

20.3. Adult effects

Adult odor releaser effects in man as embodied in sexual behavior are attractant, ancillary to more familiar signal systems, and often overridden by individual experience, though still serving to synchronize intercourse with ovulation: beside male–female attraction, or bonding during pregnancy, they may possibly, on the mammalian model, include adult male–male dominance or hostility. Wider odor communication of states of mind, as postulated by Wiener (1966), is ill-confirmed in other mammals and difficult to separate from other human sub-liminal cues. The value of seeking for the more tangible and important primer effects, which have not so far been suspected, depends on the following principal arguments:

1) Pheromonal primer effects are near-universal in social mammals, including primates.

2) Releaser pheromone effects exist in man, at least in larval form, and some involve pheromones of other mammals (musk, civetone). These in nature are rarely simple releasers, but combine priming and other effects – thus one male odor may serve to mark territory, assert dominance, repel rivals, attract females and synchronize their cycles. Unless man is a wholly special case, or his use of this potential response system has been taken over by anticipation, as part of infantile rather than adult psychosexual mechanics, then similar effects are to be looked for in man also.

3) In mammals as against insects, functional and species specificity do not seem to depend on a multiplicity of special substances. Cross-specific reactions are common (humans react to musk; bulls, goats and monkeys to the odor of women): interspecific bars between near species (dog–fox) are probably effected by addition or by concentration, the basic effector molecules being widespread. The physiological effect of similar molecules is likely to be similar between man and other mammals in which priming is known to occur.

4) Humans have a complete set of organs which are traditionally described as non-functional, but which, if seen in any other mammal, would be recognized as part of a pheromone system. These include apocrine glands associated with conspicuous hair tufts, some of which do not produce sweat and most presumably produce some other functioning secretion (Kligman and Shehadeh 1964); a developed prepuce and labia, and the production of smegma (the sebaceous secretion that collects beneath the prepuce or around the clitoris). This system in adults seems over-elaborate for the relatively small releaser role of odor in most cultures. The amputatory assault on these recognizable pheromone-mediating structures in many human societies implies an intuitive awareness that their sexual function goes beyond the decorative. A conspicuous and apparently unused antenna array presupposes an unsuspected communications system.

20.4. Patterns of response

The nature and function of such possible communications can be inferred from mammalian models, to indicate the types of priming which might be expected in humans. For instance, Le Magnen (1952) showed that women's ability to smell musks varies with the estrus cycle. It is known that women have the greater olfactory sensivity to most mammal odor, that this is estrogen-dependent and, in the case of exaltolide, cyclical (Kloek 1961; Vierling and Rock 1967). Thus women detect, and react to, boar taint in pork far more readily than men (Griffiths and

Patterson 1970), the substance detected being apparently 5α-androst-16-en-3-one (Patterson 1968). A similar material occurs in human male urine, and in female urine during the luteal phase (Brookbank and Hazelwood 1950).

The detection of this effect seems, however, to depend on the choice of olfactometric method. According to Amoore (Amoore and Venstrom 1966; Amoore personal communication) there is no true change of threshold, but women under the influence of estrogen are more inclined to react psychologically to musky odors and to describe them as 'strong'.

True anosmia, both for a musk (pentadecalactone) and for *iso*-valeric acid, has been reported in man (Whissell-Buechy and Amoore 1973). Musk anosmia was found in 7.2% of Caucasians but not in Black subjects; *iso*-valeric acid anosmia was found in 9.1% Blacks and 1.4% Caucasians. The anosmias are heritable, but the samples were not broken down by age, sex, or ingestion of hormones such as oral contraceptives. Anosmia for a potential pheromone is of biologic interest, but there is no evidence that *iso*-valeric acid anosmia, or the suppression of acid vaginal components by the Pill, overtly affect human sexual behaviors.

Since human male sexual behavior is non-cyclical and not dependent on female receptivity, the female>male influence may well be releaser only, except possibly in infancy, or in accelerating puberty, and relatively non-specific. It is not clear why odor release should be enhanced at the infertile time of menstruation, unless it overrules an infantile anxiety. The most likely true primer effects would be female>female or male>female – McClintock's chief example, if it is pheromonal, would be of the first kind: in this event male>female effects could also be sought with virtual certainty. The most likely of these, judging from mammalian form, are cycle modification or initiation (Lee and Boot 1956), seen in mice, most herding animals (sheep, pigs) and, among primates, in lemurs (Jolly 1966); and acceleration of puberty (Vandenbergh 1969). Human puberty certainly regressed to a late age during the height of Victorian purdah, and has since got steadily earlier (Tanner 1962): this has occurred in both sexes and may well involve social factors – a pheromonal effect would be impossible to isolate. If it existed, it must presumably, in view of human family structure, depend on reinforcement by strangeness, and the presence of non-familial individuals. A pheromone effect triggered only during sex play or coitus could not easily be separated from the effects of direct stimulation, though there are such pheromones in primates (Michael and Saayman 1967; Michael and Keverne 1970), and human sex play has a large, though tabooed, orogenital component. Natural pheromone effects on fertility, implantation and the like (Bruce and Parkes 1961) seem more remote in man, though they might be produced by synthetics and would be of great importance if found. The conceptuant and abortefacient effects of odor figured in mediaeval medical folklore, and musk and civet were among substances so credited.

A male>male effect cannot be ruled out. Its most likely form, on mammalian analogy, would be the release of aggression or submission, but distaste for foreign male odor seems to be reversible, for example in homosexuals (Ellis 1905), and the fact that human male bonding is prominent could suggest that other interactions, such as puberty-timing in the male group, might be expected. The work of Kalogerakis (1963) implies a dominance effect between mature and immature males.

20.5. Chemical substances

Beside the collection of considerable knowledge of insect pheromones, little has been done on mammalian smell components. The known candidates for pheromonal roles are those 'self-selected' by man and used in perfumery (muskone, civetone, castoreum, and synthetics such as exaltolide), those derived from steroids and observed incidentally, such as boar taint, and a few special cases: *cis*-4-hydroxydodeca-6-enoic acid lactone in deer tarsal gland odor (Brownlee et al. 1969; Müller-Schwarze 1969): response of some cat strains to valerianic acid and nepetalactone (Todd 1962).

Michael's team (Curtis et al. 1971) has now identified the excitant substances for the male in the vaginal secretion of the female monkey and evoked a response with the synthetic mixture. The chief components are acetic, propionic, *iso*-butyric, *n*-butyric and *iso*-valeric acids. The same substances are present in the human vagina and contribute to its attractant odor, but do not make up its main subjective component, which is musky rather than acidic. The sexually excitant component of human genital odor is complex, involving both musk-like notes and odors akin to trimethylamine ('fishy') and is enhanced by alkaline fixatives. This 'alkaline' odor component, which is not present in or compatible with the fatty-acid mixes effective in monkeys, is closely simulated both in certain plants recognized as sexual in folklore (*Chenopodium vulvaria*, *Adoxa moschatellina*) and in amine-rich hydrolized food extracts of yeasts ('Marmite') – the second of these has a fairly strong attractant effect on many cats. An alkaline component of the human male genital odor resembles another amine, 1,5 diaminopentane (cadaverine). Both these and the musky genital odor are enhanced by alkaline soaps and muted by acidic lotions. There may be a distinction here between subliminal releasers, which may well be fatty acids, and attractants, which may be cycloketonic, steroid or both. For humans, odors recognised as 'sexual' are most commonly musk-like, though the axillary odor, and that of the feet (which in many animals are provided with tracking scent glands) are both excitant for many individuals and partly acidic. Odor fixed from foot apocrine glands may well play a part in the substitutional symbolism which erotises the human foot.

Michael's findings apart, the substances of initial choice as probable releasers and possible primers in man are all musk odors (steroids, large-ring cycloketones and lactones) (Sink 1967). The part played by 6, 8, and 10-carbon acids and lactones is unknown, but like the accessory non-steroid components of sweat, of smegma and of boar odor (Nitta and Ikai 1953; Patterson 1967, 1968) they probably have to do with detailed specificity. On this model the pheromone molecule is the key, and the subsidiary 'notes', the wards adapting it to a particular biological lock, and possibly needed for reinforcement. Application of pheromones would probably require us to take account of both systems – the degree of functional specificity is likely to be as high in mammals as in insects, but more complex, involving, for example, individual recognition. To this end the odor fingerprint approach of Dravnieks seems more promising than classical chemistry. Known musks might well serve as initial markers: the musky odor of human urine appears to be due to the -3-ol precursor of boar taint (Lederer 1950) and nearly all 5α and 5β androstenones, as well as progesterone, have musky odor (Radt 1959). The identity of mouse primer pheromones could be simply attacked by the methods of concentration used with insects – so far no article on these lines has appeared.

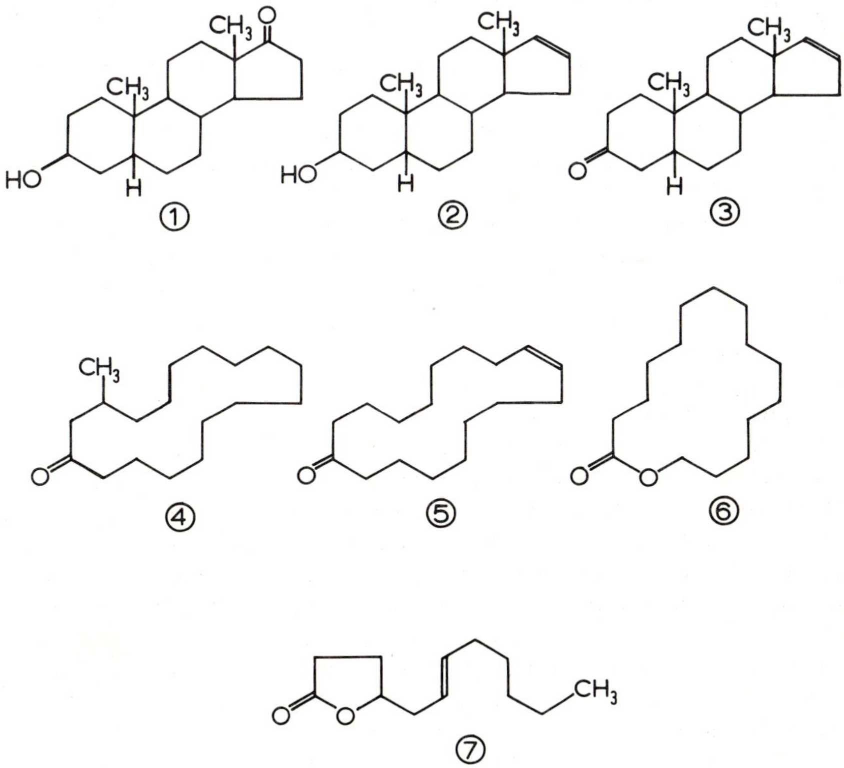

Fig. 1. Mammalian sex odors and related substances. 1) testosterone; 2) musk odor human urine; 3) 'boar taint' substance; 4) muskone; 5) civetone; 6) exaltolide; 7) blacktail deer odor. The female ability to smell compounds 3) 6) and probably 5) is far greater than the male and is hormone dependent. Compound 3) is probably formed from 2) by action of bacteria in the preputial gland secretion of the mature boar.

20.6. Source of pheromones

Many mammalian pheromones seem to be urinary, though specialized secretions are also common. Contact with urine plays little part in human relations, though it may be emphasized in paraphilias. More likely vehicles in man are the skin, including axillary and pubic apocrine glands and hair tufts, which resemble the deer's tarsal organ, and the smegma. The function of this secretion has been little studied, apart from its possible role in carcinogenesis. In the boar, its function seems to be to acquire odorous substances, either by secretion or fixation from preputial-sac urine, and 'hold' them, possibly for conversion to an active state by bacterial action. Excision of the preputial glands reduces boar taint (Dutt et al. 1959) although the source of the steroid precursor is the gonad and adrenal (Sink 1967). Humans lack the preputial sac, but male smegma contains a number of fixatives, including squalene (Sobel 1949) and β-cholestanol esters, as well as other uncharacterized steroids (Kamat et al. 1960). Some odorants may be directly secreted, others fixed from urine or a partner. Odorous drugs, for example phenylethylhydrazine, are rapidly detectable in the human male genital odor. Deer musk is a direct preputial gland secretion and a fixative for secondary odors. Apocrine glands contribute to total body odor, but a smegma pheromone would be exposed precoitally with exposure of the glands, and would thus be analogous to the 'response' substance in male moths; that is, a direct stimulus to receptivity. Odors fixed from a partner might also have a 'playback' function, as in offspring labelling. Human female genital odor components have been studied by gas chromatography, but only in relation to the elimination of bacterial odor (Dravnieks et al. 1970).

The axillary secretion is a far more likely source of human social pheromones – possibly specialized, in view of the erect posture of man (Fitzherbert 1959; Kloek 1961). Odorous steroids such as progesterone are rapidly transferred to objects handled by a pregnant woman through the sweat generally, and the large human apocrine glands may be centers of such a function. The hair tufts probably serve as odor diffusers, as in deer, and may harbor activating bacteria (Shelley et al. 1953). Many substances are probably involved, including long-chain acids and lactones. Caproic, caprylic and capric acids were named from their 'hircine' odor. Research in this field has been largely limited to deodorants and to identification of mosquito attractants in sweat (Skinner et al. 1965; Dravnieks et al. 1968). The peculiar odor of schizophrenics' sweat has been traced to *trans*-3-methyl hexanoic acid (Smith et al. 1969) – its significance is unknown.

There is a characteristic, powerful and pleasant axillary odor emitted only by women – some of them at all times, so that their presence in a room can be recognized, and others only occasionally. This odor, which resembles cumarone, appears to be unrelated to sexual excitement, but is itself attractant. It does not appear to be produced by males.

Apocrine sweat is almost wholly responsible for the normal odor of the clean human body, which differs markedly not only between 'races' but between complexions within a polytypic population; 'saucy and sometimes tiring in brunettes and black-haired women, sharp and fierce in redheads, it is heady and pervasive in blondes like the 'nose' of some flowery wines: you could almost say that it fits exactly with their manner of using the lips in kissing: firmer and more possessive in brunettes, more personal perhaps in blondes' (J. K. Huysmans *Croquis parisiens* 1880). Such literary descriptions refer to the female/male modality, but mediaeval authorities discriminate also the odor of chastity in both sexes (resembling ionone) and that of unchastity (resembling boiling starch). The odor of apocrine sweat appears to be released by bacterial action at the skin surface. That it changes with sexual excitement is a matter of common experience. Both in smegma and in apocrine hairtufts, bacteria may be true functional symbionts upon whose action odor release depends.

Prostaglandins, finally, may serve as non-olfactory pheromones. They are secreted in high concentrations in semen, and may stimulate uterine contractions which aid sperm transportation (H. A. Bern, personal communication, U. C. Berkeley).

20.7. Model for effects

A model of possible human pheromone effects can be plausibly constructed. The responsible substances are likely to occur in apocrine sweat and in smegma. They are likely to include odorous steroids, large-ring ketones, or other substances perceived as musk-like. Accessory odors probably determine behavioral specificity rather direct physiological action. Primer effects are most likely to be seen in the female; female–male effects may be limited to attraction, erection and so on and male–male effects may include dominance and attraction (bonding).

Odors fixed from a receptive partner may serve a 'play-back' function. Reinforcement by strangeness may occur. There may be an extensive biology of imprinting and so on by odor in infant–parent and child–parent relations, which later undergoes repression or modification. Releaser and primer effects probably depend on the same materials, and may include substances fixed from urine, semen, or the sexual secretions of the other sex by smegma. The existence of primer effects in humans is unproven but likely. Odor fingerprinting and gas chromatography render the testing of these hypotheses immediately practicable.

The complexity of the 'override' in human sexual behavior is such that, as in lemurs, menstrual synchrony and the like might well be subject to a mixed stimulus, involving both pheromones and visual or social interaction. What strikes the biologist is that humans seem to possess a range of organs which we assume to be 'vestigial' or non-functional, but which if we saw them in lower mammals, we should recognize as mediating odor exchange. They include strategically placed hairtufts associated with apocrine glands; and that ethnographically persecuted appendage the foreskin, which permits the accumulation of a powerful fixative and brings it into contact with traces of urine, vaginal secretion and semen.

Platyrrhine monkeys use the sternal apocrine gland, analogous to our axilla, to mark out territory, and size is a measure of male dominance. The human tendency to attack and remove both body hairs and the prepuce as unesthetic may conceivably reflect an unconscious awareness of a biological association which we have missed at the conscious level. No biologist could now rule out, for certain, the possibility that these amputative practices have behavioral effects. At least, the belief that developed organs such as the appendix and tonsil 'do nothing' and can be cut off without physiological effect is a naive one belonging to the last century.

It may be in for another shock. The time may be at hand when one can no longer tell an Alitalia plane by the fact that it has hair under its wings, and when deodorants, intimate and otherwise, rate with environmental pollution, as they already do among the sexually experienced. The notion of pheromonal influences on Man has often been mooted. It is still highly speculative, but could be important for medicine and psychiatry. We may live to see 'odor therapy' move out of the realm of fringe medicine, into a field with wider implications, some beneficial, some frankly disquieting. The extreme economy of the effect compared with the use of systemic hormones (some pheromones in insects operate at the single-molecule level) makes it well worthy of examination in a culture which urgently needs all the control over its reproductive processes that it can get.

References

Amoore, J. E. and J. Venstrom (1966) Sensory analysis of odor qualities in terms of the stereochemical theory. J. Food Sci. 31, 118–128.

Bieber, I. (1959) Olfaction in sexual development and adult sexual organisation. Am. J. Psychotherap. 13, 851–859.

Brill, A. A. (1932) The sense of smell in the neuroses and psychoses. Psychoanalytic Qu. 1, 7–42.

Brooksbank, B. W. L. and G. A. D. Hazelwood (1950) The nature of pregnanediol-like glucoside. Biochem. J. 47, 36–43.

Brownlee, R. G., R. M. Silverstein, D. Müller-Schwarze and A. G. Singer (1969) Identification, isolation and function of the male tarsal scent in blacktailed deer. Nature (London) 221, 284–285.

Bruce, A. M. and A. S. Parkes (1961) An olfactory block to implantation in mice. J. Reprod. Fert. 2, 195–196.

Curtis, R. J., J. A. Ballantine, E. B. Keverne, R. W. Bonsall, and R. P. Michael (1971) Identification of primate sexual pheromones and the properties of synthetic attractants. Nature (London) 232, 396–398.

Daly, C. D. and R. S. White (1930) Psychic reactions to olfactory stimuli. Brit. J. Med. Psychol. 10, 70–87.

Dravnieks, A., B. K. Krotoszynski, W. E. Lieb and E. J. Jungermann (1968) Influence of an antibacterial soap on various effluents from axillae. J. Soc. Cosmet. Chem. 19, 611–612.

Dravnieks, A. and B. K. Krotoszynski (1970) Detection and identification of chemical signatures. U.S. Sci. Tech. Bull. Info. 1967 AD/691738.

Dravnieks, A., B. K. Krotoszynski, L. Keith and I. M. Bush (1970) Odor threshold and gas-chromatographic assays of vaginal odors: changes with nitrofurazone treatment. J. Pharm. Sci. 59, 495–501.
Dutt, R. H., E. C. Simpson, J. C. Christian and C. E. Barnhardt (1959) Identification of preputial glands as the site of production of sexual odor in the boar. J. Anim. Sci. 18, 1557–1558.
Ellis, H. (1905) Sexual Selection in Man. v.4 (Davis, N.Y.)
Fitzherbert, J. (1959) Scent and the sexual object. Brit. J. Med. Psychol. 32, 806–809.
Gleeson, K. K. and J. H. Reynierse (1969) The behavioral significance of pheromones in primates. Psychol. Bull. 71, 58–73.
Griffiths, N. M. and R. L. S. Patterson (1970) Human olfactory responses to 5α-androst-16-en-3-one, principal component of boar taint. J. Sci. Food Agr. 21, 4–6.
Groddeck, G. (1925) The Unknown Self (Daniel, London) 207 pp.
Jolly, A. (1966) Lemur Behavior (Chicago Univ. Press) 187 pp.
Kalogerakis, M. G. (1963) The role of olfaction in sexual development. Psychosom. Med. 25, 420–432.
Kamat, V. N., T. B. Panse and V. R. Khanolkar (1960) Constituents of human smegma. Proc. Indian Acad. Sci. B. 52, 1–8.
Kligman, A. M. and N. Shehadeh (1964) Pubic apocrine glands and odor. Arch. Dermatol. 89, 461–463.
Kloek, J. (1961) The smell of some steroid sex hormones and their metabolites. Folia Psychiat. Neurol. Neurochir. Neer. 64, 309–344.
Lederer, E. (1950) Odeurs et parfums des animaux. Fortschr. Chem. Org. Naturst. 6, 87–153.
Lee, S. van der and Boot, L. M. (1956) Spontaneous pseudo-pregnancy in mice II. Acta Physiol. Pharmacol. Neer. 5, 213–215.
Le Magnen, J. (1952) Les phénomènes olfactosexuels chez l'Homme. Arch. Sci. Physiol. 6, 125–160.
McClintock, M. K. (1971) Menstrual synchrony and suppression. Nature (London). 299, 244–245.
Michael, R. P. and E. B. Keverne (1970) Primate sex pheromones of vaginal origin. Nature (London). 225, 84–85.
Michael, R. P. and G. Saayman (1967) Sexual performance index of male Rhesus monkeys. Nature (London). 214, 425–626
Müller-Schwarze, D. (1969) Complexity and relative specificity of a mammalian pheromone. Nature (London). 223, 525–526.
Nitta, H. and H. Ikai (1953) Studies on the body odor. I. Separation of the lower fatty acids of the cutaneous excretion by paper chromatography. Nagoya Med. J. 1, 217–224.
Patterson, R. L. S. (1967) A possible contribution of phenolic components to boar odor. J. Sci. Food Agr. 18, 8–10.
Patterson, R. L. S. (1968) 5α-androst-16-en-3-one: Compound responsible for taint in boar fat. J. Sci. Food. Agr. 19, 31–38.
Radt, F., ed. (1959) Elseviers Ency. Org. Chem. Series III, 4, Suppl. 23955 seq. (Springer, Berlin).
Shelley, W. B., H. J. Harley and A. C. Nichols (1953) Axillary odor: an experimental study of the role of bacteria, apocrine sweat and deodorants. Arch. Dermatol. Syph. N.Y. 68, 430–446.
Sink, J. D. (1967) Theoretical aspects of sex odor in swine. J. Theor. Biol. 17, 174–180.
Skinner, W. H., H. Tong, T. Pearson, W. Strauss and H. Maibach (1965) Human sweat components attractive to mosquitoes. Nature (London). 207, 261–262.

Smith, K., G. F. Thompson and H. D. Koster (1969) Sweat in schizophrenic patients: identification of the odorous substance. Science 166, 398–399.

Sobel, H. (1949) Squalene in sebum and sebum-like materials. J. Invest. Dermatol. 13, 333–338.

Tanner, J. M. (1962) Growth at Adolescence (Blackwell, Oxford) 325 pp.

Todd, N. B. (1962) Inheritance of the catnip response in domestic cats. J. Hered.63, 54–56.

Vandenbergh, J. G. (1969) Effect of the presence of a male on sexual maturation in female mice. Endocrinology 84, 658–660.

Vierling, J. S. and J. Rock (1967) Variation in olfactory sensitivity to exaltolide during the menstrual cycle. J. Appl. Physiol. 22, 311–315.

Welch, L. and R. F. Hayes (1957) Elements in conditioning of normal and pathological human behaviour. J. Genet. Psychol. 91, 263–293.

Whissell-Buechy, D. and J. E. Amoore (1973) Odor-blindness to musk. Nature (London) 242, 271–273.

Wiener, H. (1966) External chemical messengers: I. Emission and reception in man. N.Y. State J. Med. 66, 3153–3170.

Wiener, H. (1967a) External chemical messengers: 2. Natural history of schizophrenia. N.Y. State J. Med. 67, 1144–1165.

Wiener, H. (1967b) External chemical messengers: 3. Mind and body in schizophrenia. N.Y. State J. Med. 67, 1287–1310.

Wilson, E. O. (1963) Pheromones. Sci. Am. 208, 100–114.

Section III

Pheromones in manipulation of populations

CHAPTER 21

Pheromones in insect population management

James P. TETTE

21.1. *Introduction*

Man has long struggled to control the insects which compete with him for food and fiber or endanger his health. Unfortunately, many of the methods used in this struggle have become increasingly uneconomic and ineffective, or have detracted in many ways from the quality of man's environment. New concepts, such as the use of pheromones, are now being extensively experimented with in an attempt to bring about better insect population management and to regain this loss of environmental quality.

The first section of this book clearly indicated how important pheromones are as part of the language of insects – an essential means for communication. As man understands and begins to interpret this language he can begin to use it to manipulate insect populations in such ways as to direct an insect to a given site where it is trapped and killed; to overload the receptor system of the insect in some way so that it cannot perceive the correct signal; or by continuously monitoring a population using chemical stimuli, man can determine when insect populations are reaching an economic threshold level and apply other control measures.

Even before the sex pheromones were chemically identified, ideas had been developed on how insect populations might be affected by these materials. The attractant pheromones as a class of biologically active compounds possess several important characteristics which predispose them to consideration as practically useful compounds. These characteristics are: activity in minute quantities (see Payne ch. 3); relative specificity; low-toxicity; minimal adverse effects on non-target organisms, such as beneficial insects, since they are naturally occurring biological products; and potential low costs of development. About the time that the first chemical structures were determined, Wright (1964, 1965) recognized the need for non-toxic pest control agents and coined the term 'metarchon' for any stimulus introduced into the environment that modified the insect's behavior by inhibiting a correct response or by eliciting an incorrect one. This includes factors such as repellants, attractants, light and sound, which interfere with the insect's ability to communicate. Pheromones clearly fit into this concept. It was also proposed at an early stage that permeation of the atmosphere with pheromones could prevent reproduction and colonization (Babson 1963; Beroza and Jacobson 1963). Similarly, many early predictions and attempts were made to trap out an insect population using natural sources or extracts of pheromones (for a review see Jacobson 1972; for theoretical basis see Knipling and McGuire 1966). In the late 1960's synthetic pheromones became increasingly more available and with their advent began the true test of the early predictions.

21.2 Survey and detection

Entomologists have always wanted to understand the reasons why a particular insect appeared at a certain time or in a given area since early detection of an insect pest was often the key to effective management. Such information was, however, difficult to obtain and was based on data from many sources (e.g. emergence cages, light traps, bait pails, field collections, etc.). When pheromones and attractants were discovered one obvious application was the possibility of incorporating these materials into some type of survey or detection device, thus eliminating many of the earlier, time-consuming methods. In many instances the natural source of pheromone, the virgin (attractive) female, was, and still is being used effectively (Butt and Hathaway 1966; Jacobson 1972 for review).

In general, it has been found that a particular pheromone can be utilized in a survey device very soon after its isolation, identification and synthesis. This may seem rather surprising in view of the many factors involved and their interdependence. However, after one, or at the most two, years of field evaluation most pheromones can be put into practical application as part of a survey program.

21.2.1. Technology of deployment

In considering survey and detection programs it must be kept in mind that pheromones are only one part of a device which must capture and retain the insect so that its presence can be recorded. In order to be maximally effective, the trap should simulate the natural attractive source as closely as possible or supersede it in attractiveness. Factors such as trap design, chemical attractiveness of the pheromone and rate of pheromone release must be considered before a reliable survey trap is obtained.

The ingenuity, simplicity and extent of insect trap designs can be readily appreciated by examining the files of the United States Patent Office on insect traps. The trap not only has to retain the insect, but its particular design may be vitally important for success, since, in the final approach to the pheromone source, an insect may respond to cues other than chemical (Shorey 1970). Vision is important in attracting the gypsy moth (Doane 1968) and the cabbage looper (Shorey and Gaston 1970) and without a doubt the size, shape and color of a trap can affect the response of many insects attracted by pheromones. Design features can be incorporated into the trap to compensate for lack of visual cues (e.g. Killinen and Ost 1971; Kaae and Shorey 1972). Height and placement of the traps with regard to the insect's preferred environment can also make a big difference in the catch (Sharma et al. 1971; Hardee et al. 1972; Klein et al. 1972; Roach et al. 1972). At the present time, the least expensive and most widely used traps are those which retain an insect on a sticky surface, although light traps, electrocuting grid traps and others have been used.

The effectiveness of a pheromone in the field is greatly dependent on its purity and stability. Purity is essential, at least in the early stages of evaluation. For example, presence of small quantities of geometrical isomers has been found to reduce or eliminate attractiveness of some pheromones (Roelofs and Comeau 1968; Roelofs et al 1972); precursors carried over from the preparative stages can also inhibit attractiveness (Green et al. 1972; Tumlinson et al. 1972); and instability of pheromones in the field can lead to impurities which inhibit attractiveness (Toba et al. 1970). Use of anti-oxidants or free-radical scavengers can prevent polymerization or degradation in the field (Neumark et al. 1972; Wolf et al. 1972). Although purity can be evaluated in the laboratory the true test of any pheromone's attractiveness must rely on field testing.

A third important consideration here is the rate and means of pheromone release. Choice of a release substrate is critical (Gaston et al. 1971b). Clearly, the underlying factor here is that the pheromone must be delivered to the insect at the right concentration to evoke the desired response and not to inhibit it through overdosage or to evoke a behavior different to that desired (Klun et al. 1972; Kaae et al. 1973). Pheromone(s) have been incorporated into a slow-release substrate (polyethylene caps, rubber, open glass vials, sticky coatings, etc.), and choice of a substrate with the optimum release rate can be critically important (Gaston et al. 1971b; McKibben et al. 1971; Kuhr et al. 1972). The situation is complicated when the pheromone is a mixture of three or four components each of which requires its own subtle release rate. In addition, the release substrates will change character with the temperature and humidity. All these variables must be maximized to compete with the virgin female, to prolong the field lifetime to several weeks and to reduce expenses involved in manufacturing and servicing. Some of the problems encountered and various solutions to them will be found in the case-histories (ch. 22).

21.2.2. Chemical spray timing and reduced spray schedules

In certain geographical areas and on certain crops, the insect-pest complex is sometimes centered round a relatively few insect species. For example, in the western United States and Canada apple and pear growers currently contend with only one or two major pest problems. The most important pest is the codling moth (*Laspe-*

rysia pomonella (L.)). For the most part growers in these areas have vague and sometimes meaningless background information on the appearance of this insect in their orchards. Even when emergence is published in a state or federal extension agency information bulletin the grower may still not face a codling moth problem. His orchard may differ from the one in which emergence was noted in rainfall, exposure, abundance of natural enemies or in use of insecticides. In this dilemma growers have resorted more and more to preventive spray programs leading to greatly increased costs for chemicals and application, and upsetting the predator-prey relationships of other potential pests. Pheromone survey traps improve the grower's ability to assess the threat of this pest to his orchard, to pin-point incipient infestations and to provide more precise timing of chemical sprays.

The appearance of the pest insect in a pheromone trap is really only the first information which enters into a decision on spray application. Other inputs, such as previous emergence patterns, weather records before and after appearance, correlation of weather with egg hatch and consideration of the environment surrounding the sampling area, go into the final determination of when to spray. Further, the appearance of an insect in a pheromone trap is often quite early, and in the case of the codling moth in some growing areas, first brood appearance may appear to be out of synchrony with the crop. Thus, intelligent interpretation of the appearance of an insect in a trap is very necessary. Information such as the relationship of the numbers of captured insects to the potential economic threat to the crop is still not available in most cases. An approach where trap catches are related to continuous visual inspection of the crop (Madsen and Davis 1971; Madsen and Vakenti 1972) will hopefully provide this needed information in the future.

Significant results have, however, been obtained by working with existing crop/pest information (Bethel et al. 1972). Not only has this approach eliminated 'spraying-by-calendar', but it has created a flexible approach to choice and rate of pesticide to be used (Batiste 1972). This aim is to provide control of the harmful pest and, at the same time, permit a build-up of beneficial insects that control other potential pests.

The codling moth is cited here as one example. Similar programs are also underway with insects such as the boll weevil (ch. 22.5), redbanded leafroller (ch. 22.2), European corn borer, oriental fruit moth, pink bollworm (ch. 22.4), and various bark beetles (ch. 22.8).

A pheromone survey strategy can also be applied to crops which face a multitude of insect problems. As an example, apples in the eastern half of the United States (in contrast to the west) face a situation in which the insect complex is quite formidable with as many as five or six insects being major pests.

In a situation like this it is often difficult to time sprays according to the appearance of a particular insect. However, there is still room for spray schedules to be reduced or altered in a manner which is beneficial to both the grower and the environment. Here, a pheromone survey trap can best be used as an early warning by indicating a situation that might get out of hand. As more pheromones are discovered, the potential of monitoring more than one pest of a particular crop will be realized.

21.2.3. Expansion of range

Countries and states have long waged a continuing battle against the possible invasion of new insect pests. In many cases the problems of a new pest only become apparent after a certain amount of economic damage has been done, and unless tremendous eradication programs are undertaken, the insect soon becomes part of the local insect pest problem. The key factor in keeping an insect out is early detection, which in most cases consists of manual inspection and searching for infestations. Not only is this a costly undertaking, but if the insect is present in very low numbers, inspection might often not detect it. A pheromone survey trap would clearly be of immense value in such situations. Pheromones have successfully been used to detect the California red scale (Shaw et al. 1971); this cryptic insect could be detected in areas where visual inspection had not picked it up. The gypsy moth is a prime example of the need for early detection. This insect is continually expanding its range with the help of man (Beroza and Knipling 1972) and can inhabit areas of forest and woodland where visual inspection would be out of the question. Once again, a sensitive survey device such as the pheromone trap could give the early warning. Similarly, pheromone traps are being used to detect the potential movement of the boll weevil towards the weevil-free cotton areas of the far western United States (Hardee et al. 1970).

21.2.4. Sterile insect release

Many programs using sterile insect release to combat a particular pest have used pheromone traps as survey devices to help follow the release, dispersal and competitiveness of sterilized insects (Proverbs et al. 1966; Butt et al. 1970; White and Huff 1971). In many instances, pheromone traps pinpoint the areas which require and benefit from immediate further releases of sterile insects.

21.3. Control

A great deal has been written about the use of pheromones for controlling, i.e. suppressing or eradicating, insect populations (e.g. Beroza and Jacobson 1963; Shorey and Gaston 1967; and Jacobson 1972 for a review). The input of much new information from programs now underway should help to evaluate the various methods of pheromonal control. Technological advances in formulation, microencapsulation and fabrication of materials have assisted greatly, as has the synergistic interaction of the fields of chemistry and entomology. Basic to all the various control techniques, however, is a fundamental understanding of the biology, especially the behavior and population dynamics of the target insect. As a minimum such information must include data on emergence patterns of adult insects; habits and development of the immature stages; migration of adults from hedgerows, cover crops, woodlands or distant hosts to the crop in question; frequency of mating and flight capabilities of the gravid female. Environmental and physiological effects on production, release, reception and response to pheromone need to be determined (see Shorey ch. 4) together with the behavior of both sexes as influenced by the pheromone and the possible input of visual or auditory cues. Predators and parasites of the pest may also be attracted to the pheromone (Vite 1970; also Borden Ch. 8.5) and be unwittingly removed from the population along with the pest insect. All this biological information is incomplete unless based on *both* laboratory and field studies.

At the present time efforts to control insect populations by manipulating their pheromone systems are based on one of two strategies: 1) disruption of the insect's communication system so that mating is not accomplished, and 2) removal of a large proportion of the adult population by mass trapping.

21.3.1. Disruption of chemical signals

This concept is based on continuous disruption of the pheromone communication system used in reproduction. Usually a high concentration of the sex or aggregation pheromone is broadcast into the environment with the aim of habituating the male's central nervous system through continuous exposure to a pheromone source above the threshold level (Bartell and Lawrence 1973, and references therein), causing adaptation of the male's receptors so that he cannot physiologically respond to a female, or of producing such a high background concentration of pheromone that the male is behaviorally incapable of locating the smaller amount released by a receptive female. Similarly, other chemicals which effectively block the pheromone response could be used to the same effect. Whatever strategy is employed, the aim is the same, to prevent successful mating. One of the problems of this approach is that to have a significant impact on the next generation it may be necessary to achieve at least 99% disruption of mating (Shorey 1970; Beroza and Knipling 1972); otherwise the reproductive potential of the insect can overcome the effect of the treatment. It has so far proved very difficult to prevent all but one or a few percent of the males from finding a female and mating successfully.

Any program of this type requires extensive information on the biology, especially behavior, of the insect. A sufficient quantity of pheromone must be delivered to cover the required area for as long as adults are flying. Slow release substrates have been developed to ensure a continuous steady release of pheromone whenever the insects are present. Direct broadcast of pheromone onto vegetation is not usually effective since foliage absorbs the compounds and often accelerates their breakdown: resulting higher dosage levels increase application costs.

Unless the test area is an isolated population, migration of gravid females into the area may cause damage even though disruption of mating was completely successful (McLaughlin et al. 1972). In spite of the difficulties, however, a number of pheromone disruption experiments have been attempted with, for example, Douglas fir beetle (Furniss et al. 1972); pink bollworm (McLaughlin et al. 1972); cabbage looper (Shorey et al. 1972); gypsy moth (Stevens and Beroza 1972; Cameron 1973). Results are promising and detailed published information is still forthcoming. Meanwhile Kaae et al. (1972) have shown that a single pheromone (*cis*-7-dodecenyl acetate) has a disruptive effect on the chemical communication of six different insect species. This is clearly also attractive from a manufacturing point of view.

As Shorey et al. (1968) point out, the eventual use of an 'impure' pheromone could still produce the desired effect, and once initial tests are complete it may well be found that highly pure chemicals are not essential. A final chemical product may very well contain only 70% of the desired pheromone and some 10–25% of a behavioral inhibitor or masking agent. The cost of producing a material of this purity would be much less than chemicals now used. Other chemicals, the parapheromones (chemicals closely related to pheromones in structure and sometimes in activity) (Gaston et al. 1971a) and pheromone inhibitors (Roelofs and Comeau 1971; Carde et al. 1973), also effectively disrupt an insect's communication system and may be far less expensive to manufacture. The prospects are very bright.

21.3.2. Mass trapping

Pheromones per se do not kill the pest insect, but they can be used to lure the insect to a trap where it is then killed. The trap may be a physical restraint on the insect, such as a sticky surface, or it may be a combination of pheromone and insecticide. Whatever strategy is used, the aim is to remove a significant proportion, or all, of the target insects from a given population.

Although the principle is quite simple, the practice is very difficult. The pheromone must not only be released into the environment but it must be released in such a way as to out-compete the virgin adult and yet prevent 'disruption'. The attempt to create a superattractive source is complicated by the fact that many pheromone systems have so far been defined in terms of only one or two compounds. Even in the Lepidoptera, where sex pheromones have long been thought to be single compounds, there is mounting evidence that other components are present and are necessary to duplicate the insect's pheromonal system. Only when this system can be reproduced synthetically can we expect efficient attraction (see Roelofs and Cardé ch. 6). It is clear that pheromones of high purity are initially obligatory in order to determine exactly how the behavior is being modified and to evaluate the effectiveness of this type of program. With some species, plant–host odors are an integral part of the pheromone and must be incorporated to create a potent competitor to the natural source (Wood 1970, 1972). Attractiveness can also be increased by using synergists (materials which have no activity in themselves but which enhance a pheromone's attractiveness) (Roelofs and Comeau 1971), or keepers (Beroza et al. 1971b), which assist in controlling evaporation of a pheromone. Further, the trap should ideally incorporate any essential visual cues for orientation and provide for temporal variations in chemical concentration of pheromone, or other variables. In essence trap design and placement are much more critical for success than they are in survey programs. It is not enough to trap one or two insects as indices of population emergence, but enough insects must be trapped to make a significant reduction in the next generation (or to trap almost every insect of at least one sex, if eradication is being attempted). Use of simple sticky traps seems to provide the greatest biological effect with lowest cost at this time. The principle is now being extensively tested in the programs of Roelofs et al. (1970) with orchard pests, and Hardee et al. (1971) for the boll weevil amongst others (see also ch. 22).

A different type of mass trapping program involves combining the pheromone with an insecticide to maximize the effectiveness of two control methods. No less input is required about the population dynamics of the insect or the effect of various release rates on aggregation. For the most part this strategy has taken advantage of aggregation pheromones by creating an aggregation site at a point of insecticide application (e.g. Copony and Morris 1972. with the southern pine beetle; Lloyd et al. 1972. with the cotton boll weevil). With bark beetles, the beetles can be induced to aggregate on a host tree which is then physically removed by logging (Knopf and Pitman 1972) and the insects destroyed during processing of the timber. Care must be taken to insure against aggregation at points other than those desired.

21.4. Discussion

The true potential of pheromones, as part of survey devices and as control agents, will probably never be realized without the input of commercial technology. This includes a combination of established and new techniques plus an exchange of information between the developers (mostly industrial) and those conducting research (at this time, mostly academic). This interchange of ideas and information, which has characterized the pheromone field so far, is essential before one of the biggest hurdles can be overcome: namely, that of educating the end user. The extensive information developed by many different scientific sources must be translated into simple and reliable products for final application.

Along with translation of current information into a commercial product, a commercial pheromone developer must continually update information, often requiring alterations in production standards. As examples, one might cite the effects of impurities on the performance of a particular pheromone. Investigations can lead to more, or less, expensive materials, depending upon the type of effect desired. Problems of manufacturing formulations (substrates plus pheromones) which are very sensitive to contamination by other chemicals, may require different machinery and facilities for each pheromone formulation, separate storage areas, where even air exchange is at a minimum, and stringent regulations regarding work habits of production staff. Such factors directly affect the eventual cost of a product. Current estimates of the cost of broadcasting a pheromone (Beroza and Knipling 1972; Shorey et al. 1972), or of mass trapping an insect (Beroza and Knipling 1972) are within feasible economic limits. It appears that the prospects are bright since these estimates for the most part center around current technology with minimal commercial input.

If pheromones are to be used directly or indirectly in insect control programs, a registration protocol must be established for permitting such use. In the United States, most pheromones are considered as pesticides. The United States Department of Agriculture is currently attempting to establish with the federal Environmental Protection Agency the necessary requirements and regulations for registration of pheromones. Some commercial companies are also moving in this direction and are hopeful that current requirements may be somewhat alleviated in view of the suspected low mammalian toxicity (Beroza and Knipling 1972).

In summary, pheromones and related substances are currently being applied to a variety of problems facing agriculture and forestry. As a survey and detection device, they have already become an important tool in the overall management of certain insect pests. Their potential use in population control has been realized only to a very small extent, but efforts in this area are increasing. As the number of manufacturers of these chemicals grows, almost every known pheromone is being made available either in pure form for initial investigations or in the form of a delivery system for more direct applications. In a true sense, then, the early predictions of the potential of pheromones are slowly being realized.

References

Babson, A. L. (1963) Eradicating the gypsy moth. Science 142, 447.

Bartell, R. J. and L. A. Lawrence (1973) Reduction in responsiveness of males of *Epiphyas postvittana* (Lepidoptera) to sex pheromone following previous brief pheromonal exposure. J. Insect Physiol. 19, 845–855.

Batiste, W. C. (1972) Integrated control of codling moth on pears in California: A practical consideration where moth activity is under surveillance. Environ. Entomol. 1, 213–218.

Beroza, M. and M. Jacobson (1963) Chemical insect attractants. World Rev. Pest Control 2, 36.

Beroza, M. and E. F. Knipling (1972) Gypsy moth control with the sex attractant pheromone. Science 177, 19–27.

Beroza, M., B. A. Bierl, E. F. Knipling and J. G. R. Tardif (1971) The activity of the gypsy moth sex attractant Disparlure vs. that of the live female moth. J. Econ. Entomol. 64, 1527–1529.

Bethel, R. S., L. A. Falcon, W. C. Batiste, G. W. Morehead and E. P. Delfino (1972) Sex pheromone traps aid in determining need for codling moth control in apples and pears. Calif. Agr. 26, 10–12.

Butt, B. A. and D. O. Hathaway (1966) Female sex pheromone as attractant for male codling moths. J. Econ. Entomol. 59, 476–477.

Butt, B. A., D. O. Hathaway, L. D. White and J. F. Howell (1970) Field releases of codling moths sterilized by tepa or gamma radiation. J. Econ. Entomol. 63, 912–915.

Cameron, E. A. (1973) Disparlure: A potential tool for gypsy moth population manipulation. Bull. Entomol. Soc. Am. 19, 15–19.

Cardé, R. T., W. L. Roelofs and C. C. Doane (1973) Natural inhibitor of the gypsy moth sex attractant. Nature (London) 241, 474–475.

Copony, J. A. and C. L. Morris (1972) Southern pine beetle suppression with Frontalure and cacodylic acid treatments. J. Econ. Entomol. 65, 754–757.

Doane, C. C. (1968) Aspects of mating behavior of the gypsy moth. Ann. Entomol. Soc. Am. 61, 768–773.

Furniss, M. M., L. N. Kline, R. F. Schmitz and J. A. Rudinsky (1972) Tests of three pheromones to induce or disrupt aggregation of Douglas-fir beetles (Coleoptera: Scolytidae) on live trees. Ann. Entomol. Soc. Am. 65, 1227–1232.

Gaston, L. K., T. L. Payne, S. Takahashi and H. H. Shorey (1971a) Correlation of chemical structure and sex pheromone activity in *Trichoplusia ni* (Noctuidae). In: Olfaction and Taste, 1972, vol. IV; ed.: D. Schneider (Wissenschaftliche Verlagsgesellschaft MBH Stuttgart 1972) pp. 167–173.

Gaston, L. K., H. H. Shorey and C. A. Saario (1971b) Sex pheromones of Noctuid moths. XVIII. Rate of evaporation of a model compound of *Trichoplusia ni* sex pheromone from different substrates at various temperatures and its application to insect orientation. Ann. Entomol. Soc. Am. 64, 381–384.

Green, N., J. D. Warthen and C. L. Mangum (1971) Analysis of Hexalure as related to its attractancy to pink bollworm moths. J. Econ. Entomol. 64, 1381–1384.

Hardee, D. D., W. H. Cross, P. M. Huddleston and T. B. Davich (1970) Survey and control of the boll weevil in West Texas with traps baited with males. J. Econ. Entomol. 63, 1041–1048.

Hardee, D. D., W. H. Cross, E. B. Mitchell, P. M. Huddleston and H. C. Mitchell (1972) Capture of boll weevils in traps baited with males: Effect of size, color, location and height above ground level. Environ. Entomo. 1, 162–166.

Hardee, D. D., O. H. Lindig and T. B. Davich (1971) Suppression of populations of boll weevils over a large area in West Texas with pheromone traps in 1969. J. Econ. Entomol. 64, 928–933.

Jacobson, M. (1972) Insect Sex Pheromones (Academic Press, New York and London) 382 pp.

Kaae, R. S. and H. H. Shorey (1972) Sex pheromones of Lepidoptera. XXIV. An improved double-cone trap for males of *Trichoplusia ni*. Environ. Entomol. 1, 675–677.

Kaae, R. S., J. R. McLaughlin, H. H. Shorey and L. K. Gaston (1972) Sex pheromones of Lepidoptera. XXXII. Disruption of intraspecific communication in various species of Lepidoptera by permeation of the air with Looplure or Hexalure. Environ. Entomol. 1, 651–653.

Kaae, R. S., H. H. Shorey and L. K. Gaston (1973) Pheromone concentration as a mechanism for reproductive isolation between two Lepidopterous species. Science 179, 487–488.

Killinen, R. G. and R. W. Ost (1971) Pheromone-maze trap for cabbage looper moths. J. Econ. Entomol. 64, 310–311.

Klein, M. G., T. L. Ladd, Jr. and K. O. Lawrence (1972) The influence of height of exposure of virgin female Japanese beetles on capture of males. Environ. Entomol. 1, 600–601.

Klun, J. A. and J. F. Robinson (1972) Olfactory discrimination in the European corn borer and several pheromonally analogous moths. Ann. Entomol. Soc. Am. 65, 1337–1340.

Knipling, E. F. and J. U. McGuire (1966) Population models to test theoretical effects of sex attractants used for insect control. U. S. Dept. Agr. Inform. Bull. 308, 2–4.

Knopf, J. A. E. and G. B. Pitman (1972) Aggregation pheromone for manipulation of the Douglas-fir beetle. J. Econ. Entomol. 65, 723–726.

Kuhr, R. J., A. Comeau and W. L. Roelofs (1972) Measuring release rates of pheromone analogues and synergists from polyethylene caps. Environ. Entomol. 1, 625–627.

Lloyd, E. P., W. P. Scott, K. K. Shaunak, F. C. Tingle and T. B. Davich (1972) A modified trapping system for suppressing low-density populations of overwintered boll weevils. J. Econ. Entomol. 65, 1144–1147.

Madsen, H. F. and W. W. Davis (1971) A progress report on the use of female–baited traps as indicators of codling moth populations. J. Entomol. Soc. B. C. 68, 11–14.

Madsen, H. F. and J. M. Vakenti (1972) Codling moths: Female-baited and synthetic pheromone traps as population indicators. Environ. Entomol. 1, 554–557.

McKibben, G. H., D. D. Hardee, T. B. Davich, R. C. Gueldner and P. A. Hedin (1971) Slow-release formulations of Grandlure, the synthetic pheromone of the boll weevil. J. Econ. Entomol. 64, 317–319.

McLaughlin, J. R., H. H. Shorey, L. K. Gaston, R. S. Kaae and F. D. Stewart (1972) Sex pheromones of Lepidoptera. XXXI. Disruption of sex pheromone communication in *Pectinophora gossypiella* with hexalure. Environ. Entomol. 1, 645–650.

Neumark, S., N. Green and I. Teich (1972) The pink bollworm attractant hexalure: Improvement by formulation with antioxidant. J. Econ. Entomol. 65, 1709–1711.

Proverbs, M. D., J. R. Newton and D. M. Logan (1966) Orchard assessment of the sterile male technique for control of the codling moth *Carpocapsa pomonella*. Can. Entomol. 98, 90–95.

Roach, S. H., H. R. Agee and L. Ray (1972) Influence of position and color of male-baited traps on captures of boll weevils. Environ. Entomol. 1, 530–532.

Roelofs, W. L. and A. Comeau (1968) Sex pheromone perception. Nature (London) 220, 600–601.

Roelofs, W. L. and A. Comeau (1971) Sex pheromone perception: Synergists and inhibitors for the redbanded leaf roller attractant. J. Insect Physiol. 17, 435–448.

Roelofs, W. L., R. J. Bartell, A. S. Hill, R. T. Cardé and L. H. Waters (1972) Codling moth sex attractant-field trials with geometrical isomers. J. Econ. Entomol. 65, 1276–1277.

Roelofs, W. L., E. H. Glass, J. Tette and A. Comeau (1970) Sex pheromone trapping for redbanded leaf roller control: Theoretical and actual. J. Econ. Entomol. 63, 1162–1167.

Sharma, R. K., R. E. Rice, H. T. Reynolds and H. H. Shorey (1971) Seasonal influence and effect of trap location on catches of pink bollworm males in sticky traps baited with hexalure. Ann. Entomol. Soc. Am. 64, 102–105.

Shaw, J. G., D. S. Moreno and J. Fagerlund (1971) New red scale detector. Citrograph 56, 149–150.

Shorey, H. H. (1970) Sex pheromones of Lepidoptera. *In*: Control of Insect Behavior by Natural Products; eds.: D. L. Wood, R. M. Silverstein and M. Nakajima (Academic Press, N.Y.) pp. 249–284.

Shorey, H. H. and L. K. Gaston (1967) Pheromones. *In*: Pest Control: Biological, Physical and Selected Chemical Methods; eds.: W. W. Kilgore and R. Doutt (Academic Press, N.Y.) pp. 241–265.

Shorey, H. H. and L. K. Gaston (1970) Sex pheromones of Noctuid moths. XX. Short-range visual orientation by pheromone-stimulated males of *Trichoplusia ni*. Ann. Entomol. Soc. Am. 63, 828–832.

Shorey, H. H., L. K. Gaston and R. N. Jefferson (1968) Insect sex pheromones. *In*: Advances in Pest Control Research, vol. 8; ed. R. L. Metcalf (Interscience Publishers, N. Y.) pp. 57–126.

Shorey, H. H., R. S. Kaae, L. K. Gaston and J. R. McLaughlin (1972) Sex pheromones of Lepidoptera. XXX. Disruption of sex pheromone communication in *Trichoplusia ni* as a possible means of mating control. Environ. Entomol. 1, 641–645.

Stevens, L. J. and M. Beroza (1972) Mating-inhibition field tests using Disparlure, the synthetic gypsy moth sex pheromone. J. Econ. Entomol. 65, 1090–1095.

Toba, H. H., N. Green, A. N. Kishaba, M. Jacobson and J. W. Debolt (1970) Response of male cabbage loopers to 15 isomers and cogeners of the looper pheromone. J. Econ. Entomol. 63, 1048–1051.

Tumlinson, J. H., E. R. Mitchell, S. M. Browner, M. S. Mayer, N. Green, R. Hines and D. A. Lindquist (1972) *Cis*-7-dodecen-1-ol, a potent inhibitor of the cabbage looper sex pheromone. Environ. Entomol. 1, 354–358.

Vité, J. P. (1970) Pest management systems using synthetic pheromones. Contrib. Boyce Thompson Inst., 24, 343–350.

White, L. D. and R. B. Huff (1971) Codling moth catches in sex and light traps after exposure to 0, 25, or 40 krad of gamma irradiation. J. Econ. Entomol. 64, 1249–1250.

Wright, R. H. (1964) Metarchon: A new term for a class of non-toxic pest control agents. Nature (London) 204, 603–604.

Wright, R. H. (1965) Finding metarchons for pest control. Nature (London) 207, 103–104.

Wolf, W. W., H. H. Toba, A. N. Kishaba and N. Green (1972) Anti-oxidants to prolong the effectiveness of cabbage looper sex pheromone in the field. J. Econ. Entomol. 65, 1039–1041.

Wood, D. L. (1970) Pheromones of bark beetles. *In*: Control of Insect Behavior by Natural Products; eds.: D. L. Wood, R. M. Silverstein and M. Nakajima (Academic Press, N. Y.) pp. 301–316.

Wood, D. L. (1972) Selection and colonisation of ponderosa pine by bark beetles. *In*: Insect/Plant Relationships; ed.: H. F. van Emden, Symp. Roy. Entomol. Soc. (London) 6, 101–117.

CHAPTER 22

Programs utilizing pheromones in survey or control

M. BIRCH, K. TRAMMEL, H. H. SHOREY, L. K. GASTON, D. D. HARDEE, E. A. CAMERON, C. J. SANDERS, W. D. BEDARD, D. L. WOOD, W. E. BURKHOLDER and D. MÜLLER-SCHWARZE

22.1. General considerations

by Martin Birch

No system based on pheromones has yet been developed to the extent that it can be called a successful technique for practical pest control, in spite of a decade or more of very intensive research effort in the field and considerable speculation on the potential of pheromones as a tool for pest management or even as a solution to some pest problems. Pheromones, along with other intriguing new approaches to pest management, hormones, genetic techniques and various other biochemical determinants of behavior, have excited the imaginations of entomologists looking for a new impetus in pest control. Much of the interest has stemmed from a desire to break away from total reliance on broad spectrum chemical pesticides, particularly in the increasing number of cases where these have been shown to have economically and biologically disastrous consequences. To an agricultural system now heavily dependent on chemicals, the prospects of insect resistance, diminishing returns on investment and loss of environmental quality are portents of imminent disaster. The new techniques, such as pheromones, offer some relief, and research funding has steadily increased to investigate their potential.

In this atmosphere much has been written in the last decade on the promise of insect pheromones in pest control (Jacobson 1965, 1972; Shorey and Gaston 1967; Wood et al. 1970; inter alia), but the way in which they might be employed for managing any specific insect is still not at all clear. Outstanding advances have been made in pheromone chemistry to the extent that sex pheromones have been identified for many of the major insect pests. Identification of a pheromone compound is, however, by no means the end point of research. It must be accompanied or followed by extensive research in pest population dynamics and the technology of pheromone deployment, face the rigors of registration and be backed up by a sound biological understanding of the role the compounds play in the life of the insects. Nevertheless, preliminary results from several diverse agricultural systems are promising and the purpose of this chapter is to examine some large scale pilot programs now underway that are designed to assess the effectiveness of pheromones. All the program case-histories contributed here have been developed in the U.S.A., where virtually all the practical work has been undertaken at this time.

Some background information on application of pheromones is presented first, but each program described in this chapter has its own approach and degree of effectiveness.

22.1.1. Use of pheromones

Tette (ch. 21) has discussed the various methods for deploying pheromones. There are two basic strategies: 1) the use of pheromones to monitor or survey population emergence, density and location; and 2) deployment of pheromones in order to suppress population levels (the so-called 'control' use). The monitoring and survey role is now a well-established practice to the extent that private industry is involved. For example, Zoëcon insect monitoring systems* are now used to considerable economic benefit by fruit growers in order to concentrate sprays in infested areas and to aid timing of spray applications within an orchard. The survey principle has also worked very successfully using synthetic attractants for fruit flies (Diptera: Tephritidae). The biological basis for attractiveness is unknown, but certain chemicals, which are not insect produced and therefore not pheromones, are extremely potent as lures for several fly species. They are routinely used in quarantine survey traps to detect possible introduction of pest species and have been used in conjunction with insecticide to eradicate the oriental fruit fly from one island in the Pacific Ocean (Bateman 1972, reviews this work).

Pest control strategies tend to follow either a preventive (eradicative) approach or a containment (corrective) approach (Smith 1972). A treatment is used in a preventive manner if used prophylactically or by calendar dates, and in a containment manner if used only when pest densities are above a certain threshold. All the arguments for and against eradication cannot be enumerated here. The concept has strong proponents (Knipling 1972) who argue that a concerted attack on the total population of an insect is one of the best ways to tackle some of the major species. It may be attractive to think of the many new techniques as an arsenal to be deployed against the insect enemy with destruction the aim. The realization by a large body of entomologists, however, that disruptive approaches to pest control can intensify rather than solve a problem, or induce new problems, has led to the approach of managing a pest population using a variety of methods. In this integrated control method no attempt is made to eradicate a pest, but rather to maintain its population below an economic threshold level.

* Pherocon™ attractants, insect traps and kits marketed by Zoëcon Corporation, Palo Alto, CA 94304.

Several different approaches are described in this chapter. The boll weevil program, for example, is an attempt to eradicate the insect from a large area using a variety of techniques. Other pilot studies are attempting to demonstrate whether or not pheromones are capable of manipulating pest populations to effect satisfactory control.

22.1.2. Evaluating the effectiveness of pheromone tests

As with any treatment to suppress an insect pest population, it is not enough to count the number of insects trapped as indicative of the efficacy of the method. Some independent estimate is necessary of the percentage mortality caused by the treatment on the population. Ideally, life table information should also be available to evaluate what percentage mortality will have a significant effect on subsequent population levels.

Research on population dynamics of pest insects hand-in-hand with control methods is one of the most needed areas of applied research. This type of research is time consuming and expensive and as a consequence is often neglected. In examining the various case histories it may be illuminating to ask how much is known about the populations they are working with. Economic thresholds need to be established to determine whether it is really necessary to reduce the pest population to a minimal level, and economic thresholds have still not been adequately determined for a majority of pest species. To compound the problem, current marketing regulations set injury levels for many crops at a level that can hardly be justified on any rational basis.

In all pheromone field tests there is a severe problem in providing a check situation against which to assess the effects of the treatment. One method is to measure the trend of the population over time and to evaluate how much the imposed treatment deflects the population level from this trend. A second way is use of an untreated plot. However, if this is close enough to the treatment plot to be part of the same population, the effects of pheromone on the population of the check plot could be very real. If a remote population is chosen to avoid this effect, there is no basis for assuming that the population trend will be in the same direction as that in the treatment area: its use as a control may very well give specious information. Thirdly, checks can be, and frequently are, omitted altogether saving expense and ensuring treatment 'success' whatever the result.

22.1.3. Biology of the pest

One reason why pheromones have not developed more rapidly towards use as a practical control measure is a result of limited understanding of insect behavior as related to these materials. It does not necessarily follow that all chemically identified sex pheromones will be suitable for development as tools for pest control.

Apart from the chemical factors involved, such as stability, volatility and reactivity of the compounds, which may well affect their use, the effectiveness depends on the biology of the insect (Shorey 1972). The behavior may not be amenable to manipulation by synthetic chemicals, particularly if the response to a pheromone source is synergized by or dependent on, visual or auditory cues from the source. Presence of the pheromone could serve to release visual searching behavior which is merely intensified when man introduces pheromone into the environment. A sex pheromone that releases a totally dependent response to the source may be rare. Only a great deal of experience and research will answer these questions. The point here is that the practicality of pheromone use is heavily tied up with the biology of the insect.

If eradication is attempted using pheromones alone, strong selection pressure is being imposed which will favor the development of 'resistance', i.e. a population could rapidly evolve that relies more on other methods of communication for mating. There is no evidence that resistance is any less likely to develop against 'natural compounds', like pheromones, than against chemical pesticides, if the two are used in the same indiscriminate way.

Although sex or aggregation pheromones are the only pheromones currently being considered for use in pest management or integrated control programs, other areas of chemical communication may also hold considerable promise for the future. Concentration of predators or parasites using kairomones is one prospect, use of chemical oviposition stimuli is another. Larval forms are in many cases less discriminating than the adults and will, within limits, eat whatever substrate they are laid on. The adult egg-laden female, on the other hand, has highly selective sensory capabilities and may well be more amenable to manipulation.

Some parasitic insects are capable of selecting non-parasitized hosts over previously parasitized ones. One way in which females do this is by detecting a pheromone left by a previous female on the host or substrate (or in the host after inserting the ovipositor), thus avoiding superparasitism when neither may survive (Price 1970; Vinson 1972; Guilot and Vinson 1972). A potentially practical parallel to this behavior occurs in the apple-maggot fly, *Rhagoletis pomonella* (Walsh), where the female marks the surface of the fruit (apple or cherry) with a pheromone after laying an egg on it. This apparently deters other females from egg laying and helps to ensure that the egg laid develops to maturity (Prokopy 1972).

Another promising area is with pheromones of social insects, where alarm pheromone communication or caste differentiation may be subject to change within the confines of the nest. Very small quantities of pheromone may be needed to disrupt colony reproduction and survival. Such an approach has enormous potential if applied, for example, to the areas of Africa where termites constitute the dominant biomass.

22.1.4. *Registration*

Government approval must be obtained in the United States before any chemical can be marketed or recommended as a control method. Natural products, such as pheromones, are no more exempt from these registration procedures than are chlorinated hydrocarbon insecticides, and pheromones in fact qualify as insecticides for the purposes of registration. In the United States, the Environmental Protection Agency* is in charge of administering and enforcing registration. According to E.P.A. guidelines: 'pesticides are registered in the United States to insure that quality products are available to the public and that when properly used these products will provide consumers with effective pest control without hazard to health or significant adverse effects upon the environment'.

The applicant for registration, usually the manufacturer or formulator, is responsible for providing the information required for registration and the cost involved adds substantially to the cost of developing a new chemical. Details of experimental testing procedures must be produced giving evidence on: efficacy as a control agent; physical and chemical properties of the chemicals and of all formulations to be used; persistence in the environment; build-up of residues in non-target organisms (particularly aquatic) and food chains; soil, plant and animal metabolism studies and a hazard review, including any immediate or delayed physiological effects that could affect the welfare or reproductive potential of exposed man and beneficial animals. The review includes extensive acute and sub-acute toxicity, mutagenicity and teratogenicity tests on mammals, and reproductive studies on birds, fish and crustacea.

Registration must be approved before any product can legally be recommended for routine control purposes on a country-wide basis. Experimental use by university or federal agencies is not affected by registration. Use or sale within a state or local area may be affected by further regulations, but these have tended to be more lenient than the federal requirements. Other developed countries have similar legal requirements, but many of the developing countries of the world do not.

With products, such as pheromones, particularly where these are natural products, the E.P.A. guidelines are not yet rigid and are still open to negotiation in the light of research data and experience of use.

22.1.5. *Conclusion*

Clearly pheromones are no panacea for pesticide plagued agriculture. They are still not available for regular use, but their promise for practical use in the near future has not diminished. Whether pheromones prove to be of agricultural value as a control technique, or not, their study should produce a lot of valuable biological information about pest species and their use as a survey tool is already of great

* E.P.A., Pesticides Regulation Division, Washington, D. C. 20250.

value. Pheromones will probably take their place, along with other new techniques, as part of a broad spectrum of control strategies to provide additional and optional inputs into the pest control decision making apparatus. The future emphasis will be on a multi-faceted approach with flexibility as the key note.

22.2. *Orchard pest management*

by Kenneth Trammel

Near total reliance on chemical pesticides for controlling orchard pests has given way in recent years to the concept of 'integrated control'. As the term implies, two or more control methods are combined in a pest management program. In practice, integrated programs usually develop through modification of the chemical insecticide program to favor natural predators of phytophagous mites. However, most orchard insect pests, especially fruit-infesting species, are not adequately controlled by natural means, and other alternatives must be sought. Identification of sex pheromones or other synthetic sex attractants of several major orchard insect pests now provides a tool with considerable promise for supplementing chemicals in orchard pest management. These major pest species, all tortricid moths, include codling moth (*Laspeyresia pomonella* (L.)), oriental fruit moth (*Grapholitha molesta* (Busck)), lesser appleworm (*Grapholitha prunivora* (Walsh)), redbanded leafroller (*Argyrotaenia velutinana* (Walker)), oblique-banded leafroller (*Choristoneura rosaceana* (Harris)), tufted apple bud moth (*Platynota idaeusalis* (Walker)), fruit tree leafroller (*Archips argyrospilus* (Walker)), grape berry moth (*Paralobesia viteana* (Clemens)), summer fruit tortrix (*Adoxophes orana* (Fischer von Röslerstamm)), and *Clepsis* (=*Ancyclis*) *spectrana* (Treitschke).

Perhaps the most valuable use of sex pheromones in orchard pest management is in pest population monitoring and assessment. A second use for pheromones is for direct control of pest populations through disruption of the mating process. Both applications are under evaluation at the New York State Agricultural Experiment Station.

22.2.1. *Population monitoring*

Precision in orchard pest management programs depends on accuracy in assessing pest population pressure. Efficiency in the use of pesticides is greatly increased if applications are based on actual need rather than on a strictly preventive schedule. To determine the need for pesticides a reliable system for monitoring population levels is required. Since pheromones are one of the most potent and specific attractants available for insect detection, our current research program is attempting to develop a pheromone-based pest monitoring system that will provide a sound basis for applying chemical or other control measures.

Three years of research have indicated that a system of peripheral and internal orchard monitoring is experimentally feasible. Currently, Sectar® insect traps* are used, lined with adhesive and charged with the appropriate pheromone dispenser. Pheromone trap stations are spaced at 160 m intervals on the periphery of the orchard and one per two hectares internally. Additional research experience is expected to indicate a reduction in trap density and thus increase the efficiency of the monitoring system. Several factors must be evaluated separately for each pest species. These include pheromone purity, possible synergism, design of pheromone dispensers, release rates of pheromone attractiveness under varying climatic conditions, trap design and trap placement. In addition, an economic threshold must be determined for each pest species so that trap catch can be related to this threshold as a basis for sound pest management decisions.

Experience has shown that pest population levels vary from orchard to orchard and that pest problems can be either indigenous or exogenous depending on orchard conditions and surroundings. Orchards with a history of good pest control practices are likely to be relatively pest-free and the influx of pests from outside the orchard is then of primary concern. Orchards under marginal or poor pest control can be plagued by both internal and external pest pressure. Our monitoring and detection system is aimed at indicating the source of pest problems.

Bionomics of individual pests must also be considered. Redbanded leafroller (RBLR) has a very broad host range (Chapman and Lienk 1971) and capture of male moths in pheromone traps is usually quite high. Both internal and peripheral trapping is necessary to assess the problem. On the other hand, codling moth has a very narrow host range and relatively low trap catches are common in our area. Proximity to abandoned orchards, wild apple trees and other unsprayed host plants influences codling moth pressure on the monitored orchards and traps should be placed accordingly. Knowledge of the host range of pest species and proximity of alternate hosts to the orchard is essential for successful application of pheromones in both monitoring and control programs.

Research in pheromone monitoring of insect populations is far from complete, but the potential use of sex attractants to assess specific pest problems is very promising. The tortricid moths are an important part of the total orchard pest spectrum and pheromones in conjunction with detection devices for other pests can provide a reliable monitoring system that will indicate actual orchard pest population levels, and hence potential damage, to the pest management specialist.

22.2.2. Direct control

In the tortricid moths, the pheromone is emitted by the female and attracts the male for mating. This communication system is a potentially vulnerable point in the

* Manufactured by the 3-M Company, St. Paul, Minnesota 55101.

life cycle and can be altered to prevent sexual encounter. One way of doing this is to lure the male moths to an artificial source of pheromone and remove them from the population prior to mating (mass-trapping). Another approach is to saturate the environment with enough pheromone to prevent male orientation to any specific pheromone source, i.e., a virgin female (confusion). A further possibility is based on the fact that after males react to a pheromone stimulus, further response is suppressed for some time afterwards (habituation). An artificial source of pheromone could accomplish just this, either by constant exposure to a high level of pheromone or by periodic release into the environment. Confusion and habituation will be considered under one heading of mating inhibition because of the difficulty in distinguishing one from the other in field experiments.

Mass-trapping: Redbanded leafroller is an important pest of apples in the eastern U. S. and was the initial orchard pest species on which pheromone research was conducted. The pheromone was isolated (Roelofs and Feng 1967) and identified (Roelofs and Arn 1968) as *cis*-11-tetradecenyl acetate. The synthetically prepared chemical, 'RiBLuRe' (Roelofs and Comeau 1968), was used in an initial mass-trapping test in the summer of 1968 (Glass et al. 1970). A heavily infested 8-hectare orchard was blanketed with 1700 ice-cream carton traps lined with adhesive and baited with the attractant in polyethylene dispensers. Although the pheromone traps captured about 4000 males, larvae developed abundantly and fruit injury was extensive. Traps baited with live female moths also captured males, indicating that mating was still occurring. Concurrently with the test, synergism was discovered to be an important factor in increasing the attractancy of RiBLuRe (Roelofs and Comeau 1968, 1971). A 60:40 solution of dodecyl acetate: *cis*-11-tetradecenyl acetate was far more attractive than RiBLuRe alone and the synergized attractant has been used in all subsequent trapping work.

Mass-trapping experiments were continued in 1969. A second orchard of ca 6 ha, about 800 m from the first, at the Cohn farm on the southern shore of Lake Ontario, was selected as an additional test site. Population levels were relatively low due to an effective chemical spray program the previous season. Fruit injury was 0.1%, indicating successful control, in spite of the fact that only 800 male moths were captured during both the spring and summer flights. A second attempt to control the heavy infestation in the original test orchard was made by trapping during the summer flight, using a new commercial fold-up trap from the 3M Company. Over 17,000 males were captured by 2400 traps deployed three per tree, but resulting fruit injury averaged 32%. A model for theoretical control was applied to both sets of data (Roelofs et al. 1970), indicating that an impractical number of about 5000 traps per ha, or 50 per tree, were needed to achieve 95% control of the heavy population. However, only about 25 traps per ha were calculated to be necessary for control under the low infestation level. It was concluded that mass-trapping for control would be practical only under relatively low population levels and this principle has been adhered to in subsequent mass-trapping control experiments.

The scope of the RBLR mass-trapping program was expanded in 1970 (table 22.1). The orginal test orchard was dropped because of its continuing high populations and the second test orchard was enlarged to 16.2 ha. In addition, mass-trapping was initiated in a 10 ha orchard on the Red Jacket Fruit Farm at Geneva. Both test sites were under relatively low population pressure. Synergized RiBLuRe dispensed from polyethylene vial caps was used in the new 3M traps (Glass et al. 1970). Trap density was set at one per tree (about one per 93 sq m), except in areas of suspected heavy pressure, e.g. near wooded areas. Although trap density could have been reduced according to the model discussed above, it was decided to maintain relatively high trap density until the *principle* of mass-trapping was thoroughly evaluated.

The experiments were continued in 1971 and 1972 through the entire season of RBLR activity (table 22.1). In 1971, a check block was established on the Cohn Farm, ca 1.2 km from the trapping area, to determine what level of injury might be inflicted by the RBLR population in the absence of all control measures and to provide a base for the control obtained by mass-trapping. In 1972, peripheral trapping was intensified to minimize the influx of redbanded leafroller moths from outside the trapped areas. Traps were deployed before the spring emergence of

TABLE 22.1

Summary of results from redbanded leafroller mass-trapping control programs, New York State Agricultural Experiment Station, Geneva, 1970–72.

	Cohn Farm, Sodus, N. Y. (16.2 ha)			
		No. RBLR ♂♂ trapped		
Year	No. of traps	Spring flight	Summer flight	% injured fruit
1970	2020	1852	700	.40
1971	2809	1876	2637	2.34
1972	2008	777	376	.09
	Check Block, Cohn Farm (6.5 ha)			
1971	8	600	312	12.40
1972	4	196	66	8.48
	Red Jacket Fruit Farm, Geneva, N. Y. (10 ha)			
1970	1661	632	3692	.14
1971	2216	1331	1406	.18
1972	1328	844	1652	.39

RBLR and pheromone dispensers were replaced after the spring flight period and once during the summer flight. Moths were periodically counted and removed from the traps. Control was assessed by periodic inspection of foliage and fruit for larval activity and by examining representative fruit samples at harvest for larval injury. Data for the 1970–72 trapping experiments are presented in table 22.1. With the exception of the 1971 data from the Cohn Farm, all fruit injury data from both trapping sites support the conclusion that good commercial control was obtained. The comparatively high degree of fruit injury at the Cohn Farm in 1971 indicates weak RBLR control, but the entire control picture that season was complicated by an outbreak of two other leafroller species, *Pandemis limitata* (Robinson) and *Choristoneura rosaceana*, and much of the injury attributed to RBLR is now known to have been caused by these other species.

The traces of injury observed throughout the testing period might be attributed to one or more of the following: 1) chance matings were actually occurring inside the trapped area; 2) gravid female moths flew into the orchard from outside the trapped area; or 3) individual wind-borne first-instar larvae drifted into the orchard. Fruit injury was usually very spotty and on individual fruits or fruit clusters, indicating (3). If egg masses, which average 40 eggs each, had been deposited, as would occur in (1) and (2), injury would be expected to be more extensive in the general vicinity of the oviposition site. However, the flight activity of gravid female moths is not known and matings occurring some distance from the trapped area could influence the control picture in the orchard. This was the basis for intensifying peripheral trapping in 1972.

Monitoring traps in the check block at the Cohn Farm indicated similar RBLR pressure on both areas of the farm and depicted potential injury levels. Replication of check blocks has not been feasible in commercial orchards for economic reasons. However, past experience in RBLR control supports our conclusion that mass-trapping did effect good commercial control and in the absence of the trapping program, the level of fruit injury would have been comparable to that of the check block.

So far, the mass-trapping program appears to have succesfully controlled RBLR under moderate population pressure. Because of its wide host range and relative abundance in nature, RBLR provides a rather stringent test control technique. A species restricted to apple and/or a narrow range of host plants or a species that occurs rather sparsely would perhaps be more amenable to this type of control. Codling moth falls into this category. While being one of the universally important orchard pests, it occurs in relatively low numbers in our area because of a very successful chemical control program in the past. Since population pressure is generally very low in commercial orchards, the mass-trapping technique should fit this species and research is underway to determine if codling moth can be controlled by this method.

Mating inhibition: Our experience with this application of pheromones is limited, but preliminary work with RBLR in grape vineyards has produced some encouraging results (Taschenberg, Roelofs and Cardé, personal communication).

Two adjacent vineyards near Fredonia, New York were mass-trapped for RBLR control in 1971, under relatively high population pressure. Blocks A (ca 0.4 ha) and B (ca 0.2 ha) yielded 2900 and 2400 male moths, respectively. Previous experience in apple orchards indicates this to be excessive population pressure for successful mass-trapping, and, in fact, 5–6% berry injury was recorded. In 1972 mating inhibition was tried in Block A and Block B was maintained as a check. Pheromone release stations, discharging > 100 μg/hr, were distributed throughout Block A on a 13.4 x 7.9m spacing (91 release points/ha). Both blocks were monitored with synthetic pheromone traps releasing ca 5.0 μg/hr and with live-female traps. One fault in the experimental design was the close proximity of the two blocks, separated only by a 12 m service lane, but this was dictated by the limited availability of vineyards for the experiment. Only six males were captured by the monitoring traps in Block A while Block B yielded 429. Although this difference is highly significant, moth catch in Block B was probably affected by the pheromone release in Block A. It is very likely that over the short distance separating the two blocks some male inhibition occurred in Block B also. Fruit injury was 3.8% in Block A and 9.2% in Block B, but some of the damage in both blocks may be due to gravid females flying in from outside the area.

Future work with mating inhibition is planned for both RBLR and codling moth. It is known that other leafroller species utilize the same basic attractant as does RBLR and the possibility exists that a complex of tortricid pests could be inhibited by release of 'RiBLuRe' alone. At this stage it appears that control of multiple species of orchard pests by pheromones may be feasible. If so, the need for several chemical pesticide applications during part of the growing season can be alleviated.

22.3. *The cabbage looper*

by H. H. Shorey and Lyle K. Gaston

The cabbage looper, *Trichoplusia ni* (Hübner) (Noctuidae), is a pest of a wide variety of important agricultural and floricultural crops. Berger (1966) identified the sex pheromone, extracted from females of *T. ni*, as *cis*-7-dodecenyl acetate ('looplure'). This chemical was the first sex pheromone identified for any agricultural pest species.

Early biological observations (Shorey 1964, 1966; Shorey and Gaston 1964, 1965) indicated that *T. ni* has a sophisticated, noctural premating communication-system based primarily on the female sex pheromone. The pheromone guides the male to the vicinity of the female and activates his copulatory behavior. In fact, *T. ni* males will not respond to a female as a potential mating partner if they cannot perceive the pheromone released by her. This was demonstrated in a laboratory experiment in which groups of virgin males and females were enclosed in 2-liter glass jars (Shorey et al. 1967). Sufficient looplure was placed in some of the jars several hours before the time of mating to approach saturating the air. Under these conditions, no males mated with the females, even though the confined conditions restricted all moths to within 15 cm of one another and numerous females were observed in the supposed receptive position, with sex pheromone glands extruded and wings vibrating. Apparently the males remained unresponsive because they could not detect the small additional increment of pheromone released by the females when in the presence of the relatively massive prevailing concentration of synthetic pheromone. In jars not saturated with looplure, many males oriented to and mated with receptive females.

In principle, if males of *T. ni* in the laboratory can be rendered incapable of responding to the natural female pheromone following their continued exposure to looplure, the same phenomenon should be capable of operation as a behavioural insect control in the field.

Between 1966 and 1972, experiments were conducted to investigate the feasibility of disrupting *T. ni* pheromone communication in the field (Shorey et al. 1967, 1971, 1972; Gaston et al. 1967; Kaae et al. 1972, 1973a). In all experiments, looplure was released into the air from evaporators held at one m above the soil surface on wooden stakes. No attempt was made to use evaporation substrates that would be practical in commercial practice; instead, evaporators were designed in such a way that their rate of looplure release could be measured accurately. Most evaporators were based on the principle of a liquid film of pure looplure being exposed to the air. Evaporation rates were determined by direct weighing in the laboratory under conditions of controlled temperature and airflow. (Gaston et al. 1971).

Most experiments were designed to answer the question: if a given amount of looplure is to be maintained in the air above a certain land area, is it better that the pheromone evaporate from many sources, placed closely together, with each source releasing the chemical at a fairly low rate; or would better disruption result from a few widely separated sources, each releasing at a relatively high rate? Evaporation sources spaced 1, 3, 10, 30, 100, and 200 m apart were evaluated with evaporation rates from the sources ranging from 0.001 to 20 μg of looplure per min (table 22.2). The evaporators were placed in square, checkerboard arrays in the field, ranging from 6 x 6 (36 evaporators total) to 10 x 10 (100 evaporators total).

The experiments were evaluated by placing a trap baited with virgin *T. ni* females in the center of each array. The number of *T. ni* males caught in the trap, relative to the number caught in an identical control trap in a nearby untreated area, was used as the indication of the amount by which communication had been disrupted. No optimum evaporation rate or separation between evaporators was found (table 22.2). The important characteristic appears to be the total amount of looplure released into the air per given surface area of land. This amount can be

TABLE 22.2

A summary of 38 experiments, each designed to evaluate the disruption of sex pheromone communication in *Trichoplusia ni* by evaporators placed a specified distance apart in the field and releasing looplure at a specified rate.

Release rate/evaporator/min (μg)		Distance between evaporators (m)					
		1	3	10	30	100	200
0.001	% disruption*	3					
	mg/hectare/night**	7					
0.003	% disruption	95,93	0				
	mg/hectare/night	20	2				
0.01	% disruption	95,96	98,89,84	85,79	0,0,88		
	mg/hectare/night	70	7	0.7	0.07		
0.03	% disruption		98,91	99,88,97	97,88,94	31,36,88	
	mg/hectare/night		20	2	0.2	0.02	
0.1	% disruption		100	97,96	92,100,100	22,34	
	mg/hectare/night		70	7	0.7	0.07	
1	% disruption		100,100	100		99	
	mg/hectare/night		700	70		0.7	
20	% disruption						82
	mg/hectare/night						3

* Note that 1,2, or 3 percentages of disruption are given for each combination of release rate and distance between evaporators tested. This reflects the fact that variable numbers of experiments * (1, 2, or 3) were conducted for each combination.

** Mg of looplure evaporated into the air over a hectare during a 10-hr night.

obtained by various combinations of evaporator spacings and release rates. Disruption above 90% appears to be obtainable with the expenditure of about 10 mg looplure per hectare per night. About 100 mg per hectare per night will apparently give close to 100% disruption. At an anticipated cost of looplure of less than \$1.00 per gram, the 100 mg rate would cost less than \$0.10 per hectare per night. The cost of producing and servicing substrates and of 'wasting' looplure, due to evaporation during the heat of the day when the moths are not active and to irreversible adsorption in the substrates, may be considerably higher.

Disruption was obtained at lower looplure release rates in a cool, low wind, coastal environment than in a hot, erratically windy, desert environment (Shorey et al. 1972). The degree of disruption attained appeared to be no better in low than in relatively high density moth populations (Shorey et al. 1972). This density-independent effect was not anticipated. We expected that disruption would be more effective in the low density populations in which the average male and female presumably must communicate over greater distances.

These experiments with *T. ni* were not evaluated by direct measurements of reduction in fertile eggs, and thus larvae, of the next generation. It is likely that *T. ni* females fly long distances, possible many miles, between the time of mating and the time some days later when they complete oviposition. Therefore, the minimum-sized plot for accurate evaluation of the effect of communication disruption on the next generation will probably have to be several miles in radius. Such large plots have not yet been used.

Experiments were also conducted to determine whether the disruption of male orientation to virgin females caged in traps is truly indicative of an inability of the males to find pheromone-releasing females in the open field (Shorey et al. 1972). Virgin females were tethered in the field by lengths of thread glued to their thoraxes. The degree of prevention of mating among these tethered females when placed in looplure-impregnated plots agreed closely with the degree of communication disruption indicated by the standard trapping technique.

It is unfortunate that we do not understand the exact mechanism by which male:female communication is disrupted, as this knowledge would enable us to develop more intelligently based and effective behavioral control systems. Probably much of the disruption effect is due to adaptation of the olfactory sensory neurons and/or habituation in the central nervous system following exposure of the males to the continually present synthetic pheromone. Also, with much more pheromone probably being released into the air from the synthetic sources than from wild females, any tendency of males to orient toward pheromone sources would only serve to increase their state of adaptation and habituation.

Males of the alfalfa looper, *Autographa californica* (Speyer), and the soybean looper, *Pseudoplusia includens* (Walker), were also prevented from orienting to their females when in looplure-treated plots (Kaae et al. 1972). This is not surprising, since *Autographa californica* and *Pseudoplusia includens* are in the same subfamily (Plusiinae) as *Trichoplusia ni*, and the natural pheromone of each of these species is identical or very similar to looplure (Tumlinson et al. 1971; Kaae et al. 1973a). However, looplure also caused a high degree of disruption of intraspecific pheromone communication in the bollworm, *Heliothis zea* (Boddie), the tobacco budworm, *H. virescens* (F.), the yellow-striped army-worm, *Spodoptera ornithogalli* (Guenée), and the pink bollworm, *Pectinophora gossypiella* (Saunders). These latter four species exhibit little or no overt behavioral response to looplure. Possibly, as more data become available on the chemical structures of natural sex pheromones, a few key chemicals will be found that will disrupt male:female communication in a wide variety of pest species. On the other hand, when a number of chemicals related to looplure were evaluated for communication disruption in *Trichoplusia ni*, none of them approached looplure in effectiveness (Kaae et al. 1974). The whole research area concerning the disruptive effect of chemicals other than the natural pheromone of a given species deserves considerably more attention.

Further important research must be conducted before looplure can be used in practical cabbage looper control programs. The minimum size area needed to prevent mated females from migrating into the center of treated plots must be determined. Practical substrates, which release looplure efficiently under various conditions of air movement and temperature, must also be engineered.

22.4. *Cotton – the pink bollworm*

by Lyle K. Gaston and H. H. Shorey

The pink bollworm, *Pectinophora gossypiella* (Saunders) (Gelechiidae), is a worldwide pest of cotton. There are several reasons why the pink bollworm is probably an excellent candidate for experimental attempts to develop a pest-control technique based on disruption of pheromone communication: 1) the insect has few host crops other than cotton; thus, control measures can be directed almost exclusively at that crop. 2) Although the extent of within-field and between-field movements by the moths has not been determined, their relatively weak flight behavior probably restricts their normal wanderings to within the bounds of a single cotton field. 3) Propylure (10-*n*-propyl-*trans*-5,9-tridecadienyl acetate), the chemical previously reported to be the sex pheromone of this species (Jones et al. 1966), is apparently not biologically active in the laboratory or the field (Eiter et al. 1967; Jones and Jacobson 1968; Hummel et al. 1973). However, a second chemical, hexalure (*cis*-7-hexadecenyl acetate), is available that operates as a selective pink bollworm male attractant (Green and Keller 1968; Green et al. 1969; Keller et al. 1969). Unfortunately, hexalure is considerably less active than the natural pheromone* (Hummel et al. 1973). 4) The economic importance of cotton and of the pink bollworm stimulate federal, state, and corporate organizations to provide the necessary funding for this research.

McLaughlin et al. (1972) conducted a series of experiments to evaluate whether sex pheromone communication between male and female moths of the pink bollworm could be disrupted when the air in cotton fields was permeated with hexalure. Hexalure was evaporated from open reservoirs at rates of approximately 0.01, 0.1, and 0.3 μg/min. The reservoirs were placed at the level of the top of the foliage and were spaced at 1, 3, 10, or 30-m intervals in 8 x 8 or 10 x 10 grids. Regardless of the evaporation rate or spacing of the reservoirs, the ability of wild males to locate virgin females, used as bait in traps located in the centers of the grids, was reduced 90%, when the amount of hexalure entering the air was equal to, or greater than, 20 mg/hectare each night.

The possible utility of the communication disruption concept was then tested on a large scale. Hexalure was distributed throughout a cotton field during 2.5 months of the 1972 growing season (Shorey et al. 1974). Each substrate on which the hexalure was dispensed for placement in the field was a knot tied in a short loop of cotton string. Ten mg of hexalure was applied to each knot. Approximately 30,000 of the substrates were distributed per week in 4.8 hectares of cotton: a loop was placed around a leaf near the top of a cotton plant in every 1.6 square meters of the field. The evaporation rate of the hexalure was approximately 400 mg/ha each night. Under these conditions, male moths were almost completely prevented from locating virgin females; a seasonal total of over 11,000 males per female-baited trap were captured in two untreated, control fields, whereas only 38 males per trap were captured in the hexalure-treated field. Toward the end of the growing season, the untreated fields had an average infestation of 6.9 larvae per boll, whereas the treated field had an average of only 0.6 larvae per boll. Thus, the hexalure treatment apparently reduced the larval infestation by reducing mating communication to such an extent that few viable eggs were laid in the treated field. The authors speculated that a large proportion of the eggs were laid by fly-in females that had already mated elsewhere. If such were the case, then a scaling up of this experiment to a larger geographic area might reduce the pink bollworm population to such a low level that no insecticides would be needed for their control.

* The natural pink bollworm sex pheromone has been identified (Hummel et al. 1973) as a mixture of *cis, cis* and *cis, trans* isomers of 7,11-hexadecadienyl acetate. The isomeric-mixture sex pheromone was designated 'gossyplure'.

22.5. *Cotton – the boll weevil*

by D. D. Hardee*

Since its introduction into the United States about 1892 (Hunter and Hinds 1905), the boll weevil, *Anthonomus grandis* Boheman, has been the most costly insect in the history of American agriculture, causing losses in cotton production estimated at an average of $200 to 300 million annually. To prevent even greater losses, growers spend an estimated $70 million each year (Knipling 1964) for its control, about one-third of all insecticides used for agricultural purposes (Rainwater 1962). The extensive use of insecticides for boll weevil control may not only cause a serious problem of environmental pollution, but often causes a drastic reduction of natural biological agents that would otherwise hold other agricultural pests in check. The adverse effect on natural insect parasites and predators often leads to a subsequent increase in populations of such insects as the tobacco budworm and the bollworm (*Heliothis* spp.). The resulting intensive and increasingly ineffective use of insecticides jeopardizes cotton production.

State and Federal agencies have directed considerable resources in the past decade toward the development of ways to eliminate the boll weevil from all infested cotton growing areas in the United States and perhaps later in Mexico. A special study committee on boll weevil eradication, formed by the National Cotton Council in 1968, suggested in a meeting on May 6, 1969 that suppression techniques had been developed to the extent that eradication might be achieved if they could be applied in an integrated program. A pilot experiment, the Pilot Boll Weevil Eradication Experiment (PBWEE), was proposed to determine if eradication could be attained before a large-scale program should be initiated. The primary test site was centered in south Mississippi and extended into southeast Louisiana and southwest Alabama. Several agencies agreed to make substantial contributions to the planned experiment, but first the 1970 and then the 1971 target date for initiating the experiment were abandoned because of inadequate assured funds, and the new target date of 1972 was set.

The attempt at total suppression of the boll weevil was based on considerable research experience in several entomological disciplines over the previous decade. One area of research that had shown a great deal of promise in manipulation of populations of the boll weevil during this period was the use of pheromones.

When it was shown that the pheromone produced by the male boll weevil is not only a sex pheromone for females (Cross and Mitchell 1966), but also acts as an aggregating pheromone for bringing both sexes together for mating in the cotton

* Programs conducted in cooperation with the Mississippi State University Agricultural and Forestry Experiment Station, Mississippi State. I thank T. B. Davich, W. H. Cross and E. P. Lloyd of this laboratory and F. J. Boyd, APHIS, USDA, Prentiss, Mississippi for reviewing the manuscript.

field (Hardee et al. 1969), its potential in survey, control, and eradication of the boll weevil was immediately investigated. This potential was studied in detail in west Texas in 1968 (Hardee et al. 1970) and 1969 (Hardee et al. 1971) and in Mississippi in 1969 (Lloyd et al. 1972a). Conclusions from these studies were that: 1) live male boll weevils in traps could give 60 – 80% suppression of boll weevils in the spring following an effective reproduction-diapause control program (Lloyd et al. 1966) in the previous fall; and 2) 2.5 or 5 traps per hectare (1 or 2/acre) of cotton were more effective in terms of number of boll weevils captured per number of traps in the field than 10 or 20 traps per hectare (4 or 8/acre).

The identification and synthesis (Tumlinson et al. 1969) of the four components of the male pheromone, commonly known as grandlure (Hardee et al. 1972a), and the development of a more effective trap for the boll weevil (Leggett and Cross 1971) added more impetus to the importance of the pheromone principle in suppression of the boll weevil. Moreover, Lloyd et al. (1972b) showed the effectiveness of males and grandure in conjunction with the systemic insecticide, aldicarb, in a modified trapping system for suppressing low density populations of overwintered boll weevils. Subsequently, the effectiveness of grandlure in relation to males in short-lived (Hardee et al. 1972a) as well as slow-release formulations (Hardee et al. 1973; Bull et al. 1973; McKibben, Boll Weevil Research Laboratory, personal communication) was demonstrated in field tests as well as in the PBWEE in southern Mississippi (Boyd, personal communication).

Suppression measures to be used in the first year (1972) of the PBWEE included the use of insecticides in a reproduction-diapause control program and cultural practices (such as defoliants, desiccants, and destruction of cotton stalks) in the fall of 1971. These measures were followed in the 1972 growing season by use of grandlure, either in traps, according to the regime recommended by Hardee et al. (1972b), or in aldicarb-treated trap crops, as recommended by Lloyd et al. (1972b), followed by a single application of insecticide at the pinhead square (initial flower bud) stage, and the release of sterilized male boll weevils, all carried out successively in the same area. In early June 1972 it became obvious, through large numbers of boll weevils captured in traps and field counts of overwintered weevils higher than expected, that numbers of boll weevils in the PBWEE area were too high for eradication to be attempted. These high numbers were attributed to four factors: 1) little or no in-season control of boll weevils by growers; 2) extremely high populations in the field when the reproduction-diapause program was initiated in 1971; 3) a very mild winter in 1971–72 resulting in little or no winter kill of overwintering boll weevils; and 4) extremely late emergence in the spring of 1972. The very dry spring that year resulted in the emergence of high numbers of overwintered boll weevils after the cotton had initiated squaring and after traps, trap crops, and the spring application of insecticides had lost their effectiveness. Accordingly, releases of sterile male boll weevils were terminated and efforts concentrated on reducing the number of overwintered and reproductive boll weevils in the field and preparation for eradication in the second year of the program in 1973. These suppression measures included a thorough inseason control program with insecticides, to be followed in 1972–73 by the same steps outlined previously for 1971–72. As of December 1, 1972 numbers of boll weevils in the area, as measured by captures in traps, field counts, and preliminary woods trash examination for hibernating boll weevils, were extremely reduced in comparison to numbers in the same area in 1971 and in areas outside the PBWEE at the same time in 1972 (Boyd, personal communication).

Specifically the eradication area of the PBWEE consists of about 1200 hectares of cotton in six counties in southern Mississippi and one parish in Louisiana (fig. 22.1). Surrounding the eradication area are three buffer areas totalling about 6520 hectares (first buffer – 1560 hectares; second buffer – 1200 hectares; third buffer – 3760 hectares) with increasing populations of boll weevils resulting from decreased insecticide usage moving away from the eradication area. Strategy used in

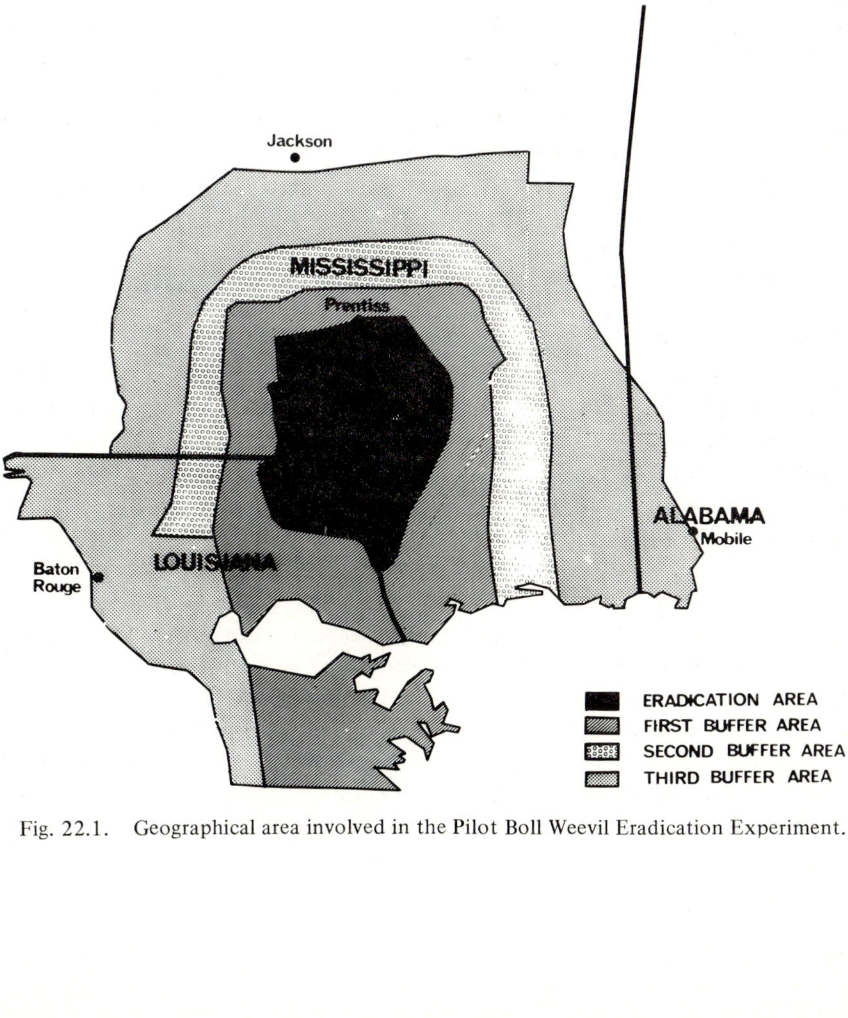

Fig. 22.1. Geographical area involved in the Pilot Boll Weevil Eradication Experiment.

1972 and planned for 1973 in employing pheromones consisted of: 1) operating five Leggett pheromone traps (Leggett and Cross 1971) per hectare of cotton from about April 1 to about July 1; the traps were serviced once per week with the most effective formulation of grandlure and were placed on stakes about one m above ground level between the edge of the cotton field and hibernation sites; and 2) baiting with grandlure, strips of an early-planted, early-fruiting variety of cotton (3–5% of total area of field) at the time of planting (about April 1) with the systemic insecticide aldicarb with an infurrow application (2.5#/hectare) and a sidedress application (5#/hectare) about five weeks later. The treated trap crops were four rows wide and were baited at 30–100 m intervals once weekly with grandlure. The strategy employed was based on the principle that overwintered boll weevils emerging from hibernation quarters in the spring detect the grandlure in traps or in the larger cotton in the trap crops. Responding weevils are captured in the traps and die from starvation or desiccation or feed on the treated cotton in the trap crops and die. The pheromone principle has worked well in programs in previous years with traps (Hardee et al. 1970, 1971; Lloyd et al. 1972a) and trap crops (Lloyd et al. 1972b), and in the first year of the PBWEE; thus there is every reason to predict that the same will be true in 1973.

Grandlure has great value in a number of survey, detection, monitoring and research programs (Hardee 1972). From the standpoint of future usage in control, suppression, and pest management, grandlure has tremendous potential in programs other than traps and trap crops. For example, field observations show clearly that boll weevils aggregate in the late fruiting plants which continue to grow in moist places within fields after the crop is mature. Boll weevils also respond to grandlure in the fall after the crop reaches maturity. These observations suggest that the reproduction-diapause control procedures could be streamlined and insecticide usage reduced by restricting treatment to the late fruiting cotton baited with grandlure rather than applying the insecticide treatment to the entire field. The confusion or inhibition technique for behavioral control of Lepidoptera (Shorey and Gaston 1964; Gaston et al. 1967; Shorey et al. 1967) has not been investigated satisfactorily in the boll weevil. Combining grandlure in a bait containing a feeding stimulant and small quantities of chemosterilant, insecticide, or pathogens is also planned. Using grandlure alone or in traps to manipulate diapausing boll weevils into a natural or artificial hibernation site to be destroyed during the winter has shown promise in west Texas where hibernation sites are somewhat limited (Bottrell, Texas A & M University, personal communication). Finally, we hope eventually to correlate numbers of boll weevils captured in traps with potential damage to cotton, so that when a given number of boll weevils are captured per trap per hectare, farmers are alerted to initiate control measures for boll weevils. This would reduce the farmer's need for early season scouting of his crop for boll weevils at a time when he is so busy. Admittedly, these systems (and undoubtedly others not discussed here) will require a great deal of research before they can be used on a grower basis, but they do have potential. In the meantime grandlure in traps and trap crops is one of the most promising of the known pheromones as a tool for detection, suppression and possible elimination of any insect species.

22.6. *The gypsy moth*

by E. Alan Cameron*

The gypsy moth, *Porthetria dispar* (L.) (Lepidoptera: Lymantriidae), a native of Eurasia and North Africa, was carried to North America in 1869 in an attempt to establish a silk industry. A few larvae accidentally escaped from the laboratory in Medford, Massachusetts, became established, and, within 20 years, had caused severe tree defoliation in the local area. It has been estimated that in excess of $100 million have been spent combating the insect since it was introduced (Beroza 1971) and expenditures continue at a multi-million dollar annual rate. Forest defoliation in the northeastern United States over the past ten years has averaged 198,801 hectares annually, with a high of 582,433 hectares in 1971 (Anon 1973).

It has long been known that the normally flightless female moth emits a chemical signal to which males respond. Beroza and Knipling (1972) briefly reviewed the history of attempts to isolate, identify and synthesize the responsible chemical(s), which work culminated with the determination of *cis*-7,8-epoxy-2-methyloctadecane, called 'disparlure', as the sex attractant (Bierl et al. 1970). Since then, this material has undergone field testing for use in survey and detection, and as a tool with which to manipulate populations both by physical capture of male moths in traps and by otherwise disrupting chemical communication between the sexes.

Results so far have demonstrated the value of disparlure for survey and detection, particularly when formulated with 'keepers' to regulate the rate of volatilization and thus prolong the action of the lure (Beroza et al. 1971). In both 1971 and 1972, small numbers of male moths were captured in baited traps in a number of states south and west of the generally infested northeast area. It is probable that many of the moths were transported as larvae or pupae on recreational vehicles or on commodities shipped to these outlying areas, and that very few represent incipient populations of the pest. However, the potential for spread has been clearly demonstrated. Establishment of the gypsy moth in valuable hardwood forests, especially those with a large oak component, would be a serious blow to currently uninfested regions.

The potential of the lure for population evaluation has not yet been adequately investigated. We are not yet able to derive estimates of population density from the

* Most of our studies at Penn State are supported by Cooperative Agreement 12-14-100-10, (946) 33 between the Agricultural Experiment Station of The Pennsylvania State University and ERD-ARS-USDA.

capture of one or more male moths in a trap or, perhaps more practically, to derive estimates of the magnitude of potential defoliation the following year. Although several investigators are working with disparlure in this context, no comprehensive program to evaluate the lure for population evaluation and prediction is currently underway.

It has been demonstrated that traps baited with as little as one nanogram of disparlure are capable of capturing male moths (Beroza et al. 1971). Since the lure is so potent, and through the use of appropriate keepers activity may be extended over periods of at least six weeks, there is optimism that disparlure may be used for gypsy moth control, not just monitoring. Beroza and Knipling (1972) discussed this possibility, and presented a model showing the theoretical effects of using disparlure-baited traps in suppression of an incipient population. They also discussed the use of the lure for 'confusion' of male moths and consequent disruption of mating success. These two approaches have been field-tested since 1971 in both natural and simulated populations, and using both wild and laboratory-reared insects (Cameron 1971, 1973 and unpublished; Cameron et al. 1973a; Schwalbe et al. 1973; Stevens and Beroza 1972).

If disparlure is shown to be capable of disrupting mating so that populations can be manipulated, it is potentially useful in the following ways:

1) To establish a barrier zone wide enough to preclude the establishment of new infestations in currently uninfested areas immediately in advance of the expanding front of infestation.

2) To eradicate isolated infested spots which may be detected outside the generally infested area.

3) To apply final suppression after other agents, such as parasites, predators, pathogens, chemical insecticides, or others, have reduced populations to very low levels.

4) To reduce the total area of general infestation.

Let us examine the results so far.

During April, 1971, the first broadcast applications of disparlure were applied under the direction of F. M. Philips, USDA, and E. A. Cameron to two 16-hectare plots on Dauphin Island, Alabama. The formulations* consisted of:

1) a spray consisting of 1000 mg disparlure in 100 cc nujol (a mineral oil keeper) diluted into 18.93 liters (5 U.S. gallons) of xylene and applied by aircraft at the rate of 62.5 mg disparlure in 1.18 liters xylene per hectare; and

2) 0.635 cm squares of hydrophobic paper impregnated with disparlure, each square containing approximately 2.5 μg disparlure, at the rate of ca 20,000 pieces (= 50 mg disparlure) per ha. Traps baited with 10 μg disparlure, approximately equal to one female in attractive power, were placed throughout the plots to recapture

* Developed and prepared by M. Beroza, Leader, Organic Chemical Synthesis Laboratory, AEQI, USDA, Beltsville, MD 20705.

released males. In the plot treated with disparlure-impregnated hydrophobic paper, none of the released males was recaptured in releases as long as 25 days after treatment. Similarly encouraging results were obtained in subsequent pre-season tests on Cape Cod, Massachusetts, this time using virgin female moths as bait in some traps and disparlure in others (Stevens and Beroza 1972). However, field tests in naturally infested areas of eastern Pennsylvania in the summer of 1971 failed to demonstrate suppression of mating through application of disparlure on either the hydrophobic paper or on granular cork. It is probable that study sites supported gypsy moth populations which exceeded the upper level at which the disruption technique may eventually be shown to be operational (Cameron 1971). In addition, these tests convinced us that we needed much more knowledge of behavior of adults of both sexes of the insect.

Following further successful pre-season testing on Dauphin Island in 1972 by USDA personnel, larger field tests of the disruption technique were undertaken in central Pennsylvania during the normal flight season in the summer of 1972. Wild insects were placed in 100-hectare study areas, treated with disparlure-impregnated granular cork applied by aircraft, to simulate incipient populations. Approximately 622 g cork, containing either 7.5 or 25 g disparlure, were applied per hectare. In all tests, the proportions of female moths fertilized were reduced, and in two of the four tests these reductions, compared with untreated check plots, were statistically highly significant (Cameron 1973). However, because of the reproductive potential of the gypsy moth, the reductions were not considered to be *biologically* significant since they would not cause a downward trend if a natural population of the same size had been allowed to persist through another year.

Late in August, yet another test of the disruption technique was conducted. A microencapsulated formulation of disparlure was aerially applied to two 100-hectare test plots at a rate of 5 g disparlure per hectare*. A sticker was incorporated into the formulation to achieve stratification of the microcapsules throughout the vertical profile of the forest. Laboratory-reared pupae were placed as before to simulate an incipient infestation. During the 12 days of the test, we were unable to detect evidence that even one female in a treated plot was mated. When compared with results from the untreated check plots, these differences were both statistically and biologically significant. Post-season tests with microencapsulated formulations on Cape Cod by USDA personnel gave similarly encouraging results. Tests in 1973, using both laboratory-reared and wild insects, and applying microencapsulated disparture at rates of 2.5–15 g per hectare, substantiated results obtained during 1972 (Cameron et al. 1973a; Schwalbe et al. 1973).

Behaviorally, we know far too little about adult gypsy moths of both sexes. At this point, we do not understand the mechanism by which disruption of response

* The formulation was developed by M. Beroza, using a microencapsulation process developed by the Capsular Products Division of National Cash Register Co., Miamisburg, Ohio 45342.

may be achieved, although several avenues might be postulated:

1) Permeating the treated area with pheromone molecules may cause the males' pheromone receptors to become habituated, and so to be non-receptive to releases of lure from females.

2) Males may investigate large numbers of discrete, attractive points (i.e., individual microcapsules), each as competitively attractive as a virgin female moth, and so reduce the probability of locating females.

3) Females themselves may be capable of monitoring the background concentration of pheromone and be inhibited from releasing lure if this concentration exceeds a certain threshold.

Recent studies have demonstrated that there are significant behavioral differences between wild and laboratory-reared gypsy moth adults (Richerson and Cameron 1973 and unpublished). Continuous monitoring of the lure output throughout the lifetime of individual females has revealed that: approximately 35% of the reared females emitted no detectable amounts of pheromone at any time, vs. a 4% rate for wild females; there is a diel periodicity of release from wild females which is not evident in laboratory insects; and laboratory females release pheromone at a rather constant rate of ca 5 ng in 30 min (range 0–19), never emitting a 'burst', while wild females produce a 'burst' of up to 841 ng in a 30 min period once in their life, and have a background release rate of ca 8–10 ng in 30 min. Wild virgin females are more attractive to both wild and lab-reared males than their lab-reared counterparts, and wild males are more responsive to either wild or lab-reared females than are lab-reared males. In addition, ca 30% of the lab-reared males failed to orient to any pheromone source in a series of tests vs ca 6% of the wild males.

All these behavioral phenomena bear directly on an assessment of the progress in translating disparlure into an operational tool. Laboratory-reared insects were used in all field tests through 1972 in which suppression of mating or recapture of released males exceeded the levels postulated as necessary to reduce the gypsy moth population in the succeeding generation (Cameron 1973). It has now been demonstrated that parallel results can be obtained using wild insects in plots treated with microencapsulated disparlure (Cameron et al. 1973a; Schwalbe et al. 1973). Future efforts will be directed towards continued behavioral studies, as well as how best to apply the lure, and a determination of the upper limits of gypsy moth population density against which the mating disruption technique may be effective. With this information in hand, it will be possible to make a more effective attempt to integrate the use of disparlure into a comprehensive pest management program directed at the gypsy moth.

Beroza (1967) and Cardé et al. (1973) have recorded the phenomenon of inhibition or masking of response to the gypsy moth sex attractant. Beroza did not identify the non-persistent inhibitor with which he worked. Cardé et al. presented evidence that an olefin, 2-methyl-*cis*-7-octadecene, present in the female pheromone gland, suppressed or almost totally inhibited male attraction to traps baited with either disparlure or virgin female moths. They suggest that, if the olefin causes mating inhibition at the central nervous system level, it could potentially be more effective in disrupting mating than the attractant itself. In field tests during 1973, in which a microencapsulated formulation of the olefin was used, we were unable to demonstrate reduced mating among test insects (Cameron et al. 1973b). The work done to date with inhibitors must be considered preliminary: much more extensive testing must be conducted before the use of the pheromone precursor can justifiably be considered as a promising avenue through which gypsy moth mating can be disrupted.

Disparlure is a valuable tool for survey and detection; it has potential use as an aid in estimating population densities or evaluating populations remaining after chemical or other suppression treatments, in estimating defoliation in subsequent years, and, perhaps most importantly, as a direct agent for population manipulation. There is clear evidence that its potential may be realized over the next several years.

22.7. *Forest Lepidoptera – the spruce budworm*

by C. J. Sanders

The name spruce budworm is commonly applied to a group of lepidopterous defoliators of the family Tortricidae, native to North America, whose larvae feed in the expanding buds and new foliage of conifers. Periodically their numbers increase dramatically to cause devastating outbreaks which collapse only after causing defoliation and tree mortality over millions of acres.

The single most important species is *Choristoneura fumiferana* (Clemens), the eastern spruce budworm, which is found throughout the range of balsam fir and white spruce from the Yukon, the northern forested areas of the Prairie Provinces and throughout Ontario, Quebec, the Maritimes, and northern New England, extending down the Appalachians into West Virginia. In the West the species of greatest economic importance is *C. occidentalis* Free., the western one-year cycle budworm which feeds primarily on Douglas fir and white fir, extending from southern British Columbia, South to New Mexico and Arizona. Three other spruce-fir feeding species are recognized in the west; *C. biennis* Free., the two-year cycle budworm; *C. viridis* Free., the green budworm, and *C. orae*, the coastal budworm. However, these three species are restricted in range and are of limited economic importance. Other *Choristoneura* species feed on pine, notably *C. pinus* Free., the jack-pine budworm in the east, and a group of species in the west, including *C. lambertiana* Bsk., whose taxonomy is still unresolved.

The mono-unsaturated aldehyde, *trans*-11-tetradecenal has been identified as a major component of the sex pheromone communication system of *C. fumiferana* and field trials have demonstrated its attractiveness to both *C. fumiferana* and *C. occidentalis* (Weatherston et al. 1971), and subsequently to male *C. biennis* (Sanders et al. 1974), three species which had earlier been shown to have similar, if not identical, sex pheromones (Sanders 1971). *C. viridis* is strongly attracted by the corresponding acetate, *trans*-11-tetradecenyl acetate (Sanders et al. 1974), a compound suspected of being a major component in the sex pheromone systems of *C. pinus* and *C. orae*, although the males of neither species are attracted by the acetate alone (Sanders, unpublished). Two compounds have been shown to inhibit the response of male *C. fumiferana* to the aldehyde, *trans*-11-tetradecenyl acetate (the compound featured in the sex pheromone system of the *C. pinus*, *C. orae* group) and the corresponding alcohol, *trans*-11-tetradecenol (Sanders et al. 1972). However, the response of male *C. occidentalis* is not inhibited by the acetate (Daterman, personal communication). Thus for the eastern spruce budworm, *C. fumiferana*, we have an attractant and two inhibitors, while for the most important of the western species, *C. occidentalis*, we have an attractant, but as yet no inhibitor.

Spruce budworm outbreaks are a natural phenomenon, the consequence of favorable climatic conditions coinciding with large uniform areas of mature host. Once an outbreak is underway it has proved impossible to regulate the numbers of budworm sufficiently to cause its collapse. Extensive aerial spraying operations using convential insecticides have been successful in keeping trees alive, but there is mounting evidence that preserving the insects' food supply in this way also prolongs the outbreak. A factor complicating attempts to control the budworm is the dispersal potential of the partially gravid females. Not only are enormous numbers concentrated and passively transported over hundreds of kilometres by storm cells and frontal systems, but there is mounting evidence of a continual downwind emigration from densely populated areas (Greenbank, personal communication), which may carry females 30 km in a night and as far as 150 km in their life-span. This means that control operations to reduce populations in portions of an outbreak must be carried out every year the outbreak persists, since the area is re-invaded by females each year.

22.7.1. Estimation of population levels

Apart from the creation of a less budworm susceptible forest which must come with future more intensive management practices, future trends in the control of these insects must move in the direction of early detection of the beginnings of outbreaks when it may prove possible to check the rate of population increase until natural factors take over. This becomes an even more attractive proposition if outbreaks start in discrete, relatively, small areas of forest, termed epicenters, for this would reduce the areas requiring treatment. However, the existence and characteristics of epicenters have yet to be described.

TABLE 22.3

Numbers of male *Choristoneura fumiferana* captured throughout the flight period in traps baited with single virgin females compared to larval counts obtained by examining foliage.

Year	Northwestern Ontario		Northern New Brunswick	
	Adults/trap+	Larvae/branch	Adults/trap*	Larvae/branch
1966	4.2	0.01	3.6	0.02
1967	31.6	0.09	3.8	0.13
1968	13.7	0.03	16.4	0.80
1969	–	0	5.5	0.49
1970	2.2	0	14.9	1.09
1971	1.6	0.01	49.1	3.54

+ Average of 10 traps.
* Average of 25 traps, C.A. Miller, unpublished data.

Between outbreaks budworm populations are extremely sparse, only a few hundred per hectare compared to several million per hectare during outbreaks. To detect fluctuations in the endemic populations, survey methods must be extremely sensitive as well as cheap in material and labor costs. For several years traps baited with virgin female budworm have been operated in endemic populations of budworm in eastern Canada (table 22.3). The traps captured male budworm in every year of operation; in other words there were no zeros, which are always problematical in the analysis of survey data. Similar results can be obtained by collecting foliage for examination for larvae, or by beating the foliage to cause the late instars to drop onto mats. However, the sex attractant traps represent a considerable saving in manpower and it is probable that the traps give a more accurate estimate of population density in endemic situations since they are effective over distances of up to 35 m and therefore can be arranged to sample a wide area. One shortcoming of the trap is that the catch each day is affected by weather, especially temperature and humidity. However, if trapping is continued throughout the whole flight period, 3–4 weeks in late June and July, daily differences are probably compensated for. Trap location also affects their efficiency, catches are highest at the top of the tree canopy, an inconvenient location for placement and retrieval. However, provided catches are adequate at lower levels there is no need to strive for maximum catches. The same consideration applies to trap design; cost and ease of handling are of prime importance and, if a simple inexpensive trap provides adequate results, costly design improvements are unnecessary.

* 3-M Co., St. Paul, Minnesota.
** Zoëcon Corporation, Palo Alto, California 94304.

TABLE 22.4

Numbers of male *Choristoneura fumiferana* captured in traps baited with different quantities of *trans*-11-tetradecenal compared with numbers captured by a virgin female.

Quantities of attractant (mg/stopper)	No. males captured per trap per night
0.1	6.8
1.0	9.4
10	13.1
100	17.8
Single virgin female	10.5

The discovery of *trans*-11-tetradecenal as a synthetic attractant provided the opportunity to test the feasibility of using sex attractant traps in extensive surveys in 1972. Green Sectar 1* traps were placed out in 272 permanent sample plots in eastern Canada. Larval population estimates are made annually in these plots by beating foliage, allowing comparisons to be made between the two sampling methods. Each trap was baited with a polyethylene vial stopper containing 2 mg Sprudamone (Zoëcon** trade name for *trans*-11-tetradecenal), which should have approximated the attractiveness of a single virgin female (table 22.4). Results showed a poor correlation between the larval counts and adult male catches. With a log–log transformation a straight line of the equation $\log Y = 0.46 + 0.49 \log X$ (where Y = moths per trap, X = larval counts) gave a correlation coefficient of 0.54. However, which method gave the better estimate could not be resolved. Results were disappointing, in that too many of the plots gave zero catches (80 out of 272), a situation which the earlier adult female trapping indicated should not have happened. Concurrent tests showed that the bait used was only about 10% as effective as a virgin female, and reasons for this discrepancy are being investigated. A shortcoming of the polyethylene vial stoppers is that the release-rate of the aldehyde (as determined by weight-loss studies) falls off very quickly over time, giving a tenfold difference over a three week period. Although preliminary results indicate that the response of the male budworm is fairly constant over a considerable range of release-rates, this is a variable which can confound the interpretation of the results. There is therefore a definite need in the future for a wick which provides a more uniform release rate throughout the budworm flight period.

22.7.2. *Prospects for control*

Investigations into the use of sex attractants and inhibitors in the control of spruce budworm populations have barely begun. It is considered unlikely that they will ever be of use in high density populations. Trapping would require an impractical number of traps, and mating disruption would be unlikely to succeed where there is a high probability of insects encountering each other by accident. Control strategy will have to involve the early detection of an ominous increase in endemic numbers followed by immediate treatment to check the increase. Possibly as few as 70 traps per hectare would be required to give 50% reduction in mating success at endemic population densities; but this is still a large number if applied to thousands of hectares. Because the spruce budworm are active throughout the canopy, traps would also have to be distributed in a vertical plane throughout the foliage which presents problems. The extensive areas involved, and their inaccessibility, necessitates the use of aircraft, and traps large enough to capture sufficient insects are relatively bulky and would involve the inefficient use of aircraft space. Thus far no tests have been made of the feasibility of using traps in population regulation of the spruce budworm, interest has moved more in the direction of mating disruption which lends itself more readily to aerial application over large areas than do traps. Preliminary tests indicate that the sex attractant and the acetate inhibitor do reduce mating success when disseminated in the atmosphere. In laboratory experiments, newly emerged, unmated male and female budworm were placed in a wind tunnel, measuring 0.6 x 0.6 x 1.8 m long, with a wind speed of about 15–18 m/min. Sixteen pieces of filter paper were suspended on threads in a 4 x 4 grid in the upwind opening of the tunnel. The treatment consisted of one mg quantities of chemicals placed on the filter paper. The insects were left overnight and collected the following morning when each female was dissected to determine if a spermatophore was present, which was taken as an indication of mating. Controls, in which no chemical was used, were alternated with the treatment. Four controls gave the percent of females mating as 62, 53, 51 and 68% an average of 58%. Four interspersed treatments with the aldehyde gave 19, 33, 42 and 59% for an average of 38% or a reduction of 34% in number of matings. A single test of the acetate inhibitor gave 50% mating with a subsequent control of 75%, a 33% reduction. There is therefore an indication that the presence of these chemicals does disrupt mating. Preliminary field trials were conducted in two 2.5 m cube screen cages located about 200 m apart in woodland near Sault Ste. Marie, Ontario in July and August 1972. Around each cage, equally spaced in a circle of radius five m, eight stakes were driven into the ground from which were hung open-ended containers housing a small polyethylene dish containing chemical. The containers were hung at heights of one and two m, making a total of 16 sources of chemical so placed that the cage would be permeated by the chemical, no matter the direction of the wind. Weight loss studies in the laboratory at 70 °F and a prevailing wind speed of about 15–18 m/min. indicated a very constant release-rate of the aldehyde at 1.2 mg per day per container. On each night of experimentation one cage was surrounded by chemical, the other cage was left untreated as a control. The following night the treatment was reversed. In this way it was hoped that variations in insect behavior due to the

TABLE 22.5

Percentages of females mated after equal numbers of virgin male and female *Choristoneura fumiferana* were left for 24 hr in an outdoor cage exposed to sex attractant (aldehyde) or inhibitor (acetate), compared to numbers mated in an untreated control cage.

Expt.	Date	Treatment	Treated cage	Control cage
1	12 July	Aldehyde	22	60
2	13 July	Aldehyde	26	33
3	20 July	Aldehyde	0	12
4	21 July	Aldehyde	39	28
5	3 August	Aldehyde	7	9
6	4 August	Aldehyde	4	22
	Average		16.3	27.3
7	17 August	Acetate	20	30
8	19 August	Acetate	44	52
9	21 August	Acetate	72	61
10	23 August	Acetate	27	32
	Average		40.8	43.8

location of the cages would be compensated for. Numbers of insects placed in the cages depended upon their availability, and varied between 35 pairs and 100 pairs. The insects were placed in the cages near mid-day, left overnight and collected the following day around mid-day. The females were subsequently examined for spermatophores.

The percentages of females containing spermatophores (table 22.5) indicated a positive effect with the aldehyde, as in the wind tunnel experiments, for a mating reduction of 41%. However, results were again less convincing with the acetate, with only 7% reduction. In both laboratory and field experiments the test populations were abnormally high, and many insects must have encountered each other accidentally. Indications of the chemicals having any effect at all are very encouraging, since in a field situation, especially at low population densities, the insects undoubtedly rely more on long-range communication, which is more easily disrupted. Experiments have also been conducted in New Brunswick (Miller, personal communication) in which groups of trees were festooned with string, soaked in solutions of the aldehyde or the acetate or alcohol inhibitors. Reductions in the numbers of male budworm captured in traps placed among the treated trees again indicate disruption of the insects' communication system. The next step in the trials must be under natural conditions in which the chemicals are applied by aircraft. Such field trials require some formulation of the chemicals to ensure their stability, coupled with a uniform release rate for a duration of at least four weeks, and which can be applied by aircraft and made to adhere to the foliage so that the chemical diffuses throughout the tree canopy.

22.8. *Bark beetles – the western pine beetle*

by William D. Bedard and David L. Wood*

Pheromones of bark beetles release an attractant response that results in the location and colonization of trees, where the insects feed, mate and oviposit. In tree-killing species, such as the western pine beetle (*Dendroctonus brevicomis* LeConte) these attractant compounds elicit a synchronized invasion by several thousand beetles (Wood 1972). The female beetles inoculate the tree with pathogenic fungi (Whitney and Cobb 1972) that rapidly inactivate natural host resistance mechanisms. As a result, the tree quickly dies and its tissues are exploited by adult beetles and their progeny. Beetles that fail to aggregate successfully do not reproduce. Thus attractant compounds derived from natural substrates have great potential for pest management. No suppression methods using pheromones are now registered for use, but many programs are under way to develop such methods.

Three suppression methods have been attempted with bark beetles. These are:

1) *Trap-out*: Insects are attracted to sticky traps baited with attractant compounds and killed (Bedard and Wood 1970; Gustafson et al. 1971, 1972).

2) *Baited-tree*: a) Living trees are baited with attractants. Those trees attacked by beetles and killed are removed by logging before emergence of the new generation (Knopf and Pitman 1972; Pitman 1973); b) Living trees unsuitable for beetle reproduction (e.g. trees with thin phloem tissue) are baited (Rasmussen 1972); beetles mass attack them, but broods are reduced; c) Living trees are poisoned with an herbicide (e.g. cacodylic acid) and baited with attractants so that the attacking beetles and their progeny are killed by the changed host substrate (Vité 1970); and d) Living trees are treated with an insecticide that has a long residual life (e.g., lindane) and baited with attractants so as to kill incoming beetles over a long period (Pitman 1971).

3) *Interruption*: The mass aggregation is reduced below the threshold number required to kill the tree (Wood 1972), either by increasing the concentration of

* We thank the following persons for their contributions to the work reported in this chapter: C. J. De Mars (evaluation of within-tree populations, aerial photography, computerization of data), Robert C. Heller (aerial photography, photo interpretation) and Paul E. Tilden (on-site field work) of the Pacific Southwest Forest and Range Experiment Station, Forest Service; Robert W. Gustafson (administration and field work) of the California Region, Forest Service; Lloyd E. Browne (technical developments), Donald L. Dahlsten (evaluation of within-tree populations and natural enemies), Bland Ewing (data processing and statistical methodology) and Peter Rauch (data processing and file management) of the University of California, Berkeley; and J. Otto Rodin and Robert M. Silverstein (chemical analyses) formerly of the Stanford Research Institute.

attractant in the area, or by introducing a compound(s) that causes a reduced catch at pheromone baited traps (Rudinsky et al. 1972). Although the latter compounds have been called anti-attractants (Wright et al. 1971), blockers, confusants, and other terms, the behavioral mechanisms that cause a reduced catch are still unknown.

In addition to suppression attempts, survey of bark beetle populations has also been attempted by using attractant-baited sticky traps (Bedard and Wood 1970; Vité 1970; Vité and Pitman 1970; Gustafson et al. 1971, 1972).

The value of both suppression and survey trials for pest management programs cannot adequately be judged from the accounts in the literature and elsewhere. Rarely have these treatments been evaluated in terms of either their effect on trend of damage, or their effect on the population of the pest and its natural enemies.

The case history described here illuminates some of the problems in attempting to develop a survey and suppression method that utilizes attractant compounds. This program is an ongoing cooperative effort involving: the Pacific Southwest Forest and Range Experiment Station and the Forest Pest Control Branch of the California Region, both of the United States Forest Service; the State of California Division of Forestry; the Department of Entomological Sciences, University of California at Berkeley (UCB); and the College of Environmental Sciences and Forestry, State University of New York. The studies were carried out from 1966 to 1972 at these locations; laboratory behavior at UCB; chemistry at Stanford Research Institute, Menlo Park, California; and field behavior and efficacy in the Sierra National Forest, Madera County, California.

The pest, the western pine beetle, *D. brevicomis*, kills 0.5 to 3.5 billion board feet (b.f.)* of commercial timber annually (Miller and Keen 1960). The value of 3.5 billion b.f. at 1972–73 prices was $280 million for trees on the stump ($80/thousand b.f.) and $600 million for lumber ($170/thousand b.f.).

22.8.1. Rationale

We selected the 'trap-out' method for these reasons:

1) Attractant compounds that are highly selective in their activity are used to kill the pest. At most, only a few species of natural enemies are attracted by these synthetic compounds, thus permitting the remaining natural enemies to concentrate on the surviving pest population.

2) Trees do not have to be sacrificed a priori, although they may be killed close to traps.

3) Timing of application is simplified. For example, a second visit to the control site before the emergence of the brood is required when logging attractant-baited trees. Logging also removes natural enemies along with the tree.

* 1 board foot = 1 ft. x 1 ft. x 1 in. (= 30 cm x 30 cm x 2.4 cm)

4) Pesticides are not necessary for success in using these compounds; thus non-target organisms, such as natural enemies, need not be sacrificed.

22.8.2. Potency of synthetic attractants

Success of a 'trap-out' strategy depends principally on the potency and deployment of the attractant compounds. These compounds must duplicate as closely as possible the potency of the natural substrate. Only in this way can the baited traps compete successfully with natural sources of attractants.

Two of the attractant compounds for *D. brevicomis*, *exo*-brevicomin and myrcene, had previously been found to be attractive in the field (Bedard et al. 1969). *exo*-Brevicomin was active alone; myrcene was not. The combination was much more attractive than *exo*-brevicomin alone, but it was still not competitive with natural sources. Seven behaviorally active compounds (*exo*- and *endo*-brevicomin, frontalin, myrcene, 3-carene, *trans*-verbenol, and verbenone) had been implicated in the attraction of *D. brevicomis* (Renwick 1967; Silverstein et al. 1968; Vité and Pitman 1969b; Bedard et al. 1970; Wood 1972).

We therefore tested all these compounds for both laboratory and field activity. The studies were conducted during 1968–70 (Browne and Wood, unpublished; Bedard and Wood, unpublished; Tilden et al., unpublished). Trapping methods for these studies are described in Bedard and Browne (1969). We found that *exo*-brevicomin, frontalin, and myrcene in a 1 : 1 : 1 ratio was the most attractive chemically defined mixture (Bedard et al. 1970; Wood 1972). Various absolute concentrations of this mixture were tested to determine their effect on catch, both at the release site and at various distances from this site. Tree killing caused by beetles attracted into the vicinity of traps was also assessed. Catch on the traps increased as evaporation rate increased; up to 20 mg of each compound per day at the release site and up to 200 mg per day 18 m from the release site. Tree killing near the release site also increased as concentration increased. Catch increased as the trapping surface was increased.

22.8.3. Design of large-scale tests

After these extensive, small-scale field trials were completed, we conducted a large-scale test to assess the potential of the attractants in the suppression and survey of *D. brevicomis*. The following considerations were of primary importance in determining the experimental design:

1) The area had to be large enough to account for population movement beyond the immediate area around each trap. The scale of the test area proved to be the most difficult parameter to assess. Although flights of ten to thirteen km from brood trees to newly-attacked trees had been reported earlier (Miller and Keen 1960), our knowledge of the flight behavior and movement of bark beetles was

generally inadequate. The same was true for predators and parasitoids.

2) An elevated concentration of attractants released simultaneously from many sites could produce such area effects as: a) mass tree killing in or along the border of such an area; b) interruption of aggregation behavior on trees, so that they are not successfully mass-attacked and killed, resulting in tree-induced beetle mortality; or c) interruption of aggregation behavior on traps.

3) The fate of natural enemies in any pest suppression effort is of critical importance with respect to pest resurgence and pest replacement by other species. Synthetic attractants could influence natural enemies by: a) Trapping them selectively. In the case of *D. brevicomis* one predator, *Temnochila chlorodia* Mann. (Coleoptera: Trogositidae), is strongly attracted to *exo*-brevicomin (Bedard et al. 1969; Vité and Pitman 1969a): b) Relocating and concentrating the prey (i.e., *Dendroctonus brevicomis*) population: c) Changing the post-treatment community structure of *D. brevicomis*. One such change could be increased predator-prey ratios as a result of selective removal of both *D. brevicomis* and *Temnochila chlorodia*. This change would result in a concentration of natural enemies on the remaining *Dendroctonus brevicomis* populations: d) Interfering with their normal host finding behavior.

4) The long term effects of a completely new treatment had to be determined so that standards of efficacy and safety could be established. The location, extent and structure of pre- and post-treatment generations were a minimum requirement to set such standards.

5) The selection of an appropriate check plot was complicated by our lack of understanding of the movement of populations and the area of attractant effects. We know little about the comparability of widely-separated *D. brevicomis* populations such as in adjoining drainages. The traditional view of a checkerboard of treatment and check plots was placed in doubt by this lack of understanding. It was possible that attractant-baited traps in treatment plots would attract insects from check plots and that trees in the treatment plots would be attacked and killed by these beetles. Such a process would result in a decrease of *D. brevicomis*-caused mortality in the check plots with a concomitant increase in the treatment plots.

6) The need to have results that can be compared to other tests dictated a limited number of treatment variables and a commitment to examine these same variables in future testing. By electing to place attractive traps in a grid configuration, both suppression and survey grids become comparable treatments in a series of tests that included as variables: a) surface area of the trap; b) number of traps per unit area; c) attractant evaporation rate; and d) location of traps with respect to infested and uninfested trees. Deployment of traps in a fixed pattern also allowed us to study the effects of trap position on size of the catch in relation to physiographic and vegetative features of the site. Such data should assist in deploying traps in locations where catch can be maximized and tree-killing minimized.

22.8.4. *The Bass Lake test*

The test was conducted during the 1970 field season. For the test site a large area, ca 65 square km, was selected within a single drainage area and bordered on most sides by forest types which contained few *D. brevicomis*, e.g., brush and non-host type. We reasoned that emigration and immigration would be minimized by the relative physiographic and ecological isolation of the area. Somewhat arbitrarily we chose two suppression plots, each 2.56 square km and two check plots, each 2.56 square km with the qualifications that each plot contain: 1) currently infested trees; 2) forests comprised principally of ponderosa pine; and 3) land as level as possible in order to facilitate access. At the outset the suppression plots were split in half, and one check plot was assigned an irregular shape (fig. 22.2) so as to meet the above requirements. Traps baited with attractants were located on 161 m centers for a total of 66 traps per 1.3 square km suppression plot. The treatment was started April 6 through 30 before the overwintering generation emerged. Suppression traps were removed June 25 to 30 after the spring flight had terminated. Other traps placed on a 0.8 km grid throughout the test site were maintained for the entire flight season (May through October) to test their potential in relating the

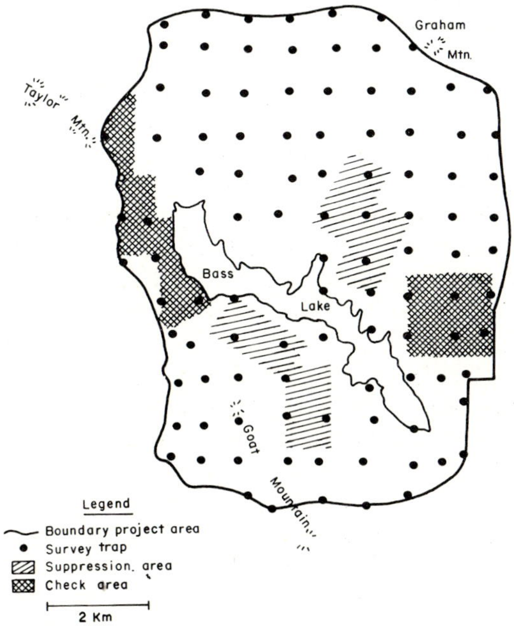

Fig. 22.2. Location and spatial relationship of survey traps, suppression plots and check plots within the Bass Lake test area, California, 1970.

magnitude and location of in-flight populations with present and subsequently infested trees, i.e., a survey role.

Test outcome was evaluated in terms of changes in the abundance and distribution of trees killed by *D. brevicomis* and changes in the numbers and distribution of populations of *D. brevicomis* and its principal natural enemies.

The important requisites for this test and its evaluations include: 1) methods to determine location of trees killed by *D. brevicomis*; 2) methods to determine the abundance of *D. brevicomis* and its principal natural enemies within trees; 3) an effective trap; 4) a device to deliver attractants; 5) a sufficient supply of attractants at a high level of purity, so that only the effects of known compounds are assessed; 6) methods to handle efficiently the diverse and abundant data; 7) trained personnel; and 8) adequate financing.

Methods to determine the location of trees killed by *D. brevicomis* and to estimate within-tree populations of *D. brevicomis* (Berryman et al. 1970; DeMars 1970) and its natural enemies (DeMars et al. 1970a, b) were known before we began the test. These methods had, however, never been applied to the evaluation of a pest suppression program. Consequently, considerable modification and innovation was required. The number and location of killed trees were estimated by using sequential aerial photography and then subsequently verified on the ground (Caylor and Thorley 1970).

The distribution and abundance of *D. brevicomis* and its principal natural enemies were estimated by using a combination of the aerial photographs and intensive within-tree sampling at three periods during brood development. Species, stage of development and estimates of numbers were determined from the within tree samples. Sample trees were located in all suppression and check plots and throughout the remainder of the study site.

A trap was designed that was easily portable and erectile in the forest and inexpensive to produce in large numbers, and that provided a maximum trapping surface. It consisted of four plastic coated, fiberglass screen panels, (2.2 x 0.5 cm mesh), each 0.76 by 2.0 m, coated with Stickem Special®*. It was erected by joining one side of each panel to a vertical metal pipe along the long axis, and at right angles to one another. The trap was then raised 2.3 m above the ground and the pipe telescoped over a second metal pipe driven into the ground. Equipment was also designed and built to wash the insects from the screen and dry-clean them for counting (Browne, unpublished).

A sequential sampling method was developed for estimating the number of *D. brevicomis* and predators caught on suppression traps at the end of the treatment period (Ewing, unpublished). Survey trap catches were estimated biweekly by

* Michael and Pelton, Emeryville, California. Trade names and commercial products and enterprises are mentioned solely for information. No endorsement by the U.S. Department of Agriculture or by the University of California is implied.

counting and removing the insects from a predetermined 9.3 square dm area on each vane.

The stability of each compound was evaluated under field conditions. Delivery devices were developed to evaporate each compound at 2 mg per day for survey traps and 20 mg per day for suppression traps (Silverstein and Rodin, unpublished). In addition, up-scaled syntheses of the attractant compounds were developed to produce the amounts required for the test (Rodin et al. 1971).

Data management specialists worked with all investigators to design forms and protocols for efficient and accurate data input to computers for storage, file management and analysis (Rauch and Ewing, unpublished). About two-thirds of the first year costs of this test were met with existing project funds. The remainder were new funds obtained from the Forest Service's California Region. Subsequent costs have been shared by the Forest Service's Pacific Southwest Forest and Range Experiment Station and the California Region, by the University of California, by the Rockefeller Foundation, and by the International Biological Program – National Science Foundation through Grant No. NSF:GB 34718.

22.8.5. Results and conclusions

From our preliminary analyses, we have concluded that pheromone-induced mortality of *Dendroctonus brevicomis* contributed substantially to the reduction of tree mortality caused by this bark beetle throughout the test area. Suppression traps caught an estimated 405,000 *D. brevicomis* while survey traps caught an estimated 189,000 beetles during the same period (table 22.6).

Tree mortality declined from 227.1 ± 23.6 trees immediately before the test (i.e., 1969–70 overwintering infested trees) to 73 ± 8 trees killed during the suppression

TABLE 22.6

Response of *Dendroctonus brevicomis* and *Temnochila chlorodia* to attractant compounds deployed over 65 square km at Bass Lake, California, May–June 1970.

Traps		No trapped during suppression period	
Type	No.	*D.b.*	*T.c.*
Suppression	242	405,000	74,000
Survey	99	189,000	12,000
Total	341	594,000	86,000

period. The high catch on survey traps relative to the low number of infested trees indicates that these traps actually played an important role in population suppression.

Detailed analyses of the effects of the treatment are underway to determine:

1) Total population produced by the 1969–70 overwintering generation and by all subsequent generations up to, and including, emergence and attack by the 1970–71 overwintering generation.

2) Community structure within trees infested by *D. brevicomis* for each generation.

3) Distribution of *D. brevicomis* and its natural enemies, and trees killed by *D. brevicomis* through the entire evaluation period.

4) Survey and suppression trap catch in relation to trees killed by *D. brevicomis* and to vegetative and physiographic characteristics of the trap site.

The approach and many of the techniques described in this case history are applicable to other bark beetle species where population suppression with attractant pheromones is desired. Regardless of the specific technique used, i.e., 'trap-out', 'baited tree', or 'interruption', intensive evaluation of the treatment effects over large areas will be necessary. Methods of population and damage assessment must be available to make these evaluations of efficacy. Such evaluations are difficult and costly, and require the efforts of many individuals with a diversity of skills.

22.8.6. *Future*

We are repeating (1971–74) this 'trap-out' technique, at McCloud Flats, Siskiyou County, California, together with full population evaluation to determine: 1) the effectiveness of the technique under population levels 10 times that occurring at Bass Lake; 2) how the technique can be modified to be effective over larger areas; and 3) how to improve and hopefully simplify the population evaluation methods.

We envision that future efforts leading to the operational use of the 'trap-out' method for *D. brevicomis* will include the development of a model(s) to assist in determining the combination of treatment variables that should be applied to reduce a population of known size. The model(s) will also provide prescriptions appropriate to specific pest situations, e.g., a small, high-value recreation area with a moderate pest population or a large, low-value area with a high population. The development of such models will be an iterative process wherein data from large-scale field tests and population studies of *D. brevicomis* will be used to predict pest abundance, given specific manipulations. As more data from field tests become available, the specific model can be tested and refined.

Key treatment variables will include: 1) density, distribution, and trend of the *D. brevicomis* population(s); 2) distribution of susceptible host trees; 3) host mortality caused by other agents, i.e., other bark beetles, flatheaded borers, root diseases, etc., and 4) competing sources of natural attraction (from windfalls, lightning strikes, logging, road construction, etc.).

The development of such models, requires estimates of the number of infested trees and their location and estimates of the number of attacking and emerging beetles per unit of bark area before and after each treatment. These critical parameters can be used to determine the treatment design for a given pest population and to assess the success of the treatment.

22.9. *Stored product pests*

by Wendell E. Burkholder*

Early awareness of insect presence is the key to effective and economic control of insect damage and infestation of stored products. Thus, the concept of prevention rather than the control of infestation is important with such commodities, especially since regulatory agencies today do not usually allow any insects or insect fragments in marketed food products. Many warehousemen, plant sanitarians and other personnel responsible for preventing insect infestations are often not aware of the existence of an insect infestation until it is too late. One undetected stored product insect can cause a greater loss than a large population of insects in other commodities. Burkholder and Dicke (1966) indicated the possibility of using sex pheromones to develop more effective and desirable ways of detecting and controlling dermestid beetles, important stored product pests, and it may soon be possible to use pheromones for such detection. Then, as the presence of insects is monitored, controls can be selectively applied when and where they are needed. Problem areas could be located by luring insects from their hiding places to trapping devices. The risk of contamination and cost of control would be considerably lessened by localised rather than routine blanket application of pesticides. Pheromone traps could also be used by warehouse managers and pest control operators to assess their pest control programs. Records indicating presence or absence of infestation could be valuable for future reference by inspectors or in the event of claims of insect damage against a company when species identification is important.

22.9.1. *Coleoptera*

The principal insect pests of stored products are Coleoptera and Lepidoptera and of these, beetles are by far the most important and most numerous (Hinton 1945). Pheromone studies have been concerned primarily with the Dermestidae, which

* Contribution from the Stored Product and Household Insects Laboratory, Agricultural Research Service, USDA, and the College of Agricultural and Life Sciences, University of Wisconsin, Madison.

includes the destructive khapra beetle (*Trogoderma granarium* Everts). Pilot control studies have utilized the principal sex attractants of the black carpet beetle, *Attagenus megatoma* (F.), and *Trogoderma inclusum* LeConte. The black carpet beetle sex attractant has been identified as *trans*-3,*cis*-5-tetradecadienoic acid, synthesized and given the trivial name megatomoic acid (Silverstein et al. 1967; Rodin et al. 1970). The primary sex attractant of *T. inclusum* was discovered to be 14-methyl-*cis*-8-hexadecen-1-ol and has also been successfully synthesized (Rodin et al. 1969; Degraw and Rodin 1971). Several species of *Trogoderma* respond to this compound.

In one of the first studies to evaluate these pheromones under practical conditions male black carpet beetles were attracted to traps treated with from 0.01 to 0.25 mg of megatomoic acid (Burkholder 1970). In a subsequent study (Burkholder 1973), megatomoic acid was used in an enclosed space (a 208-liter drum of 102 kg dry capacity) in order to evaluate the effects of the pheromone on the mating activity of black carpet beetles. A high vapor concentration was produced by placing 0.25 mg of megatomoic acid (ca 500 female equivalents) on a strip of paper inside each of 10 drums in a warehouse. Ten untreated drums served as controls. One male and one female black carpet beetle were released on opposite sides of the drum and the female was examined after 24 hours for presence of sperm. In the first series of tests during the late summer and fall only 28% of the females mated in the treated drums compared to 87% in the controls. The drums, without further treatment, were retested the following spring and summer and were still effective in reducing mating from 70% in the controls to 30% in the treatment. The initial response of these males to high pheromone concentration is usually an intense excitation, copulatory and searching behavior. Failure to mate on prolonged exposure to pheromone may be due to habituation.

In another series of pilot scale tests, unmated males of either *T. inclusum* or the black carpet beetle were released in the center of a confined area of 3 or 1.5m square. Two pheromone traps and two control traps were placed near the corners. These traps consisted of four 9 cm square single-face corrugated papers stacked together and were treated with the pheromone alone, or with pheromone plus an insecticide. The number of captured males was recorded 24 hours after release. Relatively high concentrations of pheromone (10 mg of megatomoic acid for *Attagenus megatoma* and 2.5 mg of the *Trogoderma* synthetic attractant for *T. inclusum*) were necessary, but the effective doses resulted in the capture of 70% of the released males by their respective pheromone traps vs. 20% capture in the control traps. Traps treated with both pheromones lured both species of males (Burkholder and Ma, unpublished data).

Other field tests were made in areas of warehouses with the traps treated with: 0.25 mg megatomoic acid together with an insecticide (A); 0.25 mg *Trogoderma* synthetic pheromone with an insecticide (B); an insecticide only (C) and a blank control (D). The traps were collected and replaced with fresh traps weekly for surveillance of native species of stored product insects (personal communication – A. J. Gilbert, Calif. Dept. of Agric.). In this preliminary test the traps were found to be attractive to both adults and larvae of beetles from the Dermestidae and adults of Curculionidae, Cucujidae and Tenebrionidae in sizable numbers, while adults of Bostrichidae, Nitidulidae, Ostomidae and Mycetophagidae were captured in small numbers. The ratio of adults in the traps was: 2.7(A): 2(B): 2.5(C): 1(D). The ratios of 338 larvae caught were: – 3.6(A): 2.6(B): 1(C): 1.4 (D). The structure of the trap appeared to provide an ideal hiding place for the insects. The traps with insecticide only had an average of two and one half times the number of adult insects of all families when compared to the untreated control. Concentration of pheromone appeared to be too low in these tests, but it was interesting that no larvae other than dermestid larvae were caught in the traps; that 98.2% were *Attagenus* sp. and of these 47.6% were caught in the megatomoic acid traps. This suggests, contrary to our expectations, that *Attagenus* sp. larvae are stimulated by megatomoic acid.

22.9.2. Lepidoptera

In the work with Lepidoptera, *cis*-9, *trans*-12-tetradecadienyl acetate was isolated and identified as the principal component of the sex pheromone of the almond moth, *Cadra cautella* (Walker) and the Indian meal moth, *Plodia interpunctella* (Hübner) (Brady et al. 1971a; Kuwahara et al. 1971a). It has also been isolated from the Mediterranean flour moth, *Anagasta kühniella* (Zeller) (Brady et al. 1971b; Kuwahara et al. 1971b), the tobacco moth, *Ephestia elutella* (Hübner) (Brady and Nordlund 1971) and the raisin moth, *Cadra figulilella* (Gregson) (Brady and Daley 1972). Small-scale tests using this compound were conducted in an isolated and dark room (42.4 m^3) using four traps (one liter volume paper cylinders with open ends, coated inside with a sticky compound) treated with 10 ng of the compound, and one control (Brady et al. 1971a). In tests with *Plodia interpunctella*, an average of 46% of males released in the darkened room were trapped. In similar tests, an average of 27% of *Cadra cautella* males released were trapped.

In a more extensive study, the pheromone was used in three separate buildings known to be infested with stored food moths (personal communication, D. Grant, Zoëcon Corporation). Eleven traps, each baited with 0.2 μ of the synthetic pheromone in a polyethylene cap, and four control traps, were distributed about 7 m and 2.5–3 m above the floor in the three buildings. Four species of moths were captured in these traps: *Plodia interpunctella*; *Ephestia elutella*; *Cadra figulilella* and *C. cautella*. All moths in a representative sample were males except for the raisin moth (130 males and one female). In contrast, a sample of 60 *Cadra* sp. taken in a light trap contained a 1.5:1 ratio of males to females. The light traps captured more moths than the pheromone traps (1.3:1) but they were more expensive and more difficult to set up and maintain. The pheromone traps placed at high levels caught considerably more moths than those at low levels probably because of the stratified temperatures which facilitated flying at the higher levels.

22.9.3. Prospects for success

Based on preliminary field testing it appears that sex pheromones will be useful for insect detection and survey purposes, but their use alone as a control measure is not promising unless low numbers of insects are involved. Large numbers of small inexpensive pheromone traps distributed throughout food processing plants and warehouses may be particularly useful in locating sites of infestation, so that control measures might be concentrated in areas of need. The use of pheromones to induce confusion and habituation in males shows promise. However, the large quantities of pheromone involved present several problems. For example, insects may be attracted from outside the food plant or warehouse. The commodities would probably absorb the pheromone and actually attract insects to them after leaving the warehouse and passing through the marketing channels. Unwanted pheromone residues are another potential problem area which is totally uninvestigated.

However, pheromones may soon be used in another way. They may enhance the effectiveness of existing light traps and food bait traps, particularly those of a corrugated construction which are favored by insects as pupation, oviposition, and hiding sites. Insecticides, sticky compounds or insect pathogens in combination with pheromones could also enhance the effectiveness of the pheromone traps. Pheromones could be used to bring the males to a source of disease, which they subsequently spread by mating with females. Both sexes would carry the disease to potential infestation sites and the disease could also spread when the infected insects died and were consumed by young larvae.

The basic promise of pheromone research is that its application to insect control will make it possible to reduce both our use of pesticides and our reliance on this method of control. Whatever the immediate use, pheromone research has encouraged study of insect behavior and thus will inevitably produce sounder approaches to insect control.

22.10. Application of pheromones in mammals

by Dietland Müller-Schwarze

Most of the knowledge or assumptions about applications of pheromones in mammals are still at a pre-scientific stage. For lack of work with true pheromones, this review will also cover interspecific odors. The main possibilities for using intra- and interspecific odors are in trapping, crop protection, wildlife management, and animal husbandry.

22.10.1. Trapping

Trappers' tales about large distances over which coyotes, for instance, are attracted to artificial 'scent posts', seem exaggerated. Pimlott et al. (1969) observed packs of wolves passing within 10 m of experimental scent posts without investigating them. However, coyotes have been shown to visit experimental posts treated with coyote urine four to five times as often as blanks (Linhart, personal communication).

For many centuries trappers have used concoctions containing urine and scent gland material, among other things, to attract and trap animals like beavers or coyotes. Information on the composition of the 'attractants' was (and is) traditionally secret or at least not documented, and the 'success rate' has mostly remained a matter of personal opinion. Aleksiuk (1968) caught beavers (*Castor canadensis*)* with a mixture of castoreum (a product of preputial glands) from freshly killed beavers, glycerin and anise oil. For coyotes (*Canis latrans*), urine, gall and anal glands of coyotes are mixed with glycerine. For foxes, fox urine, zinc valeriate and beaver castor are used, while for a number of canids, putrefied fish with glycerine and beaver castor are in use (Taber and Cowan 1969).

22.10.2. Crop protection and wildlife management

Owners of gardens and orchards often try to deter herbivores, especially deer, by placing droppings of carnivores next to the crop to be protected. The success again is a matter of subjective judgment. Laboratory experiments showed that naïve black-tailed deer fed significantly less than usually, or not at all, near droppings of predators. The most effective droppings were those of cougar (*Felis concolor*) and coyote, both of which occur in the range of black-tailed deer (Müller-Schwarze 1972). New opportunities may arise with the isolation and identification of the alarm pheromones of deer, which are known to inhibit feeding (Müller-Schwarze 1971). Recently, biologically quite remote extracts of rotten salmon carcasses have been demonstrated (by the U.S. Fish and Wildlife Service in cooperation with the Weyerhaeuser Company) to repel deer. Protection from black-tailed deer browsing was reported to be 'greater than that of other contact repellents available' (Rochelle 1973). So far no true pheromones but only scents or decomposition products of other species have been used in field tests. These odors may be effective by mimicking alarm pheromones or predator odors. One problem with using predator odors is that droppings and scent marks are examined by herbivores at close range (a few centimeters). Such repellents would keep herbivores from feeding on treated plants but would not keep them out of an entire area (no 'fence function').

* Author's names omitted: see footnote ch. 16.2.

22.10.3. Animal husbandry

In farm practice, odors have been used to facilitate maternal behavior. An ewe can be made to accept a strange lamb if the lamb is covered with the hide or the birth fluid of her own lamb. On the level of the species, Alpaca (*Lama pacos*) and Vicuña (*Lama vicugna*) can be crossbred by killing a newborn alpaca and using its hide to cover newborn male vicuña. A lactating alpaca female will then accept the vicuña, which in this way becomes sexually imprinted on alpacas and will later mate with alpaca females to produce desired hybrids. The cross, called 'paco-vicuña' has wool of almost the quality of the vicuña, and in the quantity typical of the alpaca (Hodge 1946).

Farmers and breeders know that sniffing and licking play an important role in the reproductive behavior of domesticated animals. However, the domestic pig is the only species for which pheromone research has yielded applicable results. Patterson (1968) identified an odoriferous compound (3α-hydroxy-5α-androst-16-ene) which occurred only in the submaxillary gland of the boar. Signoret (1970a) described a higher frequency of head-to-head approaches than of sniffing the genitalia (70 vs. 30%) in encounters between boars and oestrous gilts. An aerosol containing the steroid identified by Patterson was subsequently developed and tried in breeding programs. The aerosol was blown into the face of sows that had not assumed the typical, rigid 'mating stance', which is a prerequisite for mating. Forty-six per cent of formerly unresponsive females assumed the mating stance after treatment, while none of the individuals treated with a blank aerosol did so (Melrose et al. 1971). In the same study, a spray with preputial fluid and urine had a similar effect. Signoret (1970b) reported similar results: 48.3–52.5% of the sows responded with the mating stance to warm preputial secretion, but only 22.5% to the cold secretion. When placed in a pen where a boar had been, the figure increased to 62.2%. Perry et al. (1972) showed that removal of the submaxillary glands from males early in life results in a later inability to release the mating stance in sows, and induces aggressivity by the females toward the male.

References

Aleksiuk, M. (1968) Scent mound communication, territoriality and population regulation in the beaver. J. Mammal. 49, 759–762.

Anon (1973) Final environmental statement on the cooperative 1973 gypsy moth suppression and regulatory program. (USDA-USFS & APHIS, Washington, D.C.) 164 pp.

Bateman, M. A. (1972) The ecology of fruit flies. Ann. Rev. Entomol. 17, 493–518.

Bedard, W. D. and L. E. Browne (1969) A delivery-trapping system for evaluating insect chemical attractants in nature. J. Econ. Entomol. 62, 1202–1203.

Bedard, W. D. and D. L. Wood (1970) Administrative Study. Field evaluation of synthetic pheromones for the suppression and survey of the western pine beetle. Unpublished report on file U.S. Department Agriculture, Forest Service, Pacific Southwest Forest and Range Experiment Station, P.O. Box 245, Berkeley, CA. 94701.

Bedard, W. D., P. E. Tilden, D. L. Wood, R. M. Silverstein, R. G. Brownlee and J. O. Rodin (1969) Western pine beetle: Field response to its sex pheromone and synergistic host terpene, myrcene. Science 164, 1284–1285.

Bedard, W. D., R. M. Silverstein and D. L. Wood (1970) Bark beetle pheromones. Science 167, 1638–1639.

Berger, R. S. (1966) Isolation, identification, and synthesis of the sex attractant of the cabbage looper, *Trichoplusia ni*. Ann. Entomol. Soc. Am. 59, 767–771.

Beroza, M. (1967) Non-persistent inhibitor of the gypsy moth sex attractant in extracts of the insect. J. Econ. Entomol. 60, 875–876.

Beroza, M. (1971) Insect sex attractants. Am. Sci. 59, 320–325.

Beroza, M. and E. F. Knipling (1972) Gypsy moth control with the sex attractant pheromone. Science 177, 19–27.

Beroza, M., B. A. Bierl, J. G. R. Tardif, D. A. Cook and E. C. Paszek (1971) Activity and persistence of synthetic and natural sex attractants of the gypsy moth in laboratory and field trials. J. Econ. Entomol. 64, 1499–1508.

Berryman, A. A., C. J. DeMars, Jr. and R. W. Stark (1970) The development of sampling methods for 'within-tree' populations of the western pine beetle. *In*: Studies on the population dynamics of the western pine beetle, *Dendroctonus brevicomis* LeConte (Coleoptera: Scolytidae); eds.: R. W. Stark and D. L. Dahlsten, (Univ. of California, Division of Agricultural Sciences), pp. 33–36.

Bierl, B. A., M. Beroza and C. W. Collier (1970) Potent sex attractant of the gypsy moth: Its isolation, identification, and synthesis. Science 170, 87–89.

Brady, U. E. and D. A. Nordlund (1971) *Cis*-9, *trans*-12-tetradecadien-1-yl acetate in the female tobacco moth *Ephestia elutella* (Hübner) and evidence for an additional component of the sex pheromone. Life Science 10, 797–801.

Brady, U. E. and R. C. Daley (1972) Identification of a sex pheromone from the female raisin moth, *Cadra figulilella*. Ann. Entomol. Soc. Am. 65, 1356–1358.

Brady, U. E., J. H. Tumlinson III, R. G. Brownlee and R. M. Silverstein (1971a) Sex stimulant and attractant in the Indian meal moth and in the almond moth. Science 171, 802–803.

Brady, U. E., D. A. Nordlund and R. C. Daley (1971b) The sex stimulant of the Mediterranean flour moth, *Anagasta kuehniella*. J. Ga. Entomol. Soc. 6, 215–217.

Bull, D. L., J. R. Coppedge, D. D. Hardee, D. R. Rummel, G. H. McKibben and V. S. House (1973) Formulations for controlling the release of the synthetic pheromone (grandlure) of the boll weevil. III. Laboratory and field evaluations of three slow-release preparations. Environ. Entomol. (in press)

Burkholder, W. E. (1970) Pheromone research with stored product Coleoptera. *In*: Control of Insect Behavior by Natural Products; eds.: D. L. Wood, R. M. Silverstein and M. Nakajima, (Academic Press, New York) pp. 1–20.

Burkholder, W. E. (1973) The Black Carpet Beetle; Reduction of mating by megatomoic acid the sex pheromone. J. Econ. Entomol. (in press)

Burkholder, W. E. and R. J. Dicke (1966) Evidence of sex pheromones in females of several species of Dermestidae. J. Econ. Entomol. 59, 540–543.

Cameron, E. A. (1971) Field tests of disparlure in Pennsylvania. Paper read at Annual Meeting, Entomol. Soc. Am., Los Angeles, CA.

Cameron, E. A. (1973) Disparlure: A potential tool for gypsy moth population manipulation. Bull. Entomol. Soc. Am. 19, 15–19.

Cameron, E. A., C. P. Schwalbe, M. Beroza and E. F. Knipling (1973a) Disruption of gypsy moth mating with microencapsulated disparlure Science (in press).

Cameron, E. A., C. P. Schwalbe, L. J. Stevens and M. Beroza (1973b) Field tests of the olefin precursor of disparlure for suppression of mating in the gypsy moth (in preparation).

Cardé, R. T., W. L. Roelofs and C. C. Doane (1973) Natural inhibitor of the gypsy moth sex attractant. Nature (London) 241, 474–475.

Caylor, J. A. and G. A. Thorley (1970) Sequential aerial photography as an aid in the evaluation of bark beetle population trends in west-side Sierra Forests. *In*: Studies on the population dynamics of the western pine beetle, *Dendroctonus brevicomis* LeConte (Coleoptera: Scolytidae); eds.: R. W. Stark and D. L. Dahlsten, (Univ. of California, Division of Agricultural Sciences) pp. 8–32.

Chapman, P. J. and S. E. Lienk (1971) Tortricid fauna of apples in New York. Special Publication, New York State Agricultural Experiment Station, Geneva. 122 pp.

Cross, W. H. and H. C. Mitchell (1966) Mating behavior of the female boll weevil. J. Econ. Entomol. 59, 1503–1507.

Degraw, J. L. and J. O. Rodin (1971) Synthesis of methyl 14-methyl-*cis*-8-hexadecenoate and 14-methyl-*cis*-8-hexadecen-l-ol. Sex attractant of *Trogoderma inclusum* LeConte. J. Org. Chem 36, 2902–2903.

DeMars, C. J. Jr. (1970) Frequency distributions, data transformations, and analysis of variations used in determination of optimum sample size and effort for broods of the western pine beetle. *In*: Studies on the population dynamics of the western pine beetle, *Dendroctonus brevicomis*, Le Conte (Coleoptera: Scolytidae); eds.: R. W. Stark and D. L. Dahlsten (University of California, Division of Agricultural Sciences) pp. 42–65.

DeMars, C. J. Jr., A. A. Berryman, D. L. Dahlsten, I. S. Otvos and R. W. Stark (1970a) Spatial and temporal variations in the distribution of the western pine beetle, its predators and parasites, and woodpecker activity in infested trees. *In*: Studies on the population dynamics of the western pine beetle, *Dendroctonus brevicomis* LeConte (Coleoptera: Scolytidae); eds.: R. W. Stark and D. L. Dahlsten (Univ. of California, Division of Agricultural Sciences) pp. 80–101.

DeMars, C. J. Jr., D. L. Dahlsten and R. W. Stark (1970b) Survivorship curves for eight generations of the western pine beetle in California, 1962–1965, and a preliminary life table. *In*: Studies on the population of dynamics of the western pine beetle, *Dendroctonus brevicomis* LeConte (Coleoptera: Scolytidae); eds.: R. W. Stark and D. L. Dahlsten (Univ. of California, Division of Agricultural Sciences) pp. 134–146.

Eiter, K., E. Truscheit and M. Boness (1967) Synthesen von D,L-10-acetoxy-hexadecen-(7-*cis*)-ol-(1), 12-acetoxy-octadecen-(9-*cis*)-ol-(1)('Gyplure') und 1-acetoxy-10-propyl-tridecadien-(5-*trans*-9). Liebigs Ann. Chem. 709, 29–45.

Gaston, L. K., H. H. Shorey and C. A. Saario (1967) Insect population control by the use of sex pheromones to inhibit orientation between the sexes. Nature (London) 213, 1155.

Gaston, L. K., H. H. Shorey and C. A. Saario (1971) Sex pheromones of noctuid moths. XVIII. Rate of evaporation of a model compound of *Trichoplusia ni* sex pheromone from different substrates at various temperatures and its application to insect orientation. Ann. Entomol. Soc. Am. 64, 381–384.

Glass, E. H., W. L. Roelofs, H. Arn and A. Comeau (1970) Sex pheromone trapping red-banded leaf roller moths and development of a long-lasting polyethylene wick. J. Econ. Entomol. 63, 370–373.

Green, N. and J. C. Keller (1969) Attractant for pink bollworm moths, U.S. Patent Application filed Dec. 2, 1968, Serial no. 780–596.

Green, N., M. Jacobson and J. C. Keller (1969) Hexalure, an insect attractant discovered by empirical screening. Experientia 25, 682–683.

Guillot, F. S. and S. B. Vinson (1972) Source of the substances which elicit behavioral response from the insect parasitoid, *Campoletis perdistinctus*. Nature (London) 235, 169–170.

Gustafson, R. W., W. D. Bedard and D. L. Wood (1971) Pilot control study. Field evaluation of synthetic pheromones for the suppression and survey of the western pine beetle, McCloud Flats, Shasta-Trinity National Forest. Unpublished report on file U.S. Department Agriculture, Forest Service, Branch of Forest Pest Control, 630 Sansome St., San Francisco, CA. 94111.

Gustafson, R. W., W. D. Bedard and D. L. Wood (1972) 1972 supplement to: Pilot Control Study. Field evaluation of synthetic pheromones for the suppression and survey of the western pine beetle, McCloud Flats, Shasta-Trinity National Forest, Unpublished report on file U.S. Department Agriculture, Forest Service, Branch of Forest Pest Control, 630 Sansome St., San Francisco, CA. 94111.

Hardee, D. D. (1972) A review of literature on the pheromone of the boll weevil, *Anthonomus grandis* Boheman (Coleoptera: Curculionidae). USDA Coop. Econ. Inst. Rpt. 22, 200–207.

Hardee, D. D., W. H. Cross and E. B. Mitchell (1969) Male boll weevils are more attractive than cotton plants to boll weevils. J. Econ. Entomol 62, 165–169.

Hardee, D. D., W. H. Cross, P. M. Huddleston and T. B. Davich (1970) Survey and control of the boll weevil in west Texas with traps baited with males. J. Econ. Entomol. 63, 1041–1048.

Hardee, D. D., O. H. Lindig and T. B. Davich (1971) Suppression of populations of boll weevils over a large area in west Texas with pheromone traps in 1969. J. Econ. Entomol. 64, 928–933.

Hardee, D. D., G. H. McKibben, R. C. Gueldner, E. B. Mitchell, J. H. Tumlinson and W. H. Cross (1972a) Boll weevils in nature respond to grandlure, a synthetic pheromone. J. Econ. Entomol. 65, 97–100.

Hardee, D. D., W. H. Cross, E. B. Mitchell, P. M. Huddleston and H. C. Mitchell (1972b) Capture of boll weevils in traps baited with males: Effect of size, color, location, and height above ground level. Environ. Entomol. 1, 162–166.

Hardee, D. D., T. M. Graves, G. H. McKibben, W. L. Johnson, R. C. Gueldner and C. M. Olsen (1973) A slow-release formulation of grandlure, the pheromone of the boll weevil. J. Econ. Entomol. (in press)

Hinton, H. E. (1945) A Monograph of the Beetles Associated with Stored Products (British Museum, London) 443 pp.

Hodge, W. H. (1946) Camels of the clouds. Nation. Geogr. Mag. 89, 641–656.

Hummel, H. E., L. K. Gaston, H. H. Shorey, R. S. Kaae, K. J. Byrne and R. M. Silverstein (1973) A clarification of the chemical status of the pink bollworm sex pheromone. Science 181, 873–875.

Hunter, W. D. and W. E. Hinds (1905) The Mexican cotton boll weevil. USDA Bur. Entomol. Bull. 51, 181 pp.

Jacobson, M. (1965) Insect Sex Attractants (Wiley, Interscience; New York) 154 pp.

Jacobson, M. (1972) Insect Sex Pheromones (Academic Press, New York and London) 382 pp.

Jones, W. A. and M. Jacobson (1968) Isolation of *N,N*-diethyl-*m*-toluamide (Deet) from female pink bollworm moths. Science 159, 99–100.

Jones, W. A., M. Jacobson and D. F. Martin (1966) Sex attractant of the pink bollworm moth: Isolation, identification, and synthesis. Science 152, 1516–1517.

Kaae, R. S., J. R. McLaughlin, H. H. Shorey and L. K. Gaston (1972) Sex pheromones of Lepidoptera. XXXII. Disruption of intraspecific pheromone communication in various species of Lepidoptera by permeation of the air with looplure or hexalure. Environ. Entomol. 1, 651–653.

Kaae, R. S., H. H. Shorey and L. K. Gaston (1973a) Pheromone concentration as a mechanism for reproductive isolation between two lepidopterous species. Science 179, 487–488.

Kaae, R. S., H. H. Shorey and L. K. Gaston (1973b) Sex pheromones of Lepidoptera. XLIII. Disruption of pheromone communication in *Trichoplusia ni* and *Pectinophora gossypiella* by permeation of the air with non-pheromone chemicals. Environ. Entomol. (in press)

Keller, J. C., L. W. Sheets, N. Green and M. Jacobson (1969) *cis*-7-hexadecen-1-ol-acetate (hexalure), a synthetic sex attractant for pink bollworm males. J. Econ. Entomol. 62, 1520–1521.

Knipling, E. F. (1964) The potential role of the sterility method for insect population control with special reference to combining this method with conventional methods. USDA ARS-33-98, 54 pp.

Knipling, E. F. (1972) Entomology and the management of man's environment. J. Aust. Entomol. Soc. 11, 153–167.

Knopf, J. A. E. and G. B. Pitman (1972) Aggregation pheromone for manipulation of the Douglas-fir beetle. J. Econ. Entomol. 65, 723–726.

Kuwahara, Y., C. Kitamura, S. Takahashi, H. Hara, S. Ishii and H. Fukami (1971a) Sex pheromone of the almond moth and the Indian meal moth: *cis*-9, *trans*-12-tetradecadienyl acetate. Science 171, 801–802.

Kuwahara, Y., H. Hara, S. Ishii and H. Fukami (1971b) The sex pheromone of the Mediterranean flour moth. Agr. Biol. Chem. 35, 447–448.

Leggett, J. E. and W. H. Cross (1971) A new trap for capturing boll weevils. USDA Coop. Econ. Inst. Rpt. 21, 773–774.

Lloyd, E. P., F. C. Tingle, J. R. McCoy and T. B. Davich (1966) The reproduction-diapause approach to population control of the boll weevil. J. Econ. Entomol. 59, 813–816.

Lloyd, E. P., M. E. Merkl, F. C. Tingle, W. P. Scott, D. D. Hardee and T. B. Davich (1972a) Evaluation of male-baited traps for control of boll weevils following a reproduction-diapause program in Monroe County, Miss. J. Econ. Entomol. 65, 552–555.

Lloyd, E. P., W. P. Scott, K. K. Shaunak, F. C. Tingle and T. B. Davich (1972b) A modified trapping system for suppressing low-density populations of overwintered boll weevils. J. Econ. Entomol. 65, 1144–1147.

McLaughlin, J. R., H. H. Shorey, L. K. Gaston, R. S. Kaae and F. D. Stewart (1972) Sex Pheromones of Lepidoptera. XXXI. Disruption of sex pheromone communication in *Pectinophora gossypiella* with hexalure. Environ. Entomol. 1, 645–650.

Melrose, D. B., H. C. B. Reed and R. L. S. Patterson (1971) Androgen steroids associated with boar odour as an aid to the detection of oestrus in pig artificial insemination. Br. Vet. J. 127. 497–502.

Miller, J. M. and F. P. Keen (1960) Biology and Control of the Western Pine Beetle. See section on 'Summary of Information on Flight Behavior'. USDA Misc. Publ. 800, p. 57.

Müller-Schwarze, D. (1971) Pheromones in black-tailed deer. Anim. Behav. 19, 144–152.

Müller-Schwarze, D. (1972) Responses of young black-tailed deer to predator odors. J. Mammal. 53, 392–394.

Patterson, R. L. S. (1968) Identification of 3α-hydroxy-5α-androst-16-ene as the musk odour component of boar submaxillary salivary gland and its identification to the sex odour taint in pork meat. J. Sci. Fd. Agric. 19, 434–438.

Perry, G. C., R. L. S. Patterson and G. C. Stinson (1972) Submaxillary gland involvement in porcine mating behavior. Proc. VIIth Internat. Congr. Reprod. Artif. Insem. Munich.

Pimlott, D. H., J. A. Shannon and G. B. Kolenosky (1969) The ecology of the timber wolf in Algonquin Provincial Park. (Ontario Dept. of Lands and Forests) 92 pp.

Pitman, G. B. (1971) *Trans*-verbenol and alpha-pinene: their utility in manipulation of the mountain pine beetle. J. Econ. Entomol. 64, 426–430.

Pitman, G. B. (1973) Further observations on Douglure in a *Dendroctonus pseudotsugae* management system. Environ. Entomol. 2, 109–112.

Price, P. W. (1970) Trail odors, recognition by insects parasitic on cocoons. Science 170, 546–547.

Prokopy, R. J. (1972) Evidence for a marking pheromone deterring repeated oviposition in apple maggot flies. Environ. Entomol. (in press)

Rainwater, C. F. (1962) Where we stand on boll weevil control and research. *In*: Proc. Boll Weevil Research Symposium, State College, Mississippi. March 21, 1962. USDA pp. 10–19.

Rasmussen, L. A. (1972) Attraction of mountain pine beetles to small-diameter lodgepole pine baited with *trans*-verbenol and alpha-pinene. J. Econ. Entomol. 65, 1396–1399.

Renwick, J. A. A. (1967) Identification of two oxygenated terpenes from the bark beetles *Dendroctonus frontalis* and *Dendroctonus brevicomis*. Contrib. Boyce Thompson Inst. 23, 355–360.

Richerson, J. V. and E. A. Cameron (1973) Differences in pheromone release and sexual behavior between laboratory reared and wild gypsy moth adults. Environ. Entomol. (Submitted for publication).

Rochelle, J. A. (1973) Wildlife damage control with chemicals. *In*: Forest pesticides and their safe use. A short course. Oregon State Univ. and Washington State Univ. Coop. Ext. Services, and U.S. Forest Service, Region 6, Feb. 6 and 7, 1973. Portland, Oregon.

Rodin, J. O., R. M. Silverstein, W. E. Burkholder and J. E. Gorman (1969) Sex attractant of female dermestid beetle *Trogoderma inclusum* LeConte. Science 165, 904–906.

Rodin, J. O., M. A. Leaffer and R. M. Silverstein (1970) Synthesis of *trans*-3, *cis*-5-tetradecadienoic acid (megatomoic acid), the sex attractant of the black carpet beetle, and its geometric isomers. J. Org. Chem. 35, 3152–3154.

Rodin, J. O., C. A. Reece, R. M. Silverstein, V. H. Brown and J. I. Degraw (1971) Synthesis of brevicomin, principal sex attractant of western pine beetle. J. Chem. Eng. Data. 16, 380–381.

Roelofs, W. L. and H. Arn (1968) Sex attractant of the red-banded leaf roller moth. Nature (London) 219, 513.

Roelofs, W. L. and A. Comeau (1968) Sex pheromone perception. Nature (London) 220, 600–601.

Roelofs, W. L. and A. Comeau (1971) Sex pheromone perception; synergists and inhibitors for the red-banded leaf roller attractant. J. Insect Physiol. 17, 435–448.

Roelofs, W. L. and K. C. Feng (1967) Isolation and bioassay of the sex pheromone of the red-banded leaf roller, *Argyrotaenia velutinana* (Lepidoptera: Tortricidae). J. Econ. Entomol. 60, 1199–1203.

Roelofs, W. L., E. H. Glass, J. Tette and A. Comeau (1970) Sex pheromone trapping for red-banded leaf roller control; theoretical and actual. J. Econ. Entomol. 63, 1162–1167.

Rudinsky, J. A., M. M. Furniss, L. N. Kline and R. F. Schmitz (1972) Attraction and repression of *Dendroctonus pseudotsugae* (Coleoptera: Scolytidae) by three synthetic pheromones in traps in Oregon and Idaho. Can. Entomol. 104, 815–822.

Sanders, C. J. (1971) Sex pheromone specificity and taxonomy of budworm moths (*Choristoneura*). Science 171, 911–913.

Sanders, C. J., R. J. Bartell and W. L. Roelofs (1972) Field trials for synergism and inhibition of *trans*-11-tetradecenal, sex pheromone of the eastern spruce budworm. Can. Dept. Env., Bi-mon. Res. Notes. 28, 9–10.

Sanders, C. J., G. E. Daterman, R. F. Shepherd and H. Cerezke (1974) Sex attractants for two species of western spruce budworm, *Choristoneura biennis* and *C. viridis* (Lepidoptera: Tortricidae) Can. Entomol. (in press).

Schwalbe, C. P., E. A. Cameron, D. J. Hall, J. V. Richerson, M. Beroza and L. J. Stevens (1973) Disruption of gypsy moth mating with microencapsulated disparlure under field conditions. Environ. Entomol. (submitted for publication).

Shorey, H. H. (1964) Sex pheromones of noctuid moths. II. Mating behavior of *Trichoplusia ni* (Lepidoptera: Noctuidae) with special reference to the role of the sex pheromone. Ann.

Entomol. Soc. Am. 57, 371–377.

Shorey, H. H. (1966) The biology of *Trichoplusia ni* (Lepidoptera: Noctuidae). IV. Environmental control of mating. Ann. Entomol. Soc. Am. 59, 502–506.

Shorey, H. H. (1972) Use of pheromones in pest Control. Proc. North Central Branch, Entomol. Soc. Am. 27, 30–34.

Shorey, H. H. and L. K. Gaston (1964) Sex pheromones of noctuid moths. III. Inhibition of male responses to the sex pheromone in *Trichoplusia ni* (Lepidoptera: Noctuidae). Ann. Entomol. Soc. Am. 57, 775–779.

Shorey, H. H. and L. K. Gaston (1965) Sex pheromones of noctuid moths. V. Circadian rhythm of pheromone-responsiveness in males of *Autographa californica, Heliothis virescens, Spodoptera exigua*, and *Trichoplusia ni* (Lepidoptera: Noctuidae). Ann. Entomol. Soc. Am. 58, 597–600.

Shorey, H. H. and L. K. Gaston (1967) Pheromones. *In*: Pest Control: Biological, Physical and Selected Chemical Methods; eds.: W. W. Kilgore and R. Doutt (Academic Press, New York) pp. 241–265.

Shorey, H. H., L. K. Gaston and C. A. Saario (1967) Sex pheromones of noctuid moths. XIV. Feasibility of behavioral control by disrupting pheromone communication in cabbage loopers. J. Econ. Entomol. 60, 1541–1545.

Shorey, H. H., L. K. Gaston and L. L. Sower (1971) The male inhibition technique . . . cabbage looper control by confusing sex pheromone communication. Calif. Agric. 25 (12), 11.

Shorey, H. H., R. S. Kaae, L. K. Gaston and J. R. McLaughlin (1972) Sex Pheromones of Lepidoptera. XXX. Disruption of sex pheromone communication in *Trichoplusia ni* as a possible means of mating control. Environ. Entomol. 1, 641–645.

Shorey, H. H., R. S. Kaae and L. K. Gaston (1974) Sex pheromones of Lepidoptera. LXVII. Development of a method for pheromonal control of *Pectinophora gossypiella* in cotton. Environ. Entomol. (submitted for publication).

Signoret, J. P. (1970a) Reproductive behaviour of pigs. J. Reprod. Fert. Suppl. 11, 105–117.

Signoret, J. P. (1970b) The mating behaviour of the sow. Symposium 70.0 on 'Effect of diseases and stress on reproductive efficiency in swine'. Univ. Nebraska College of Agriculture, June 1970, pp. 295–313.

Silverstein, R. M., J. O. Rodin, W. E. Burkholder and J. E. Gorman (1967) Sex attractant of the black carpet beetle. Science 157, 85–87.

Silverstein, R. M., R. G. Brownlee, T. E. Bellas, D. L. Wood and L. E. Browne (1968) Brevicomin: principal sex attractant in the frass of the female western pine beetle. Science 159, 889–891.

Smith, R. F. (1972) Management of the environment and insect pest control. Presented at the FAO conference on 'Ecology in Relation to Plant Pest Control', Rome.

Stevens, L. J. and M. Beroza (1972) Mating-inhibition field tests using disparlure, the synthetic gypsy moth sex pheromone. J. Econ. Entomol. 65, 1090–1095.

Taber, R. D. and I. McT. Cowan (1969) Capturing and marking wild animals. *In*: Wildlife Management Techniques. (The Wildlife Society , Washington, D.C.) pp. 277–317.

Tumlinson, J. H., D. D. Hardee, R. C. Gueldner, A. C. Thompson, P. A. Hedin and J. P. Minyard (1969) Sex pheromones produced by male boll weevils: isolation, identification and synthesis. Science 166, 1010–1012.

Tumlinson, J. H., E. R. Mitchell, S. M. Browner and D. A. Lindquist (1972) A sex pheromone for the soybean looper. Environ. Entomol. 1, 466–468.

Vinson, S. B. (1972) Competition and host discrimination between two species of tobacco budworm parasitoids. Ann. Entomol. Soc. Am, 65, 229–236.

Vité, J. P. (1970) Pest management systems using synthetic pheromones. Contrib. Boyce Thompson Inst. 24, 343–350.

Vité, J. P. and G. B. Pitman (1969a) Insect and host odors in the aggregation of the western pine beetle. Can. Entomol. 101, 113–117.

Vité, J. P. and G. B. Pitman (1969b) Aggregation behavior of *Dendroctonus brevicomis* in response to synthetic pheromones. J. Insect Physiol. 15, 1617–1622.

Vité, J. P. and G. B. Pitman (1970) Management of western pine beetle populations: Use of chemical messengers. J. Econ. Entomol. 63, 1132–1135.

Weatherson, J., W. L. Roelofs, A. Comeau and C. J. Sanders (1971) Studies of physiologically active arthropod secretions. X. Sex pheromone of the eastern spruce budworm, *Choristoneura fumiferana* (Lepidoptera: Tortricidae). Can. Entomol. 103, 1741–1747.

Whitney, H. S. and F. W. Cobb, Jr. (1972) Non-staining fungi associated with the bark beetle *Dendroctonus brevicomis* (Coleoptera: Scolytidae) on *Pinus ponderosa*. Canadian J. Bot. 50, 1943–1945.

Wood, D. L. (1972) Selection and colonization of ponderosa pine by bark beetles. *In*: Insect/Plant Relationships; ed.: H. F. van Emden. Symp. Roy. Entomol. Soc. (London) 6, 101–117.

Wright, R. H., D. L. Chambers and I. Keiser (1971) Insect attractants, anti-attractants, and repellents. Can. Entomol. 103, 627–630.

Subject index